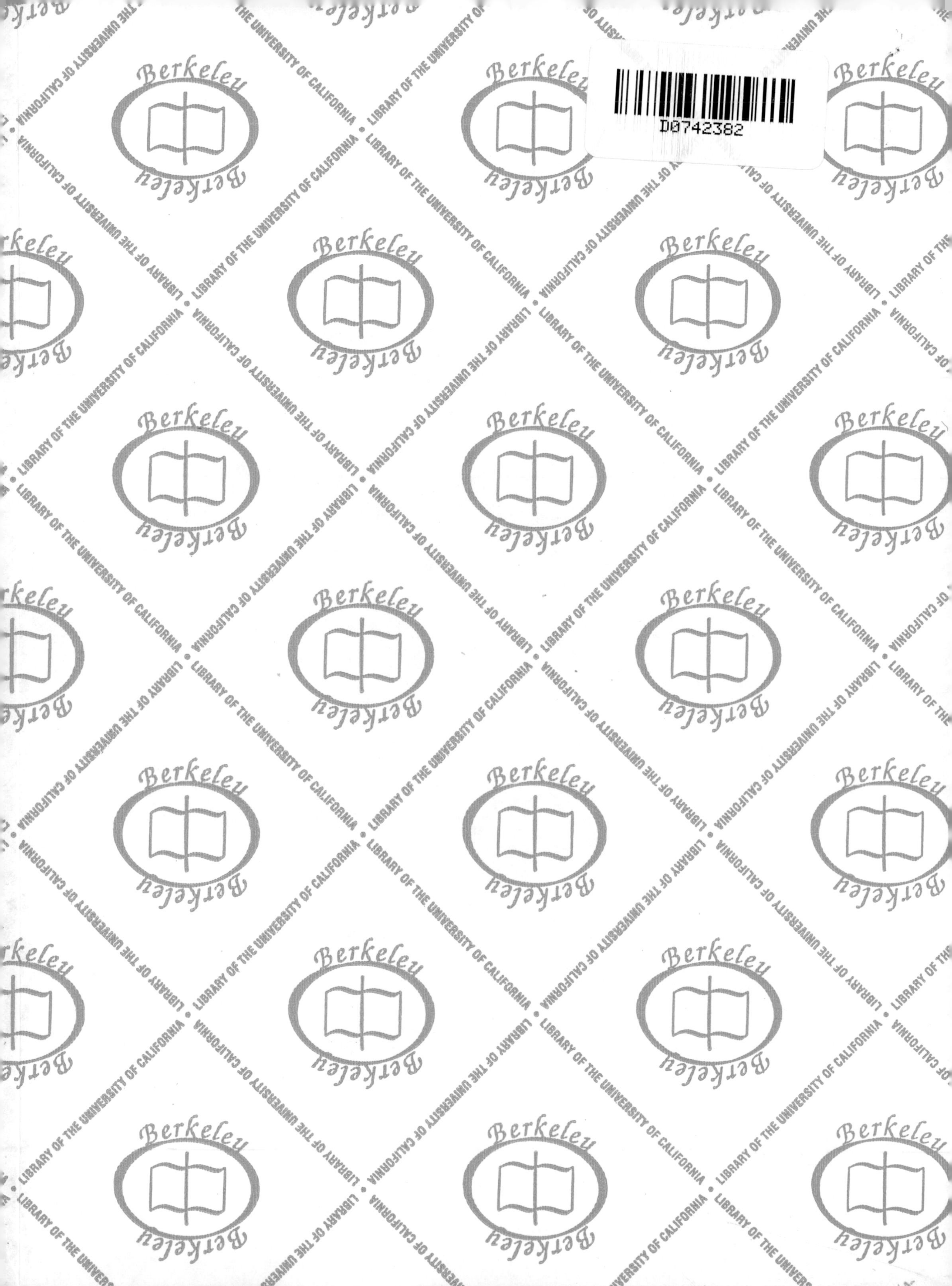

ATLAS OF ADULT PHYSICAL DIAGNOSIS

Dale Berg, MD

Director of Curriculum, Rector Clinical Skills Center
Jefferson Medical College
Director Advanced Physical Diagnosis Course
Jefferson Medical College and Harvard Medical School
Visiting Faculty, Harvard Medical School
Associate Professor of Medicine
Jefferson Medical College
Philadelphia, Pennsylvania

Katherine Worzala, MD, MPH

Director, Rector Clinical Skills Center
Jefferson Medical College
Assistant Professor of Medicine
Jefferson Medical School
Philadelphia, Pennsylvania

LIPPINCOTT WILLIAMS & WILKINS
A **Wolters Kluwer** Company
Philadelphia • Baltimore • New York • London
Buenos Aires • Hong Kong • Sydney • Tokyo

Acquisitions Editor: Sonya Seigafuse
Managing Editor: Julia Seto
Production Manager: Bridgett Dougherty
Senior Manufacturing Manager: Benjamin Rivera
Marketing Manager: Kathy Neely
Design Coordinator: Holly McLaughlin
Compositor: Nesbitt Graphics, Inc.
Printer: Quebecor World

351 West Camden Street
Baltimore, MD 21201

530 Walnut Street
Philadelphia, PA 19106

Printed in the United States of America

0-7817-4190-4
Library of Congress Cataloging-in-Publication Data
available upon request

To purchase additional copies of this book, call our customer service department at (800) 638-3030 or fax orders to (301) 824-7390. International customers should call (301) 714-2324.

Visit Lippincott Williams & Wilkins on the Internet: http://www.LWW.com. Lippincott Williams & Wilkins customer service representatives are available from 8:30 am to 6:00 pm, EST.

10 9 8 7 6 5 4 3 2 1   06 07 08 09

To Stephanie, Sara, Brian, Michael and Christopher,
and to all of our students, and their students.

Coauthors

Coauthor of Chapter 4:
Cardiovascular Examination

Ajit Babu, MBBS, MPH, FACP

Professor of Medicine
Amrita Institute of Medical Science
Kerala, India
Emeritus Associate Professor of Medicine
St. Louis University School of Medicine

Coauthor of Chapter 6:
Abdomen Examination

David Axelrod, MD

Assistant Professor of Medicine
Jefferson Medical College

Contents

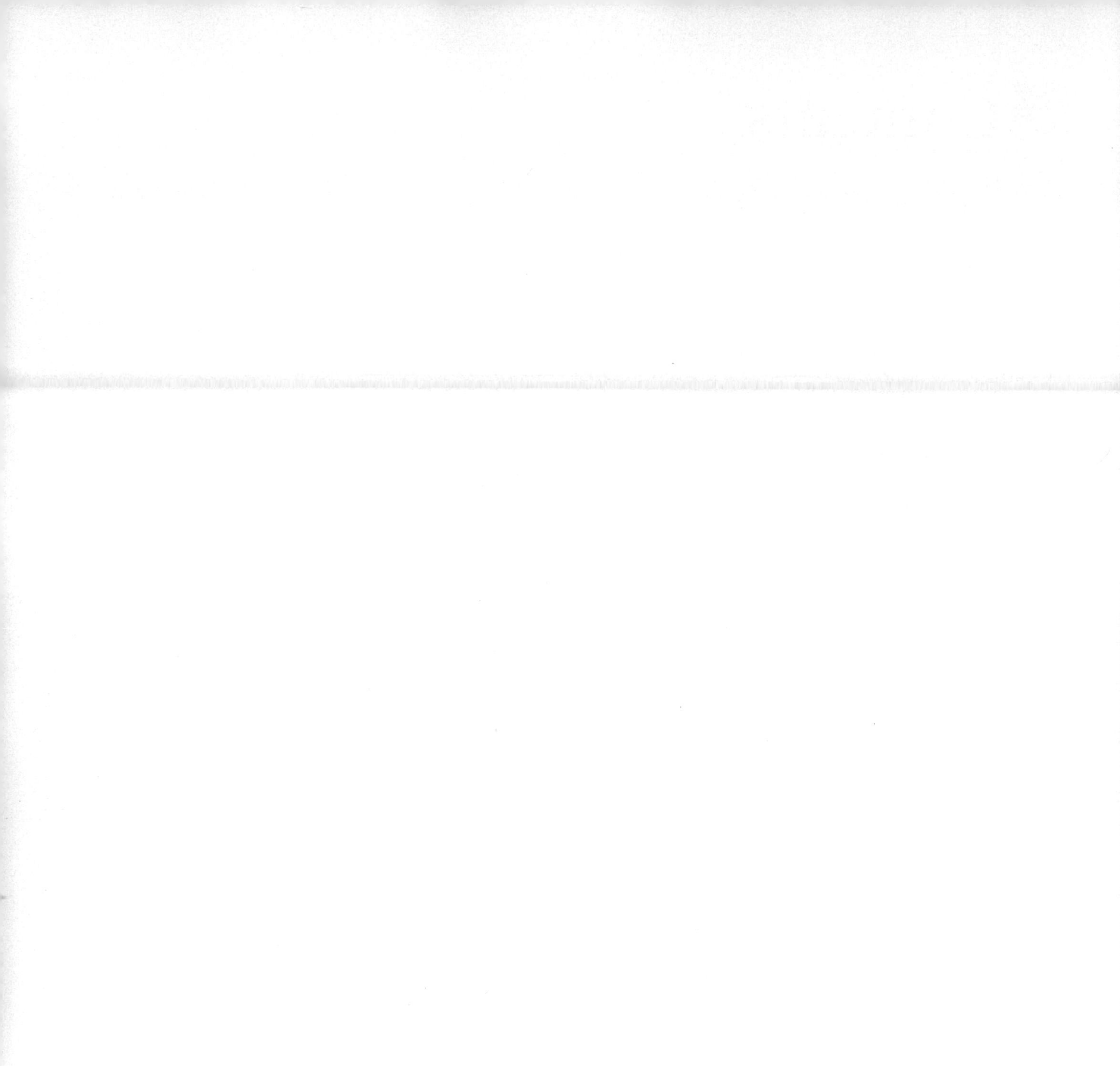

Contributors

Clara Callahan, MD
Professor of Pediatrics
Senior Associate Dean
Jefferson Medical College

Jeannie Hoffman-Censits
Chief Medical Resident
Instructor of Medicine
Jefferson Medical College

Lindsey Lane, MD
Associate Professor of Pediatrics
Clerkship Director, Pediatrics
Jefferson Medical College

Hector Lopez, MD
Assistant Professor of Anatomy
Jefferson Medical College

Joseph Majdan, MD, FACP
Assistant Professor of Medicine
Faculty, Rector Clinical Skills Center
Jefferson Medical College

Bernardo Menajovsky, MD
Associate Professor of Medicine
Jefferson Medical College

Thomas Nasca, MD
Professor of Medicine
Dean
Jefferson Medical College

Susan Rattner, MD
Associate Professor of Medicine
Associate Dean for Education
Jefferson Medical College

Richard Schmidt, PhD
Professor of Anatomy
Course Director Human Form and Development
Jefferson Medical College

John Spandorfer, MD
Associate Professor of Medicine
Jefferson Medical College

Preface

Sir William Osler, perhaps the finest clinician and teacher of the 19th and 20th centuries, wanted his epitaph to read, "I taught medical students on the wards." In this, he states what each of us as practicing and teaching physicians already know: that one of the most challenging and rewarding endeavors is being a teacher of medicine. The teacher himself must be a student of medicine: intellectually curious, exploring new methods, scientifically questioning current methods and studying data. Furthermore, the clinician must be a role model for the student physician; he must use the principles he teaches day to day in his other Oslerian charged roles. All this must be done in a way that keeps a patient-centered focus and in a manner so that every student receives a reproducible curriculum. Perhaps there is no other set of knowledge in teaching or practice that requires as much hands-on, patient-centered instruction as the physical examination. This set of skills requires a clinician and teacher who in addition to having clinical expertise and experience in the field, must be able to be a coach and to provide the student with detailed feedback.

The technologic advances of modern medicine have been extraordinary. Imaging techniques that allow a clinician to see within the body without surgery are nothing less than spectacular for clinician, student and patient. But these tools require time and modern facilities (like electricity). As such, a physician practicing outside of a modern clinic or hospital remains the constant, he remains a physician. Physical examination is a clinical skills set that allows a physician to practice in all environments.

Physical examination is a set of skills that allows the practicing physician the ability to derive objective data from a physician patient encounter in the office. As all clinicians know, these skills, when mastered, allow the clinician to define, delineate, describe and even diagnose the patient. In addition to knowledge of how to define the primary attributes of a problem, the "company it keeps" provides a wealth of further data and information that is very powerful in patient diagnosis and follow-up. In addition, physical examination data allows the clinician the opportunity to perform, as clinically indicated, a well thought out and refined evaluation paradigm. Finally, as anyone who has practiced in the third world knows, without electricity, a CT scanner does not work. Thus a physician must be able to return to his roots to diagnose in the field.

Teaching medicine requires time, skill, and patience, and fall primarily on practicing physicians. The teacher should have available a set of tools with which to work. These tools make the teaching more effective but do not decrease the need of time for teaching. They include the bedside teaching, clinical patient-centered teaching, the use of "patient extenders" including some of the fascinating teaching tools of Harvey and Sim-man. Furthermore, it is of great import to be able to assessment the student's skills and evaluate any teaching activities or curricular interventions. Hence a program using an Objective Standardized Clinical Examination (OSCE) should be intimately tied to this endeavor. To facilitate the goals of teaching and bring together the tools described above, centers of education like our Clinical Skills Center at Jefferson Medical College have been developed. In these centers, all of the tools are placed in one location so that they may be mixed with students and dedicated faculty to reform and reshape medical education. These centers provide a fertile environment for new curricula and are of tremendous value and potential.

A significant deficit in this set of tools is that although there are many textbooks on physical examination for students, there is no text or manual written for the practitioner or teacher who is teaching physical examination. We write this book to fill that void. This book has been written by teachers for teachers and clinicians in practice. It is and will be useful for them to teach each other, themselves and their students the tenets of physical examination. It has been written to set goals for teachers and for students so that they know what is expected of them not only for testing, but for their practice of medicine.

The work is divided into 15 discrete chapters, each an anatomic site of the examination. Each chapter is reproducibly formatted in the following fashion:

- A discussion of the surface anatomy of the site with emphasis on the practical clinical aspects of anatomy.

- Methods to teach and to refresh the knowledge learned in the dissection lab are stated. The discussion of surface anatomy and anatomy itself serves as a foundation for the teaching of the physical examination itself.
- Methods to teach the fundamentals, that is aspects of the examination that every second year student should know and be to perform are described in detail.
- A discussion of methods to teach physical diagnosis features used to describe, define, delineate and thus diagnose discrete medical problems.

There are a large number of images to aid the teacher in teaching the techniques and describing the examination points of pathology. The vast majority (>95%) of these images are from our personal collection; others are from *The Wills Eye Hospital Atlas of Clinical Ophthalmology, 2nd Edition,* the *Atlas of Pediatric Physical Diagnosis, 2nd edition,* the *Bates' Guide to Physical Examination, 8th edition* and *Clinically Oriented Anatomy, 4th edition.* Sections and tables on associated findings, i.e. "the company it keeps" are given throughout the text so that the teacher may further demonstrate the whole and not only the parts in clinical diagnosis. This also complements a work that we wrote for medical students in their 3rd and 4th years entitled *Advanced Clinical Skills.* "Tips for teachers of medicine" accompany each illustration so that the teacher may use each image as a teaching example. There is a thorough state of the science set of evidence to form the basis for many physical examination findings. All of these points are required for the effective and credible teaching of physical diagnosis. At the end of each section of the chapter, there is a set of "teaching points" to help the teacher plan the lesson and thus set some goals and objectives. Finally there is an annotated bibliography at the end of each chapter that supports effective and quality teaching.

This work is a compilation of what we have learned and what we practice here at Jefferson Medical College. It has been and continues to be a work in progress, influenced by the pithy questions of the students and colleagues who teach us while we are teaching and the patients who teach us as we practice. We have gained insights from literally thousands of medical students with whom we have worked and taught at Medical College of Wisconsin, University of Minnesota, Harvard Medical School, Boston University School of Medicine and Jefferson Medical College. It also is based on the incredible altruism of many patients throughout the years who have consented to have their images taken so as to teach others physical examination and medicine itself. They are the true professors of medicine from whom we all learn how to teach and to whom we are so deeply indebted.

We believe that this work will be useful to teachers and practitioners of medicine and hopefully will foster improvement of medical education, faculty development, and teaching by residents and faculty. We believe that it will serve to foster this reform, nay, revolution in medical education. Forward!

Dale Berg
Katherine Worzala
Ajit Babu
Thomas Nasca

1

The Head, Ears, Nose, and Throat (HENT) Examination

PRACTICE AND TEACHING

EAR

Anatomy (Fig. 1.1 and Fig. 1. 2)

The **auricle** is the external ear appendage. It consists of the helix—the peripheral rim, the antihelix—the concave area inside the rim, the tragus—a triangular-shaped structure found anterior to the external opening of the ear, the external canal orifice, and the lobe. With the exception of the lobe, the entire structure is composed of cartilage. The **preauricular lymph node**, immediately anterior to the tragus, drains the periorbital structures and the tragus. The **posterior auricular lymph node** behind the auricle drains the auricle. The **external canal**, which extends from the auricle to the tympanic membrane, is lined with stratified squamous epithelium. The **tympanic membrane**,

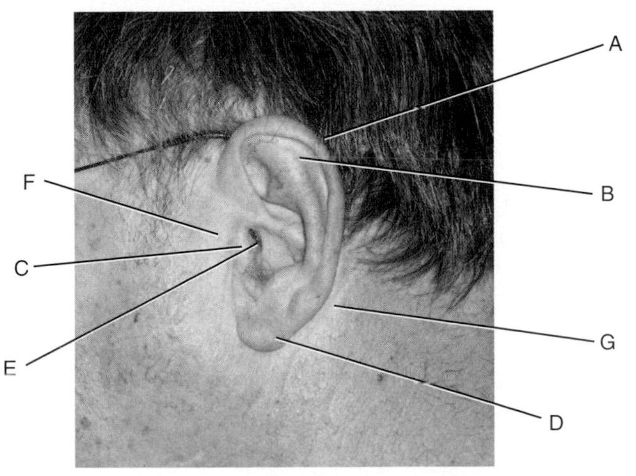

Figure 1.1.

External ear structures. **A.** Helix. **B.** Antihelix. **C.** Tragus. **D.** Lobe. **E.** External auditory orifice. **F.** Preauricular node site. **G.** Posterior auricular node site.

TIPS

- Helix: the peripheral rim
- Antihelix: concave area inside the peripheral rim
- Tragus: triangular-shaped structure mid-anterior
- Lobe: no cartilage in the structure
- External auditory orifice often with cenumen
- Preauricular node and posterior auricular nodes drain the area

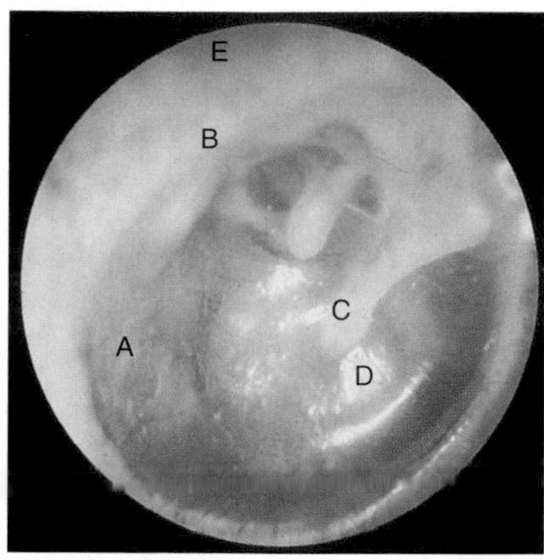

Figure 1.2.

Tympanic membrane features. **A.** Pars flaccida. **B.** Pars tensa. **C.** Umbo. **D.** Reflex cone of light. **E.** Annulus tympanicus. (From Moore KL, Dalley AF. *Clinically Oriented Anatomy*, 4th ed. Philadelphia: Lippincott Williams & Wilkins, 1999:966, with permission.)

TIPS

- Pars flaccida and tensa: both components of the membrane itself
- Umbo: tip of the malleus
- Light reflex: cone-shaped on inferior tympanic membrane
- Annulus tympanicus: rim of the membrane, minimal in superior aspect of TM

located between the external canal and the middle ear, vibrates with sound waves. Features on the surface of the tympanic membrane include the umbo, i.e., the evagination of the malleus; the cone of light reflex; the **pars flaccida** and the **pars tensa**, both of which are components of the membrane itself, and the rim, which is called the annulus tympanicus. The **light reflex** is normally cone-shaped and located on the inferior tympanic membrane; the **annulus tympanicus** is at the rim of the membrane and minimal in the superior aspect of the membrane.

Auricle

Darwin's tubercle is a nontender, benign papule found on the superior surface of the helix **(Fig. 1.3)**. It is inherited autosomal dominant and can be found either unilaterally or bilaterally. Among its numerous colloquial synonyms are "Pixie" ear, "Spock" ear, or "Vulcan" ear, given the appearance of Spock's auricles on the television show Star Trek.

Auricular tophi manifest with one or more non- to minimally tender yellow papules on the helix and antihelix **(Fig. 1.4)** in a patient with gout. Look for tophi in any patient recently diagnosed with gout or suspected of having gout. Thus, patients presenting with a sore toe at first metatarsophalangeal (MTP) joint should have their ears checked. Auricular tophi occur primarily in mid to upper latitudes. In the northern hemisphere, they are more

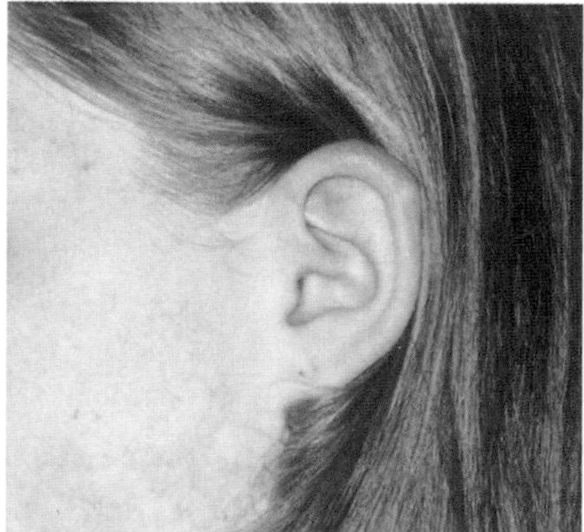

Figure 1.3.

Darwin's tubercle in an adolescent girl.

TIPS

- Darwin's tubercle: nontender papule on the superior surface of the helix
- Congenital, benign

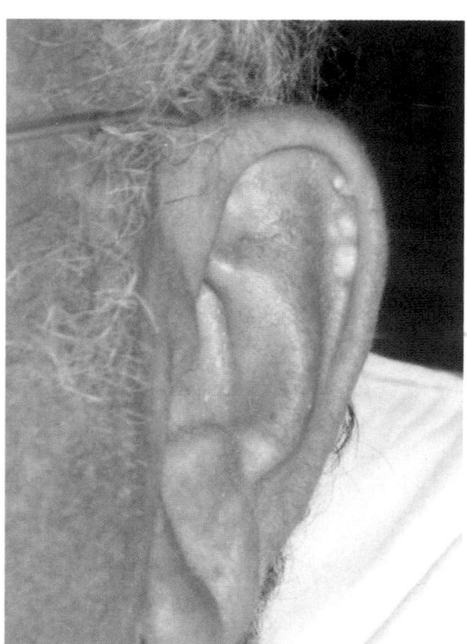

Figure 1.4.

Tophi on auricle.

TIPS

- Tophi: one or more nontender, yellow papules present on the helix and antihelix
- Antecedent monoarticular arthritis, including podagra not uncommon

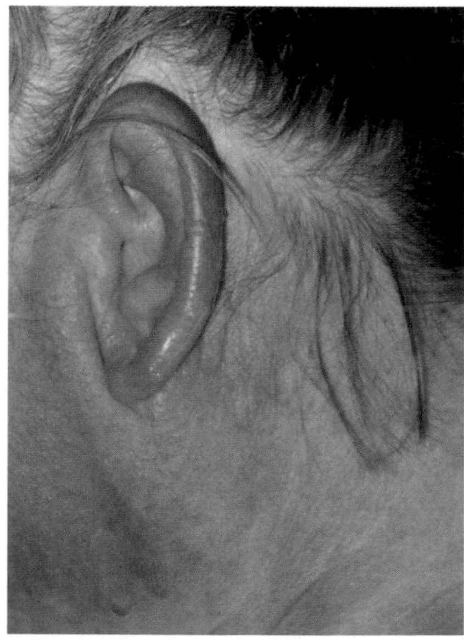

Figure 1.5.

Otitis externa malignant. The entire auricle is enlarged and tense. Blood cultures grew out *Pseudomonas*.

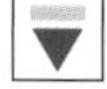
TIPS

- Otitis externa maligna: the entire auricle is diffusely swollen, red, and tender
- "Jug ear" appearance if concurrent mastoiditis
- *Pseudomonas aeruginosa* infection
- Immunocompromised patient
- Lobe is not spared

common north of the fourtieth parallel and rare south of it, probably because cold precipitates uric acid out of solution.

Otitis externa maligna manifests with an erythematous, exquisitely tender, diffusely swollen auricle **(Fig. 1.5)**. A life-threatening, emergent problem caused by a *Pseudomonas aeruginosa* infection, it is found in immunocompromised patients. Such immunocompromise can result from poorly controlled diabetes mellitus, high-dose steroid use, or absolute neutropenia. The company it keeps includes swelling of the mastoid with a "jug ear" appearance, fever, hypotension, and, if untreated death from sepsis.

Relapsing polychondritis manifests with diffuse painful swelling of the upper two thirds of the auricle **(Fig. 1.6)**, can be unilateral or bilateral and involve the alar and septal cartilage of the nose. The company it keeps includes low-grade fever and small joint polyarticular arthritis. Any structure that contains cartilage is a target for this inflammatory process. The fact that it spares the lobe of the auricle is helpful diagnostically.

Ramsay Hunt syndrome manifests with painful swelling in the lower one third of the auricle, including the external canal, and clusters of vesicles **(Fig. 1.7)**. Often, pain and dysesthesia over the area involved are antecedent to the onset of the rash. The company it keeps includes a lower motor neuron cranial nerve VII (CNVII) palsy, changes in taste, i.e., dysguesia, or both. This is due to herpes zoster of the geniculate ganglion.

Earlobe keloids manifest with one or more soft, nontender nodules in the lobe **(Fig. 1.8)**. Keloids are usually caused by trauma, specifically ear piercing. Most keloids occur on the medial (in)side of the lobe, i.e., the receiving side of the piercing. Soft or firm nodules on the lateral (out)side are less likely to be keloids. **Lipomas** usually manifest as smooth, soft nodules in the lobe. **Lepromas** of leprosy manifest as multiple, soft nodules on the antihelix, lobe, and concha. The company it keeps includes severe stocking-glove neuropathy, palpable enlarged nerves, and in several cases, a coarsening of the face (Leonine facies) **(Table 1.1)**.

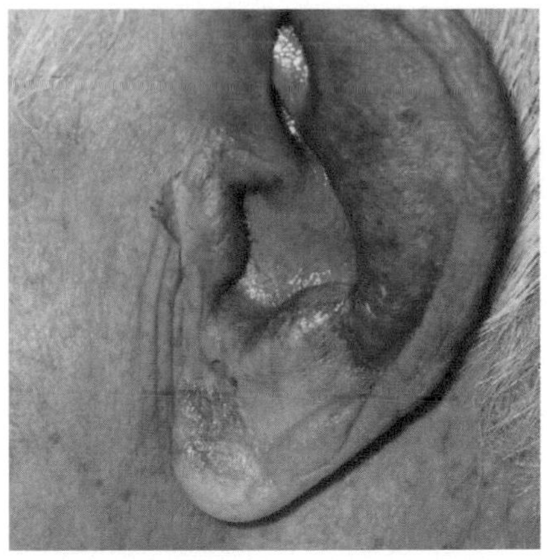

Figure 1.6.

Relapsing polychondritis. Note the absence of lobe involvement.

 **TIPS**

- Relapsing polychondritis: diffuse swelling of the upper two thirds of the auricle; relapsing
- Spares the lobe, because the lobe has no cartilage
- If severe, can lead to "cauliflower ear"
- Obviously treated differently than otitis externa maligna

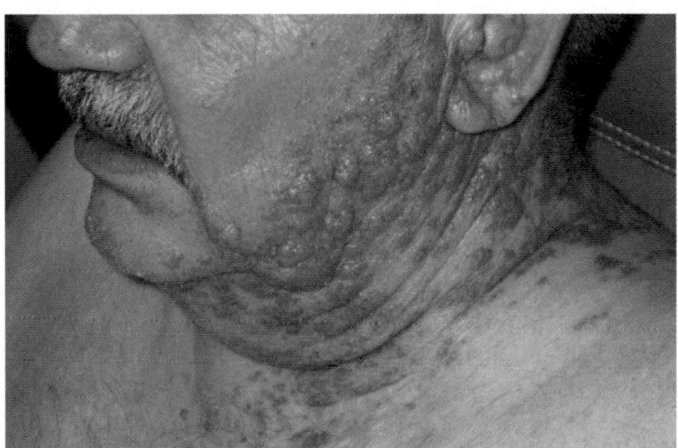

Figure 1.7.

Ramsay Hunt: Clusters of painful lesions in the distribution of cranial nerve (CN) 7. This patient was immunocompromised from Waldenström's macroglobulemia. Several cervical roots are concurrently involved in the patient.

 **TIPS**

- Ramsay Hunt syndrome: painful swelling with clusters of vesicles present in the lower one third of the auricle; the canal is involved
- Herpes zoster of the geniculate ganglion

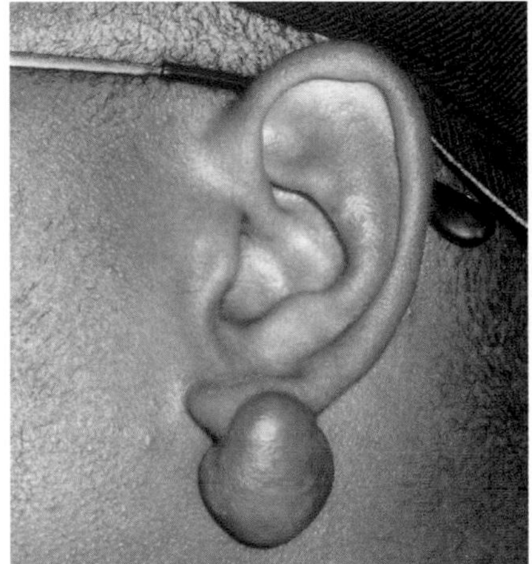

Figure 1.8.

Keloid as the result of piercing of earlobe.

 **TIPS**

- Keloid: a soft, nontender, nonerythematous nodule
- Caused by exuberant connective tissue at sites of scar, piercing, or recurrent trauma
- The keloid is on the "receiving" side of the needle during a piercing activity

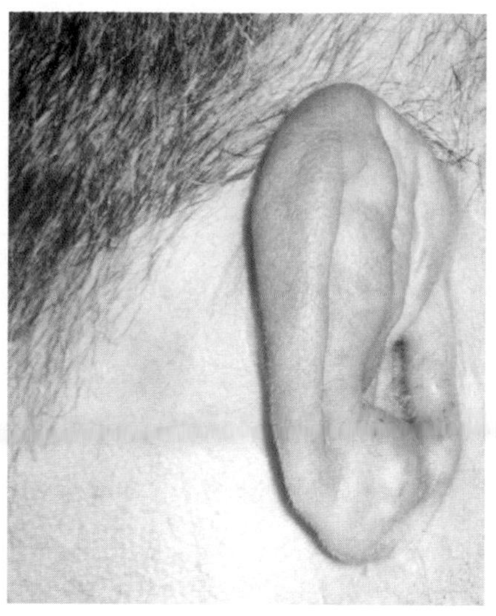

Figure 1.9.

Cauliflower ear. Patient had a remote history of severe trauma to the auricle.

 **TIPS**

- Cauliflower ear: a complete loss of structure but not volume of the auricle
- Nonspecific result of severe trauma involving the auricle

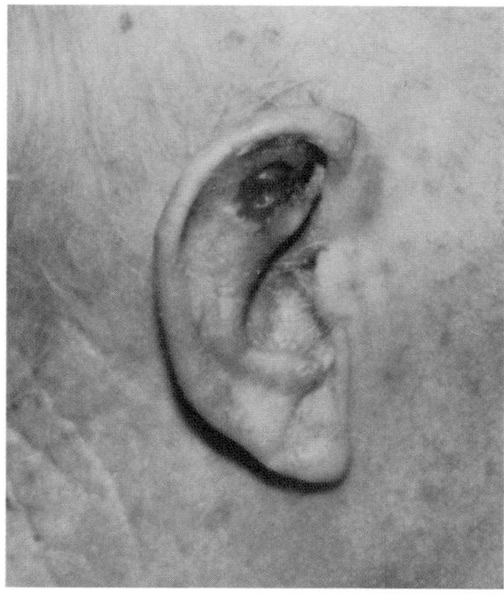

Figure 1.10.

Auricle squamous cell carcinoma.

 **TIPS**

- Squamous cell carcinoma: a painless ulcer on the auricle
- Ulcer is often remarkably clean of debris and has distinct borders
- Need to assess for posterior auricular node enlargement
- May have concurrent, adjacent cellulitis

Cauliflower ear manifests with a marked loss of structure and function of the auricle **(Fig. 1.9)**. A nonspecific, severe result of marked damage to the auricle, cauliflower ear is caused by untreated severe inflammation, infection, or trauma. If trauma-related, it most commonly results from boxing or wrestling encounters, i.e., auriculus pugilistica or gladitorium.

Squamous cell carcinoma manifests with a clean, relatively painless, distinctly bordered ulcer on the auricle itself **(Fig. 1.10)**. Squamous cell carcinoma will spread to lymph nodes around the ear, especially the posterior auricular nodes. The auricle is often overlooked on examination and by the patient. The auricle is also a part of the body often missed when an individual applies sunscreen, thus increasing the risk of ultraviolet related damage. The company it keeps includes multiple actinic and solar keratoses.

Table 1.1. Lumps, Bumps, and Swellings On and About the Auricle

Diagnosis	Auricular findings	Company it Keeps
Tophi	Multiple papules on helix and antihelix	Podagra Tophi on hands Tophi on olecranon Tophi on toes
Darwin's Tubercle	Solitary papule on top of helix	Congenital
Leproma	Multiple soft to slightly firm nodules On lobe, antihelix and concha Bilateral	Stocking-glove neuropathy, severe Damage to fingers and toes Palpable ulnar, radial, common peroneal, tibialis nerves Leonine facies
Lipoma	Solitary nodule Lobe Soft, fleshy	Nonspecific
Keloid	Soft, fleshy Adjacent to a scar On receiving side of the piercing needle	Other keloids
Cauliflower Ear	Complete loss of structure of auricle No loss of substance Old severe trauma or inflammation	Conductive hearing loss
Otitis Externa Maligna	Tense, tender swelling entire auricle, red "Jug ear" appearance, if mastoiditis present	Fever Sepsis Death, if not treated
Relapsing Polychondritis	Tender swollen auricle, spares the lobe Waxes and wanes Bilateral	Nasal cartilage involved May develop septal perforation Polyarticular small joint arthritis
Ramsay Hunt	Canal and lobe involved Vesicles and severe dysesthetic pain	Dysguesia Bell's palsy Conjunctival redness due to weakness of eye closure Ipsilateral
Mastoiditis	Swelling and tenderness over mastoid "Jug ear" appearance	Antecedent/concurrent otitis media or otitis externa maligna
Sebaceous Cyst	Tender nodule in crease between auricle and mastoid May become fluctuant	Nodular acne Rosacea

Other diagnoses include **mastoiditis**, which manifests with swelling and tenderness over the mastoid process and a "jug ear" appearance. This is caused by a primary otitis media infection or by spread of a malignant otitis externa. **Posterior auricular node** enlargement manifests with a nodule posterior to the auricle but anterior to the mastoid process. These are enlarged because of mischief involving the auricle or the external ear canal. **Sebaceous cyst enlargement** manifests as tender nodules in the area posterior to the auricle. If infected, these may be tender, markedly red, and fluctuant. (See Table 1.1).

External Ear Canal

In the normal canal, the walls are smooth and directed slightly anterior. Thus to ease otoscopy **(Fig. 1.11)**, the examiner should posteriorly retract auricle.

Furuncle manifests with an erythematous, tender nodule in the canal, often fluctuant **(Fig. 1.12)**. It may drain purulent material. Often, it is caused by an infected sebaceous cyst. Concurrent otitis externa is not uncommon.

Otitis externa manifests with the patient reporting decreased hearing and a feeling of fullness in the affected ear. On inspection, there is modest to significant swelling, erythema, and serous discharge from the canal. The swelling may occlude the canal. Often this results from a foreign body in canal or cerumen impaction or swimming in lake water—the infection is with *Staphylococcus* or *Streptococcus* sps. **Cerumen impaction** manifests with the patient reporting decreased hearing and a sense of fullness in the ear **(Fig. 1.13)**. Often, the canal is completely blocked, which precludes otoscopic visualization of the tympanic membrane. Concurrent mild otitis externa is often present.

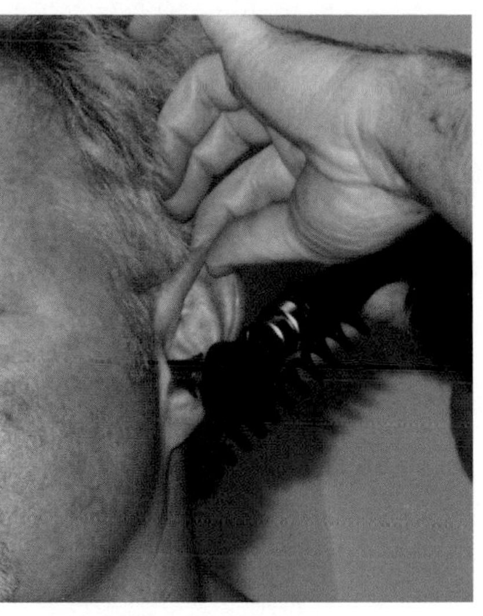

Figure 1.11.

Technique to perform otoscopy.

 **TIPS**

- Gently retract the auricle, insert the tip of the speculum into the canal, inspect the canal and the tympanic membrane
- Canal is directed slightly anterior in most individuals
- If unable to visualize, remove the speculum and slightly reposition the speculum
- Remove any foreign bodies from canal

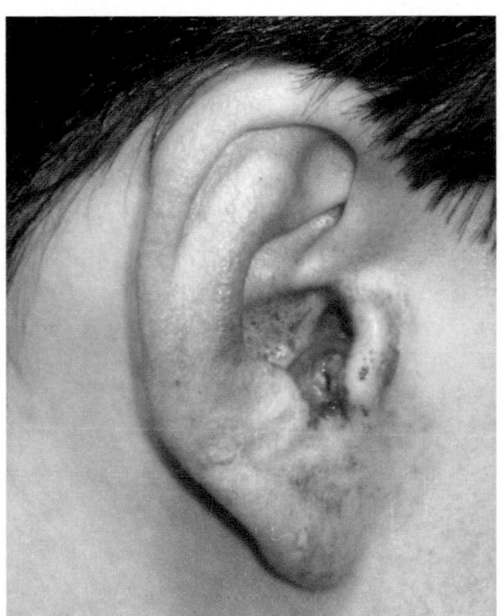

Figure 1.12.

Furuncle in the ear canal.

 **TIPS**

- Furuncle: erythematous, tender fluctuant nodule in the canal; may drain purulent material

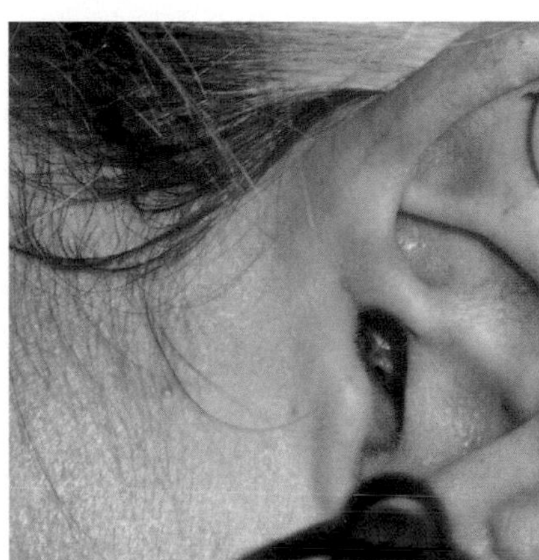

Figure 1.13.

Otitis externa caused by cerumen impaction.

 **TIPS**

- Otitis externa: modest to significant swelling; erythema and serous discharge from the canal; swelling may occlude the canal
- Often presence of cerumen or a foreign object contributes to the pathogenesis
- *Staphylococci, Streptococci* common organisms

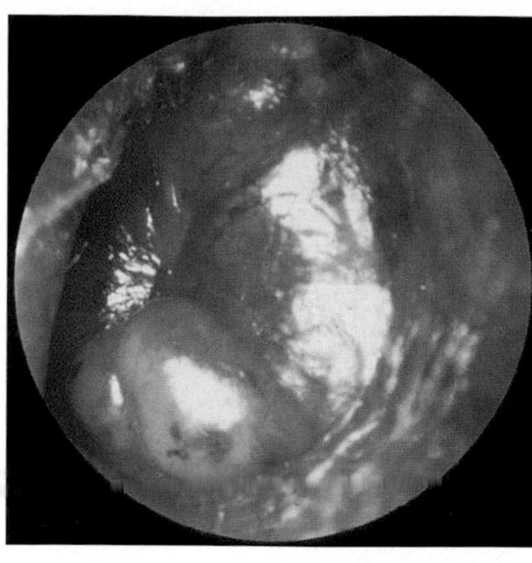

Figure 1.14.

Purulent otitis media. Marked bulging of the tympanic membrane with erythema. (From Moore KL, Dalley AF. *Clinically Oriented Anatomy*, 4th ed. Philadelphia: Lippincott Williams & Wilkins, 1999:969, with permission.)

TIPS

- Purulent otitis media: erythema with prominent vessels around the periphery of the membrane
- Bulging of the membrane, with a loss of the umbo and loss of light reflex

Table 1.2. Middle Ear Diagnoses

Diagnosis	TM findings	Company it Keeps
Serous Otitis Media	TM retraction Prominent umbo Diffuse light reflex Dull	Nasal congestion Cough Conjunctival injection Nonexudative pharyngitis
Purulent Otitis Media	TM bulging Loss of umbo Diffuse light reflex Red	Fever
Bullous Myringitis	Vesicles Dull to red	Nonproductive cough Diffuse crackles on lung examination
Tympanoplasty Tube	Plastic or metal orifice periphery of TM Inferior quarter	History of procedure
Perforation	Hole in TM periphery 1–3 mm in size Bloody or purulent drainage	Antecedent otitis media or barotrauma
Epidermoid Cholesteatoma	Warty structure Rim of the TM Superior aspect TM Perforation present	Nonspecific

TM = tympanic membrane

Tympanic Membrane and Middle Ear (Table 1.2)

The normal tympanic membrane is translucent beige, with a rim of small vessels at the periphery of the tympanic membrane; the umbo is present with a cone-shaped light reflex on its inferior side. This is best visualized by otoscopy **(Fig. 1.11)**.

Serous otitis media manifests with dullness, a loss of the translucency of the tympanic membrane, and prominence of the umbo and malleus, which is caused by retraction of the tympanic membrane. The light pattern is scattered and there are air–fluid levels present. The patient relates a decrease in hearing, a popping or crepitant sound with swallowing, and a feeling of ear fullness. Serous otitis media is caused by a viral or atopic process. The company it keeps includes rhinorrhea, coughing or sneezing, and often a serous or stringy conjunctivitis. **Purulent otitis media** manifests with marked erythema of the

TEACHING POINTS

EXTERNAL AND INTERNAL EAR

1. Several systemic disorders, including tophaceous gout, can manifest in the auricle.
2. Otitis externa maligna is a life-threatening *Pseudomonas* sp. infection of the auricle.
3. Otitis media is extremely common; it is usually serous.
4. Presence of bulging and erythema of the membrane indicates purulent otitis media.
5. Vesicles on the TM—*Mycoplasma* sp. or viral; vesicles in the canal and earlobe—Ramsay Hunt syndrome.
6. Perforation of temporomandibular (TM) with a relief of otalgia: antecedent purulent otitis media.
7. Perforation with onset of severe otalgia: usually barotrauma or sound trauma-related perforation.

tympanic membrane with prominent vessels around its periphery, i.e., the annulus tympanicus, bulging of the membrane, a loss of the umbo and malleus, and absent light reflex **(Fig. 1.14)**. The company it keeps includes decreased hearing, a moderate to severe earache (otalgia), and a feeling of ear fullness. Purulent otitis media is caused by a bacterial infection, usually *Streptococcus pneumoniae, Haemophilus influenzae,* or *Branhamella catarrhalis.*

Bullous myringitis manifests with a dull tympanic membrane; light reflex is scattered and one or more vesicles is found on the membrane. The patient reports decreased hearing, the presence of an earache (otalgia), and a feeling of ear fullness. Bullous myringitis is caused by a viral or *Mycoplasma pneumonia* infection of the middle ear. The company it keeps includes a nonproductive cough and crackles on lung auscultation if concurrent pneumonia. **Epidermoid cholesteatoma** manifests with a warty growth of epidermal tissue on the superior aspect of the tympanic membrane, often with a concurrent TM perforation. The patient reports a sensation of ear fullness, otalgia, decreased hearing, and may also have vertigo and tinnitus; the lesion is often progressive and invasive.

Another diagnosis includes a **tympanoplasty tube**, which is seen as a dull metal or plastic orifice on the inferior side of the peripheral tympanic membrane (TM). The tube, which is used for the treatment of chronic otitis media in children, usually fall out by young adulthood. **Perforation of the TM** manifests with a hole that is 1 to 3 mm in size, a loss of light reflex, and a dull tympanic membrane. If *otitis media-related,* otalgia is antecendent and is acutely diminished with acute onset of purulent discharge, often reported by the patient to be found on a pillowcase in the morning. If *barotrauma* or *sound-trauma related,* there is a bloody discharge and an acute, even precipitous, onset of severe ipsilateral ear pain, nausea, and vertigo.

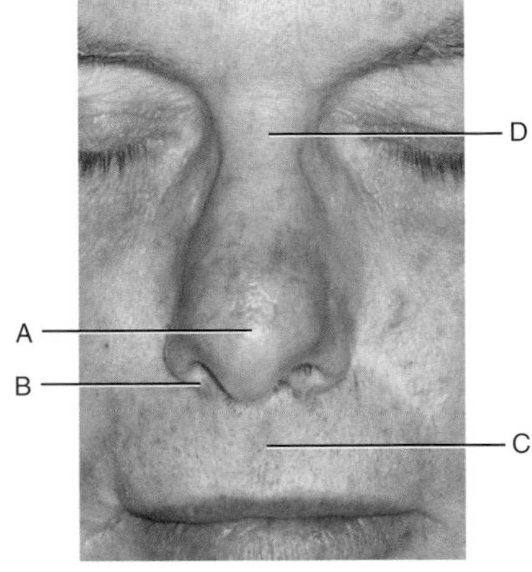

Figure 1.15.

External nose landmarks. **A.** Alar cartilage. **B.** Nares. **C.** Philtrum. **D.** Bridge (nasal bone)

TIPS

- Alar cartilage: soft, pliable; comprises most of the external nose; structure for nares and the septum
- Nares: two orifices into the nose, air flows through these openings
- Philtrum: between the nose and the upper lip—inferior to septum
- Bridge: bone, major support of the nose

NOSE

The nose is composed of the alar and septal cartilage and the midline and superiorly placed nasal bone **(Fig. 1.15)**. The nose is covered by mucosa and skin; internally, it has an excellent vascular supply; the rich venous plexus is called "Kasselbach's plexus". The **internal surface** of the nares includes the inferior, middle, and superior turbinates. For routine examination, tipping the head back and using a non-handheld light source will be adequate to see to the inferior turbinate. A Vienna speculum **(Fig. 1.16B)** is required to examine the more proximal turbinate **(Fig. 1.16A)**. It is important to know how to use the Vienna speculum and every clinic should have easy access to one.

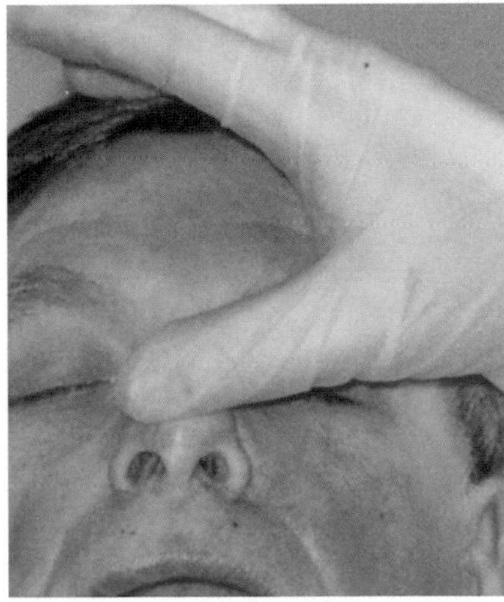

A

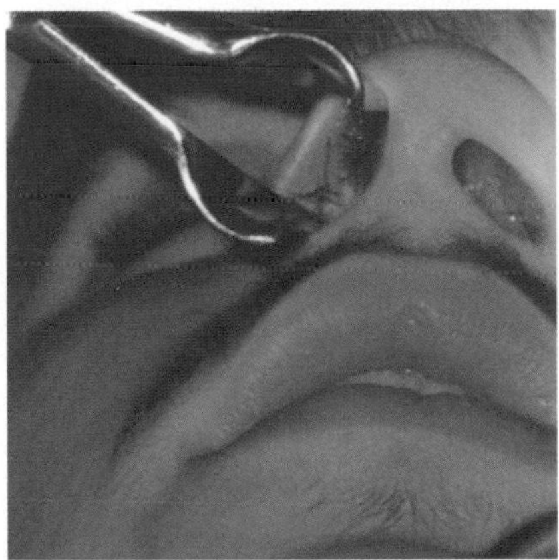

B

Figure 1.16.

Methods to inspect the nares. **A.** Standard procedure. **B.** Use of the Vienna speculum.

TIPS

- Slightly backward flexed head and neck
- Examiner presses downward on the tip of nose so as to open up the nares
- Use a non-handheld light source
- Examiner gently inserts the bill of the speculum into nares

TEACHING POINTS

NOSE

1. Nasal obstruction can be caused by polyps, congestion, foreign body, or septal deviation.
2. Using a Vienna speculum, one can easily see to the middle turbinate.
3. Complications of nasal fracture include septal deviation, septal hematoma, septal perforation, and infraorbital fracture.
4. Saddle nose is rare; it is usually caused by recurrent severe inflammatory processes, e.g., Wegener's granulomatosis.
5. Any nasal fracture requires examination of the facial bones, pupils and range of motion of the eyes.

Rhinophyma (Fig. 1.17) manifests with a painless increase in nose size, with glandular hypertrophy and telangiectasia, i.e., gin blossoms. This is caused by sebaceous gland enlargement. The company it keeps includes rosacea. An example of someone with rhinophyma is the famous Philadelphian W. C. Fields. Although the condition is reported to be associated with alcohol use, this has not been clearly defined.

Wegener's granulomatosis manifests in destruction of the nasal cartilage such that it appears saddle-shaped or beaked **(Fig. 1.18)**. The company it keeps includes anterior epistaxis from necrotizing sinusitis, renal failure, and

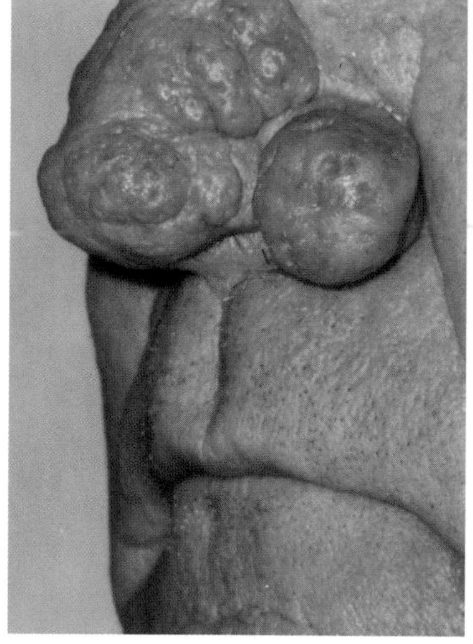

Figure 1.17.

Marked rhinophyma. Patient has concurrent rosacea.

 **TIPS**

- Rhinophyma: painless increase in size of the nose, glandular hypertrophy, and telangiectasia
- Concurrent rosacea

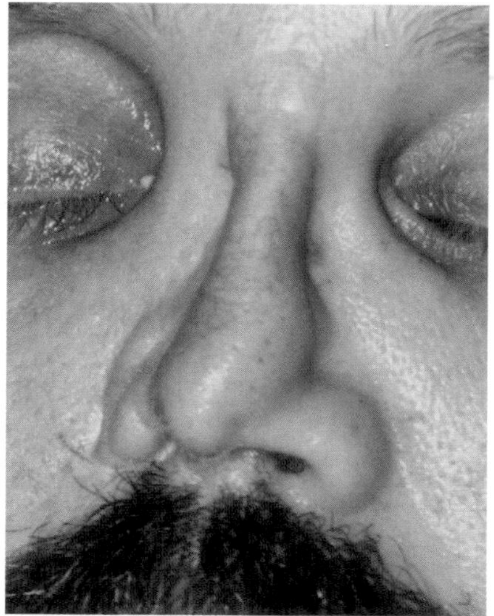

A

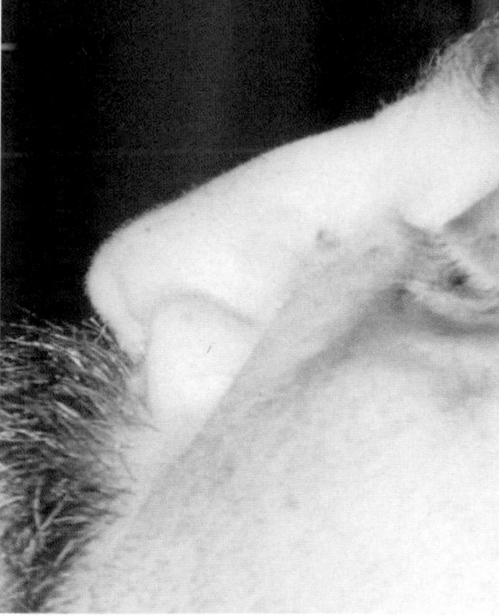

B

Figure 1.18.

The saddle-shaped or beaked nose of Wegener's granulomatosis. **A.** Front view. **B.** Side view.

 **TIPS**

- Wegener's granulomatosis: nose appears saddle-shaped or beaked necrotizing lung lesions. A saddle nose, which is also associated with relapsing polychondritis, has been classically associated with the *snuffles* of congenital syphilis, but this etiology is extremely rare today.

Nasal fracture manifests with a trauma-related onset of a painful, swollen, ecchymotic nose, with anterior epistaxis. Local complications include septal deviation, perforation, and hematoma **(Table 1.3)**. **Septal deviation** manifests with abnormal deviation of the septum from the midline, with a resultant decrease in size of one naris and increase in size of the other **(Fig. 1.19)**. **Septal perforation** manifests with a hole in the septum itself, such that the two nares are not independent. In a septal perforation, light crosses over to the other naris through the septum when light is shone into one naris. Perforation can also be caused by nasal rings, snorting of cocaine, and Wegener's granulomatosis, or result from the complication of an undrained septal hematoma. **Septal hematoma** manifests with a discrete purple colored collection of blood in the nasal septum, which obstructs or decreases the size of both nares **(Fig 1.19)**.

Allergic rhinitis manifests with mild to modest diffuse swelling of the nasal mucous membranes with serous rhinorrhea, often concurrent with conjunctivitis and sneezing. **Viral rhinitis** manifests with mild to modest diffuse swelling and congestion of the nasal mucosa; nasal discharge that is clear, white, or even yellow; mild serous conjunctivitis; nonexudative pharyngitis; and a nonproductive cough.

Nasal polyps manifest with one or more soft, red, pedunculated entities in the nasal canals, usually hanging from a turbinate or the septum **(Fig. 1.20)**. These polyps are caused by atopic rhinitis or by foreign bodies, e.g., nose rings.

Blue nose manifests with a bluish discoloration of the nose tip, which is caused by exposure to cold, or is related to sarcoidosis or to amiodarone use. In cold-related cases, it is also known as lupus pernio, which can be tender and is a form of acrocyanosis. The amiodarone use-related blue discoloration, which is painless and benign, has become more infrequent in recent years.

Table 1.3. **Complications of Nasal Fracture**

Complication	Nasal findings	Company it keeps
Septal Deviation	Septum off midline One naris larger than other	Nasal obstruction Deformity
Septal Hematoma	Septum midline Both nares obstructed Purple collection in septum	Risk for furuncle or septal perforation
Septal Perforation	Hole in septum Unable to blow nose one naris at a time Transillumination of both nares with light in one	Severe deformity Saddle nose
Skull Fracture	Deformity Serous rhinorrhea	Raccoon eyes Otorrhea Decreased level of consciousness Battle's sign
Infraorbital Rim (zygoma fracture)	Step-off of rim of infraorbital bone (zygoma)	Mild walleye: damage to inferior oblique Mild crosseye: entrapment of inferior oblique (Fig. 1.24) Entire globe inferiorly displaced (Fig. 1.24)

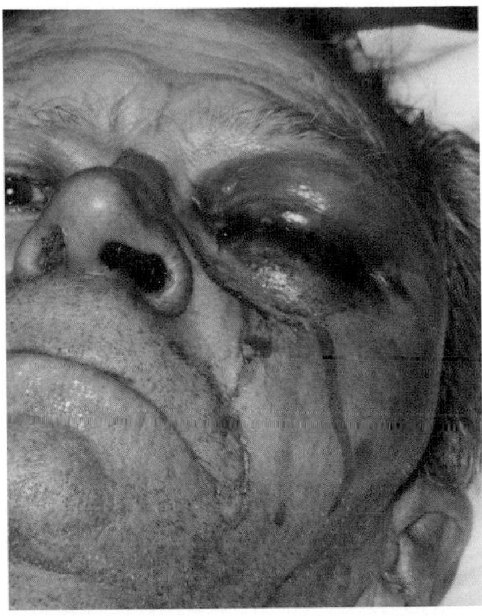

Figure 1.19.

Nasal fracture with a septal hematoma and septal deviation. Concurrent orbital contussion.

 **TIPS**

- Nasal fracture: painful swollen, ecchymotic nose
- Septal deviation: displacement of septum—one naris is smaller than the other

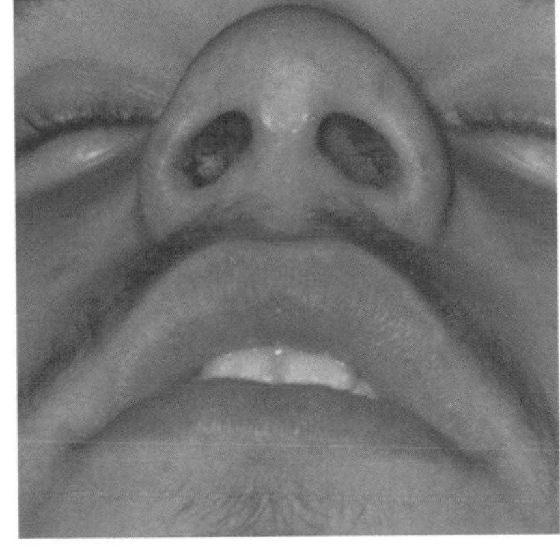

Figure 1.20.

Nasal polyps in nares hanging from inferior turbinates.

 **TIPS**

- Nasal polyps: soft, red, fleshy pedunculated nodules in the nasal canals, hanging from turbinate or septum
- Can result in nasal obstruction

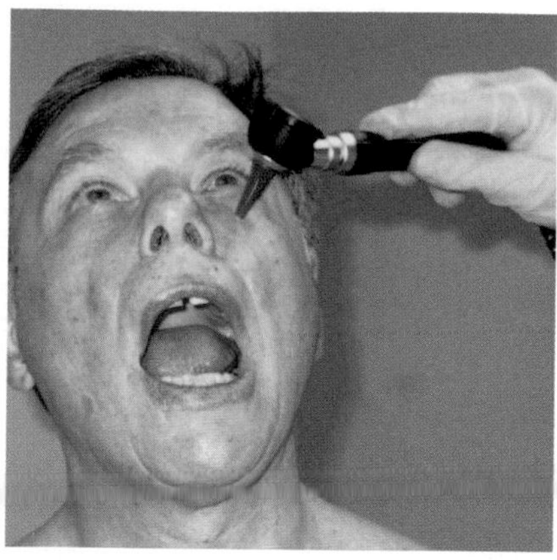

Figure 1.21.

Method to transilluminate maxillary sinus.

 **TIPS**

- Patient with mouth open
- Use a light to transilluminate the maxillary sinus; light source placed on mid infraorbital rim; note light transillumination
- Normal: sinus transilluminable
- Maxillary sinusitis: decreased transillumination in the affected sinus

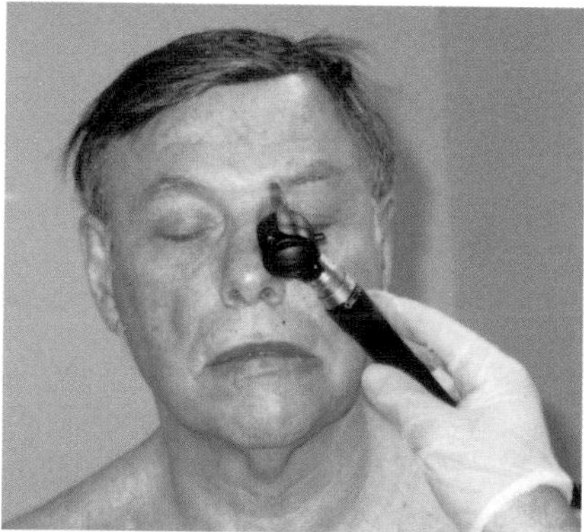

Figure 1.22.

Method to transilluminate frontal sinus.

 **TIPS**

- Use a light to transilluminate the maxillary sinus; light source placed on the medial supraorbital rim
- Normal: sinus transilluminable
- Frontal sinusitis: decreased transillumination in the affected sinus

FACE AND SINUSES*

The **frontal sinuses** are located above eyes in the frontal bone; the **maxillary sinuses** are in the maxillary bone. Other facial structures include the **parotid gland**, which is inferior and anterior to the auricle; it secretes serous saliva into the mouth adjacent to the second premolar via orifice of Stensen's duct. The **submandibular glands**, which are deep to the mandible, drain mucous saliva into sublingual area via Wharton's duct. The **muscles** of the orbicularis oris (cranial nerve [CN] 7) act in smiling; those of the orbicularis oculus (CN7) act to close eyes; and the masseter muscle (CN5) acts to close the jaw. CN7 runs through the parotid gland to provide motor to the facial and frontalis muscles.

Maxillary sinusitis manifests with the patient reporting a unilateral headache and some green nasal discharge. There is tenderness to percussion over the affected sinus and decreased transillumination in the affected sinus relative to the other side. Technique in **Fig. 1.21**.

Frontal sinusitis manifests with the patient reporting a unilateral headache, some green nasal discharge, tenderness to percussion over the affected sinus, and a decreased transillumination in the affected sinus relative to the other side. Technique in **Fig. 1.22**.

Certain signs indicate the presence of acute sinusitis **(Box 1.1)**.

Inspection of features of the patient's face may provide distinct clues to diagnosis. Certain disease processes manifest with features in the face that are so characteristic that they are diagnostic. These are the classic *facies* of disease. Although facies as a concept has been a traditional component of medical education and student-physicians often ask questions regarding specific ones, the importance of facies to clinical medicine is probably overstated. That being said, there are several facies that a physician should know. See **Table 1.4**.

Amyloidosis manifests with periorbital plaquelike ecchymosis **(Fig. 1.23)**. The company it keeps includes macroglossia caused by amyloid protein infiltration of the tongue; right ventriclular failure, including hepatomegaly, increased neck veins; full veins in the arms when forward flexed above the heart (von Recklinghausen's maneuver), an S_3 gallop and peripheral pitting edema. The right heart failure is due to amyloid infiltration of the heart. Concurrent, frothy urine and anasarca may develop, as nephrotic range loss of

Box 1.1.

Acute Sinusitis

Decreased clinical suspicion, if:

1. Absence of maxillary toothache
2. Presence of transilluminable sinus
3. Absence of purulent (green) nasal discharge

(From Williams JW, Simel DL, Roberts LR, Samsa GP. Clinical evaluation for sinusitis: making the diagnosis by history and physical examination. *Ann Intern Med* 1992;117:705–710.)

Increased clinical suspicion, if:

1. Presence of purulent or mucoid nasal discharge
2. Decreased transillumination over the sinus
3. Headache specific to eyebrow—frontal sinus
4. Headache specific to cheek—maxillary sinus

(From Herr RD. Acute sinusitis: diagnosis and treatment update. *Am Fam Phys* 1991;44(6):2055–2062.)

* See also examination for CN5 and CN7, Chapter 7: Neurology.

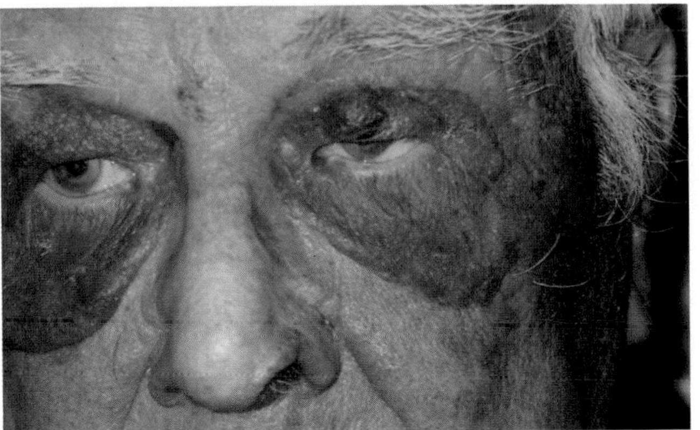

Figure 1.23.

Amyloidosis in this 84-year-old man.

 **TIPS**

- Amyloidosis: has periorbital plaque-like ecchymosis
- Concurrent findings of right ventricular failure, hepatomegaly, and macroglossia are common

albumin and renal failure may also develop. The patient is usually older than age 60 years or has a history of monoclonal gammopathy.

Acromegaly manifests with a coarsening of facial features, enlargement of the skull bones, including the mandible, the maxilla, and the frontal bones. This increase in bone size manifests as increased length of forehead ("Beetled-brow") and increased spacing between the teeth; on profile, it has been called a "lantern-shaped" face and jaw. The company it keeps includes macroglossia; increased size of feet and toes; and increased size of hands and fingers (traditionally termed "spade-shaped hands"). When asked, the patient will relate a recent need to change rings or even have a ring cut off. Acromegaly is due to pituitary adenoma producing growth hormone in an adult. The examination must *always* include visual fields.

Basilar skull fractures manifest with acute, trauma-related bilateral periorbital ecchymosis. The company it keeps includes a decreased level of consciousness, large subconjunctival hemorrhage, clear rhinorrhea of cerebrospinal fluid (CSF), clear or bloody otorrhea of CSF, hematotympanum, and Battle's sign (i.e., ecchymosis over the mastoid process). Battle's sign is the last to develop, 24 to 48 hours after the trauma event. Always palpate the facial bones, specifically the zygoma, the infraorbital rim of the maxilla **(Fig. 1.24)**, and the midline of the maxilla deep to the philtrum, because step-offs may be present in case of fractures. Boney step-offs involving both maxillas are consistent with a tripod fracture and, thus, a basilar skull fracture. Rhinorrhea of CSF can be differentiated from nonspecific serous rhinorrhea by performing a dipstick test for glucose on the fluid. In theory, the CSF rhinorrhea has measurable glucose in it, whereas, in serous rhinorrhea it is a more complex sugar. In practice, however, this procedure is not all that useful. The final component of examination is to perform an active range of motion (ROM) of the eyes because it is not uncommon to develop trauma-related entrapments or weakness of one or more of the eye muscles.

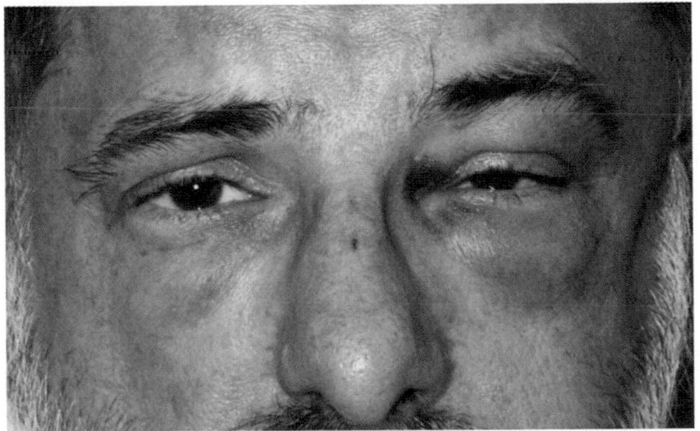

Figure 1.24.

Left zygomatic arch fracture. Note ecchymosis and mild left crosseye.

 **TIPS**

- Basilar skull fracture: periorbital ecchymosis, rhinorrhea
- Subconjunctival hemorrhage, otorrhea, Battle's sign, and hematotympanum may also be present
- Battle's sign is a late manifestation
- Palpate facial bones and perform active range of motion of the eyes and note any deficits

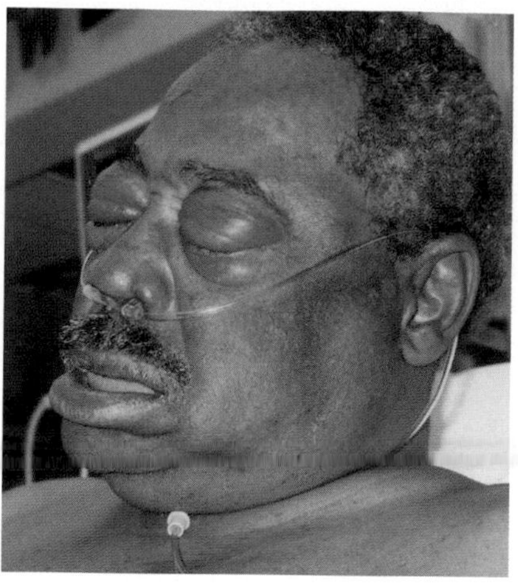

Figure 1.25.

Superior vena cava syndrome from a right apical lung carcinoma.

 TIPS

- Superior vena cava (SVC) syndrome: diffuse nonpitting edema of face and, especially, the eyelids
- Concurrent conjunctival injection
- Macroglossia so that tip of tongue protrudes
- Increased size of neck veins

Superior vena cava (SVC) syndrome manifests with a suffused, edematous face with nonpitting edema of eyelids **(Fig. 1.25)**. There is macroglossia such that the tongue may protrude slightly from the mouth. The company it keeps includes diffuse, nonpitting edema on the upper extremities, elevated jugular venous pressure (JVP), dilated upper extremity and chest skin veins, multiple varicosities in chest skin, and sublingual varices. Elevated venous pressures are also demonstrated by the maneuver described by von Recklinghausen, which is a surrogate for neck vein assessment. Inspect the veins in the upper extremity with the arm below the level of the heart; passively or actively forward flex the arm to 170 degrees; note the arm veins and angle above or below the base of the heart at which they flatten. In SVC syndrome or right ventricular failure, the veins remain full with the arm forward flexed well above the heart base (Fig 4.1). Normally, the veins collapse when the arm is forward flexed at, or slightly above, the heart base. In SVC syndrome, the patient may develop upper airway compromise and, thus, assessment of forced maximal expiration is important.

Tetany manifests with facies of a snide-appearing tight smile, i.e., Risus sardonicus, akin to that of the Mona Lisa or the Joker on "Batman". The company it keeps includes positive *Trousseau's* and *Chvostek's* signs, usually caused by **hypocalcemia. Trousseau's sign (Fig. 1.26)** appears when the examiner places the sphygmomanometer around the arm and inflates to >10 mm Hg above the systolic blood pressure for 60 seconds; the hand and fingers are inspected. There are no findings in the normal state, whereas, in tetany, spasm of flexion of the thumb at metacarpophalangeal joint (MCP), the MCP of 4 and 5; and spasm of extension at the other joints. **Chvostek's sign (Fig. 1.27)** appears when the examiner uses the index finger to gently tap immediately anterior to the parotid gland and repeats with the fingertip 10 times. Sites of spasm or twitch include the corner of mouth (level 1), maxillary area (level 2), eye, orbicularis oculus (level 3), and frontalis (level 4). In the normal state, no twitch occurs at a level 1 or 2, whereas in tetany or hypocalcemia, twitching is seen to a level 3 or 4. The examiner uses the index finger to gently tap immediately anterior to the parotid gland and repeats with the fingertip

Figure 1.26.

Technique for Trousseau's maneuver to detect tetany (often caused by hypocalcemia). A positive outcome seen here.

 TIPS

- Place the sphygmomanometer around the arm, inflate to >10 mm Hg above the systolic blood pressure for 60 seconds
- Observe the hand and fingers
- Tetany or hypocalcemia: spasm of flexion of the thumb at MCP, the MCP of 4 and 5; spasm of extension at the other joints

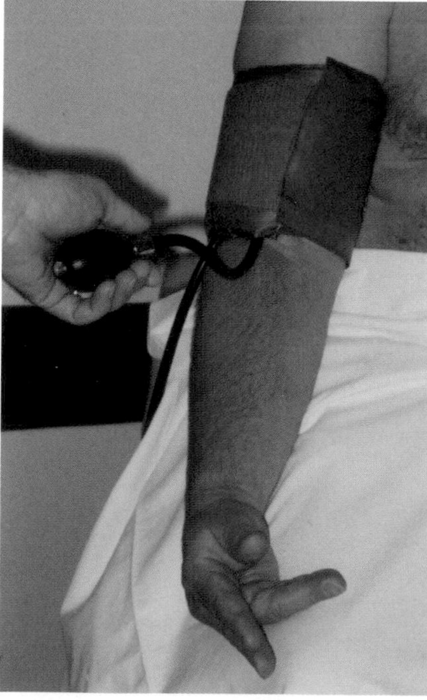

10 times. These are powerful tests when performed and interpreted fastidiously and correctly. Although rare, tetany is most commonly due to hypocalcemia. Although these tests will not be used on a daily basis, they are useful as clinical markers for emergent calcium replacement if, indeed, the patient's calcium level is low and in the evaluation of a patient with cramps, twitching, or new seizures. The company pseudohypoparathyroidism keeps includes hypocalcemia and a shortened fourth metacarpal bone and, thus, a loss of the fourth knuckle when making a fist.

Another diagnosis includes **Paget's disease**, which manifests with headaches, areas of thickened tender skull bones. The company it keeps includes frontal bossing, i.e., elongation of the forehead, and bruits over the skull bones. Auscultation of the skull bones with the bell or diaphragm is indicated for such a patient. Also, there is pain in the pelvis and hips and evidence of high output heart failure, including tachycardia and a gallop. **Bell's palsy** manifests with unilateral droop of mouth and an ipsilateral inability to smile, growl, close eye, and wrinkle forehead on the affected side due to CN7 palsy (Fig. 7.21). **Leprosy** manifests with a coarseness of facial skin features, sometimes described as a leonine appearance. The company it keeps includes significant peripheral neuropathy; the nerves that supply the neuropathic areas are markedly enlarged and palpable, and multiple soft nodules are seen on the auricles. The patient often is a visitor or recent immigrant from a Third World country. Due to *mycobacterium leprae* infection. **Rosacea** manifests with diffuse, nodular, and even pustular erythema in the face that is centered on the nose (i.e., rhinophyma). **Myotonic dystrophy** manifests with bilateral ptosis, loss of muscle, especially in the sternocleidomastoid and platysma, a sad appearance, and frontal hair loss (Fig. 7.7). The company it keeps includes proximal muscle weakness, myotonia, and congestive heart failure. **Parkinson's disease** manifests with a flat, almost emotionless face. The company it keeps includes pill-rolling tremor, bradykinesis, cogwheel rigidity, Myerson's sign, and a narrow-based shuffling gait.* The *facies of Botox* (cosmetic-related use of botulinum-toxin) manifest with a flat face, lack of wrinkles and "crow's feet" about the eyes, and the presence of mortician's perfection about the face. "Botox" decreases the specificity of various tests for CN7 activity. **Myxedema** manifests with coarsening of facial features, macroglossia, patchy hair loss, loss of the lateral eyebrow hair (i.e., Queen Anne's sign), and delayed relaxation phase of reflexes. See hypothyroidism discussion, page 29.

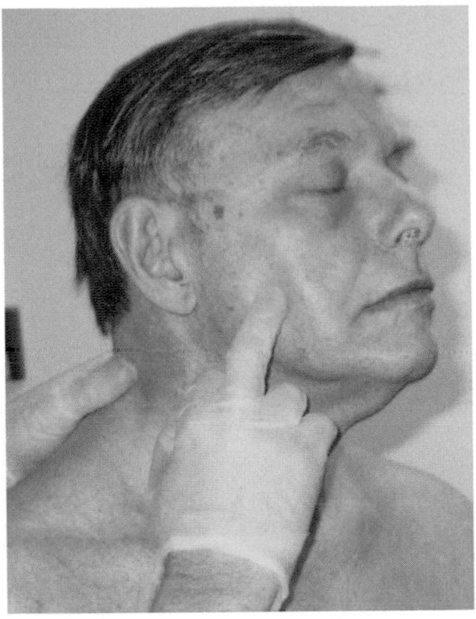

Figure 1.27.

Technique for Chvostek's maneuver to detect tetany, most often hypocalcemic-related.

TIPS

- Note site on face, immediately anterior to the parotid gland, to tap; using fingertip, repeat 10 times
- Sites of spasm or twitch include corner of mouth (level 1), maxillary area (level 2), eye, orbicularis oculus (level 3), frontalis (level 4)
- Normal: no twitch on level 1 or 2
- Tetany or hypocalcemia: level 3 or 4

TEACHING POINTS

FACE AND SINUSES

1. Specific systemic disorders can manifest with specific facies.
2. Macroglossia is associated with the facies of acromegaly, hypothyroidism, and superior vena cava (SVC) syndrome.
3. Presence of a specific facies indicates relatively advanced disease.
4. Transillumination of the sinuses has a relatively low sensitivity and specificity.
5. The best two manifestations of sinusitis are tenderness to percussion and mucopurulent discharge from the appropriate naris.

* Refer to page 161, Neurology exam.

Table 1.4. Facies in Disease

Diagnosis	Facial features	Company it Keeps
Amyloid	Periorbital ecchymosis Macroglossia	Right ventricular failure Nephrotic range proteinuria
Acromegaly	Coarsened face Increased length of forehead Macroglossia Increased hat size	Increased size of fingers and toes Increased shoe and ring size Entrapment neuropathies Visual field defects
Myxedema	Coarsened face Macroglossia Patchy alopecia Lateral eyebrow loss (Queen Anne's sign) Goiter	Diminished DTR Delay of relaxation phase of DTR Thickened skin
Basilar Skull Fracture	Periorbital ecchymosis Subconjunctival hemorrhage Rhinorrhea Otorrhea Battle's sign Nasal deformity	Decreased level of consciousness Anisocoria
Superior Vena Cava	Bilateral swelling eyelids Suffusion of face Increased JVP Sublingual varices Macroglossia Nonpitting edema of face	Increased peripheral veins chest and upper extremity akin Swelling in neck and arms Lung cancer
Tetany	Sardonic smile (Risus sardonicus) Twitching	Seizures Muscle spasms Trousseau's sign Chvostek's sign
Paget's Disease	Increased frontal skull length Bossing of frontal skull Nodules in bone	Headaches Bruits over the bone Pelvic and hip pain High output heart failure
Bell's Palsy	Inability to smile or growl on one side Inability to close eye on one side Inability to wrinkle forehead on one side	Tinnitus conjunctivitis
Leprosy	Leonine appearance Multiple soft nodule in skin overlaying auricle	Palpable peripheral nerves Significant peripheral neuropathy
Rosacea	Bilateral facial redness Multiple pustules, nodules in the erythema	Rhinophyma
Myotonic Dystrophy	Atrophy of the facial and sternocleidomastoid muscles Bilateral ptosis Frontal balding	Proximal muscle weakness Myotonia
Parkinson's Disease	Flat face Few expressions	Cogwheel rigidity Pill-rolling tremor Bradykinesia Narrow-based shuffling gait
Cushing's Syndrome	Round or rubicund shaped Like the full moon	Purple-red striae on abdomen Central obesity with bison hump Thin arms and legs

DTR = deep tendon reflex; JVP = jugular venous pressure

NECK MASSES

Two triangles are important in defining the location of neck structures and entities. These include the **anterior neck triangle**, defined by *anterior*: median line of the neck; *posterior*: sternocleidomastoid muscle, from the sternum and the clavicle to the occiput of the skull; *superior*: mandible; and *apex*: the notch of the manubrium sternum. The borders of the **posterior neck triangle** are *anterior*: sternocleidomastoid muscle; *posterior*: trapezius; *inferior*: clavicle; and *apex*: meeting of sternocleidomastoid and trapezius muscles.

Goiter manifests with a visible and palpable enlarged thyroid (Fig. 1.64), and may have concurrent manifestations of hyperthyroidism, hypothyroidism, or may be asymptomatic, i.e., euthyroid. The first step in thyroid gland examination is visual inspection. It is relatively easy to see the gland before palpation (see page 29). **Thyroglossal duct cyst** manifests with a nodule or mass in the midline anterior neck in any location between the base of the tongue and the thyroid gland **(Fig. 1.28)**. This entity moves upward when the examiner gently pulls outward on the tongue (grasp tongue tip with a 4 x 4 cotton gauze). Embryologically, the thyroid migrates inferiorly from the foramen cecum at the tongue base; a duct cyst is a tissue remnant of that migration. According to Hamilton Bailey, 5% of these cysts are transilluminable.

Cervical lymph node enlargement manifests with one or more nodules or masses in the neck. In *metastatic disease*, the nodes are stoney hard; in *lymphoma*, they are rubbery; and in *infection-related* disease, they are tender and swollen. This is one of the most commonly performed parts of the physical examination, this procedure provides significant clues about the primary complaint. We use the "Ring of Nodes" scheme to reproducibly palpate all of the cervical nodes **(Fig. 1.29)**.

Parotid gland enlargement manifests with a tender or nontender lateral neck swelling immediately inferior and anterior to the auricle. The

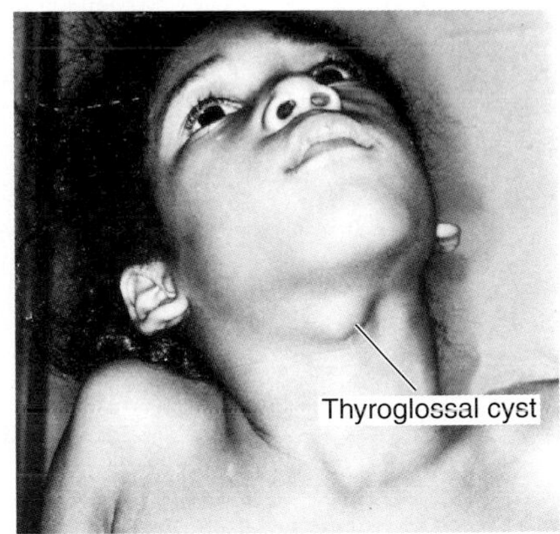

Figure 1.28.

Thyroglossal duct cyst. (From Moore KL, Dalley AF. *Clinically Oriented Anatomy*, 4th ed. Philadelphia: Lippincott Williams & Wilkins, 1999:1074, with permission.)

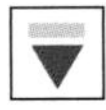

TIPS

- Thyroglossal duct cyst: fluctuant nodule or mass in the midline anterior neck
- Superior to the thyroid gland, midline

TEACHING POINTS

ANTERIOR AND LATERAL NECK

1. Lymph node enlargement is the most common reason for nodules in the neck.
2. Lateral neck and facial masses include enlarged lymph nodes, parotid gland enlargement, cystic hygroma, and branchial cleft cysts.
3. Anterior masses include enlarged lymph nodes, thyroglossal duct cysts, and goiter.
4. Goiter: look for the company it keeps—hypothyroidism or hyperthyroidism, which helps define but will not completely diagnose the underlying process.
5. Parotid enlargement with dry mouth: assess for dry eyes with Schirmer's test and look for underlying rheumatologic problem like Sjögren's disease.
6. Parotid enlargement that is nontender—think bulimia, ethanol use, anorexia, Sjögren's disease, and human immunodeficiency virus (HIV)-related disease.

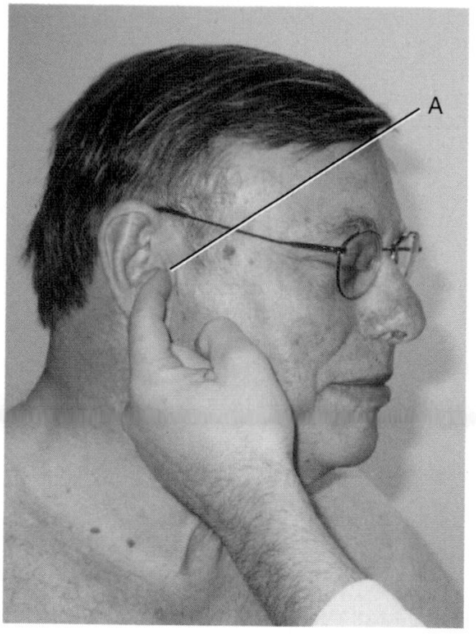

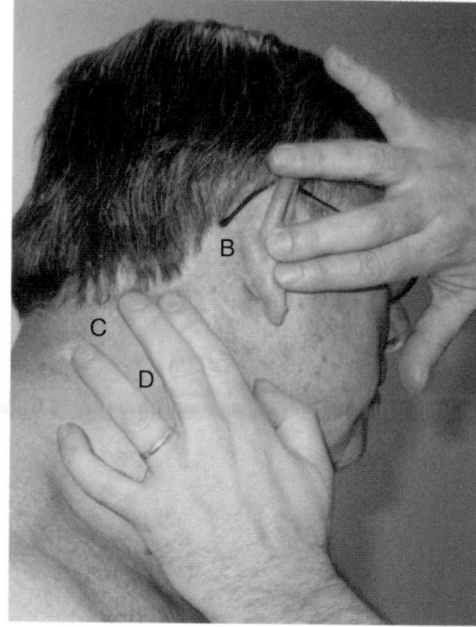

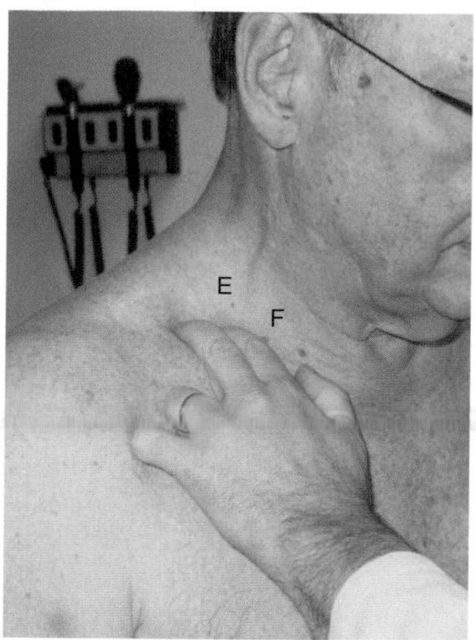

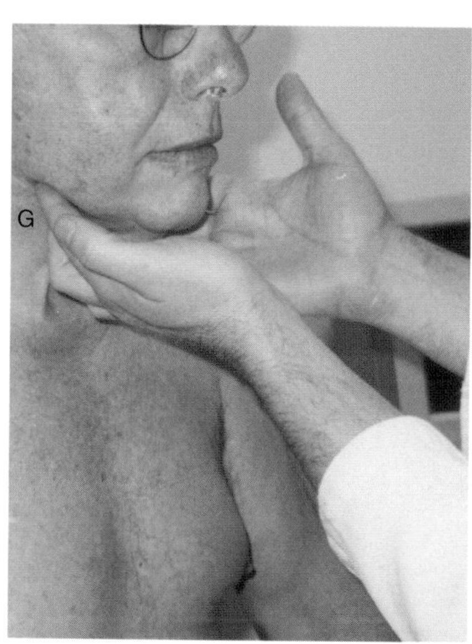

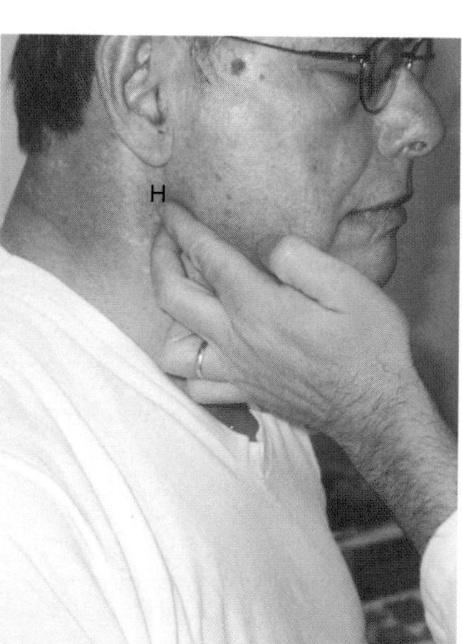

Figure 1.29.

Technique to palpate lymph nodes. Note the *Ring of Nodes* to remember the method to examine all node tissue. **A.** Preauricular nodes. **B.** Posterior auricular nodes. **C.** Occipital nodes. **D.** Posterior cervical nodes. **E.** Anterior cervical nodes. **F.** Supraclavicular nodes. **G.** Submandibular nodes. **H.** Jugulodigastric nodes.

TIPS

- Examiner uses digits 2 and 3 to palpate the *Ring of Nodes*
- Preauricular: drains the periorbital and tragus areas
- Postauricular: drains the auricle
- Occipital: drain the scalp
- Posterior cervical: nonspecific drainage
- Anterior cervical: nonspecific drainage
- Supraclavicular: drains from the breast and on the left side from the thoracic duct, i.e., the stomach and pancreas
- Submandibular: drains the mouth, mucosa, and teeth
- Jugulodigastric: drains the posterior pharynx

earlobe may be elevated because of gland enlargement. Parotid gland enlargement may result from **mumps**, which manifests with tender diffuse swelling, **bulimia**, **ethanol abuse**, and **human immunodeficiency virus (HIV) infection**, which manifests with nontender diffuse swelling. Neoplasia includes **Warthin tumor**, which manifests with nontender unilateral diffuse swelling; and **sialolithiasis**, which manifests with exquisitely tender, diffuse swelling, tenderness at Stensen's duct **(Fig. 1.31)**, and exacerbation of pain with eating. **Sjögren's disease** manifests with bilateral parotid gland enlargement, dry mouth, lacrimal gland enlargement, and dry eyes. The patient may have the paradox of significant tearing early in the course because the first lacrimal glands to be damaged are the small ones in the lids themselves. A rheumatoid arthritis-related infiltration of the salivary and tear glands, this disease is objectively assessed by performing Schirmer's test. Place a strip of sterile Schirmer's paper in the inferior conjunctival sulcus for 60 seconds. Normally, tears will wet the paper, whereas in Sjögren's syndrome the paper does not become wet.

Branchial cleft cyst manifests with a nontender, fluctuant nodule or mass in the lateral neck, anterior to the upper one third of the sternocleido-

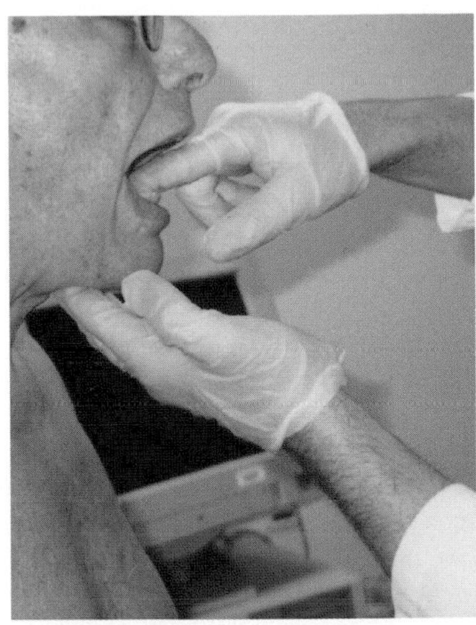

Figure 1.30.

Method to perform bimanual palpation of floor of the mouth.

TIPS

- Patient in anatomic neutral position, mouth open
- Examiner uses two fingers to palpate the submental structures, and two fingers in sublingual area for bimanual palpation
- Excellent method to define any floor of mouth lesion

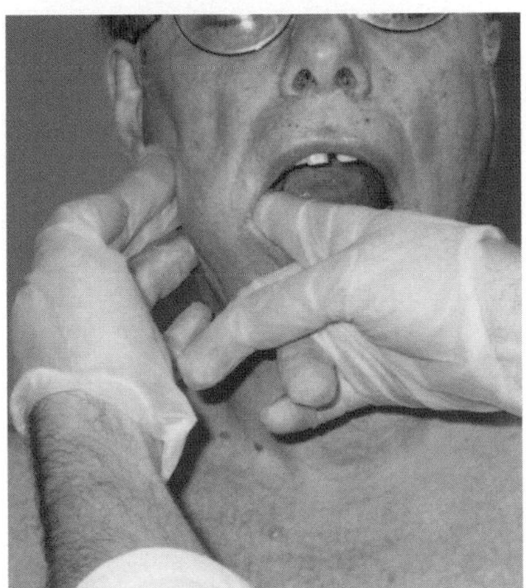

Figure 1.31.

Technique to palpate Stensen's duct.

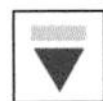

TIPS

- Patient's head neutral and in anatomic position, open mouth
- Examiner places one to two fingertips on the buccal mucosa opposite of the second maxillary premolar; palpate the duct orifice; other hand can be used to press inward (i.e., bimanual palpation)
- Sialolithiasis: marked tenderness, may have swelling of orifice and purulent discharge

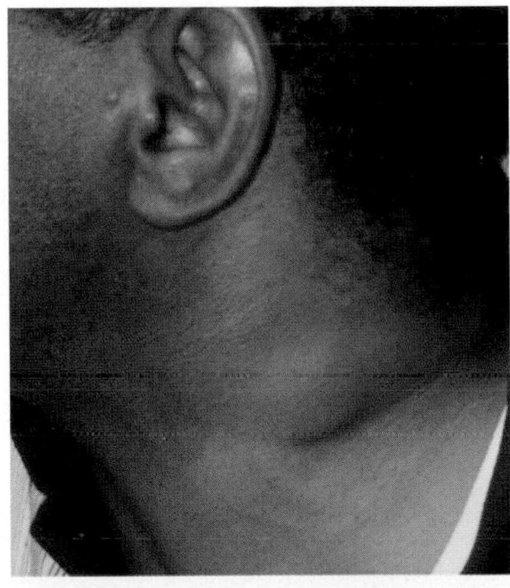

A

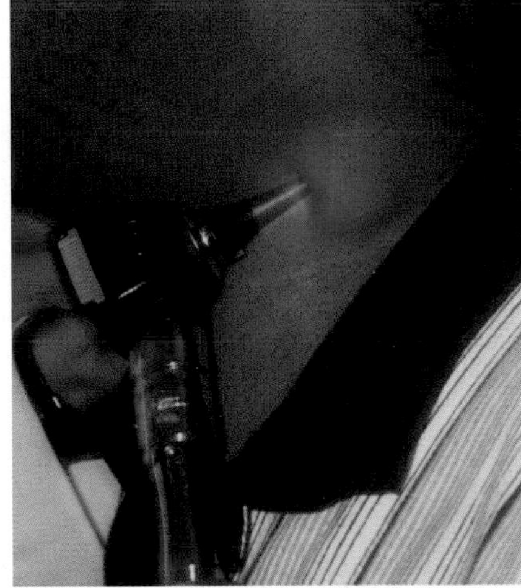

B

Figure 1.32.

Cystic hygroma. **A.** Nodule in the anterior cervical triangle. **B.** Transilluminable.

TIPS

- Branchial cleft cyst: nontender, fluctuant nodule or mass in anterior area of upper one third of the sternocleidomastoid muscle
- Cystic hygroma: nodule or mass in the anterior cervical triangle; brilliantly transilluminable

mastoid. There may be an associated sinus tract, which can become tender, but is usually not transilluminable. **Cystic hygroma** manifests with a palpable, fluctuant mass in lateral neck, which can be large, and is uniformly transilluminable **(Fig. 1.32)**. Very large cystic hygromas are found in Turner's syndrome (XO) in which they contribute to the classic neck webbing of that syndrome.

GINGIVA AND ORAL MUCOSA

The inspection of gingiva and oral mucosa is an often overlooked and undertaught component of the physical exam. Many diseases may be diagnosed by simple but thorough inspection and palpation. The best technique is the two-tongue blade approach to inspection. This procedure exposes the mandibular and maxillary mucosa **(Fig. 1.33)**. It is normal to some pigmented macules in the gingiva of African-Americans **(Fig. 1.34)**.

Gingival hypertrophy manifests with diffuse gingival thickening. Rarely will the patient present to a physician for this, rather the patient presents to a dentist. The enlargement may be tender or nontender, and may even cover the teeth. It often results from a side effect of medications such as phenytoin

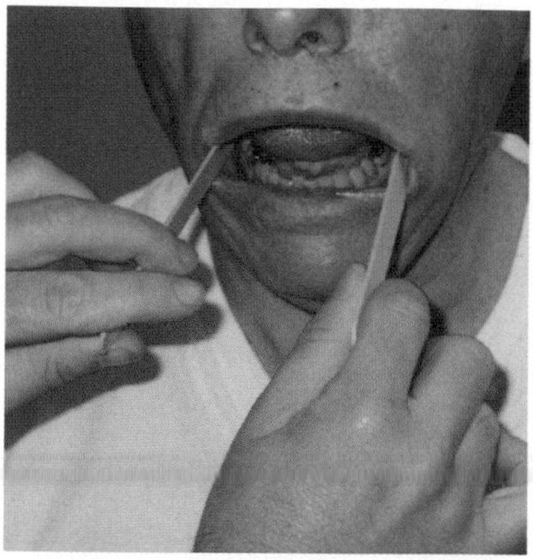

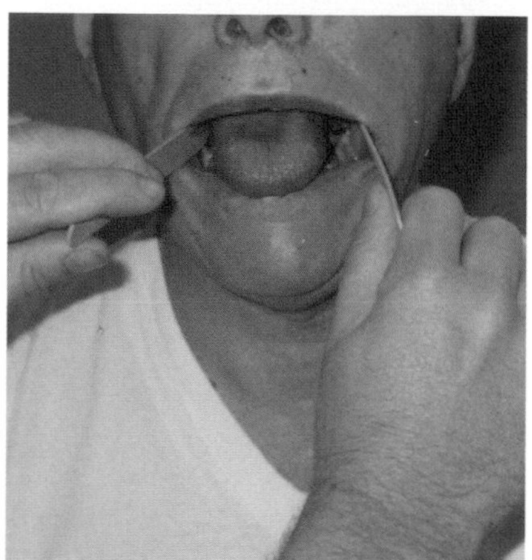

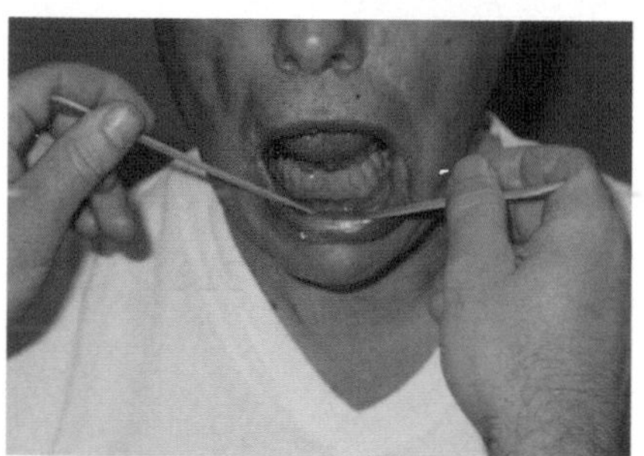

Figure 1.33.

Two-tongue blade technique to inspect the entire oral and posterior pharynx mucous membrane. Inspect the mandibular and then maxillary (not shown) mucosa.

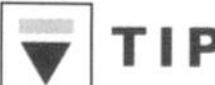

TIPS

- Place a tongue blade into the sulcus (i.e., the fold formed between the buccal mucosa and the buccal gingiva, external to teeth), place another tongue blade on other side
- Gently pull outward to inspect the entire oral mucosa
- Adequate indirect light source necessary

or cyclosporine A, or from infiltration of the gingiva with M5 acute nonlymphocytic leukemia **(Fig. 1.36)**.

Gingivitis vulgaris manifests with diffuse tender swelling, tartar and calculus at gingiva–tooth interface, and mild bleeding; in moderate cases, recession of the gingiva uncovers the roots of teeth. There are multiple root caries. In very advanced cases, purulent material is present at the gingiva–tooth interface and loss of teeth **(Fig. 1.37)**. Because of a high risk of pneumonia and of endocarditis in such cases, it is important to assess the heart and lungs of such a patient.

Localized gingivitis manifests with a hypertrophic interdental papilla **(Fig. 1.38)**. Epulis is caused by irritation, such as overzealous flossing. It is most common in the third trimester of pregnancy.

Other problems include **scurvy**, which manifests with a livid, i.e., deep purple red, gingival hyperplasia that bleeds easily. Concurrently, the teeth are loose and easily fall out. The company it keeps includes easy bruising with ecchymoses, perifollicular pectechial, especially in a saddle lower extremity distribution, corkscrew hair, and poor wound healing. **Plumbism** manifests with a set of minute black dots in the tartar at the gingiva–tooth interface (Burton's line). The company it keeps includes peripheral neuropathy and renal failure. **Amalgam tattoo** manifests with a silver colored macule in the area of gingiva or mucosa adjacent to a tooth restored with silver amalgam material. **Sinus tract of a periapical abscess** manifests with the orifice of the sinus deep to gingival–tooth interface. This often is draining purulent material, it is a not uncommon complication of advanced dental caries **(Fig. 1.35)**.

Torus mandibularis manifests with one or more mucosa covered, bony nodules, usually on the lingual side of the mandible; it is benign but needs to be clinically recognized **(Fig. 1.39)**. This can be a problem if there is a need for dentures or plates; otherwise, it is a normal variant.

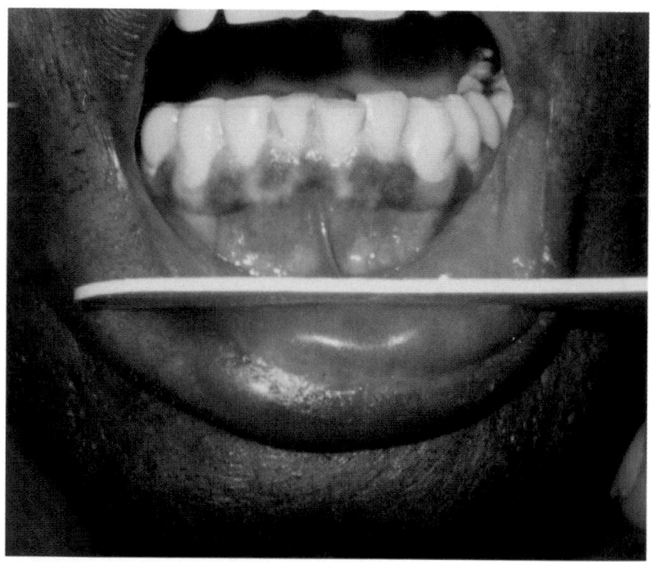

Figure 1.34.

Normal gingival pigment in African-American individual.

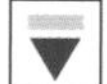

TIPS

- Inspect the gingival mucosa
- Normal: often areas of pigment in the gingival tissue are seen in individuals of African descent

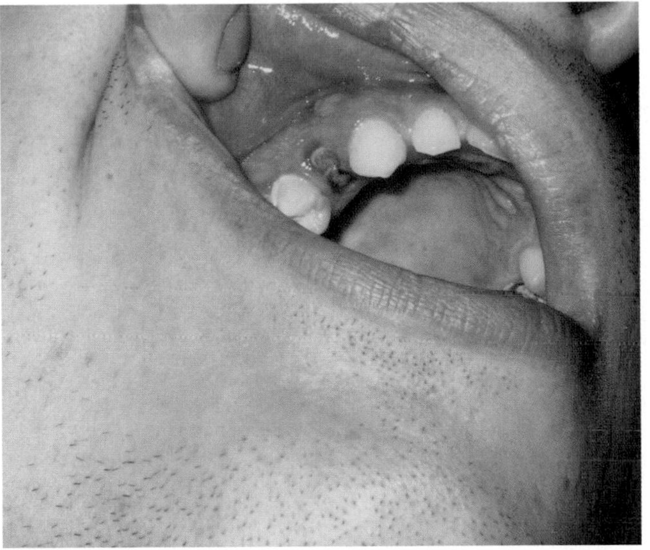

Figure 1.35.

Orifice of sinus from periapical abscess; premolar tooth.

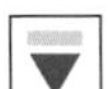

TIPS

- Caries are common
- Complications include periapical abscess

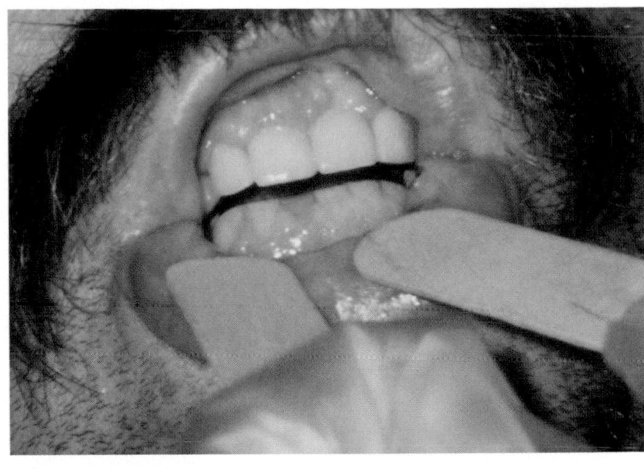

Figure 1.36.

M5 acute non-lymphocytic leukemia (ANLL) with gingival infiltration of the tumor clone.

TIPS

- Acute nonlymphocytic leukemia, M5 subtype: diffuse gingival hypertrophy
- Caused by infiltration of the leukemic cells into gingiva
- Papular appearance to surface

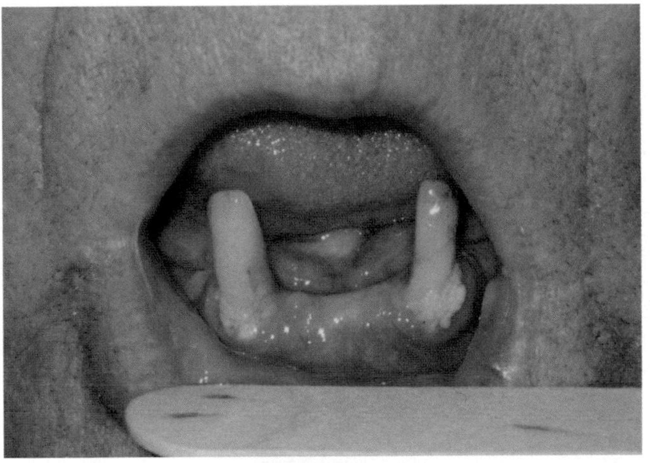

Figure 1.37.

Marked gingivitis with tooth loss.

TIPS

- Mild gingivitis vulgaris: diffuse tender swelling, with tartar and calculus at the gingival—tooth interface; mild bleeding
- Severe gingivitis vulgaris: recession of the gingiva to uncover the roots of teeth root caries and tooth loss; purulent material may be present at gum line

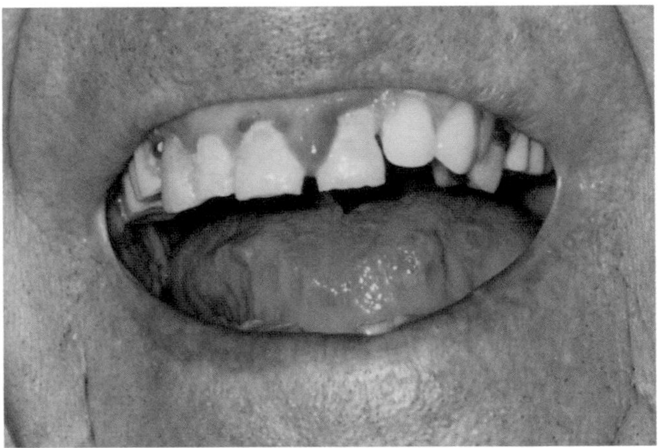

Figure 1.38.

Hypertrophy of interdental papilla between the two maxillary incisors.

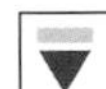

TIPS

- Hypertrophic interdental papilla
- Common in third trimester of pregnancy

TEACHING POINTS

GINGIVA AND MUCOSA

1. Gingival hypertrophy is caused by gingivitis vulgaris infiltration by tumor or inflammatory cells or is a side effect of phenytoin use.
2. Red or white mucosal plaques on mucosa may indicate carcinoma.
3. One excellent method to expose the oral cavity is the two-tongue blade approach.
4. Thrush is relatively common as a cause of white lesions in the mouth.
5. The physician must be deft at performing this exam.

Thrush manifests with white papules and plaques that appear to be akin to curdled milk. Each papule or plaque has an underlying erythematous base on the mucosa. There is often concurrent pharyngeal and tongue involvement, which is caused by infection with *Candida albicans*, usually as the result of local or systemic immunosuppression. The most common local cause is the use of topical inhaled steroids. The company it keeps includes dysphagia and perhaps odynophagia due to candida esophagitis. **Aphthous stomatitis** manifests with one or more tender erosions on the buccal mucosa, which is idiopathic and usually self-limited. If recurrent or if it involves the skin, consider a viral or systemic disorder or a chemotherapy (e.g., 5-fluorouracil) side effect. Viral etiologies include coxsackie virus (Fig. 1.42) and herpes simplex virus; systemic disorders include systemic lupus eurythematosus, Behçet's disease, Reiter's disease, and Crohn's disease. **Koplik's spots** manifest with a cluster of painless white dots on the area adjacent to both Stensen's ducts. The company it keeps includes the exanthem, rhinorrhea, cough, high fevers, and conjunctivitis of rubeola. Koplik's spots herald the onset of the rash. **Squamous cell carcinoma** manifests with a red or white ulcer or plaque on the buccal mucosa. Johnson reports that of SCCA, 30% are red, and 5% are white. **Ranula** manifests with a fluctuant mass that has a bluish hue in the floor of the mouth on the side of the lingual frenulum. On bimanual palpation, a fluctuant, nontender mass is seen on the floor of the mouth. This is due to damage to minor salivary gland. **Sialolithiasis of Wharton's duct** manifests with tender palpable area of swelling about the duct in the floor of the mouth.

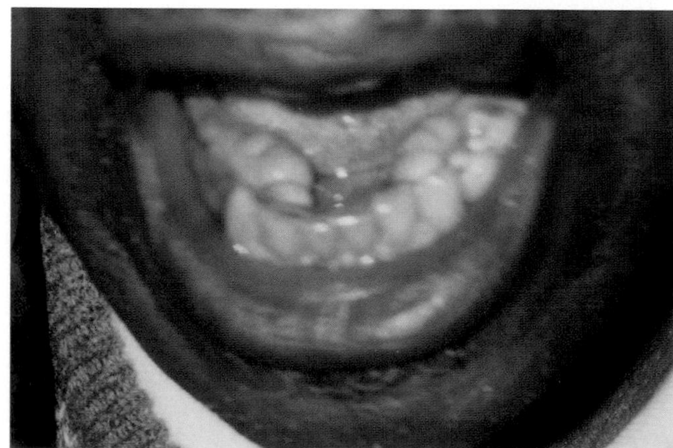

Figure 1.39.

Bilateral torus mandibularis.

 **TIPS**

- Torus mandibularis: one or more, often bilateral, gingival covered bony nodules, lingual side of the mandible
- Benign

TEETH

As with the gingiva, the teeth need to be inspected. The tongue blade approach **(Fig. 1.33)** is excellent for buccal side; the dental mirror **(Fig. 1.40)** is best for lingual side. Normally there are 4 pairs of incisors, 2 pairs of canines, 4 pairs of premolars and 4–6 pairs of molars.

Caries manifest with disruption, destruction, or both of the tooth enamel, as a brown or black discoloration on the affected tooth adjacent to sites of restoration or at the interface between gingiva and tooth. This is an extremely common process that, if untreated, can lead to significant morbidity and even contribute to mortality. It is incumbent to stress the importance of performing an adequate dental and oral examination in conjunction with a physical examination.

Tooth attrition manifests with a wearing down of the incisural, i.e., bite, surfaces of the teeth **(Fig. 1.41)**. In a young patient, consider bruxism and assess for concurrent temporomandibular joint dysfunction. **Tooth abrasion** manifests with a wearing down of the tooth in a specific site, and appears to be notched from the use of a pipe, cigarette holder, or toothpick in a specific site. **Tooth erosion** manifests with a brown discoloration and atrophy of the enamel from acid, e.g., bulimia or reflux disease in which the erosion is diffusely on the lingual side.

Congenital lues manifests with Hutchinson's incisors (peg topped and notched) and dome-shaped first molars (Moon's teeth) in the adult teeth. This is something that is decidedly rare today, and is mainly of historical import.

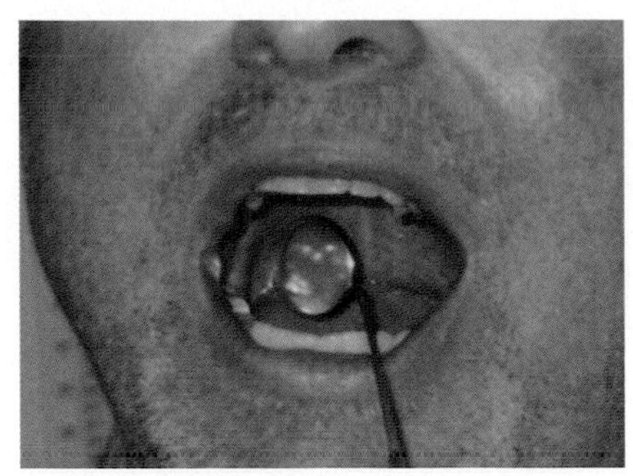

Figure 1.40.

Technique using a dental mirror to assess the buccal and lingual sides of the teeth.

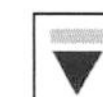

TIPS

- Visually inspect tooth surfaces, lingual and buccal, pay attention to the interface between the gingiva and the tooth and areas adjacent to restorations

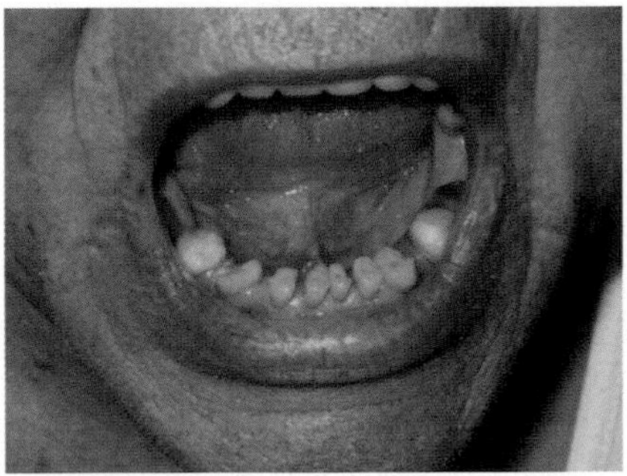

Figure 1.41.

Severe tooth attrition in a man 80 years of age.

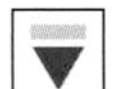

TIPS

- Tooth attrition: wearing down of the incisural surfaces of the teeth
- Caused by wear and tear of the teeth
- In young patients, consider bruxism and assess for temporomandibular joint dysfunction
- Tooth abrasion: notch that forms on the incisural side of tooth; wearing of the tooth in a specific site

TEACHING POINTS

TEETH

1. Erosion: loss of enamel on one side of the teeth—usually acid-related.
2. Attrition: wearing down of incisural surfaces of the teeth.
3. Caries: decay, disruption of the enamel, adjacent to a restoration or below the gingival–tooth interface.
4. Complications of caries include tooth fracture, abscess, and tooth loss.
5. Erosions: look for the company of calluses on fingers in bulimia; pyrosis, burping, and acid taste in mouth with reflux disease.
6. Multiple new caries: think dry mouth including Sjögren's syndrome or radiation therapy to the head and neck.
7. Examine buccal side of teeth with a tongue blade; examine lingual side with a dental mirror.

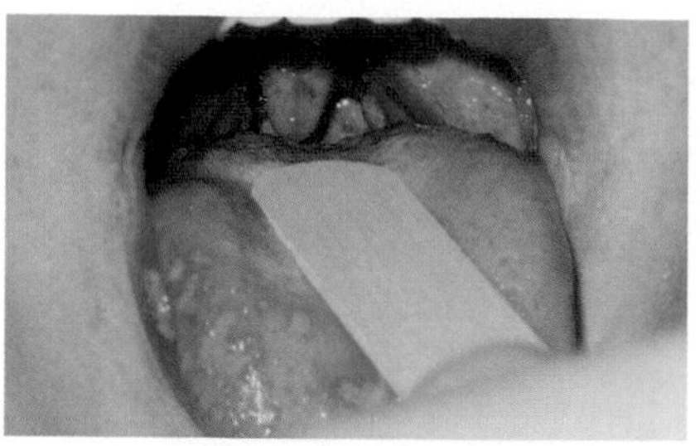

A

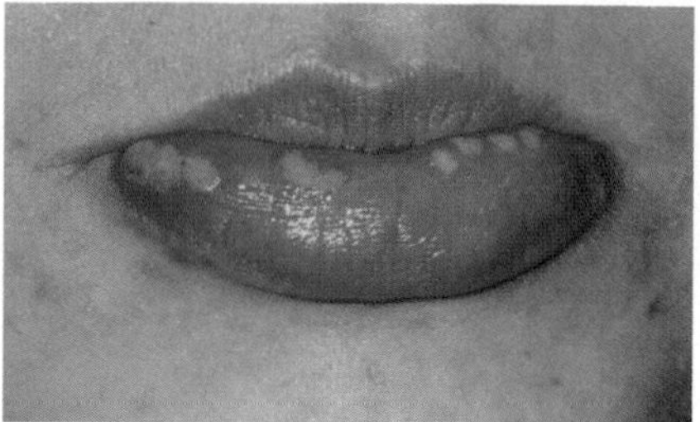

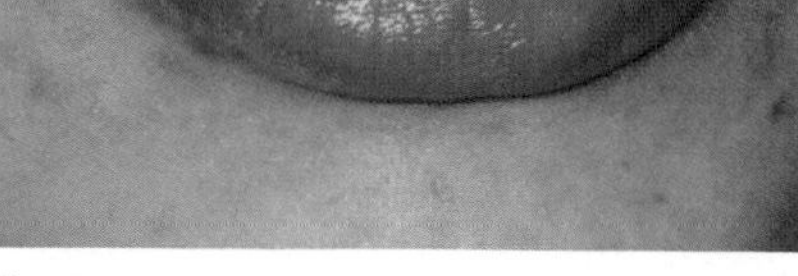

B

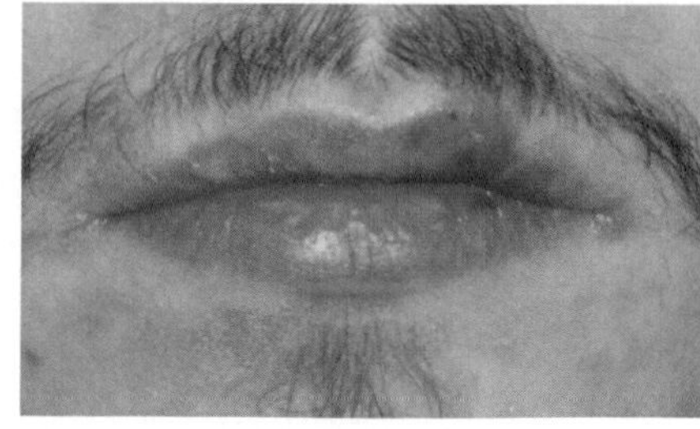

C

Figure 1.42.

Painful erosions and vesicles on mucous membranes and lips **(A, B)**. Coxsackie A-herpangina. Multiple lesions on the lips, gingiva, and posterior pharynx. **C.** Herpes labialis, here recurrent; the vesicles involve the mucous membranes and the skin across the vermillion border.

TIPS

- Visually inspect the gingiva, buccal mucosa, palate mucosa, lip, and skin adjacent to the lip
- Coxsackie stomatitis **(A** and **B):** diffuse vesicles rapidly become painful erosions and ulcers on gingiva, mucosa, lip; the posterior pharynx, does not cross the vermillion border of the lip onto skin
- Hand-foot-mouth disease: Coxsackie-related vesicles on the palms and soles
- Herpes simplex stomatitis or labialis **(C):** clusters of vesicles that rapidly become painful erosions and ulcers on gingiva, mucosa, lip, and skin outside the vermillion border
- Diffuse involvement may indicate immunosuppression

LIPS

Herpes simplex labialis or **stomatitis** manifests with clusters of vesicles that rapidly become painful erosions and ulcers on gingiva, mucosa, lip, and skin outside the vermillion border. Recurrent labialis **(Fig. 1.42C)** (also called a "cold sore") is limited and can result in only two to three vesicles on the lip and adjacent skin. Primary labialis is more intense than recurrent. **Coxsackievirus labialis** or **stomatitis (herpangina)** manifests with diffuse vesicles that rapidly become painful erosions and ulcers on the gingiva, mucosa, lips, and the posterior pharynx **(Fig. 1.42A and B)**. The lesions do not cross the vermillion border of the lip. A variant is **hand-foot-mouth disease** which manifests with herpangina and vesicles on the palms of the hands and the soles of the feet.

Other diagnoses include **squamous cell carcinoma**, which manifests with a painless papule or ulcer on the lip; lower lip most likely site. Metastases are first to local lymph nodes and then systemically **(Fig. 1.43)**. It is imperative to stress the importance of this because it is a type of squamous cell carcinoma that is increasing in incidence, which may be caused by the lack of ultraviolet (UV) protection on lips when participating in outdoor activities. **Cheilitis**, which manifests with one or more transverse fissures in the lip, is caused by dryness or exposure to UV light. This sunburn to lips is a risk factor

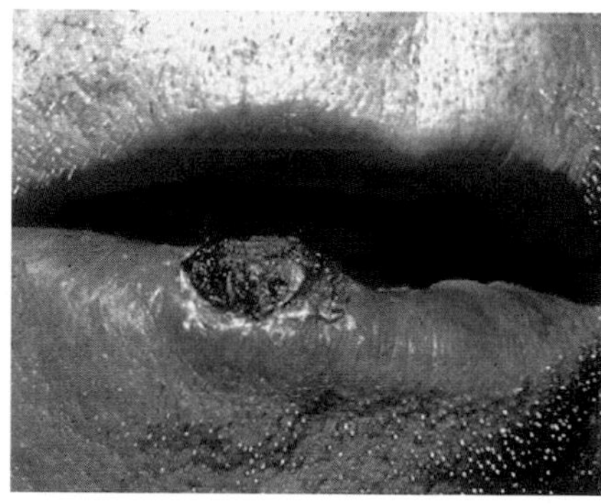

Figure 1.43.

Squamous cell carcinoma of lip. (From Moore KL, Dalley AF. *Clinically Oriented Anatomy*, 4th ed. Philadelphia: Lippincott Williams & Wilkins, 1999:869, with permission.)

TIPS

- Squamous cell carcinoma of lip: ulcer on the lip, nonhealing and nontender
- Lower lip most likely site

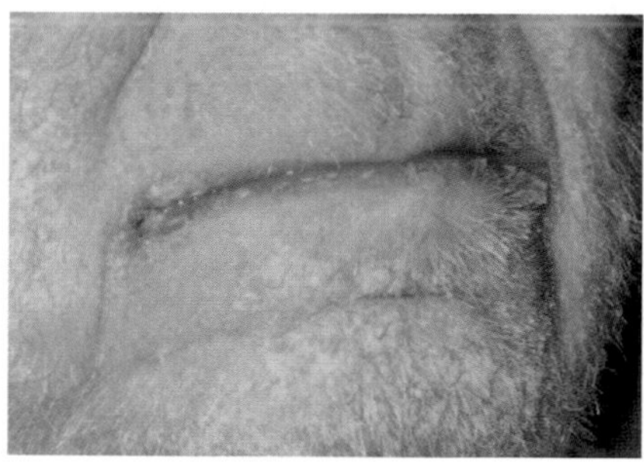

Figure 1.44.

Cheilosis or angular stomatitis. Here, caused by ill-fitting dentures—a Candidal stomatitis.

TIPS

- Cheilosis: crusty fissures on angles of the mouth caused by *Candida* sp. or iron deficiency
- Company iron deficiency keeps: anemia, koilonychia, and dysphagia

TEACHING POINTS

LIPS

1. Cold sore, if not involving the skin itself; think Coxsackie A virus infection.
2. Ultraviolet light exposure to lips: actinic cheilitis may develop.
3. Angular stomatitis: most common underlying reason is ill-fitting dentures or being edentulous, *Candida* infection.
4. Painless ulcers, irrespective of color of lesion: think squamous cell carcinoma.

for squamous cell carcinoma. **Cheilosis**, i.e., perlèche or angular stomatitis, which manifests with crusty fissures on the angles of the mouth **(Fig. 1.44)**, most often results from *Candida* organisms or iron-deficiency states. **Mucocele** manifests with a non-tender, transilluminable blue-purple papule on the lip, on buccal lower lip, due to trauma to minor salivary gland in lip.

Angioedema manifests with an acute onset of significant and pruritic swelling of the lip **(Fig. 1.45)**; it may be associated with stridor caused by angioedema of the throat and tongue or wheezing because of reversible airway disease. Look for concurrent urticaria. This can be caused by angiotensin-converting enzyme (ACE) inhibitor use or an allergy-mediated process.

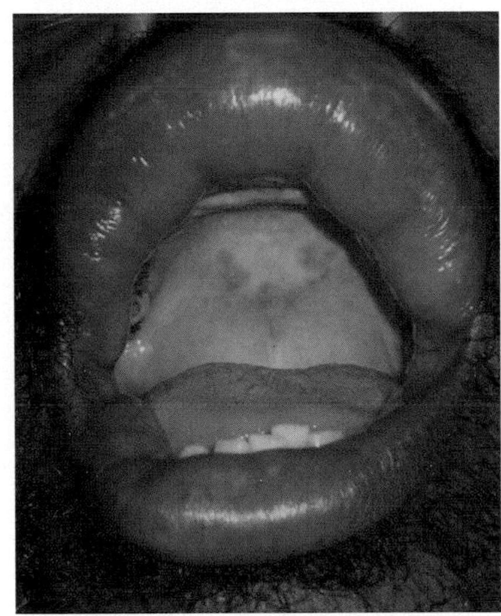

Figure 1.45.

Marked angioedema in the lip.

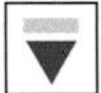

TIPS

- Angioedema: acute significant, pruritic swelling of the lip
- Look for angioedema of the throat and tongue; monitor for stridor and wheezing

TONGUE

The master physical diagnosis physician, Hamilton Bailey, stated, "Inspect the tongue out, palpate with the tongue in." The tongue is a muscular structure that is exclusively innervated by CN12. Indeed, the tongue examination requires a two-step (in and out) approach as described by Bailey **(Fig. 1.46)**. This is as important as visual inspection because early malignant lesions are often easier to palpate than to visualize.

Macroglossia manifests with an enlarged tongue with peripheral indentations from the adjacent teeth, also called, *serratoglossia*; often, there is a history of biting the tongue sides and of severe snoring. When very large, the tongue tip will protrude outside of the lips even with the mouth closed (Fig. 1.25). Macroglossia is most often caused by right ventricular failure, amyloidosis, acromegaly, or hypothyroidism **(Fig. 1.47)**. Often seen are the facies of each of these underlying processes.

Thrush manifests with white papules and plaques that appear to be akin to curdled milk **(Fig. 1.48)**. These are on the tongue, buccal mucosa, gingival surfaces, and the posterior pharynx. The tongue is often modestly swollen, which is caused by infection with *Candida albicans.* **White hairy tongue**, also known as hairy leukoplakia, manifests with a plaque on the tongue with white fronds from its surface, which is deeply adherent to the surface and cannot be scraped off **(Fig. 1.49)**. The tongue is not swollen. White hairy tongue is associated with severe immunocompromise and is an ominous sign in a patient as it indicates advanced acquired immunodeficiency syndrome (AIDS). It is rarely seen in a patient with a CD 4 count of >50. It is caused by Epstein-Barr virus (EBV) infection.

Papilloma manifests with a papular or plaquelike warty, exophytic lesion, which may secondarily ulcerate **(Fig. 1.50)**. These lesions are caused by

Figure 1.46.

Technique to **A.** inspect and **B.** palpate tongue.

TIPS

- Place a gloved finger (usually index) on lateral tongue, to the depth of the posterior pharynx; palpate surface on left lateral, sublingual and then right lateral surfaces
- Early squamous cell carcinoma: may be palpable before visible
- Often grasping tip with a 2 x 2 gauze is of aid to clinician

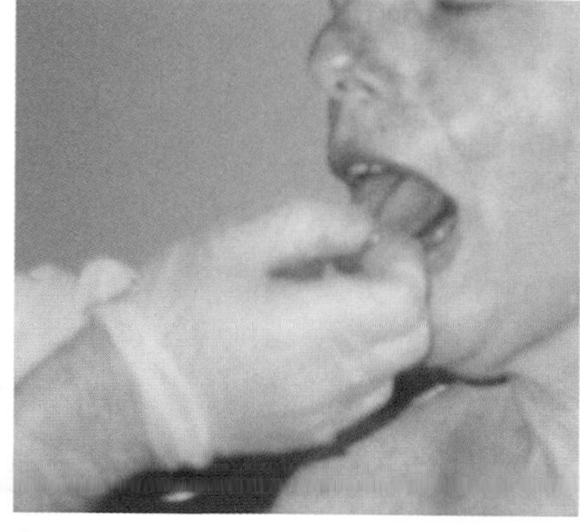

A

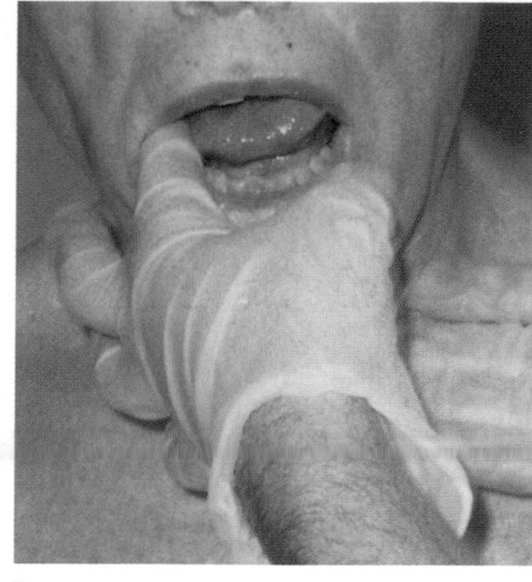

B

human papilloma virus (HPV) infection. Associated with an increased risk of squamous cell carcinoma, these HPV-related warts can occur in any area of mucosa.

Atrophic glossitis manifests with a smooth almost shiny appearing tongue **(Fig. 1.51)**. There is a loss of all fungiform and filiform papilla, with a relative prominence of the circumvallate papilla on the posterior surface, which is caused by a vitamin B_{12} or folate deficiency. There is concurrent loss

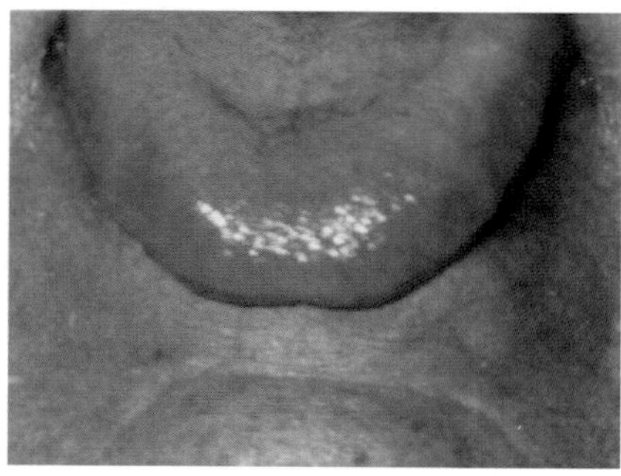

Figure 1.47.

Macroglossia caused by amyloidosis. Patient had history of snoring, signs of right ventricular failure, and chronic periorbital ecchymosis.

TIPS

- Macroglossia: diffusely enlarged tongue with peripheral indentations from the teeth
- Amyloidosis, acromegaly, or hypothyroidism
- Right ventricular failure or superior vena cava (SVC) syndrome

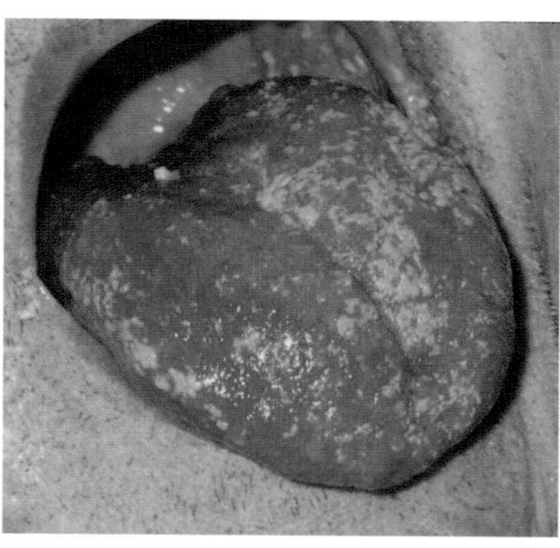

Figure 1.48.

Thrush.

TIPS

- Modestly swollen tongue
- White papules and plaques, loosely adherent on surface of tongue; can be scraped off
- Each papule has an erythematous base

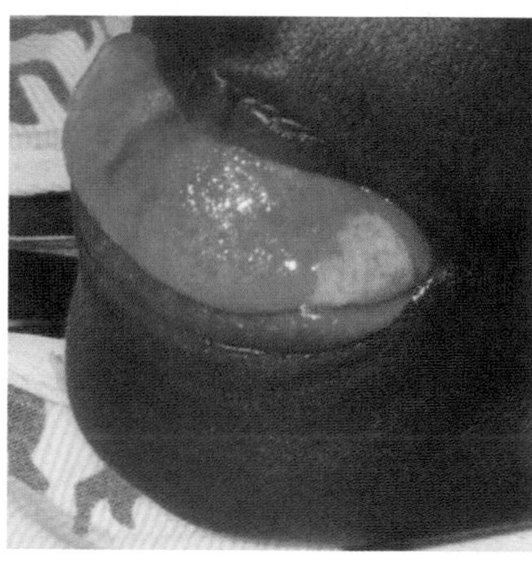

Figure 1.49.

White hairy tongue in patient with advanced acquired immunodeficiency syndrome (AIDS) with a CD 4 of <50.

TIPS

- White hairy tongue: solitary plaque with white fronds on the surface of the tongue
- Epstein-Barr virus (EBV) infection of the tongue surface
- Concurrent problems, including thrush, are not uncommon
- Associated with immunocompromise, especially advanced human immunodeficiency virus (HIV) disease; rare if CD 4 >50

TEACHING POINTS

TONGUE

1. Plaques, papules, or ulcers on tongue, irrespective of color, are suggestive of squamous cell carcinoma until proven otherwise.
2. Atrophy of papilla is the major feature of atrophic glossitis.
3. Causes of atrophic glossitis: B_{12} and folate deficiency states.
4. Palpation of the tongue is complementary to visual inspection.
5. Black tongue is usually caused by staining with nicotine or bismuth, but may result from colonization with an *Aspergillus sp.*

of fine touch and vibratory sensation if caused by B_{12} deficiency, but no such neuropathy in folate deficiency.

Geographic tongue manifests with red patches of denuded tongue epithelium, surrounded by rims of white and areas of normal tongue epithelium, which change from day to day **(Fig. 1.52)**. This is an idiopathic process that is self-limited.

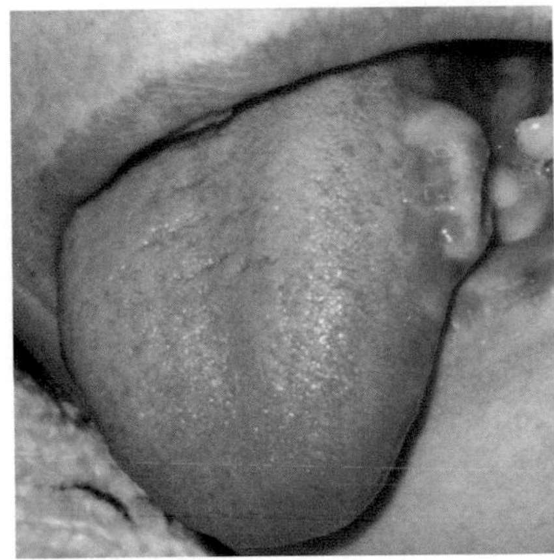

Figure 1.50.

Tongue papilloma. Large exophytic ulcerating lesion on lateral tongue.

 **TIPS**

- Papilloma: papular or plaquelike warty, exophytic lesion, caused by human papilloma virus (HPV)
- Increased risk of squamous cell carcinoma of the tongue with this lesion

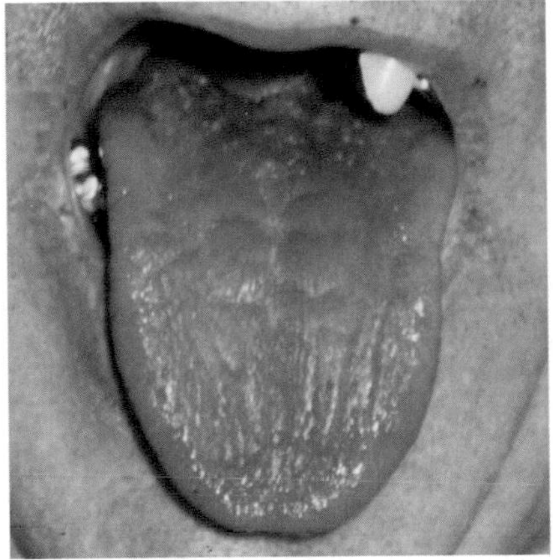

Figure 1.51.

Atrophic glossitis of B_{12} deficiency. Classic shiny, smooth surface of the tongue.

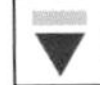 **TIPS**

- Atrophic glossitis: smooth, shiny tongue with atrophy of all fungiform and filiform papilla; prominence of the circumvallate papilla on posterior surface
- Deficiency of vitamin B_{12}, folate, or both

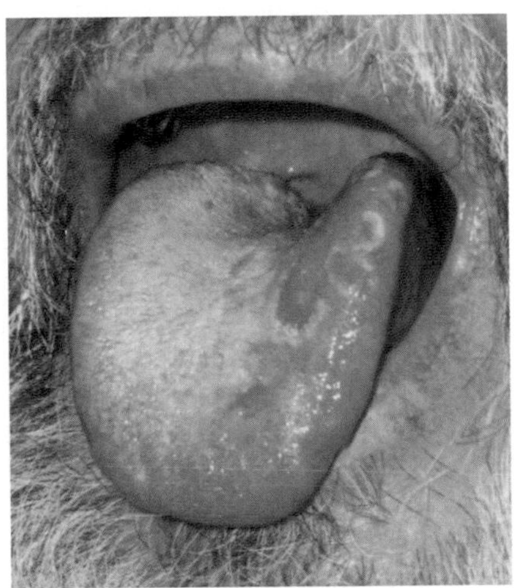

Figure 1.52.

Geographic tongue. Migratory erythema of denuded epithelium with rims of white.

 **TIPS**

- Geographic tongue: patches of denuded tongue epithelium, surrounded by rims of white; changes from day to day
- Idiopathic but benign

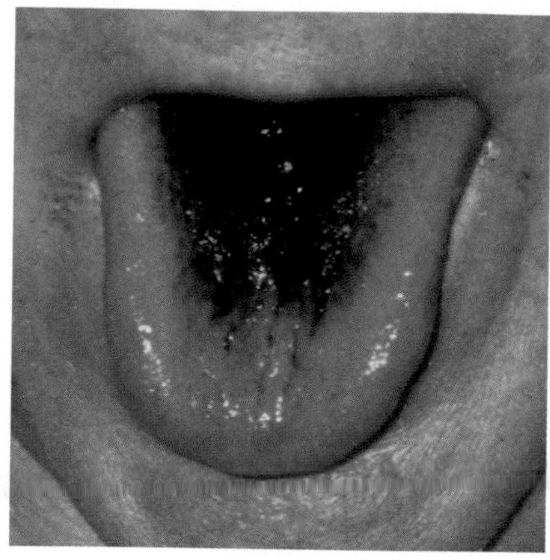

Figure 1.53.

Black tongue.

 **TIPS**

- Black tongue: black color on tongue surface, specifically on the fungiform and filiform papilla
- Caused by colonization with *Aspergillus niger* or staining with black licorice, nicotine, bismuth, or charcoal

Black tongue manifests with a black color to the surface of the tongue, specifically the fungiform and filiform papilla **(Fig. 1.53)**. The black discoloration is painless and does not scrape off. The most common reasons for this include the superficial colonization with *Aspergillus niger*, especially in a patient who has had radiation therapy to the head and neck; nicotine-staining; and use of anise-containing black licorice, or of bismuth, or oral charcoal.

Osler-Weber-Rendu, also known as hereditary telangiectasia syndrome, manifests with multiple telangiectasia in the buccal mucosa, tongue, and face **(Fig. 1.54)**. The company it keeps includes arteriovenous malformations in the GI tract, the brain, liver, or lungs. Thus, the patient is at risk for gastrointestinal bleeds, cerebrovascular accidents, infection, and high-output heart failure. One key to the diagnosis is to look for tongue telangiectasia. Telangiectasia are not uncommon in facial skin, but is decidedly uncommon in the mucosa of the tongue.

Sublingual varicosities manifest with a set of bilateral purple vessels on the sublingual surface **(Fig. 1.55)**. These manifestations are usually benign and bespeak no mischief of themselves. However, they can accompany right ventricular failure or SVC syndrome. Thus, look for sublingual varicosities in the setting of congestive heart failure (CHF), SVC syndrome, macroglossia, or clinical suspicion of increased jugular venous pressure (JVP). If SVC syndrome or right ventricular failure is suspected, sublingual varicosities may indicate increased right-sided pressures.

Squamous cell carcinoma manifests with a painless red or white exophytic papule or plaque that ulcerates on the tongue **(Fig. 1.56)**. The most common sites are at the lateral surfaces and root of the tongue. Thus, palpate and inspect the deep lateral and sublingual surfaces of the tongue. Palpation

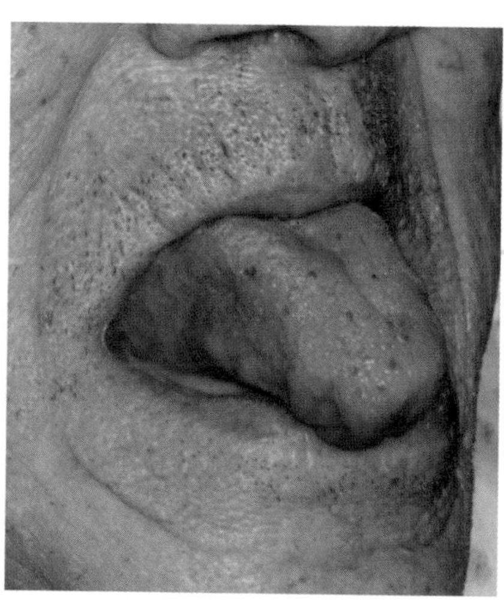

Figure 1.54.

Osler-Weber-Rendu disease. Multiple telangiectasia in the facial skin but, most importantly, in the tongue mucosa.

 **TIPS**

- Osler-Weber-Rendu disease: multiple telangiectasia in tongue and buccal mucosa
- Associated with gastrointestinal bleeding and arteriovenous malformations
- Autosomal dominant

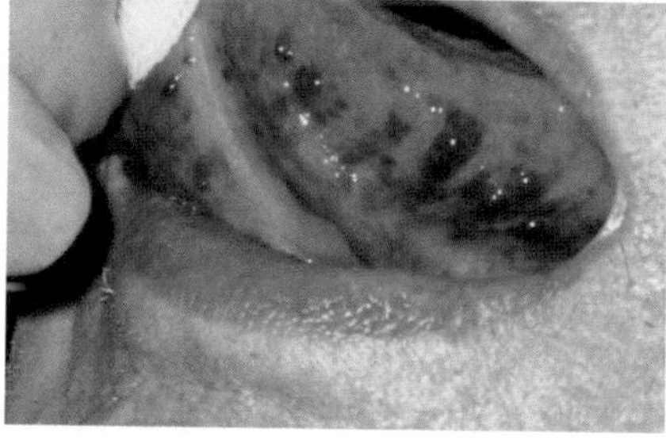

Figure 1.55.

Sublingual varicosities. This patient has had significant right ventricular failure over several years.

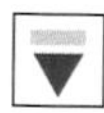 **TIPS**

- Observe the sublingual surface of the protruded tongue
- Sublingual varicosities: set of purple vessels on the sublingual surface bilaterally
- May be normal or be company with which elevated JVP keeps; indicates right ventricular failure if macroglossia concurrently present

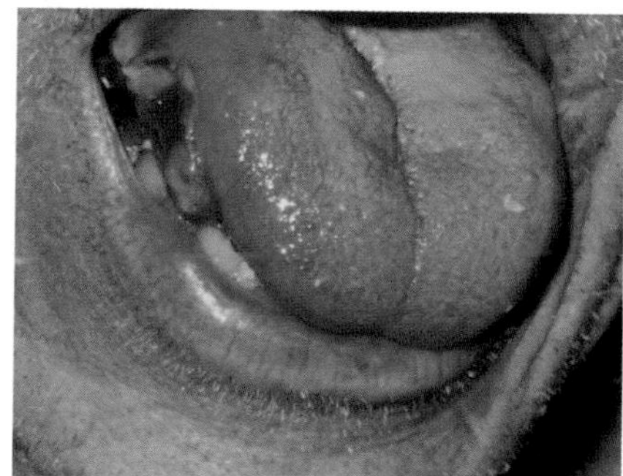

Figure 1.56.

Large exophytic carcinoma of the lateral tongue.

 **TIPS**

- Squamous cell carcinoma: painless red or white exophytic papule, plaque, or ulcer
- Must palpate submandibular nodes as a part of the physical examination, as this is the first place for metastases

and inspection are components requisite to the tongue examination. Recall, most early squamous cell carcinomas are not white but actually are red.

Strawberry tongue manifests with mild swelling of the tongue such that the filiform papillae appear enlarged and edematous. This is preceded by white strawberry tongue, in which the surface is covered with a diffuse, adherent white substance which desquamates to form red strawberry tongue. The company it keeps includes antecedent exudative pharyngitis and the diffuse erythematous rash of scarlet fever. Strawberry tongue is also associated with Kawasaki disease. **Peutz-Jeghers** manifests with multiple pigmented macules on the tongue, lips, and buccal mucosa. This is associated with colon or small intestinal hyperplastic-type polyps.

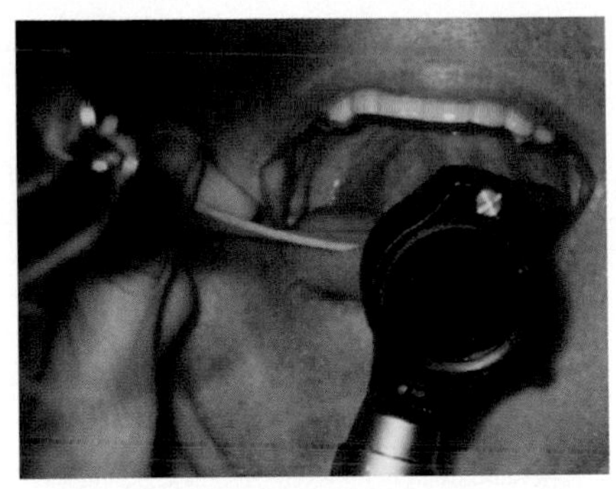

Figure 1.57.

Technique for posterior pharynx imaging, AHHHH approach.

TIPS

- Place a tongue blade on the mid posterior tongue, press downward as patient says AHHHH
- Use a light source to inspect the posterior pharynx
- Complementary to the two-tongue blade approach to oral structure and posterior pharynx inspection

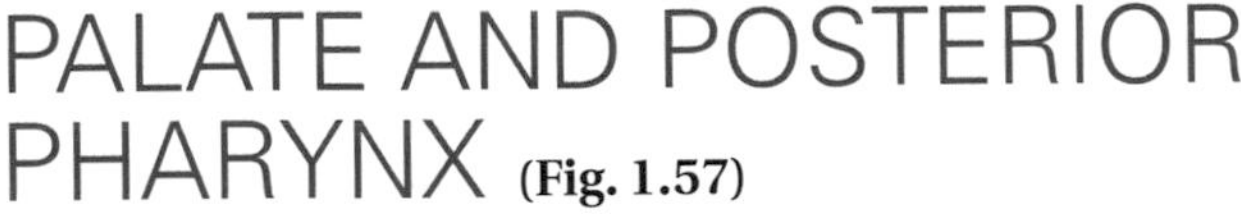

PALATE AND POSTERIOR PHARYNX (Fig. 1.57)

Torus palatinus manifests with a single nontender nodule in the hard palate covered with mucosa **(Fig. 1.58)**. This is a benign, not uncommon bony exostosis. It is important to be able to recognize this variant of normal. No symptoms are associated with it and it is a problem only if the patient ever needs dentures.

Cleft palate manifests with a defect in the midline of the hard and soft palate, so that the nasopharynx can be visualized **(Fig. 1.59)**. Often a concurrent, albeit, surgically corrected, cleft lip. It is rarely seen in adults today, but may be seen in immigrants from Third World countries. **Bifid uvula** manifests with asymptomatic bifurcation of the tip of the uvula; it is usually benign, but may be associated with a submucosal cleft palate.

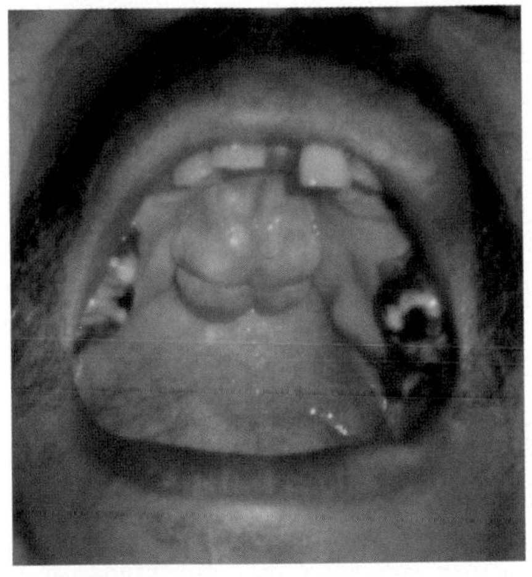

Figure 1.58.

Torus palatinus.

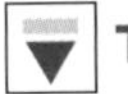

TIPS

- Torus palatinus: nontender bony nodule in the hard palate covered with normal mucosa
- Benign bony exostosis

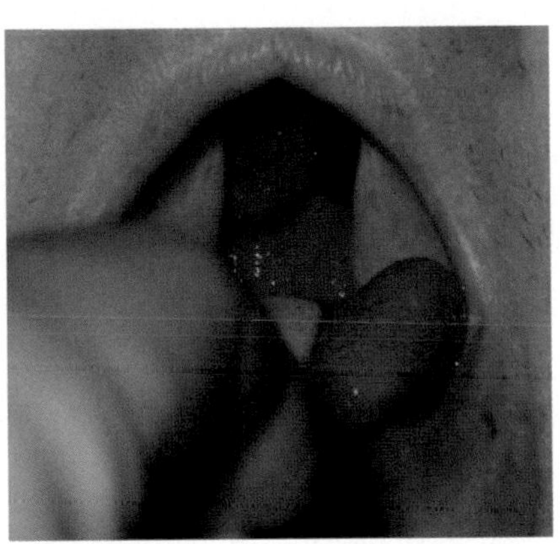

A

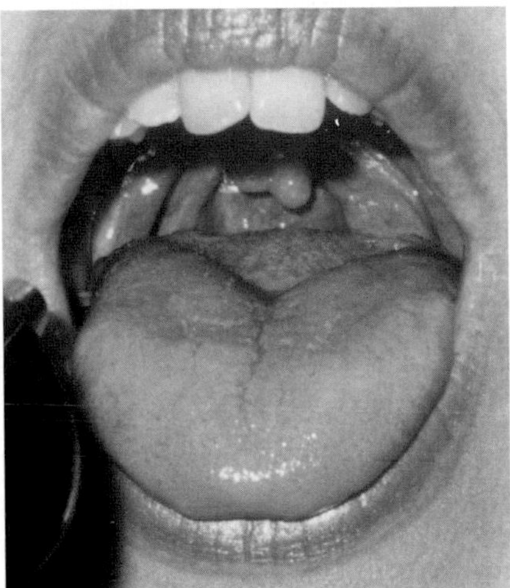

B

Figure 1.59.

A. Cleft palate. **B.** Bifid uvula, usually a normal variant but may have a submucosal cleft palate associated.

TIPS

- **A.** Cleft palate: large defect in midline of the hard and soft palate; nasopharynx can be visualized
- **B.** Bifid uvula is a normal variant. Palpate the hard palate because there may be a cleft palate that is covered with mucosa, thus occult

TEACHING POINTS

POSTERIOR PHARYNX EXAMINATION

1. Local complications of exudative pharyngitis include Ludwig's angina and peritonsillar abscess (quinsy), each of which can be life-threatening.
2. Hard palate findings include cleft palate, high arch, and torus palatinus.
3. Exudative pharyngitis has jugulodigastric node enlargement in streptococcal pharyngitis; diffuse lymphadenopathy in infectious mononucleosis.
4. Nonexudative pharyngitis: cough and rhinorrhea with diffuse cervical lymph node enlargement.

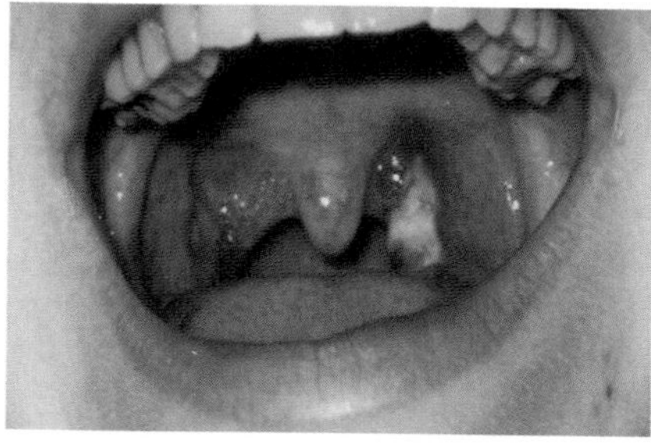

Figure 1.60.

Exudative pharyngitis.

TIPS

- Exudative pharyngitis: erythema with swelling and exudate on the posterior pharynx and uvula
- Streptococcal: exudate and jugulodigastic node enlarged
- Infections mononucleosis: exudate, petechine, diffuse lymph node enlargement

Nonexudative pharyngitis manifests with erythema and swelling of the tonsils and posterior pharynx. The company it keeps includes diffuse tender cervical lymph node enlargement, serous rhinorrhea, and serous otitis media and cough. **Exudative pharyngitis** manifests with swelling, erythema, and exudates on the surface of the posterior pharynx and uvula **(Fig. 1.60)**. The company it keeps is specific to the underlying etiology; if *streptococcal* etiology, enlarged tender jugulodigastric nodes (Fig. 1.29H) and no cough **(Box 1.2)**; if *infectious mononucleosis*, diffuse lymphadenopathy, petechial on pharynx and, potentially, splenomegaly can result.

Local complications of exudative pharyngitis include quinsy and Ludwig's angina. **Quinsy** manifests with a smooth nodule or mass in the posterior pharynx adjacent to a tonsil **(Fig. 1.61)**. This is a streptococcal abscess in the peritonsillar area. **Ludwig's angina** manifests with swelling in the mouth floor confirmed by bimanual palpation and erythema in the submental area. This extension of infection to the floor of the mouth and in the retropharynx is a life-threatening local complication of streptococcal exudative pharyngitis. Because the patient can develop airway compromise, stridor may develop.

The local complications are rare, but need to be discussed. These are complications that most patients over the age of 80 years can state and describe, because they may have known of classmates or had siblings who died of these complications in the pre-antibiotic era. Although emphasis is placed in curricula about systemic complications, little is taught about these treatable local conditions. *Systemic complications* of streptococcal pharyngitis include rheumatic fever, glomerulonephritis, and scarlet fever. These are discussed further in Chapter 14 and in Table 14.5.

Other problems include **high-arched palate**, which manifests with a diffuse upward concavity of the hard palate, i.e., an invagination. This is a normal variant or may be congenital, e.g., in Holt-Oram syndrome. **Temporomandibular joint (TMJ) dysfunction** manifests with limited opening or closing of the mouth with pain anterior to the tragus. If the TMJ problem is caused by dislocation, the jaw is locked open; if from arthritis, closure is satisfactory, but the opening is limited. If the TMJ dysfunction is trismus, it is due to spasm of masseter muscles.

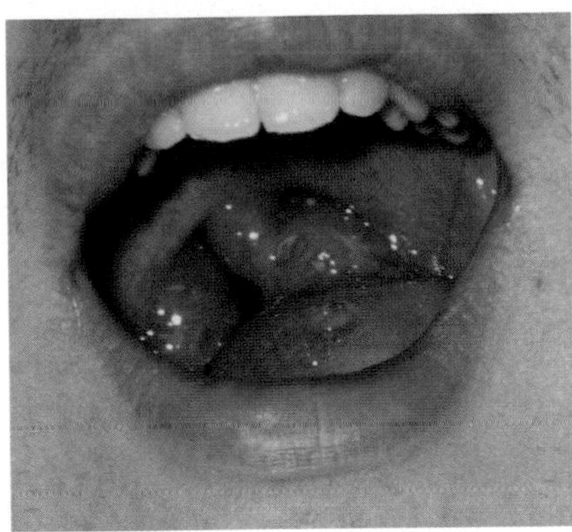

Figure 1.61.

Left peritonsillar abscess, quinsy. A potentially life-threatening complication of streptococcal pharyngitis. (Modified from Moore KL, Dalley AF. *Clinically Oriented Anatomy*, 4th ed. Philadelphia: Lippincott Williams & Wilkins, 1999:167, with permission.)

TIPS

- Quinsy: smooth nodule of mass in the posterior pharynx adjacent to a tonsil
- Complication of streptococcal pharyngitis

Box 1.2

Features of streptococcal pharyngitis

1. Presence of exudates on the posterior pharynx
2. Presence of fever
3. Presence of palpable tender anterior cervical lymph node
4. Absence of cough

(From Centor RM, Meier FA, Dalton HP. Throat cultures for diagnosis of group A streptococcal pharyngitis. *Ann Intern Med* 1986;105:892–899.)

GOITER-THYROID EXAMINATION

In the normal setting, the thyroid is a butterfly-shaped structure that is subcutaneous and the isthmus of the thyroid is adjacent to the cricoid cartilage. If you cannot find the cricoid cartilage, you cannot find the thyroid gland **(Fig. 1.62)**. **Goiter**, which is a nodular or diffuse mass in anterior neck, is thyroid gland enlargement. Look at the thyroid gland location and landmarks first, then gently palpate the structures. Apply pressure as if palpating for lymph nodes, i.e., do not apply too much pressure.

Hypothyroidism manifests with the patient reporting symptoms of being cold, constipated, gaining weight, depression, and feeling fat. Often, patchy or diffuse alopecia is seen with the specific loss of the lateral eyebrows, Queen Anne's sign **(Fig. 1.63)**. In addition, a particularly excellent test is DTR's—the DTRs are diminished and have a delayed relaxation phase. The company it keeps include bradycardia, thickened doughy skin, proximal muscle weakness, and a goiter or a thyroidectomy scar over the neck **(Fig. 1.64)**. If goiter is **retrosternal**, Pemberton's maneuver should be performed to

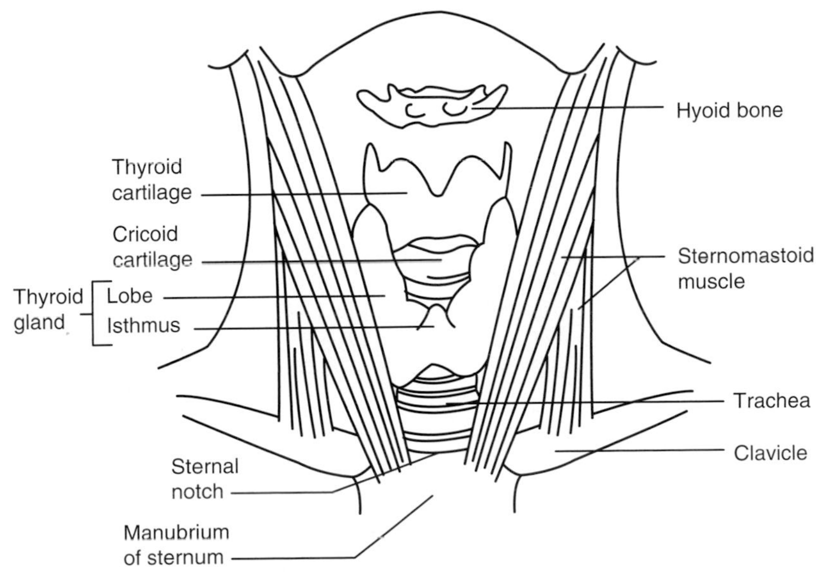

Figure 1.62.

Landmarks for thyroid examination. Inspect first, then palpate. **A.** Cricoid cartilage. **B.** Thyroid gland. **C.** Trachea. **D.** Thyroid cartilage.

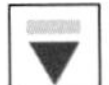

TIPS

- Note the landmarks of the cricoid and thyroid cartilage
- Look at the thyroid gland location
- Gently palpate the structures, use pressure as if palpating for lymph nodes, i.e., do not apply too much pressure

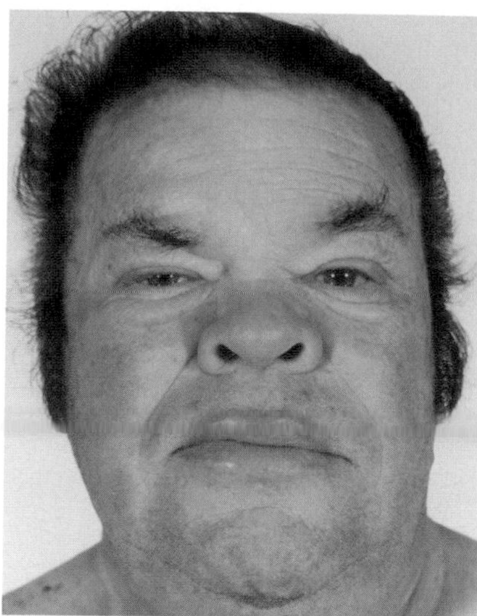

Figure 1.63.

Hypothyroidism. Classic features of coarsened skin, macroglossia, diffuse hair loss, which is coarse, and loss of lateral eyebrows, bilaterally. Thyroid-stimulating hormone (TSH) was >100.

 **TIPS**

- Hypothyroidism: patchy or diffuse hair loss; hair present coarse and thick to palpation
- Profound hypothyroidism or myxedema: note coarsening of facial features, Queen Anne's sign, and diffuse alopecia; and thickened coarse skin

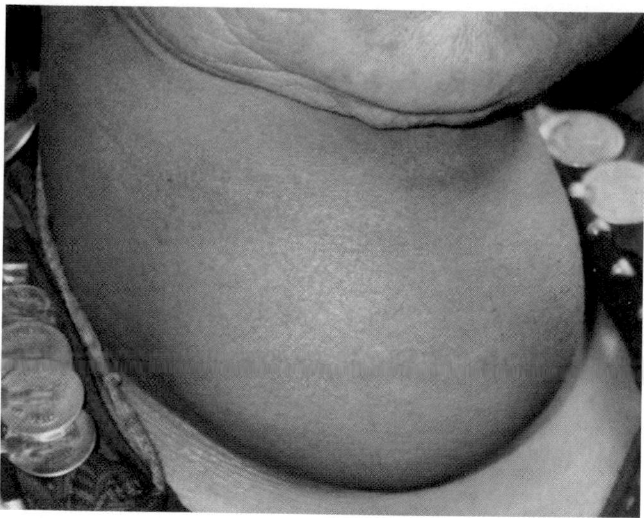

Figure 1.64.

Massive goiter in a patient with iodide deficiency, i.e., endemic goiter.

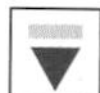 **TIPS**

- Hypothyroidism: goiter or a scar over the neck
- The goiter may be quite massive

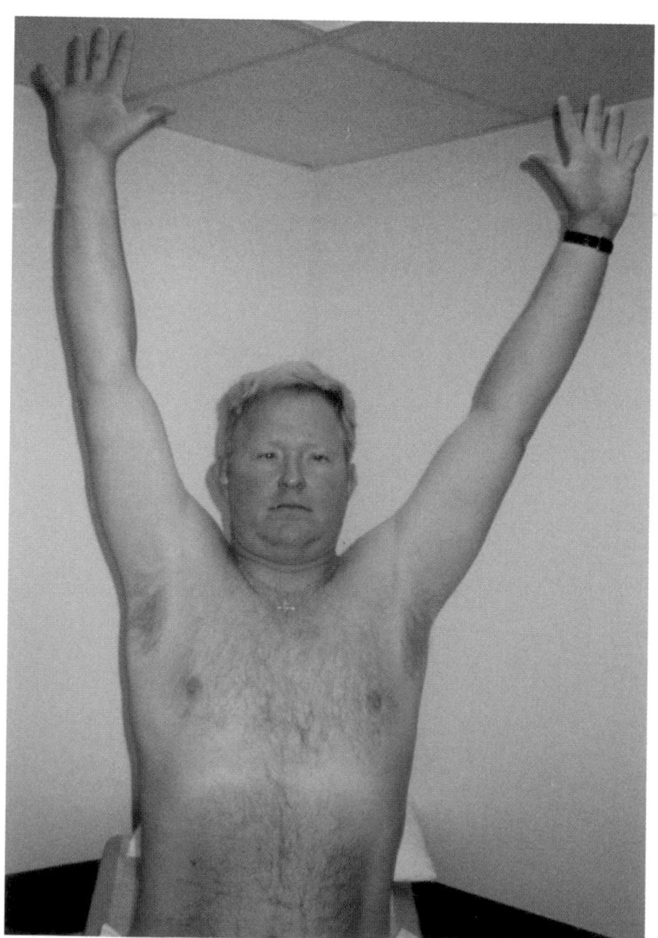

Figure 1.65.

Technique to perform Pemberton's sign for a symptomatic retrosternal goiter.

 **TIPS**

- Patient standing, forward flex both arms above the head
- Normal: no suffusion of face, no increase in jugular venous pressure (JVP)
- Retrosternal goiter: facial suffusion, increased JVP, and the development of dizziness, even syncope

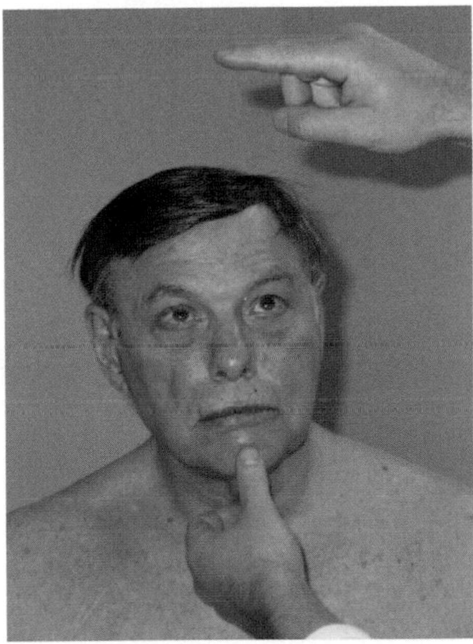
A

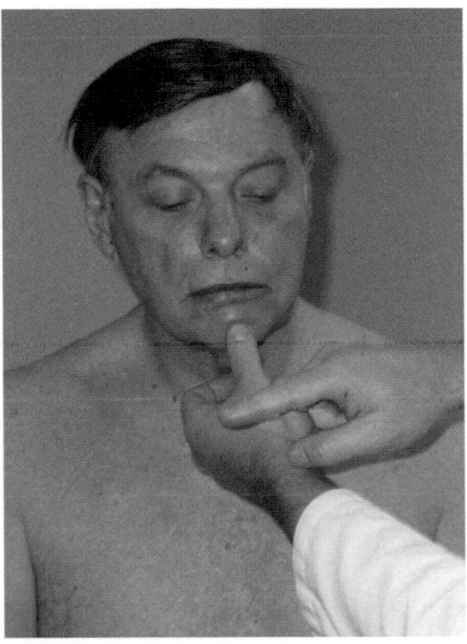
B

Figure 1.66.

Technique to assess eyes in hyperthyroidism. **A.** Baseline. **B.** Active downward gaze of the eyes.

TIPS

- Inspect the eyelid margin, relative to the sclera
- Normal: the upper lid covers the upper limbus slightly
- Hypercatecholamine excess (fear): the upper lids are not covering the limbus
- Hyperthyroidism: unilateral lid retraction (Stellwag's sign), bilateral—Dalrymple's sign
- Maintain neutral position of head with thumb placed on chin

make certain the patient is not at risk for syncope **(Fig. 1.65)**. An anonymous Mayan physician first described this technique in art; however, Dr. Pemberton received the eponym for his report.

Hyperthyroidism manifests with the patient reporting symptoms of unintentional weight loss, heat intolerance, and hyperdefecation. There is unilateral or bilateral elevation, i.e., retraction, of the upper eyelid (unilateral-Stellwag's sign, bilateral-Dalrymple's sign) on baseline gaze **(Fig. 1.66)**. This is confirmed by active lid lag of the upper eyelid with downward gaze (Von Graefe's sign) and active lower lid lag of bottom eyelid with upward gaze (Griffith sign) **(Fig. 1.67)**. These are caused by thyroid hormone or catecholamine-related spasm of Müller's muscle. In addition, a systolic rub is heard over the precordium (Mean-Lerman scratch) and noted are brisk, i.e., 3+ deep tendon reflexes that are symmetric and have short, staccato contraction and relaxation phases. The company it keeps includes a fine diffuse distal tremor, thin skin, proximal muscle weakness, and distal onycholysis, i.e., Plummer's nails in which the plates are thin and distally lifted off the nailbeds **(Fig. 1.69)**. Finally, the patient may have tachycardia and the absence of wrinkles in forehead on looking upward (Joffroy's sign).

Graves' disease manifests with findings of a diffuse goiter when the thyroid is involved, which is virtually always visible on inspection **(Fig. 1.68)**. A bruit is also heard over the goiter, especially if it is diffuse, and over a closed eye (Riesman's sign). If a goiter is present, the patient invariably has manifestations of hyperthyroidism as described above. Remember, a pa-

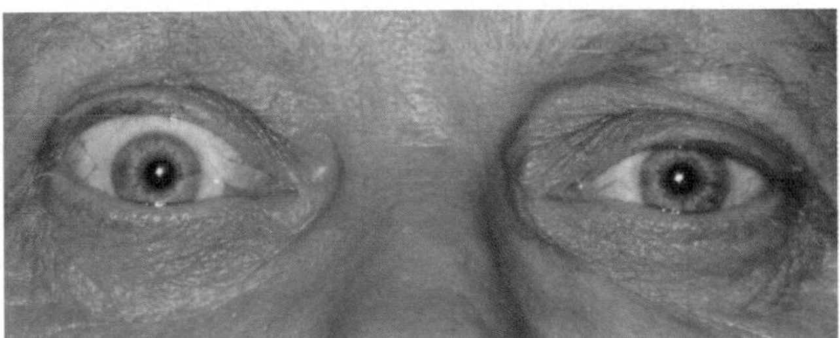

Figure 1.67.

Stellwag's sign of hyperthyroidism. Note that left eye has lid lag, right eye has normal placement of the upper eyelid. No proptosis was evident in this patient.

TIPS

- Inspect the eyelid margin, relative to the sclera
- Hyperthyroidism: unilateral lid retraction (Stellwag's sign), bilateral—Dalrymple's sign

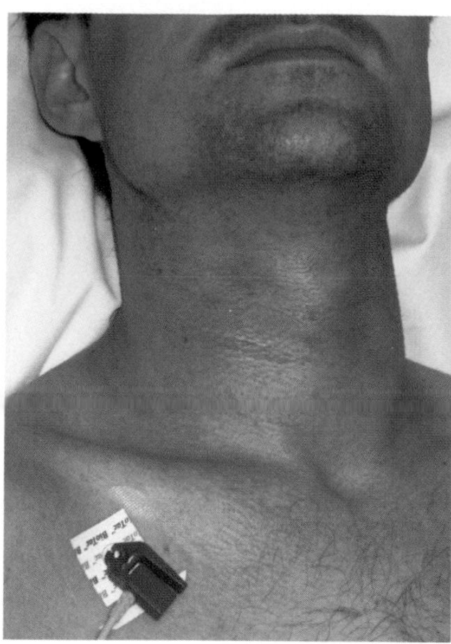

Figure 1.68.

Goiter of Graves' disease—symmetric, nontender and diffuse.

 **TIPS**

- Visually inspect the anterior neck of the patient
- Graves' disease: diffuse goiter
- Plummer's disease: multinodular goiter
- Ectopic thyroid: no goiter, may even have a scar

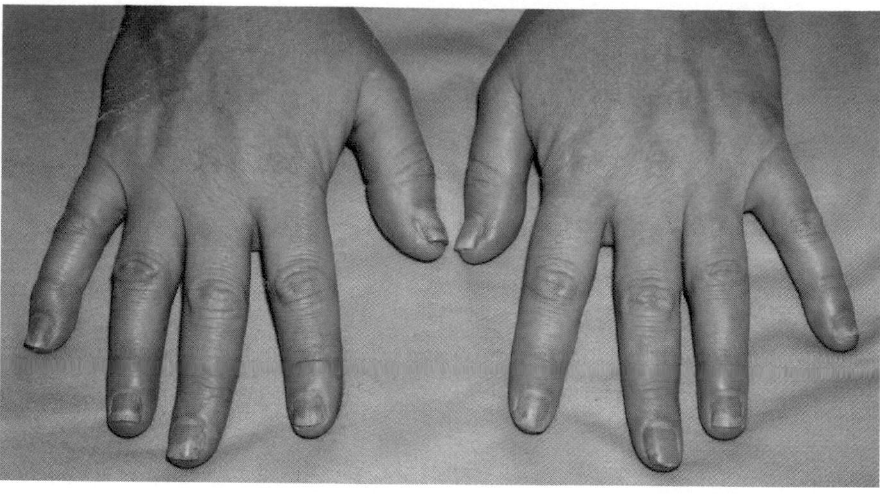

Figure 1.69.

Plummer's nails: sign of hyperthyroidism. Note that the nail plates are thin, and the distal aspects are destroyed and lifted off the underlying beds.

 **TIPS**

- Inspect the nails, specifically the distal nail plates provide clues to diagnosis
- Hyperthyroidism: nail plates are thin, the distal aspects are destroyed and lifted off the underlying beds; classic Plummer's nails; no pitting present

tient with Graves' disease may not necessarily have thyroid disease as a component and, although lid lag and exophthalmos may be present in Graves' disease, exophthalmos is specific to it, whereas, lid lag is specific for hyperthyroidism, irrespective of cause. Other two components of Graves' are **pretibial myxedema**, which manifests with red plaques on the

TEACHING POINTS

THYROID EXAMINATION

1. Goiter can be associated with normal, high, or low thyroid states.
2. Graves' disease can manifest with proptosis and skin findings without any thyroid problems.
3. Exophthalamus or proptosis specific to Graves' disease, not related to hyperthyroidism.
4. Lid lag is spasm of the Müller's muscle, specific to hyperthyroidism, nonspecific to the etiology.
5. Alopecia is associated with significant hypo- or hyperthyroidism.
6. Proximal muscle weakness is associated with significant hypo- or hyperthyroidism.
7. Relaxation phase delay in DTR is associated with hypothyroidism.

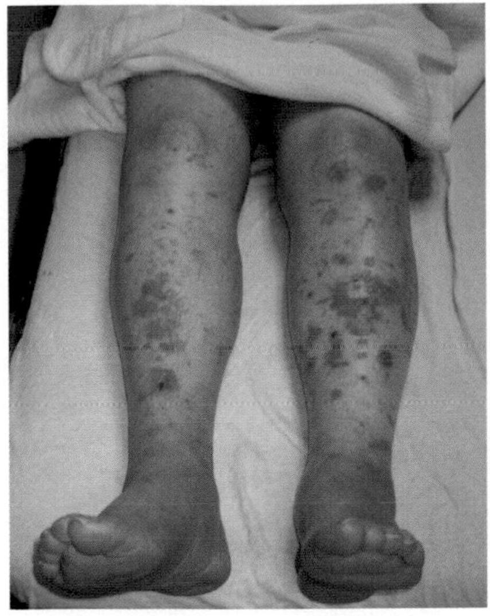

Figure 1.70.

Pretibial myxedema of Graves' disease on anterior tibial surfaces

 **TIPS**

- Graves' disease: papules and plaques in the anterior tibial skin; independent of thyroid status

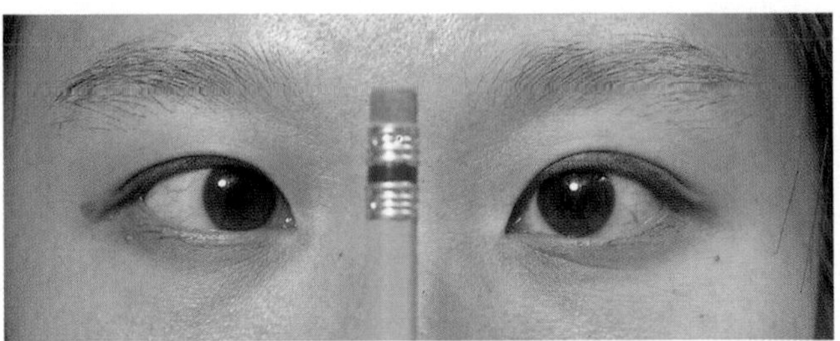

Figure 1.71.

Technique to unmask early exophthalmus, also known as proptosis. If patient can symmetrically converge eyes, proptosis is unlikely. (From Bickley LS, Szilagyi PG. *Bates' Guide to Physical Examination*, 8th ed. Philadelphia: Lippincott Williams & Wilkins, 2003:151, with permission.)

 **TIPS**

- Horizontal gaze: instruct patient to follow pencil inward so as to converge, that is the Möebius maneuver
- Normal: eyes converge
- Graves' disease: decrease in convergence bilateral

anterior tibial surface of the legs, and over time evolves into pigmented areas **(Fig. 1.70)**, and **proptosis** also known as **exophthalamus**. Exophthalamus manifests with diplopia, one or both eye globes projecting beyond the orbital rims, decreased ROM to eye movement, and the Möebius sign of decreased eye convergence **(Fig. 1.71)**. Often the exophthalmos develops after the goiter and hyperthyroidism have been effectively treated; indeed, often the patient is actually on thyroid hormone replacement. **Plummer's disease** also known as toxic multinodular goiter manifests with the signs of hyperthyroidism; the goiter is multinodular, but no dermatopathy or ophthalmopathy are present.

Annotated Bibliography

Ear and Auricle

Hawke M, Keene M, Alberti PW. *Clinical Otoscopy: A Text and Colour Atlas.* Edinburgh: Churchill Livingstone, 1984:76–77.

A good resource for images and discussion of practical aspects of otoscopic examination. A must for primary care physicians.

Iloeje UH, Schneiderman H. Chiclero ulcer of cutaneous leishmaniasis. *Consultant* 1997; 37:2920–2924.

Case report with excellent images of this rare entity. Chiclerois—a painless ulceration of the helix and antihelix caused by cutaneous Leishmaniasis (Central and South America).

Lee D, Sperling N. Initial management of auricular trauma. *Am Fam Phys* 1996;53(7): 2339–2344.

A nice anatomic discussion of the pathoanatomic underpinnings and the first-line therapy of this relatively common process, with good images of acute hematomas and end-stage cauliflower ear.

Norman LK, West PD, Perry P. Unilateral pulsatile tinnitus relieved by contralateral carotid endarterectomy. *JR Soc Med* 1999;92:406–407.
Report of a rare entity. Remember, arteriorvenous malformations (AVM) and carotid vascular problems can manifest with pulsatile tinnitus.

Ruckenstein MJ. Hearing loss. *Postgrad Med* 1995;98(4):197–208.
Overview of the first steps in the evaluation of hearing loss, including history and physical examination manifestations. Definitions of hyperacusis (sounds are overly loud), diplacusis (same sound has different pitches in different ears)—both in sensorineural deafness; paracusis (word easier to understand with a noisy ambient environment in conductive deafness); pulsatile tinnitus is with arteriorvenous malformations (AVM), carotid dehiscence, but continuous tinnitus neural etiology. Discusses otoscopy and the Rinne and Weber tests—recommends the 512 tuning fork.

Schneiderman H. Bullous myringitis: background, recognition, inferences. *Consultant* 1994;34:1181–1182.
Case based description of this relatively uncommon, but easily recognizable, entity. Nice color image and discussion—one or more bullae (vesicles) on the surface of the tympanic membrane. Points out that Mycoplasma infection is part of the differential diagnosis, but viral infections, such as EBV or influenza, are also causes.

Schneiderman H. Battle's sign and external assessment of head trauma. *Consultant* 1995;35:1529–1530.
Case-based discussion of this relatively late finding of a basilar skull fracture. Restates that the presence of Battle's sign has a high positive predictive, but its absence has a minimal, negative, predictive value.

Schneiderman H. What's your diagnosis—mastoiditis. *Consultant* 1997;37:2423–2425.
Case-based discussion and color images of a rare but important diagnosis (mastoiditis, which manifests with unilateral "jug ear," i.e., auricle displaced anteriorly because of a mastoid swelling); discusses pathogens and that further problems can develop if not adequately treated.

Uwaifo GI, Scheiderman H. Relapsing polychondritis: otic and non-otic findings. *Consultant* 1997;37:2187–2188.
Case report with excellent images of the auricular findings of relapsing polychondritis. Nice discussion of associated features, including that lobes are spared because of a lack of underlying cartilage, but that polyarticular arthritis and nasal cartilage are involved. Refreshes the reader with the fact that cauliflower ear results from trauma or inflammation of the auricle and saddle deformity of the nose is a deformity caused by chronic inflammation (lues, polychondritis, trauma, Wegener's granulomatosis).

Waitzman AA, Hawke M. Otoscopic examination. *Consultant* 1996 (June):1299–1303.
Excellent images of common entities found on otoscopic examination: purulent otitis media—TM often bulging; serous otitis media—often retracted TM; perforation of the TM; hematotympanum; and cholesteatoma (a collection of keratin and cholesterol in a sac of epithelium, slowly growing in the middle ear)—not malignant.

Zuber TJ, Dewitt DE. Earlobe keloids. *Am Fam Phys* 1994;49:1835–1841.
Discusses this relatively common entity that is increasing in incidence. Risk factors, including piercing, and some therapeutic endeavors are discussed.

Nose

DeRemee RA. Wegener's granulomatosis. *Contemporary Internal Medicine* 1994;6(2):42–48.
Emphasizes the ELK classification of findings: E = ear, nose, throat; L = lungs; K = kidneys. Describes the findings of saddle nose, sinusitis, mulberry gingivitis, conjunctivitis, and uveitis as examples of "E" manifestations. Some nice images of mulberry (hypertrophic) gingivitis.

Hocutt JE, Corey GA, Rodney WM. Nasolaryngoscopy for family physicians. *Am Fam Phys* 1990 (Nov):1257–1268.
Reviews the technique, indications, and findings (both normal and abnormal) detected when performing this technique. Makes a fair case that this is something that primary care physicians should be able to perform. Excellent images of normal structures to the true vocal cords; also, two images of pathology of the cords—polyp and carcinoma. Not truly a physical examination paper, but a nice review of the anatomy and sites of potential problems.

Ludman H. ABC's of ENT: nasal obstruction. *BMJ* 1981;282:886–888.
Discussion of location, manifestations, and pathophysiology of nasal polyps.

Face and Sinus

Battle WH. Three lectures on some points relating to injuries to the head. *BMJ* 1890;2:75–81.
The classic

Donlon WC, Jacobson AL. Maxillofacial pain. *Am Fam Phys* 1984:30(1):151–163.
A comprehensive review of syndromes that might cause facial pain, including maxillary sinusitis, frontal sinusitis, and the unilateral neuralgias of the trigeminal nerve (tic douloureux)—usually V2 or V3, sphenopalatine neuralgia (Sluder's syndrome)—lacrimation, rhinorrhea; glossopharyngeal—unilateral posterior tongue, pharynx, temporomandibular joint (TMJ), temporal arteritis, Ramsay Hunt syndrome— geniculate neuralgia—zoster; and the importance of looking for a dental source of the pain.

Herr RD. Acute sinusitis: diagnosis and treatment update. *Am Fam Phys* 1991;44(6): 2055–2062.

A well-written paper on sinusitis for the primary care physician, especially one who sees both children and adults. Reviews fact that sinuses do not develop until after birth (maxillary becomes clinically significant only after age 2 years and frontal after age 6 years). Discusses the pathogenesis and pathogens and the sites of pain (maxillary—subzygomatic over cheek, above upper teeth; frontal forehead over eyebrow and ethmoid—periorbital). Also purulent or mucoid discharge is often present from the nares or posterior pharynx. Transillumination is limited to adults and notoriously unreliable. Transillumination procedure described: frontal: light source inferior to medial border of supraorbital ridge, if transilluminates—normal; if opaque—thickened or pus filled; maxillary: light on mid infraorbital rim, mouth open, look for light through the hard palate and the maxilla of face—transilluminable—normal; opaque—thickened or pus filled. Reviews the antibiotics and referral. Overall, a good basic paper.

Melmed S. Acromegaly. *N Engl J Med* 1990;322:966–977.

An erudite and robust review of the manifestations and pathophysiology of this rare, but significant, endocrinopathy.

Uwaifo GI, Uwaifo OO, Schneiderman H. What's your diagnosis: acromegaly. *Consultant* 1998 (June):1550–1576.

A splendid review of the physical findings of advanced acromegaly based on one individual with classic facies and findings; ample old photographs for comparison. Very edifying and demonstrates that a picture is indeed worth a thousand words. Descriptions of prognathism, "beetling brows" or prominent supraorbital ridges, nasal enlargement, macroglossia, carpal tunnel syndrome, and the "numberless" physical findings. The teeth are spaced widely and the tongue has bitemarks on the peripheral surfaces, and serratoglossia.

Williams JW, Simel DL, Roberts LR, Samsa GP. Clinical evaluation for sinusitis: making the diagnosis by history and physical examination. *Ann Intern Med* 1992;117:705–710.

A review of the physical examination manifestations of sinusitis, in which the absence of findings was more predictive of ruling out sinusitis (i.e., that the absence of maxillary toothache, abnormal transillumination of the sinus, and purulent [green] nasal discharge) markedly decreased the likelihood of acute sinusitis.

Neck Masses

Ahola SJ. Unexplained parotid enlargement. A clue to occult bulimia. *Conn Med* 1982; 46:185–186.

Makes the point that bilateral parotid enlargement may be caused by bulimia.

Alter M, Steiger P, Harshe M. Mastoid ecchymosis: Battle's sign of skull fracture. *Minn Med* 1974;57:263–265.

Basilar skull fractures can manifest with ecchymosis over the mastoid process.

Andrews FFH. Dental erosion due to anorexia nervosa with bulimia. *Br Dent J* 1982; 152:89–90.

Excellent report.

Rubin MM, Ford HC, Sadoff RS. Bilateral parotid gland enlargement in a patient with AIDS. *J Oral Maxillofac Surg* 1991;49:529–531.

Parotid enlargement may be associated with AIDS.

Tongue

Grossman ME, Stevens AW, Cohen PR. Brief report: herpetic geometric glossitis. *N Engl J Med* 1993;329(25):1859–1860.

Herpes simplex virus infection of the tongue in immunosuppressed patients—longitudinal, branched, or latticelike pattern of tender linear fissures on tongue surface. Excellent image of the lesion set.

Walker JC. Serratoglossia. *N Engl J Med* 1964;271:375.

A description of indentations of the peripheral tongue in macroglossia. Inspection is indeed the key.

Oral Mucosa

Buchner A, Hansen LS. Amalgam pigmentation (amalgam tattoo) of the oral mucosa. A clinicopathologic study of 268 cases. *Oral Surg* 1980;49:139–147.

Reviews this not uncommon entity.

Burns RA, Davis WJ. Recurrent aphthous stomatitis. *Am Fam Phys* 1995;32(2):99–104.

Review of this common, if not ubiquitous process—aphthous ulcers in the mouth. Divides them into two groups, major and minor. Unknown etiology, but need to include Reiter's syndrome, Behçet's syndrome, and viral infections in the differential diagnosis.

Eisenberg E, Barasch A. Oral examination. *Consultant* 1995;(Nov):1710–1721.

Overview of the oral examination, underscoring the importance of the oral examination, including bidigital palpation, palpation of the structures, Stensen's duct, and Wharton's duct. Nice discussion of some of the common entities of the oropharynx.

Eisenberg E. Common lesions of the oral mucosa: examination and differential diagnosis. *Prime Care and Cancer* 1992;(Jan):17–40.

Very rich collection of color images that are commonly demonstrated in the examination of the oral cavity. Included are images and discussion of torus palatinus, geographic tongue, black hairy tongue, mucoceles, ulcers, squamous cell carcinoma, herpes stomatitis, herpes labialis, thrush, lichen planus, and hairy leukoplakia. Overall, an adequate discussion of inspection and description of lesions.

Galloway RH, Gross PD, Thompson SH, Patterson AL. Pathogenesis and treatment of ranula. Report of three cases. *J Oral Maxillofac Surg* 1993;22:113–115.

Overview of the physical findings, pathogenesis, and treatment of this uncommon problem.

International Study Group for Behçet's Disease. Criteria for diagnosis on Behçet's disease. *Lancet* 1990;335:1078–1080.

Authoritative statement of features used to diagnose this disorder that manifests with erosions and ulcers in the oral mucosa.

Johnson JT. Examination of the oral cavity: when, how and what to look for. *Consultant* 1999;(Jan):114–120.

Nice, practical overview of the examination for a primary care physician, which discusses the technique for use of two tongue blades to assess adequately the entire mucosa. Also documents the need for bimanual palpation of the mouth and mouth structures. Reviews the definitions of the structures: vermilion border to the circumvallate papillae = oral cavity; discussion of Wharton's duct and Stensen's duct; also states that, on the tongue buccal mucosa 5% of white lesions are malignant, whereas, 30% of red lesions are malignant. Good color images included.

Lawson W. Pigmented oral lesions: clues to identifying the potentially malignant. *Consultant* 1998;(May):1253–1260.

For the primary care physician, an overview of pigmented entities in the mouth, including the normal entity—melanoplakia—broad patches in the buccal mucosa, perfectly normal; also reviews Peutz-Jeghers pigmented macules in the lips, buccal mucous membranes, polyps in intestine, amalgam tattoo—silver amalgam adjacent to a restored tooth—the amalgam precipitates collagen, nevi, and melanoma—localized black patch with diffuse borders and secondary ulceration, lead line—on the tooth surface adjacent to gingival—lead precipitated out as lead sulfide by bacteria.

Lawson W. White oral lesions: differentiating infections, neoplasms, and signs of systemic disease. *Consultant* 1994;(Sept):1267–1278.

Practical and complete review of processes that manifest with white lesions on the mouth and tongue, including the features of hairy leukoplakia, squamous cell carcinoma, lichen planus (including Wickstram's striae), candidiasis, and angular cheilosis.

Lawson W. Erythematous oral lesions. *Consultant* 1994;(Oct):1446–1451.

Terse overview of some entities that manifest with red lesions; highlights the importance of including malignant neoplastic disorders in the differential diagnosis of these entities.

Lorber M. Dental topics for medical students. *Journal of Medical Education* (Abstract) 1976;51:342.

Brief statement of importance to medical students by a master of this component of the examination and the teaching of it.

Mizuno A, Yamaguchi K. The plunging ranula. *Int J Maxillofac Surg* 1993;22:113–115.

Describes a variant of ranula—plunging type that is palpable inferiorly through the submental area.

Peery WH. Clinical spectrum of hereditary hemorrhagic telangiectasia (Osler-Weber-Rendu disease). *Am J Med* 1987;82:989–996.

Scholarly review of the manifestations of this rare autosomal dominant disorder of vessels. Discusses the cutaneous, hepatic, mucous membrane, pulmonary, central nervous system, AVM, telangiectasia, and aneurysms. A must for anyone interested in this disorder.

Samaranake LP, Pindbourg JJ. Hairy leucoplakia: three quarters of patients develop AIDS in two to three years. *BMJ* 1989;298:270–271.

Discusses the profound prognostic impact of this specific finding.

Schneiderman H, Nzeako UC. Ranula. *Consultant* 1996;36:311–312.

Case report with excellent images of a ranula (a sac of secretions from a sublingual salivary gland that may be posttraumatic). The physical examination features, including a domed, solitary, nontender, fluctuant nodule, or mass in floor of mouth (wax and wane in size) or, if a "plunging ranula," (herniation through the mylohyoid muscle) into the submandibular space. Usually a bluish hue over the surface because of a thin mucosa. Mucocele is same process in a very small salivary gland of the lip—fluctuant nontender papule.

Spangler JG, Salisbury PL. Smokeless tobacco: epidemiology, health effects and cessation strategies. *Am Fam Phys* 1995;52(5):1421–1430.

Extremely important paper describing this all too common use of tobacco products. Excellent images demonstrating mucosal findings caused by the chewing tobacco, including white and red lesions and oral carcinoma. Reviews strategies to lead to cessation of the use of these materials.

Uwaifo OO, Schneiderman H. What's your diagnosis? Hand foot and mouth disease. *Consultant* 1998;(May):1262–1265.

Case-based discussion and color images of Coxsackie A—vesicles and erosions on mouth to lips, and then the palms and soles. Also discusses the differential diagnosis, including HSV—crosses onto skin.

Yeatts D, Burns JC. Common oral mucosal lesions in adults. *Am Fam Phys* 1991;44(6): 2043–2050.

Nice review of the most common entities of the oral mucosa. Reviews entities, including tori, hemangioma, papilloma, epulis, and varices.

Teeth

Amsterdam JT. Dental emergencies: pain and trauma. *Emerg Med* 1993;(Nov):27–43.

Rich in text; minimal images; discussion of caries, dry socket, and dental trauma.

Andrews FFH. Dental erosion due to anorexia nervosa with bulimia. *Br Dent J* 1982; 152:89–90.

Makes the point that erosions are most severe on lingual side of teeth in bulimia.

Clark MW, Album MM. Preventive dentistry and the family physician. *Am Fam Phys* 1996;53(2):619–626.

Nice overview of the practical aspects of caries preventions in young children, with images of teeth and gingival anatomy, nomenclature, and numbering of teeth. The numbering system begins with the right upper molars and proceeds in a clockwise direction from 1 to 32. Images of nursing bottle caries. Thumb sucking can lead to mild protrusion of upper incisors if it continues after permanent teeth erupt.

Greene JC, Louie R, Wycoff SJ. Preventive dentistry. II. Periodontal diseases, malocclusion, trauma and oral cancer. *JAMA* 1990;263:421–425.

Excellent reference for a commonly overlooked component of the physical examination.

Greene JC, Louie R, Wycoff SJ. Preventive dentistry. I. Dental caries. *JAMA* 1989;262: 3459–3463.

Excellent reference for a commonly overlooked component of the physical examination.

Krutchkoff DJ, Eisenberg E, O'Brien JE, Ponzillo JJ. Cocaine-induced dental erosions. *N Engl J Med* 1990;322:408.

Adds cocaine to the list of substances that can manifest with dental erosions, especially on the outer (labial) side.

Schneiderman H, Eisenberg E. Bulimia: a dangerous variant of anorexia with oral physical signs. *Consultant* 1995;35:1695–1700.

Case report, with good images of erosions on the lingual side of the teeth as a manifestation of severe bulimia. Reviews other features, including scarring on the dorsum on dominant hand and bilateral parotid enlargement.

Palate and Pharynx

Centor RM, Meier FA, Dalton HP. Throat cultures for diagnosis of group A Streptococcal pharyngitis. *Ann Intern Med* 1986;105:892–899.

Excellent paper setting the foundation for a discussion of the pretest probability using history and physical examination as a more effective way to utilize and interpret further diagnostic tests in the evaluation and management of pharyngitis. Based presumptive diagnosis by using four history and physical examination features: exudate on the pharynx, presence of fever, enlarged tender anterior cervical lymph nodes, and lack of cough. Makes recommendations that treatment should be initiated without need for culture if high probability of streptococcal pharyngitis exists based on these features.

Janjua TA, Sasaki CT. Hoarseness: just a cold or something more serious? *Consultant* 1996; (Feb):242–251.

Excellent overview of the differential diagnosis and the physical examination, with emphasis on patients who smoke cigarettes; a good description of how to examine the vocal cords using a dental mirror. Practical tips are included. Multiple images of vocal cord pathology are included, as well as a differential diagnosis of unilateral vocal cord paralysis. A well done paper.

McSherry JA. Diagnosing infectious mononucleosis. *Am Fam Phys* 1985;32(4): 129–132.

Discusses clinical manifestations of infectious mononucleosis: fever, exudative tonsillitis, generalized lymphadenopathy, splenomegaly, and petechiae.

Murray BJ. Medical complications of infectious mononucleosis. *Am Fam Phys* 1984;30(5): 195–199.

Discusses the potential sequelae of infectious mononucleosis, including localized pharyngeal swelling that results in dysphasia and even stridor; and splenomegaly, including splenic rupture. A somewhat dated paper.

Rosen CA, Anderson D, Murry T. Evaluating hoarseness: keeping your patient's voice healthy. ***Am Fam Phys*** **1998;57(11): 2775–2782.**

A robust overview of the differential diagnosis of hoarseness, with symptoms and physical diagnostic features of each. Reviews common causes including papilloma, reflux laryngitis, Reinke's edema (fluid in vocal cords—smoking and reflux), from cardiac surgery, and nodules. Also reviews history: queries include recent screaming, smoking, recent surgeries, or history of pyrosis (reflux). Less than robust physical examination—specifics are mentioned only in passing. Central to evaluation is vocal cord inspection. Mentions some features of therapy.

Yetter JF. Cleft lip and cleft palate. ***Am Fam Phys*** **1992;46(4):1211–1218.**

A practical review of the embryologic underpinnings and manifestations of cleft lip and palate, which occurs in 0.8 to 2.7/1,000 live births. Increased association with other syndromes. Reviews supportive and therapeutic endeavors to treat this not uncommon entity.

Overall

Hatton ER, Gogan CM, Hatton MN. Common oral conditions in the elderly. ***Am Fam Phys*** **1989;40(5):149.**

A well-written review of periodontal disease, caries; abrasion, attrition, and erosion of the teeth; mucosal ulcerations, angular chelosis, thrush, pemphigus, zoster; and the malignant neoplastic lesions of squamous cell carcinoma and melanoma. Deftly describes tongue entities, including varices, geographic tongue, and vitamin deficiencies with fine images included for the most common entities.

Moazzaz AH, Alvi AA. Head and neck manifestations of AIDS in adults. ***Am Fam Phys*** **1998;57(8):1813–1822.**

Nice review of the common entities that involve the ear, nose, and throat in patients with AIDS. Categorized by ear, nasal and sinus, oral, and neck. Color images. Discusses examination in the diagnosis of the more common entities. Particularly nice discussion of oral lesions, including HPV, candida, white hairy tongue (EBV), and herpes simplex infection-type 1 and 2. Neck nodules and masses are also discussed in detail, including lymphoma, mycobacterial disease, and parotid enlargement.

Replogle WH, Beebe DK. Halitosis. ***Am Fam Phys*** **1996;(Mar):1215–1220.**

Important discussion of this common, but at times a finding that has significant pathologic and diagnostic importance. Reviews specific odors, including ketones from ketoacidosis, ammonia (fishy) in renal failure, sweet amine or rotten egg, fetid odor of a lung abscess, and odor of fetor hepaticus (sulfur-containing amino acids).

2

The Male Genitourinary Examination

PRACTICE AND TEACHING

SURFACE ANATOMY

The external components of the male genitourinary system include the penis, scrotum, testes, and spermatic cords **(Fig. 2.1)**. The **penis** consists of three tubular erectile structures, the corpora cavernosa, and the corporum spongiosum. The **urethra** runs the length of the penis on its ventral side, surrounded by the corporum spongiosum. The orifice of the urethra is the **meatus**, which is at the tip of the glans. The penis is divided into two components, the **shaft** and the **glans**, which is the tip. The **corona**, which is between the shaft and glans, is easily demonstrated in circumcised patients, because it is the site of origin of the foreskin. The **foreskin**, present in uncircumcised individuals, envelopes the glans and, at its distal end, forms an opening called the prepuce.

The **scrotum** is a sac inferior to the penis. It is composed of ruggated, wrinkled, and retractible skin. The scrotum wall includes fibers of muscle called the "dartos" muscle. This muscle, innervated by sacral roots $S_{2,3,4,5}$, reflexively contracts in cold and relaxes with warmth. The scrotum contains two testes. Of some interest is the observation that the left testis usually hangs slightly lower than the right. The surface of each testis is smooth, 3.5 to 5 cm long, and has a tubular convoluted structure present on the posterior longitudinal surface. This structure is the **epididymis**, which drains into the vas deferens. These are connected to the **spermatic cords**, which include the vas deferens, testicular vein, as the pampiniform plexus and artery to each testis. The **cremasteric muscle**, which is innervated by the sacral roots $S_{2,3,4,5}$, is located here also. It contracts in the cold and relaxes in warmth to keep the testes at a relatively stable temperature. The seminal vesicles and prostate are internal structures only palpable via rectal examination. The **seminal vesicle** and the **prostate** supply secretions that, in addition to the spermatozoa from the testes, comprise semen.

Penile Examination

The penis is examined by gently grasping on the side, at the corona and lifting to inspect the surface structures. If uncircumcised, the foreskin and prepuce are inspected **(Fig 2-5A)**; the foreskin should be gently retracted **(Fig 2.5B)**. After exam, return foreskin to baseline position. Palpate inguinal lymph nodes.

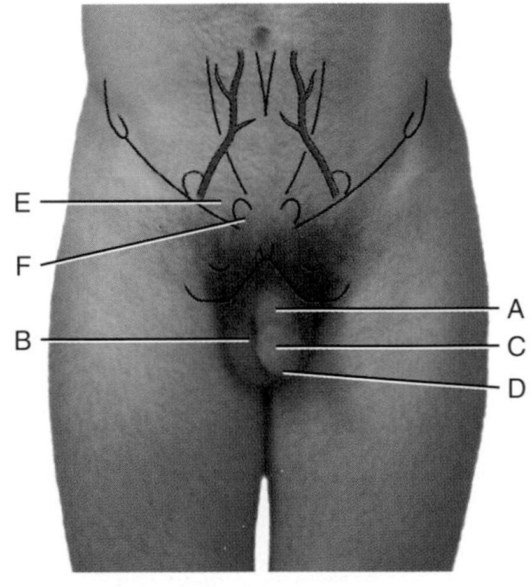

Figure 2.1.

Anterior surface anatomy. **A.** Penis. **B.** Scrotum. **C.** Glans penis. **D.** Urethral meatus. **E.** Hasselbach's triangle. **F.** Superficial inguinal ring. (From Moore KL, Dalley AF. *Clinically Oriented Anatomy,* 4th ed. Philadelphia: Lippincott Williams & Wilkins, 1999, with permission.)

TIPS

- Penis: composed of the shaft and glans, the corona is between
- Scrotum: contains the testes
- Foreskin: skin surrounding the glans, not present if circumcised
- Glans: the bulbus distal component of the penis, distal to the corona
- Prepuce: opening in the foreskin
- Urethral: meatus—opening in the tip of the glans

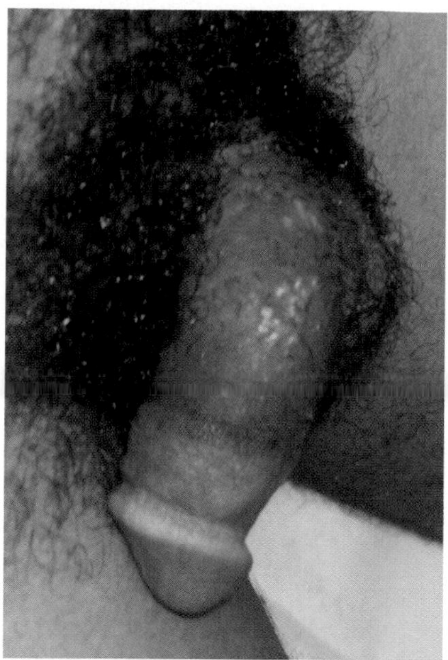

Figure 2.2.

Herpes simplex on penis.

 TIPS

- Herpes simplex: clusters of superficial vesicles or erosions; painful, clear fluid
- Bilateral inguinal node

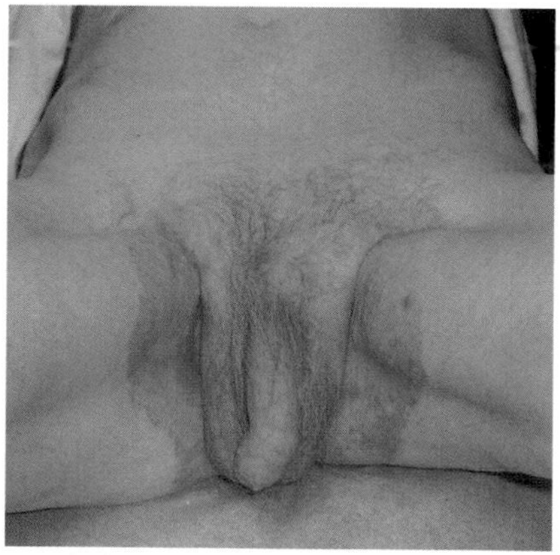

Figure 2.4.

Balanoposthitis. Note the significant inflammation of the glans and the foreskin; concurrent tinea cruris.

 TIPS

- Inspect the foreskin and glans
- Balanoposthitis: swelling of the foreskin, often with discharge, dysuria, and dribbling; caused by *Candida albicans* infection

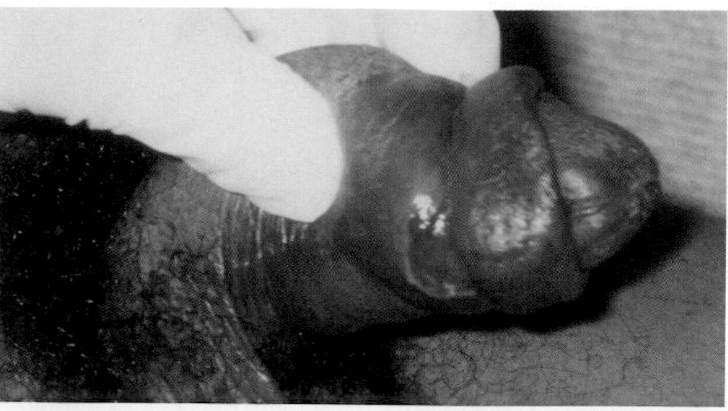

Figure 2.3.

Chancre on the corona of the penis. Relatively nontender ulcer with regular, indurated borders.

 TIPS

- Chancre: single indurated ulcer with distinct borders and serous drainage; minimally painful
- Bilateral inguinal node

Herpes simplex manifests with one or more clusters of superficial vesicles or erosions **(Fig. 2.2)**. These are painful and contain a clear fluid; the patient often has bilateral tendon inguinal nodes. An infection with *Herpes labialis* (usually type II) causes this condition. The **chancre** of primary *lues venereum* manifests with a single indurated ulcer, most often at the corona or glans, but may be on any mucous membrane site. A chancre has sharp borders and serous drainage **(Fig. 2.3)**. Concurrent bilateral inguinal lymphadenopathy, which is often present. This is caused by infection with *Treponema pallidum.* Relative to ulcer depth, there is a remarkable paucity of pain. Although the classic teaching is that a chancre is a painless solitary ulcer, the patient may have some discomfort with it. **Balanitis** manifests with redness, pain, and swelling of the glans itself. Recall that balan means glans. Patients often complain of urinary discharge, dysuria, and dribbling of urine. This inflammation of the glans is most commonly caused by *Candida albicans,* but can also result from an autoimmune disorder or Reiter's syndrome. If Reiter's syndrome, the company it keeps includes conjunctivitis and keratoderma blenorrhagica. **Balanoposthitis** manifests with inflammation of the glans and the foreskin, and the patient often presents with discharge, urinary dribbling, and dysuria **(Fig. 2.4)**. Most often, this is caused by *Candida albicans* infection, trauma, or the autoimmune disorder described in balanitis. **Phimosis** manifests with a decreased size of the prepuce, which can be to the size of a pinhole **(Fig. 2.5)**. In Greek, the term phimosis means closure. With phimosis, there is an inability to retract the foreskin; the patient may have concurrent balanoposthitis, and often reports dysuria and urinary dribbling. **Paraphimosis** manifests with an incarcerated or strangulated glans penis distal to the site of a partially retracted phimotic foreskin **(Fig. 2.6)**. The patient often presents with severe pain and significant swelling in the area distal to the paraphimosis—usually the glans and the foreskin itself. The glans may be suffused and cyanotic. If untreated, this could lead to necrosis. Of specific note, this is a potential complication of Foley catheter insertion. The foreskin may be overzealously retracted and precipitate such a crisis. Furthermore, of specific concern are patients with spinal cord injuries, in which case the paraphimosis may be painless and, thus, go unnoticed until significant harm has occurred.

Hypospadias manifests with the urethral meatus located on the ventral midline aspect of the penis **(Fig. 2.7)**. A first-degree hypospadias is distal, on

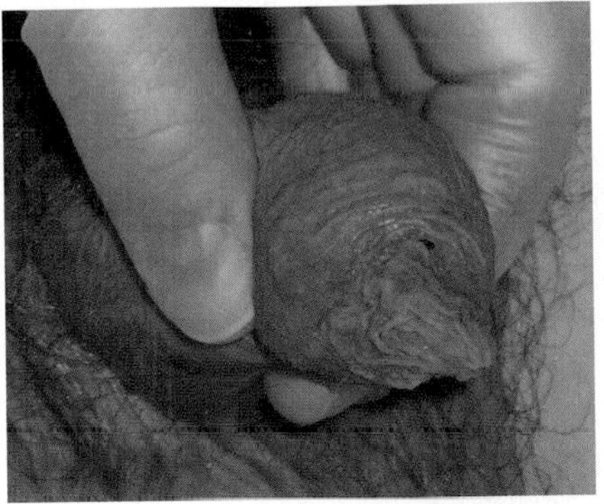

A

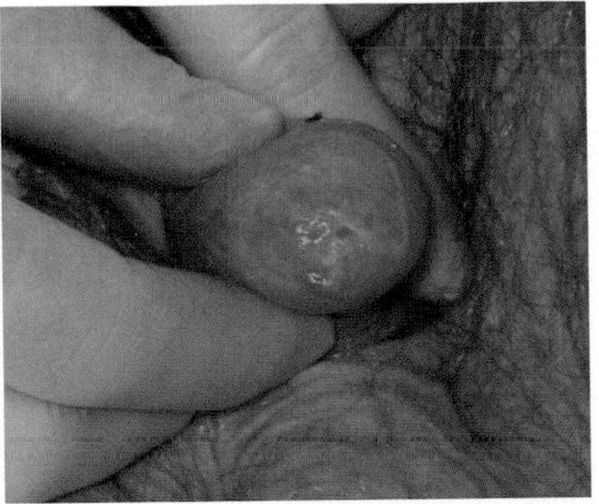

B

Figure 2.5.

Phimosis. Note the inability of the patient to retract the foreskin about the glans; the prepuce is constricted. **A.** Baseline. **B.** Retraction.

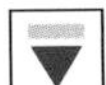

TIPS

- Phimosis: decreased size of the prepuce, inability to retract the foreskin
- Urgent condition

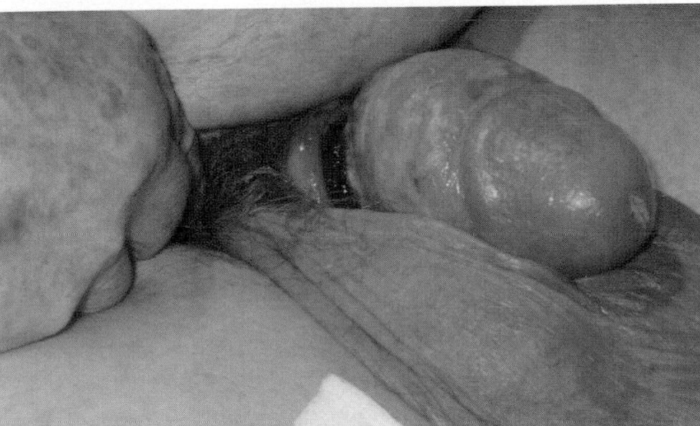

Figure 2.6.

Paraphimosis. Note that the patient had placed a band around the shaft, which caused the glans to be incarcerated and suffused with blood.

TIPS

- Paraphimosis: incarcerated or strangulated glans penis distal to site that phimotic foreskin has been retracted
- Emergent condition

the ventral glans; second-degree hypospadias is on the ventral shaft of the penis; and third-degree or complete hypospadias is at the base of the penile shaft (on the perineum). Third-degree hypospadias is an associated feature of cryptoorchitis and hermaphrodism. **Penile carcinoma** manifests with a painless ulcer that grows and destroys tissue over time. Often, inguinal lymph nodes are present, as it spreads first to local lymph nodes. Most commonly, this is squamous cell carcinoma. Risk factors for this include no circumcision and human papilloma virus (HPV) infection. **Penile warts (condylomata acuminatum)** manifest as one or more exophytic, cauliflowerlike growths on the glans, corona, or penis shaft; and the perineum, the perianal area, or both. These warts are caused by HPV infection and are a risk factor for the development of squamous cell carcinoma of the penis. (See skin examination.) **Peyronie's disease** manifests with significant painless bending of the shaft of the penis, especially evident with an erection. This is caused by fibrosis from chronic inflammation, trauma, or old priapism. **Priapism** manifests with a severely painful erection for an extended period of time. Risk factors include sickle cell disease, cocaine use, and erectile dysfunction medications, an emergency. **Urethral stricture** manifests with a diminished urinary flow and, on examination, a narrow caliber urethral meatus. This may be a sequela of urethra inflammation or infection, e.g., untreated gonococcal urethritis. In the preantibiotic era, this was not an uncommon finding. **Dorsal vein thrombosis** manifests with a tender serpiginous venous structure on the penis dorsum, most commonly caused by trauma or intercourse–related activities, often due to gonococcal infection. ***Neisseria gonorrhea*** **urethritis** manifests with acute onset of marked dysuria, pyuria, crusting on underpants, and often frankly purulent discharge from the urethral meatus. **Chlamydial urethritis** manifests with mild dysuria and discharge, but is often asymptomatic. This is concurrent with gonococcal urethritis in more than 50% of cases. **Chancroid** manifests

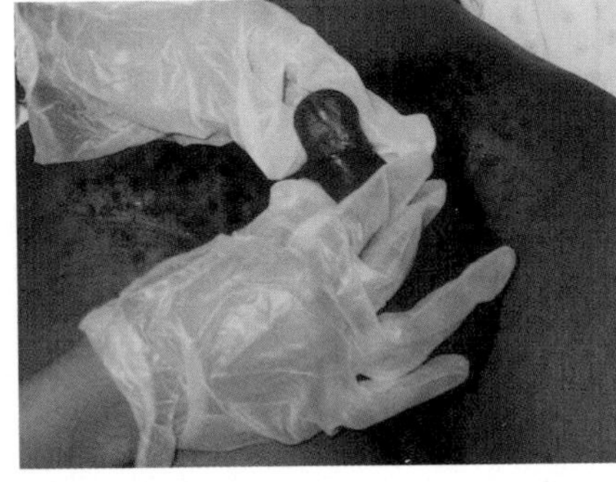

Figure 2.7.

First-degree hypospadias.

TIPS

- Inspect ventral surface of penis
- Hypospadias: an orifice on the ventral aspect of the penis, most commonly on the ventral glans

TEACHING POINTS

PENIS EXAMINATION

1. Most of the examination is inspection.
2. Carefully retract foreskin if patient is uncircumcised to inspect the glans.
3. Do not force retraction of a foreskin because it can precipitate a paraphimosis.
4. Balanitis is very common—inflammation specific to the glans.
5. Balanoposthitis is quite common in uncircumcised men: inflammation of both the foreskin and glans.
6. The simulated patient models are an excellent method for the beginner to use to learn some of the fundamental aspects of the scrotal, penile, and prostatic examination.

with one or more deep, nonindurated, irregularly bordered ulcers, each with a yellow base and unilateral, ipsilateral inguinal nodes. The nodes may be so enlarged, tender, and fluctuant that they can be called "buboes." This is a sexually transmitted disease caused by *Haemophilus ducreyi.*

Scrotum Examination

The overall examination of the scrotum includes inspection of the skin and palpation of the sac itself for any nodules or masses. Palpation of the sac is performed best by placing the patient in a warm environment, either standing or supine **(Fig. 2.8)**. Place one hand on the inferior scrotum, the other on the anterior scrotum, and use the index finger and thumb to palpate structures (i.e., the testes, tunica vaginalis [anterior], head and tail of epididymis [posterior], and the spermatic cord) with the vas deferens to the external ring. Perform the examination on the left and then the right side, and compare sides. **Normally**, the testes are 3.5–5 cm in length and nontender with a

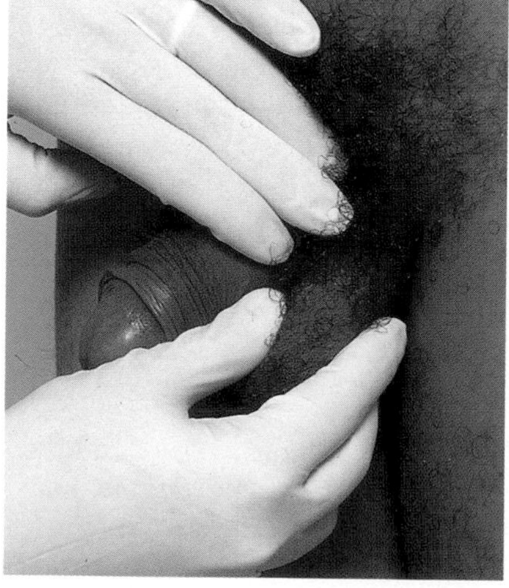

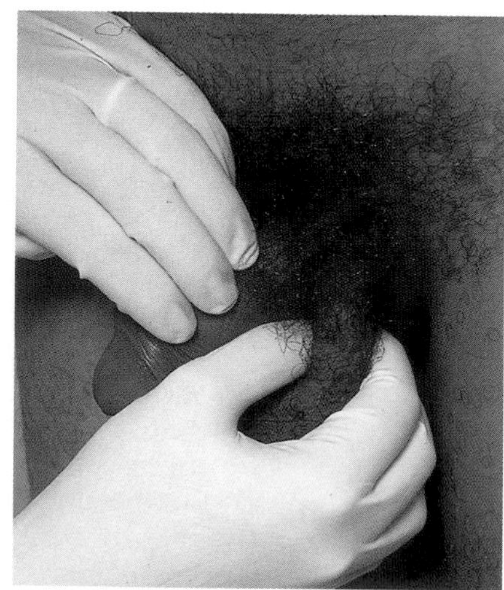

Figure 2.8.

Technique to perform bimanual examination of scrotum. (From Bates B. *A Guide to Physical Examination and History Taking*, 5th ed. Philadelphia: JB Lippincott, 1991:376, with permission.)

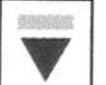 **TIPS**

- Warm environment, keep the patient relaxed
- Patient standing or supine, place one hand on inferior scrotum, other hand on anterior, use index finger and thumb to palpate structures (testes, tunica vaginalis [anterior], head and tail of epididymis [posterior]), and the spermatic cord with the vas deferens to the external ring
- Normal: testes are >3.5. cm in length, nontender with a smooth surface; the epididymis is on posterior aspect; testes are located >4 cm inferior to the pubic tubercles

Table 2.1. Scrotal Lumps and Bumps

Diagnosis	Transilluminable	Tenderness	Location	Company it Keeps
Normal Testes	No	None	Bilateral > 4 cm inferior to pubic tubercle Left lower than right	Smooth surface Epididymis posterior 3.5 to 4.5 cm long
Cryptoorchidism	No	None	One (or rarely both) testis not palpable, or is < 4 cm from the pubic tubercle	Look for concurrent hypospadias Risk for testicular carcinoma
Hydrocele	Yes	None	Anterior to the testes Mass	Fluid in tunica vaginalis testis; congenital
Spermatocele	Yes	None	Head of epididymis posterior to testes Nodule	Benign
Neoplasm	No	None, unless resultant infarction or torsion	Contiguous with testes anterior or posterior	Irregular nodule or mass
Varicocele	No	None	Posterior to testes; Left side more common than right side	"Bag of worms" in the spermatic cord Size decreases with: scrotal elevation (elevate entire scrotum); or with forward bending at trunk Size increases with: Valsalva's maneuver
Epididymitis	No	Yes	In epididymis, posterior to testes	Swelling or discrete nodule or mass Mass may be fluctuant if abscess
Torsion	No	Yes	Swelling and mass tender in and about the testis	Exquisite pain and tenderness May have concurrent testicular carcinoma
Anteverted Epididymitis	No	No	Epididymis are anterior to testes	Normal variant Changes location of any pathology 7% of males
Direct Inguinal Hernia	No	None, unless incarcerated or strangulated	Base of mass from Hasselbach's triangle floor May extend into scrotum	Reducible or Incarcerated: stuck out or Strangulated: incarcerated and ischemic
Indirect Inguinal Hernia	No	None, unless incarcerated or strangulated	A scrotal hernia Congenital Through the internal and external rings	Reducible or Incarcerated: stuck out or Strangulated: incarcerated and ischemic
Femoral Hernia	No	None, unless incarcerated or strangulated	A thigh hernia Under the medial inguinal ligament	Reducible or Incarcerated: stuck out or Strangulated: incarcerated and ischemic

smooth surface; the epididymis is on the posterior aspect and the testes are located >4 cm inferior to the pubic tubercles. **Cryptoorchidism** manifests with either an absent testis or one that is not completely descended, i.e., is <4 cm from the pubic tubercle. Specific lumps and bumps in the scrotum include those described in **Table 2.1**.

Direct inguinal hernia manifests with a mass in the lower medial aspect of the abdominal wall through Hasselbach's triangle **(Figs. 2.1** and **2.9)**. The examination is performed by direct palpation over the abdominal wall immediately superior to the inguinal ligament, with patient supine, then standing because the sensitivity for the examination increases with standing. Finally, a cough or

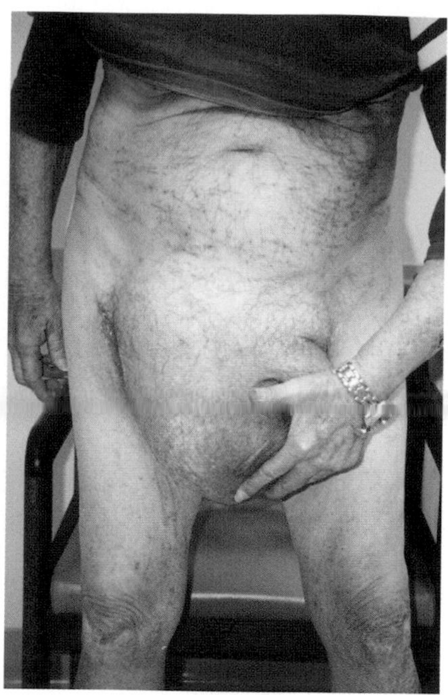

Figure 2.9.

Large direct inguinal hernia through the floor of Hasselbach's triangle.

 **TIPS**

- Direct inguinal hernia: mass in the lower medial aspect of the abdominal wall through Hasselbach's triangle; can be massive

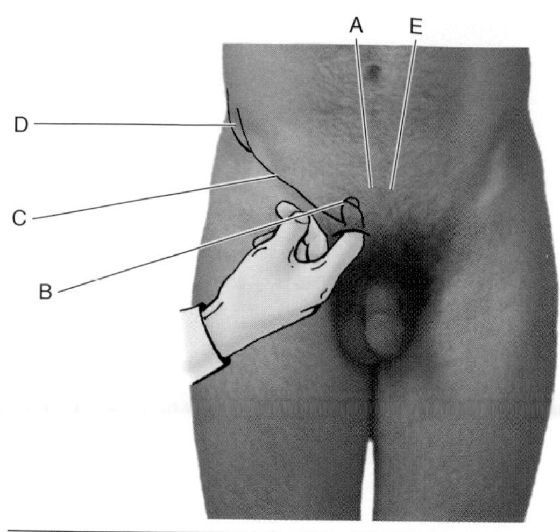

Figure 2.10.

Technique for palpation for indirect inguinal hernia. **A.** Hasselbach's triangle: direct hernia. **B.** Superficial inguinal ring: indirect hernia. **C.** Inguinal ligament. **D.** Anterior superior iliac spine. **E.** Linea alba. (From Moore KL, Dalley AF. *Clinically Oriented Anatomy,* 4th ed. Philadelphia: Lippincott Williams & Wilkins, 1999:206, with permission.)

 **TIPS**

- Patient supine or standing: palpate the testis, follow the spermatic cord proximally to site of the superficial inguinal ring; instruct patient to cough or perform Valsalva's manuever to increase sensitivity
- Indirect inguinal hernia: a defect in the ring and a mass in the scrotum that passes through the superficial inguinal ring

other method to effect Valsalva's maneuver will further increase the sensitivity of the examination. These hernias can become massive and extend into the ipsilateral scrotum **(Fig. 2.9)**, but are invariably not transilluminable. **Indirect inguinal hernia** manifests with a mass in the scrotum that passes through the superficial inguinal ring. The examination is best performed by direct palpation of each testis, then follow the spermatic cord up to the superficial inguinal ring feeling for any masses or defects **(Fig. 2.10)**. Perform the examination with the patient supine, then standing, because the sensitivity for the examination increases with standing. Finally, a cough or other method to effect Valsalva's maneuver will further increase the sensitivity of the examination. It is not transilluminable unless a hydrocele is concurrently present **(Fig. 2.11)**.

Femoral hernia manifests with a mass located in the superior aspect of the femoral triangle, immediately distal to the inguinal ligament, which is a thigh, not an abdominal, hernia. A high risk exists of incarceration or strangulation in this type of hernia. Thus, it is necessary to look for features that indicate such complications. (Please refer to the Hip and Back chapter for details.) This is the most common type of groin hernia seen in women.

If **incarcerated** or **strangulated**, it can become tender; if the hernia is composed of a loop or a portion of bowel wall (Richter's hernia), bowel sounds may be present over the mass. If **bowel obstruction** has developed,

Table 2.2. Types of Hernias

	Symptoms	Signs	Intervention
Reducible Hernia	Nontender	Easily reduced	Required
Incarcerated Hernia	Tender or nontender	Nonreducible	Urgent
Strangulated Hernia	Tender	Tender and nonreducible	Emergent

there is abdominal distension with tympany to percussion, hyperactive bowel sounds that often are high-pitched and tinkling **(Table 2.2)**.

Hydrocele manifests with a fluctuant mass or nodule adjacent to the vas deferens **(Fig. 2.11)**. It is anterior to the testis (unless an anteverted epididymis). The mass is invariably nontender and distinctly transilluminable, often with a concurrent indirect inguinal hernia.

Scrotal edema manifests with diffuse swelling of the penis and scrotum skin. Often, the edema is pitting, can be massive **(Fig. 2.12)** and thus, very troublesome for the patient. The company the edema keeps helps determine the underlying etiology and diagnosis. **Right-sided congestive heart failure** manifests with lower extremity pitting edema, an S_3 gallop, elevated jugular venous pressure, mild hepatomegaly, and cardiomegaly. **Budd-Chiari syndrome** (hepatic vein thrombosis) manifests with lower extremity pitting edema, abdominal vein collateral formation, and no heart failure manifestations. **Liver failure** manifests with ascites, abdominal venous collateral formation, lower extremity edema, and gynecomastia. **Cellulitis** manifests with scrotal or penile edema that is isolated to those areas. Absence of concurrent decompensated findings of liver or heart failure and the presence of warmth, redness, fevers, and chills should suggest cellulitis. A specific type of cellulitis called **Fournier's gangrene** manifests with tender diffuse swelling of the scrotum, perineum,

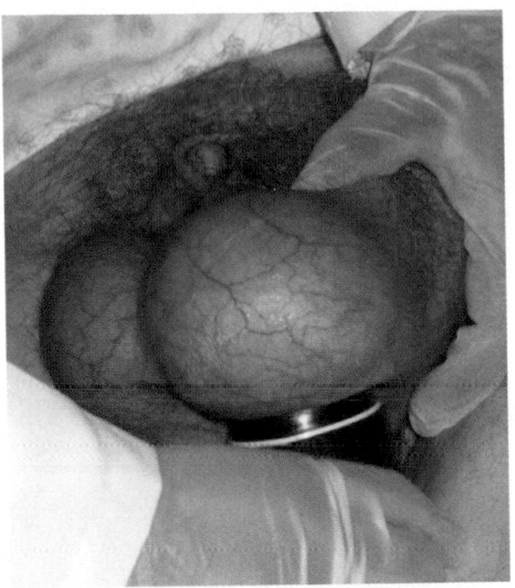

Figure 2.11.

Massive hydrocele. This is brilliantly transilluminable, nontender, and fluctuant.

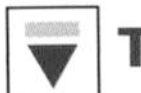

TIPS

- Apply a light source to the scrotal mass or nodule
- Hydrocele: transilluminable, fluctuant mass or nodule anterior to the testes (unless an anteverted epididymides); nontender
- The only other entity that is transilluminable is a spermatocele.

TEACHING POINTS

SCROTUM EXAMINATION

1. The acute scrotum includes the emergent conditions of testicular torsion, Fournier's gangrene, epididymitis with abscess formation, and strangulated inguinal hernia.
2. Femoral hernias are thigh hernias.
3. Inguinal hernia, indirect and direct, often extend into the scrotum.
4. Masses or nodules that are transilluminable include hydrocele and spermatocele.
5. Hydroceles are commonly associated with indirect inguinal hernia.
6. Most epididymides are posterior; 7% are anterior to the testis. These are termed anteverted epididymides.
7. Uncontrolled diabetes mellitus, high-dose steroids, and neutropenia are risk factors for development of Fournier's gangrene.
8. The simulated patient models, including the "ZACH" model, are an excellent method for the beginner to learn some of the fundamental aspects of the scrotal, penile, and prostatic examination.

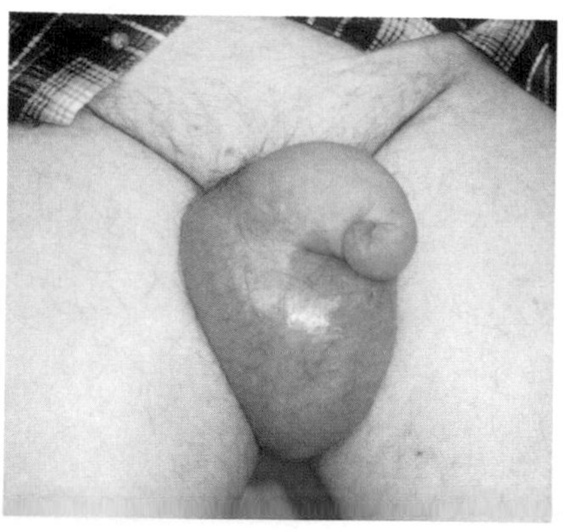

Figure 2.12.

Edema as manifestation of right ventricular failure.

 **TIPS**

- Palpate penis and scrotum
- Pitting edema of scrotum: pitting remains in the skin of the scrotum
- Right ventricular failure: pitting edema of scrotum, penis, and lower extremities; company it keeps includes S_3 gallop, increased JVP

and penis (**Fig. 2.13**). There is often palpable crepitus in the skin and soft tissues, with black color to the tissue because of necrosis. Sepsis rapidly develops in this form of acute scrotum. This life-threatening infection with several bacterial organisms, including anaerobes and gram-negative rods, is most common in patients with underlying immunocompromise, including uncontrolled diabetes mellitus, high-dose steroid use, and neutropenia. A useful rule to use and teach is to be aware of edema isolated to the penis or scrotum; if no edema is seen outside of the scrotum and penis, cellulitis may be present. (See **Table 2.3** for specific features of each.)

Torsion of the testis (spermatic cord) manifests with acute onset of a painful scrotum. A tender mass is found in the scrotum; the pain does not decrease when the scrotum is gently elevated (Prehn's sign); and no reflexive elevation (absent cremasteric reflex) of the testis occurs when gently stroking the extreme superior and medial thigh skin cremasteric reflex on the affected side with fingertip or a cotton-tipped swab. In addition, the epididymis is in a pseudonormal, posterior position: one complete rotation of 360 degrees or two complete rotations of 720 degrees will result in pseudonormal position-

Table 2.3. Etiologies of Pitting Edema in Scrotum

Diagnosis	Complications	Company it Keeps
Right Ventricular Failure	Pitting penile and scrotal edema Increased JVP Right-sided S_3 gallop Lower extremity pitting edema Ascites Mild hepatomegaly Tricuspid regurgitation	Primary pericardial, myocardial, or endocardial process
Hepatic Failure	Pitting penile or scrotal edema Normal JVP Absence of heart abnormalities Large or small liver Abdominal venous collaterals Gynecomastia Spider angiomata Palmar erythema	End-stage liver disease, irrespective of cause
Budd-Chiari	Pitting penile or scrotal edema Normal JVP Normal heart examination Large liver Pitting lower extremity edema Marked dilation of abdomen and lower extremity veins	Hepatic vein thrombosis
Fournier's Gangrene	Acute penile or scrotal edema Tender Absence of edema outside of penis and scrotum Rapidly progressive Fevers present Crepitus in soft tissues from gas Acute scrotum	Uncontrolled diabetes mellitus Steroid use Neutropenia

JVP = jugular venous pressure.

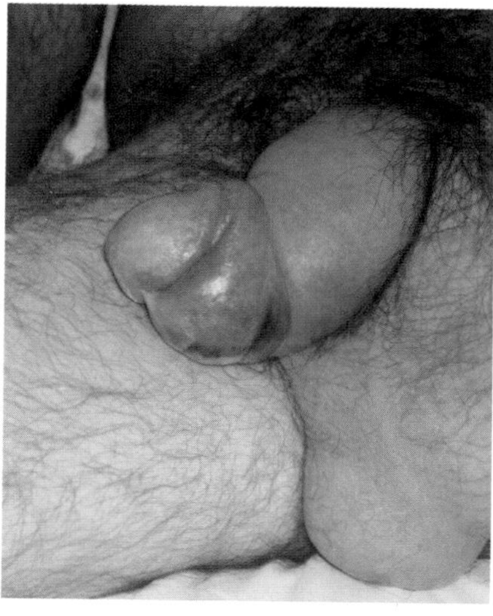

Figure 2.13.

Fournier's gangrene in a patient with uncontrolled diabetes mellitus.

 **TIPS**

- Fournier's gangrene: tender swelling in the scrotum, perineum, and penis; associated with crepitus and necrosis of the skin and tissue
- Concurrent fevers and sepsis are not uncommon
- Emergent condition

ing. In addition, urinalysis results are normal. Although the condition most commonly occurs spontaneously and is idiopathic, testicular neoplasia can cause such a torsion. **Orchitis** or **epididymitis** manifests with a gradual onset of scrotal pain, often with urethral discharge, scrotal edema, erythema, antecedent dysuria, hesitancy in urination, and, at times, pyuria. A tender mass or fullness is noted in the scrotum, and the pain decreases when the scrotum is gently elevated (Prehn's sign). There is a reflexive elevation (present cremasteric reflex) of the testis on gentle stroking of the extreme superior and medial thigh skin. An abscess cavity has formed when there is discrete fluctuance in the mass. This is caused by the same organisms that cause pelvic inflammatory disease in a woman, including gram-negative rods and **Chlamydia** organisms. **Torsion of the testicular appendix** manifests with acute scrotal pain referred specifically to a tiny tender nodule in the affected testis. An overlying **blue-dot sign**, which develops early in course of disease, is seen in the scrotal skin. This is a less severe process than the crisis of spermatic cord torsion.

These are all examples of the **acute scrotum**. The acute scrotum requires emergent evaluation and therapy, including emergent referral to a surgeon. The causes of acute scrotum include torsion of the testis, epididymitis with abscess formation, strangulated hernia, and Fournier's gangrene.

Perirectal abscess manifests with an exquisitely tender, fluctuant mass posterior and lateral to the anus in the subperineal soft tissue **(Fig. 2.14)**. The pain, which is in the anal area (proctalgia), increases with any bowel movement. Individuals who are immunocompromised, including those with poorly controlled diabetes mellitus, are at increased risk to develop this disorder.

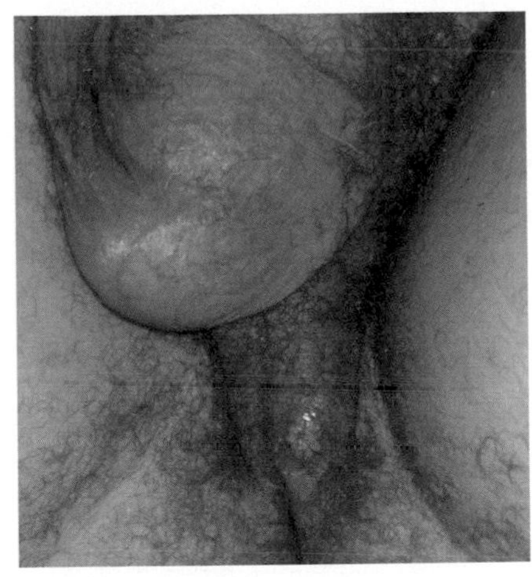

Figure 2.14.

Perirectal abscess. Large fluctuant collection in the subperineal skin most often, as here, anterior to the anus. Fistula and sinus tracts concurrent to the abscess.

TIPS

- Perirectal abscess: fluctuant tender area about the perineum and perianal area; exquisitely tender

Prostate Examination

The **prostate gland** is a structure located at the base of the urinary bladder, through which the proximal urethra passes as it enters the penis. The prostate

TEACHING POINTS

PROSTATE EXAMINATION

1. The prostate can be easily examined with the patient in either the decubital or the dorsal lithotomy position.
2. Boggy prostate indicates inflammation.
3. The absence of a prostate may indicate past radiation or surgery for prostate carcinoma.
4. Important to assess the size of urinary bladder in any case of prostate enlargement.
5. Include prostate in any man who has suprapubic abdominal discomfort, a distended abdomen, or both.
6. The simulated patient models, including the "ZACH" model, are an excellent method for the beginner to learn some of the fundamental aspects of the scrotal, penile, and prostatic examination.

gland, along with the paired and adjacent seminal vesicles and Cowper's glands, contributes secretions to the seminal fluid. The prostate examination can be performed in either the decubital position or the supine dorsal lithotomy position. Although most examinations are taught and performed using the decubital position, the dorsal lithotomy position allows for a bimanual examination of the prostate and may be useful in patients who are unable to roll onto side. Many of the simulated patient models (e.g., ZACH) are in the dorsal lithotomy position. In either position, the patient should void completely before the examination.

In the **decubital position**, the patient rolls over onto the left or right decubital position, knees flexed, and hips forward flexed; whereas in the **dorsal lithotomy position**, the patient is supine, knees flexed, hips forward flexed and abducted 30 degrees, with feet positioned on table. The bimanual component can be performed by concurrently deeply palpating over the suprapubic area. This is exactly the same position as for a bimanual pelvis examination in a woman. Perform a standard digital rectal examination (DRE), paying particular attention to the anterior midline of the rectum. Palpate across the transverse plane of the prostate first, feeling the two lateral lobes and the median prostatic furrow. Then, palpate in the cranial–caudad axis in the median furrow. Normally, the gland is in the anterior rectum, placed midline; it has a smooth surface and is the size of a small walnut. The consistency of the gland should be that of a contracted, firm muscle belly, e.g., contracted thenar eminence, without any nodules. The gland should not be tender. The seminal vesicles and Cowper's glands are not palpable normally.

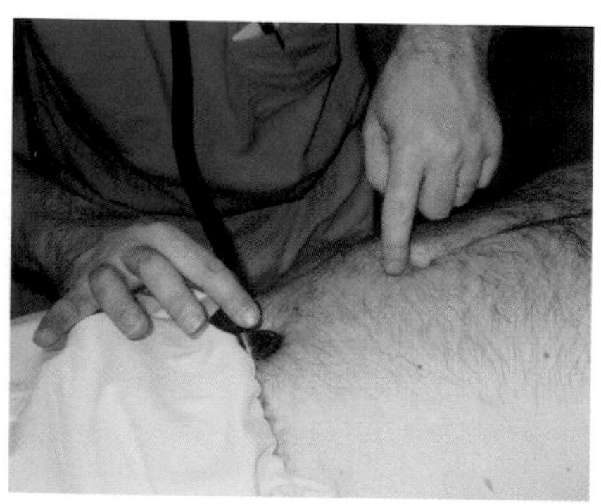

Figure 2.15.

Technique for bedside method to assess size of urinary bladder using auscultatory scratch. This is a good first-line test for bladder size in a patient with a distended bladder or any prostate problem.

 **TIPS**

- Instruct patient to void, then place him supine; place diaphragm of stethoscope over the symphysis pubis, scratch the skin in the midline from the pubis superiorly
- Normal: minimal scratch sound present
- Urinary bladder enlargement, usually caused by prostate enlargement; scratch sound clearly heard above the pubis; may extend to the umbilicus if grossly dilated

Acute prostatitis manifests with the patient complaining of an acute onset of dysuria, pyuria, fever, and pain in the low back and in the perineum. On DRE, a warm, tender, boggy prostate will be noted; the complication of urinary bladder obstruction is not uncommon. Acute prostatitis is caused by bacterial infection, usually from gram-negative rods; there may be concurrent epididymitis, cowperitis, and seminal vesiculitis. In such cases, Cowper's gland or the seminal vesicles may be palpable adjacent to the prostate gland. **Chronic prostatitis** manifests with mild dysuria, intermittent pyuria and, occasionally, hematospermia. On DRE, the gland is firm, enlarged, and moderately tender, which usually indicates a low-grade inflammation of the gland. **Benign prostatic hypertrophy** (BPH) manifests with the patient complaining of progressively worsening nocturia, urgency, hesitancy, postvoid dribbling, and double voiding. On DRE, the gland is enlarged, firm, and not tender; enlargement is symmetric. Because urinary bladder outflow obstruction is common, outflow needs to be zealously evaluated in such a patient. (See examination techniques below.) BPH is idiopathic, but increases in prevalence with increasing age. **Prostate nodules** and **carcinoma** manifest with minimal symptoms until advanced. One or more firm to rock-hard nodules may be found and the gland itself may be mildly enlarged, but not tender. In addition, it is important to assess the inguinal areas for enlarged lymph nodes. This carcinoma increases in prevalence with increasing age and may have a hormone-mediated component. African-American men are at great risk for the development of this neoplasm. After **radiation therapy** to the prostate bed or after prostate resection for carcinoma, the prostate is not palpable.

A complication of any prostate problem is urinary bladder outlet obstruction, with urinary retention. **Bladder obstruction** manifests with lower abdominal distension, **dullness** to percussion over the area of **distension**, and a scratch test with increased transmission above the pubis, even to the level of the umbilicus. For the **scratch test**, place the stethoscope over the pubis symphysis and gently scratch over the midline from pubis to umbilicus **(Fig. 2.15)**. Increased transmission indicates a fluid-filled structure, i.e., uri-

Table 2.4. Prostate Problems

Diagnosis	Manifestations	Etiology
Acute Prostatitis	Diffusely enlarged, boggy prostate Very tender May have tender, palpable seminal vesicles or Cowper's glands	Infectious
Chronic Prostatitis	Diffusely enlarged, boggy prostate Mild to moderate tenderness	Chronic infection
Benign Prostatic Hypertrophy	Diffusely enlarged, smooth, rubbery akin to cartilage Nontender	Idiopathic Increasing age
Prostate Carcinoma	One or more very hard nodules in the substance of the prostate itself	

nary bladder beneath. The patient may report a lack of voiding, but may also report the seemingly paradoxic finding of urinary incontinence, which is reflexive and caused by overflow mechanisms **(Table 2.4)**.

Annotated Bibliography

Scrotum

Cass AS. Torsion of the testis. *Postgrad Med* 1990;87(1):69–74.

Brief but complete overview of this urologic emergency. Mechanism described requires an abnormal twist in the spermatic cord often caused by excessive contraction of the cremasteric muscle. Can be associated with trauma and may spontaneously reduce with resultant venous and lymphatic blockage and ischemia. Reviews the symptoms, including acute or subacute pain in scrotum or even abdomen. Differential diagnosis includes epididymitis, torsion of the testicular appendage, and true torsion of testis. Reviews the physical examination and Prehn's sign. Emphasis on clinical suspicion, especially in young men and boys. Emergent testicular Duplex and referral for surgical intervention including orchidopexy of contralateral testis is emphasized.

Henry SA. *Cancer of the Scrotum in Relation to Occupation.* London: Oxford University Press, 112.

Carcinoma of the scrotum found to be associated with occupation.

Junnila J, Lassen P. Testicular masses. *Am Fam Phys* 1998;57(4):685–692.

An excellent primary care-based paper on the differential diagnosis and approach to the patient with this not uncommon problem. Emphasizes the emergent or urgent causes of masses, including torsion, epididymitis, acute orchitis, strangulated hernia, and testicular cancer. A robust discussion of the physical examination, including normal (testis should be >3.5 cm long), with the epididymis being posterior to each testis. Describes the standing Valsalva's maneuver while palpating the posterior testis to find a small varicocele and the cremasteric reflex. Excellent discussion of pathogenesis and manifestations of torsion: pain in scrotum, tender mass in scrotum, a positive Prehn's sign (no decrease in symptoms with scrotal elevation), an absent cremasteric reflex, epididymis in normal position (360–720 degrees of torsion), and a normal urinalysis. Also discusses torsion of the testicular appendage: a remnant of the müllerian duct, can be twisted, causing severe acute scrotal pain, and a tiny tender nodule with an overlying "blue-dot" sign is seen early in course. Refer to a urologist, but usually surgical intervention is not necessary. Epididymitis is common, with gradual onset of pain in scrotum, urethral discharge, scrotal edema, and erythema, pyuria; elevation of scrotum decreases pain; cremasteric reflex is present; acute orchitis; acute testicular tenderness, swelling, and fever, either from mumps (35% of parotiditis develops orchitis) or inguinal hernia. Testicular cancer is discussed in great detail. Other masses described and discussed include hydrocele, which is painless, communicates with the peritoneum (a new hydrocele requires ultrasound of testes given the small but finite risk of a concurrent testicular neoplasm); varicocele, a tortuous and enlarged pampiniform plexus, 20% prevalence (left more common than right); best to examine with the patient standing because supine will result in resolution of varices; spermatocele, a painless cystic nodule or mass, superior and posterior to testis, which is transilluminable. An excellent paper.

Lamb RC, Juler GL. Fournier's gangrene of the scrotum. *Arch Surg* 1983;118:38–40.

Excellent review of this devastating infection of the scrotum.

Murphy NJ, Weiss BD. Hematospermia. *Am Fam Phys* 1985;32(4):167–171.

Nice overview of this relatively uncommon (or unseen) entity. Nice differential diagnosis, including a stratification of patients into those <30 years of age in which the etiology was usually idiopathic or an inflammatory condition such as epididymitis, orchitis, or urethritis; in those >40 years of age, more malignant disorders, including prostate carcinoma or transitional cell carcinoma of the *bladder, must be considered. Also describes melanospermia, dark semenlike hematospermia, which was caused by the presence of melanin from a prostate malignant melanoma. A thorough physical examination of the genitourinary system often will reveal source.*

O'Brien WM, Lynch JH. The acute scrotum. ***Am Fam Phys*** **1988;37(3):239–247.**
Solid overview of this rare, but significant problem. Covers differential diagnosis, including testicular torsion, epididymitis, testicular appendage torsion, and strangulated hernia. Describes the features of each, including the blue-dot finding of testicular appendage torsion.

Schulze KA, Pfister RR. Evaluating the undescended testis. ***Am Fam Phys*** **1985;31(6): 133–139.**
Excellent primary care-based review of this not uncommon problem (3.4% of term babies; most descend in next 3 months, but 8/1,000 do not). Discussion of etiology: lack of testis descent in the last trimester of intrauterine development because of a lack of abdominal wall or lack of human chorionic gonadotropin (hCG) or receptors to it. On examination, the undescended testis can be located in the high scrotum, i.e., distal to the superficial ring but <4 cm from the pubic tubercle, immediately proximal to the superficial inguinal ring, in a pouch or in the inguinal canal; or in the abdomen. Approximately 90% have an associated indirect inguinal hernia. Ultrasound to localize the testis is necessary if it is not palpable; it is important to look for an underlying chromosomal abnormality if the patient has bilateral cryptoorchitis. It is also associated with a marked increase in risk of seminoma.

Tishler PV. Diameter of the testes. ***N Engl J Med*** **1971;285:1489.**
Good reference paper.

Prostate

O'Brien WM. Benign prostatic hypertrophy. ***Am Fam Phys*** **1991;44(1):162–171.**
Overview of the manifestations, evaluation, and treatment, including surgical and pharmacologic interventions. Describes the symptoms of double voiding, i.e., need to urinate again 5–10 minutes after initial void. Describes a patient encounter form to assess symptoms of BPH in which nocturia, dribbling, and urgency are all questioned and placed into a weighted scale.

Schwager EJ. Treatment of bacterial prostatitis. ***Am Fam Phys*** **1991;44(6):2137–2141.**
Although the title is "treatment," diagnostic features of various prostatitis syndromes are discussed: acute bacterial prostatitis, accompanied by acute fever, low back pain, dysuria, pyuria, perineal pain, urgency, and frequency; tender, warm, boggy gland; chronic bacterial prostatitis, accompanied by dysuria, hematospermia, and perineal pain; gland is boggy or indurated. Prostatodynia is also discussed.

Smith RA, Wake R, Soloway MS. Benign prostatic hyperplasia. ***Postgrad Med*** **1988;83(6): 79–85.**
A fairly detailed description of the potential pathogenesis of this extremely common age-related disorder. Reviews in some detail the symptoms associated with BPH: nocturia: one of first symptoms (detrusor muscle hyperactivity); urgency because of inadequate voiding in which the detrusor muscle produces pressure insufficient to overcome the obstruction, thus increased postvoid residual and urgency; hesitancy: difficulty initiating stream because of an inability of the detrusor to cause an increase in bladder pressure to move past the obstruction; postvoid dribbling and urinary tenesmus. Dysuria and fever indicate a sequela, i.e., infection has occurred. Physical examination includes digital prostate examination. Treatment with emphasis on surgical intervention is described.

Penis

Gleckman R, De La Rosa G. A practical approach to the patient with genital ulcers. ***Contemporary Internal Medicine*** **1998;10(2):17–26.**
Overview written for primary care physicians; discusses the three most common causes of genital ulcers: Treponema pallidum, Haemophilus ducreyi, and herpes simplex virus (HSV). Excellent table of manifestations of each, natural course, laboratory findings, and drug therapy. Classic description of chancre: single indurated papule with sharp border and serous drainage and bilateral inguinal lymphadenopathy; chancroid: several or one deep, nonindurated, with irregular border, yellow base, and unilateral inguinal nodes; HSV: superficial cluster of vesicle, clear secretions, and bilateral inguinal nodes. Other ulcerative disorders, including Behçet's syndrome and Crohn's disease, are discussed. Treatment, evaluation, and the risk of secondary infection, especially with HIV, are all very well described and discussed. Excellent paper for diagnosis and treatment of these common disorders. Excellent color images included.

3

Female Genitourinary Examination

PRACTICE AND TEACHING

EXTERNAL ANATOMY

The **external genitalia** includes the mons pubis, the vulva, and the perianal areas **(Fig. 3.1)**. The **mons pubis** is a hair-covered area of skin overlying the symphysis pubis. The normal adult distribution of hair over the mons is shaped as an ipsilateral triangle with its base parallel to the pubis bone and its apex the labia majora. The **vulva** includes all of the structures external to the vagina, including (and within) the labia majora. The **labia majora** (labia Latin lip) are a pair of skin-covered pads of adipose tissue. The skin of the labia majora is covered with hair and has multiple sebaceous and apocrine glands along with the hair follicles. The anterior angle or bifurcation of the labia majora is immediately posterior to the mons pubis. The labia are located on the extreme lateral aspect of the vulva and reattach posteriorly at the fourchette. The glands of **Bartholin**, which are exocrine glands, and are located in the posterior one third of the labia majora. The **labia minora** are non–hair-bearing thin ridges of tissue that parallel the labia majora. Within the labia minora are the clitoris and the vestibule. The **clitoris**, which is located anterior in the anterior bifurcation of the labia minora, consists of erectile tissue. The **vestibule** is the superficial area bounded by the posterior two thirds of the labia minora. This is the location of the urethral meatus, the **paraurethral glands** of **Skene**, and the **introitus** of the vagina. The introitus, or vaginal opening, may be covered with a thin membrane called the **hymen** in many pre-adolescent girls or nonsexually active women. The **urethral meatus** is posterior to the clitoris and anterior to the introitus. **Bartholin's glands**, although located in the labia majora, empty via ducts into the posterior vestibule (i.e., the labia minora). The labia minora and majora rejoin posteriorly to form the **fourchette**, the area of skin between the vulva and the **anus**. The external genitalia are richly innervated by branches of sacral roots 2, 3, 4, and 5, mainly by the pudendal nerve.

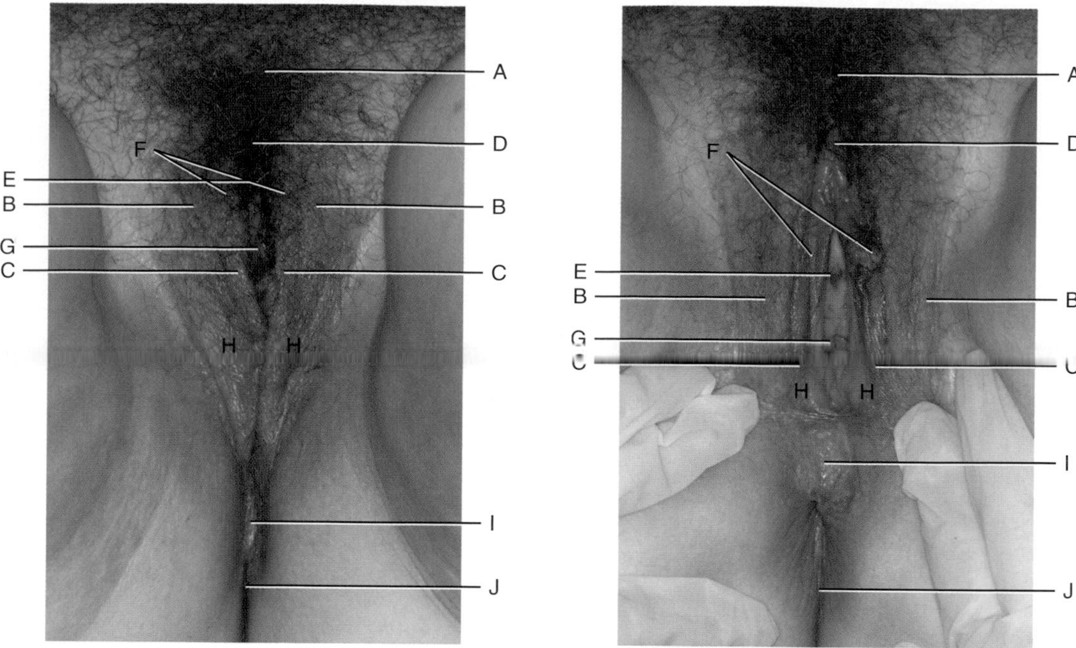

Figure 3.1.

External surface anatomy. **A.** Mons pubis. **B.** Labia majora. **C.** Labia minora. **D.** Clitoris. **E.** Urethral meatus. **F.** Paraurethral glands of Skene. **G.** Vaginal introitus. **H.** Bartholin's gland. **I.** Fourchette. **J.** Anus.

 **TIPS**

- Mons pubis: triangle-shaped area of hair
- Labia majora: hair-bearing pads of skin
- Labia minora: within and parallel to majora
- Clitoris: erectile tissue, extreme anterior
- Urethral meatus: anterior vestibule
- Paraurethral glands of Skene: anterior
- Introitus of vagina
- Bartholin's glands
- Fourchette: posterior
- Anus

Hair and Hair Distribution

An often overlooked but simple part of the examination is inspection of hair and its distribution. **Hirsutism** manifests with an increase in the quantity or distribution of hair. One of the most specific sites for an increase in hair distribution is the mons pubis. **Normal** adult hair distribution is a **triangular-shaped** area of hair, the shape specifically being an ipsilateral equilateral triangle with the base parallel to the pubis bone and the apex at the labia majora. A variant that may be normal is the **diamond-shaped** area of hair, such that the superior angle of the diamond is at the umbilicus. This diamond-shaped pattern is more typical of adult men and, thus, is an androgen-mediated distribution. **Virilization** manifests with a diamond-shaped pattern and hirsutism on back, chest, and face. The company it keeps includes an abnormal loss of hair in temporal or occipital areas, the presence of primary or secondary amenorrhea, the development of a deepened voice, and clitoromegaly. A common cause of hirsutism is polycystic ovary syndrome (PCOS), in which there is virilization, ovarian cysts, and insulin-resistant diabetes mellitus. Hirsutism can also be caused by increased androgens, e.g., in athletes taking androgens for strength or in Cushing's syndrome, or by decreased estrogen states most commonly seen in postmenopausal women.

Delayed puberty manifests with delay in menstruation, which is known as primary amenorrhea. The usual age of menarche is 12 years. If menarche is after age 14 or 15 years, look for other signs of delayed puberty, such as a diminished distribution of hair in the mons pubis. An excellent method to stage this feature of sexual development is the Tanner staging of pubic hair. This Tanner staging system uses **type** of hair—downy versus coarse—and **distribution** of hair (**Table 3.1**). The Tanner staging of breast development is a complementary method to assess the level of sexual development (see Table 3.5). The company it keeps is specific to the underlying cause. If from loss of function of the anterior pituitary, often manifestations of hypothyroidism and adrenal insufficiency are seen; if because of malnutrition, including anorexia nervosa or bulimia. The company it keeps includes weight loss, calluses on fingers, and tooth erosions. Recall, axillary hair usually develops 2 years after the growth of pubic hair.

TEACHING POINTS

EXTERNAL GENITALIA AND HAIR

1. The vestibule is the area within the labia minora.
2. The urethral meatus is posterior to the clitoris and anterior to the introitus of the vagina.
3. Skene's glands empty into area about the urethral meatus.
4. Bartholin's glands, although located in posterior labia majora, drain into posterior vestibule, i.e., the labia minora.
5. Labia majora are covered with hair, apocrine glands, and sebaceous glands.
6. Need to perform staging using the Tanner system if any suspicion of delayed puberty.
7. Need to assess for other features of virilization if diamond-shaped hair distribution on mons pubis.

Table 3.1. Tanner Staging: Pubic Hair Distribution

Stage	Description
Stage 1:	No pubic hair—preadolescent girls
Stage 2:	Long straight downy hair along the labia
Stage 3:	Darker coarser hair, curlier; spreading sparsely over mons
Stage 4:	Coarse curly hair over the entire mons
Stage 5:	Coarse curly hair over entire mons and on the extreme proximal aspect of medial thigh

Vulva: Labia Majora and Minora

Inspection of the vulva is the next step in performing a pelvic examination **(Fig. 3.2)**. This does not require any specific equipment, but provides much information that can be used to diagnose, define, and delineate specific problems. Although inspection is minimally invasive, it is important that the examiner describe each step to the patient before the procedure. Position the patient **supine**, legs in a position in which the hips are forward flexed to 45 degrees and abducted to 45 degrees, and the knees flexed to 90 degrees, also known as a **dorsal lithotomy position**, on the pelvic examination table. Wear gloves in all cases. Place the dorsal surface of the dominant hand on the

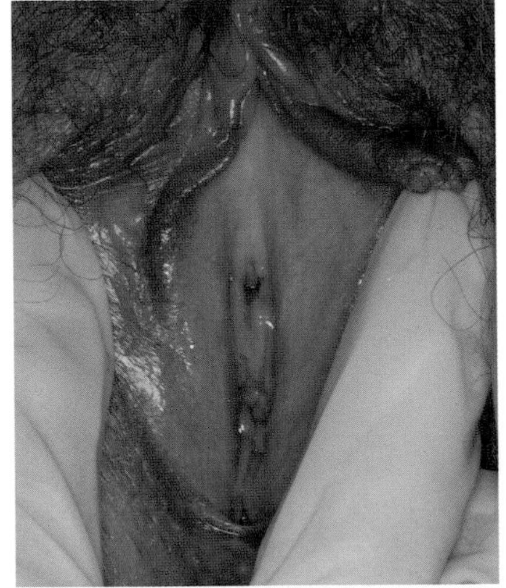

A

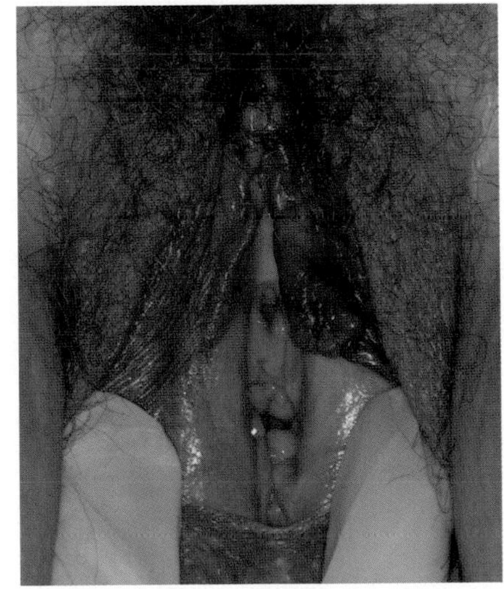

B

Figure 3.2.

A. Technique to inspect vulva. **B.** Technique to inspect for Bartholin's glands.

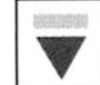
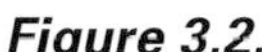

TIPS

- Supine, with legs in a position in which the hips are forward flexed to 45 degrees and abducted to 45 degrees and the knees flexed to 90 degrees; also known as a dorsal lithotomy position on the pelvic examination table
- With the dorsal surface of dominant hand on the medial thigh, use the thumb and index finger to gently open the labia majora and then the labia minora to expose the clitoris, and the structures of the vestibule (Fig. 3.2A)
- Gently palpate about the lateral labia majora and insert index finger to palpate the left and right vestibule including the Bartholin's cyst (posterior) (Fig. 3.2B)

medial thigh, and with the thumb and index finger gently open the labia majora and then the labia minora (Fig. 3.2) to expose the clitoris and the structures of the vestibule, i.e., the urethral meatus and vaginal introitus. Furthermore, inspect the fourchette and perianal skin. Finally, gently palpate about the lateral labial majora and insert the index finger to the vestibule on left and right to palpate for any adjacent nodules or fullness.

Seborrheic dermatitis manifests with one or more red patches or plaques adjacent to, or in, the hair-bearing areas of the mons and labia majora with greasy scales. Distribution on the labia majora and mons is symmetric. Often, concurrent patches and plaques are seen in other hair-bearing areas, including the scalp and eyebrows. **Acanthosis nigricans** manifests with multiple pigmented patches that can become confluent over the vulva and inguinal areas. The company it keeps include similar pigmented patches over the axilla and other folds. This is highly correlated with hyperinsulin states, e.g., insulin-resistant diabetes mellitus, including that from PCOS. **Tinea cruris** manifests with macerated erythematous, pruritic patches in the inguinal folds and on the labia majora. This is caused by Candida infection of the skin. There is often concurrent Candida vulvovaginitis and candidal infections in other areas, including the feet and axilla. This can be associated with diabetes mellitus and the use or elevated serum levels of glucocorticoids. **Candidal vulvovaginitis** manifests with moderate vulvar and vaginal pruritus, and a white, curdled milk-type vaginal discharge. The vulva itself is red and pruritic with areas of maceration; thick, white, curdled milk-type discharge from the introitus occurs. A speculum examination, as well as a wet mount of the vaginal secretions, will confirm this. A potassium hydroxide (KOH) preparation* of the vaginal secretions reveals yeast; however, the clinical appearance of candida is often so classic that a KOH preparation is necessary only for atypical presentations. **Contact dermatitis** manifests with a maculopapular erythematous rash on the entire vulva. Often, this is extremely pruritic; may have excoriations; and in severe cases, a few oozing and crusting vesicles may be present. This is caused by exposure to a topical agent. Examples include new laundry soap, new underpants, new type of sanitary pad, or new bubble bath. The rash may be in a specific distribution that matches the article of clothing or pad. History is extremely important in the assessment of contact dermatitis.

Vulvar dystrophy includes the diseases of lichen sclerosis, squamous cell hyperplasia, and mixed dystrophy, which are not uncommon processes, especially in postmenopausal women. Because of this, it is important to recognize these features and to include them in the differential diagnosis of vulvar lesions. **Lichen sclerosus et atrophicus** manifests with the patient presenting with bloody vaginal discharge, vulvar pain, pruritus, and marked dyspareunia. Often, postcoital bleeding occurs. On examination, multiple very fragile macules are seen on the vulva that, over time, increase in number and size to coalesce into large symmetrically placed patches. This classic pattern has been called a "keyhole" pattern. The company it keeps include a loss of skin appendages, including skin pigment and hair, and a shiny atrophic appearance. The affected areas are easily traumatized and often there are breaks seen in the skin and mucosa. In advanced stages, actual fibrosis and obliteration of vulvar tissue occur, which results in a decreased elasticity and size of the vaginal introitus and posterior fourchette. This advanced stage is called **kraurosis vulvae**. **Squamous hyperplasia** manifests with one or more, usually multiple, papules and plaques that are whitish or pale in color. These papules are thickened areas of keratin, which are palpable and firm to bumpy

*KOH preparation: 2 drops of potassium hydroxide added to 2 drops of secretion on a glass slide, warmed and inspected using a microscope.

on palpation. These lesions are limited to the vulva. This variant is also known as hyperplastic dystrophy. **Mixed dystrophy** is a mixture of lichen sclerosis and squamous hyperplasia. Although these dystrophies are most common in postmenopausal women, they can occur at any time during life. They are idiopathic, although some evidence indicates an autoimmune component in their pathogenesis.

Inclusion vulvar cysts manifest with one or more nontender nodules on the lateral aspects of the labia majora. The nodules often have a yellow hue to them. If the cyst erupts or has been traumatized, thick, caseous malodorous material is produced. **Follicular cysts** manifest with one or more mildly pruritic, smooth papules or nodules at the base of a hair shaft. These cysts are caused by obstruction and infection of the gland that supports the individual hair. They are limited to the mons and the labia majora. A variant of this is **Fox-Fordyce disease**, which manifests with multiple pruritic or painful papules and nodules. This is specifically caused by inflammation of the apocrine glands adjacent to the hair follicles. This can be intensely pruritic or painful to the patient and lead to great symptomatic mischief. **Bartholin's cysts (Fig. 3.3)** manifest with pain specific to the posterior vagina into the fourchette. There is also dyspareunia. There is a tender nodule present in the posterior labia majorum that protrudes into the introitus on that side, which is caused by acute obstruction of the Bartholin's gland duct. **Bartholin's gland abscess** manifests with an exquisitely tender nodule in the posterior labia with overlying erythema and warmth. There may be concurrent purulent discharge into the introitus on that side. A Bartholin's gland cyst or abscess in a postmenopausal woman should increase clinical suspicion for Bartholin's duct adenocarcinoma. ***Neisseria gonorrhea*** infection manifests with bilateral Bartholin's gland abscesses. **Skene's gland abscess**, or adenitis, manifests with a tender fluctuant nodule or papule in the anterior vestibule that is adjacent to the urethra. Patients complain of dysuria, pyruria and discharge, and dyspareunia in the anterior vagina. This is often caused by infection with *N. gonorrhea*. When these are large and multiple, the condition is called a **urethral carbuncle**.

Vulvar intraepithelial neoplasia (VIN) manifests with one or more plaques or papules on the vulva that are usually white, but can be red or flesh colored, each with associated thickened keratin. Over time, these will increase in size and develop modest local edema and ulceration. The area becomes pure white when dilute acetic acid is applied. In this examination, 10% acetic acid is applied to the area adjacent to the primary lesion. Areas of VIN or condyloma acuminatum will be white. VIN is a precancerous entity that if left untreated, may, and often will, develop into squamous cell carcinoma. The company it keeps includes the human papilloma virus-related condyloma acuminatum. VIN replaces the old nomenclature of Bowen's disease, carcinoma in situ, and vulvar dysplasia. **Condyloma acuminatum** manifests with one or more fleshy, warty, exuberant, exophytic lesions **(Fig. 3.4)**, which can be so numerous as to be confluent. Each lesion may be pedunculated. They are in an asymmetric distribution on the vulva and perianal areas. They are caused by infection with human papillomavirus, most often, serotypes 16 and 18. Condyloma acuminatum is a very common form of sexually transmitted disease. Any area that is infected, even early in the course, will turn white with the application of dilute (10%) acetic acid. The pattern of lesions that are white are often in a satellite configuration about individual warts. **Squamous cell carcinoma (SCCA)** of the vulva manifests with an ulcer that is solitary, erythematous, and often painless, with discrete margins and a relatively clean base. Evidence of adjacent VIN may be present. This ulcer slowly increases in size. Enlarged ipsilateral inguinal lymph nodes may also be seen. Risk factors for squamous cell carcinoma include exposure to ultraviolet (UV) light, working as a chimney-sweep, and human papilloma virus infection. SCCA is the

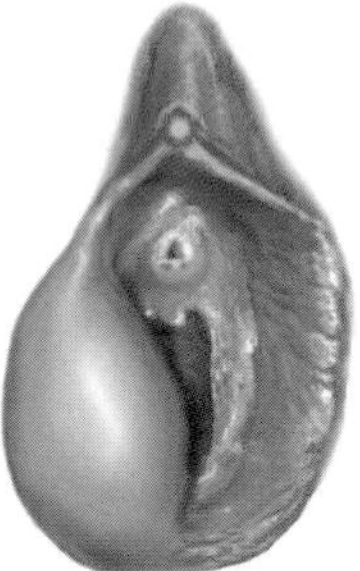

Figure 3.3.

Bartholin's cyst or abscess.

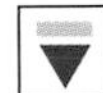 **TIPS**

- Bartholin's cyst: one fluctuant nodule on the posterior medial aspect of the labia majora
- Bartholin's abscess: markedly tender fluctuant nodule in posterior labia majora
- Abscess: think gonococcal etiology
- Postmenopausal: think adenocarcinoma

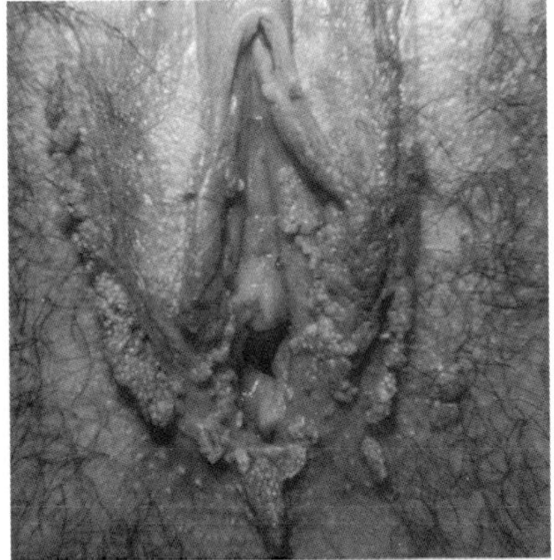

Figure 3.4.

Condyloma acuminata of the vulva. Note the exophytic, cauliflower-like papule located on the labia majora, labia minora, vaginal introitus and fourchette. Due to human papilloma virus infection.

 **TIPS**

- Condyloma acuminata: one or more warty, exophytic lesions on the vulva or perianal mucosa
- Human papilloma virus infection
- Stain white with acetic acid

most common type of vulvar carcinoma. **Malignant melanoma** manifests with a pigmented lesion that has dysplastic features using the ABCDE criteria (Fig. 14.56) discussed in Dermatology. Although it is rare, i.e., <2% of all vulvar neoplastic lesions, be aware of it because it can be overlooked by an examiner or the patient and, thus, be advanced when recognized. **Paget's disease** of the vulva manifests with one or more well-demarcated plaques with scales, each with a deeply red base. This extramammary Paget's disease is a slow growing, intraepidermal neoplasia histopathologically identical to Paget's disease of the breast. **Condyloma lata** manifests with multiple, nontender, moist-appearing papules. Each papule and plaque has a central gray-white exudate. These papules are distributed in the skin folds of the inguinal area and about the vulvar mucosa. They are caused by a systemic infection with *Treponema pallidum*, specific to the secondary phase lues venereum.

Ulcers and Erosions (Table 3.2)

Herpes simplex virus (HSV) manifests with clusters of painful vesicles. The patient reports pain and dysthesia in the area before the onset of the vesicles. After the vesicles have ruptured, these become clusters of erosions or ulcers. The primary episode is more severe than the recurrent. These are caused by infection with herpes simplex virus, most commonly type II, a sexually transmitted infection. **Chancroid** manifests with one or more painful ulcers; very few, if any, symptoms are antecedent to the onset of the ulcers. Not well demarcated, the ulcers have irregular borders, significant exudate and debris in each base. Their borders are termed, "soft." A classic location for these ulcers is

Table 3.2. Erosions and Ulcers on Vulva

Diagnosis	Ulcer	Pain	Lymph nodes	Company it Keeps	Organism
Herpes Simplex	Clusters of erosions/ Ulcers Antecedent vesicles	Yes	Bilateral mild	Recurrent Antecedent pain	HSV II
Chancroid	One or more Irregular border Soft border Exudate at base Often at fourchette	Yes	Buboes: large fluctuant nodes	Sinuses Fistulas	*Haemophilus ducreyi*
Chancre	Solitary Smooth border Firm border Clean base	No	Minimal	Progression to secondary and tertiary lues	*Treponema pallidum*
Granuloma Inguinale	Solitary Irregular border Granular, friable base	No	Firm, inguinal Nodes with granulomas Pseudobuboes	Progressive May destroy large areas of tissue	*Calymmato-bacterium granulomatis*
Lymphgran-uloma Venereum	Solitary Clean borders Clean base Superficial	Yes	Ipsilateral	Develops from a papule	*Chlamydia trachomatis*
Behçet's Syndrome	One or more superficial ulcers	Yes	Bilateral	Aphthous ulcers Conjunctivitis Keratoderma Blenorraghicum	Autoimmune
Squamous cell Carcinoma	Solitary Red	No	Early: none Late: bilateral	Condyloma acuminata VIN	Neoplastic

HSV = herpes simplex virus.

TEACHING POINTS

VULVAR EROSIONS AND ULCERS

1. Ulcers on the vulva always require further assessment.
2. Most ulcers are painful; the ones that are not include chancre and granuloma inguinale.
3. The huge fluctuant lymph nodes of chancroid are called buboes.
4. Granuloma inguinale, if untreated, can result in a marked loss of skin and tissue.

on the fourchette. Furthermore, an ulcer on one labium minora will often be present at the same location on the other labium, a "kissing-ulcer" effect. Invariably, the inguinal lymph nodes are enlarged. The nodes can become large, fluctuant, and tender—called "buboes." Chancroid is caused by infection with *Haemophilus ducreyi,* a sexually transmitted infection. Although relatively uncommon in the United States, it is common worldwide. A **chancre or primary lues** manifests with an ulcer that is solitary, painless relative to the depth, located usually on the mucous membrane surfaces. No symptoms are antecedent to the ulcer. The ulcer itself is well demarcated, and has firm indurated borders, hence the classic term "hand chancre," and a clean base without significant debris or exudates. Chancre is a primary infection with *Treponema pallidum.* **Granuloma inguinale** manifests with a solitary painless ulcer. The ulcer border is indurated with raised borders; its base has a friable granulation tissuelike appearance that bleeds easily with minimal trauma. Few, if any, antecedent symptoms are present. If untreated, it will slowly enlarge in circumference and in depth to invade and destroy the adjacent vulvar, perineal, and groin tissue. The ulcer can reach the depth of the underlying deep fascia. The development of firm, non- to mildly-tender inguinal lymph nodes is not uncommon. These nodes are called "pseudobuboes" in that they are filled with granulomas and develop in up to 25% of cases. Granuloma inguinale is caused by the gram-negative pleomorphic bacterium, *Calymmatobacterium granulomatis.* This is a decidedly rare cause of sexually transmitted disease in the United States, but is not uncommon worldwide. **Lymphogranuloma venereum** manifests with a solitary painful ulcer that is superficial. The ulcer develops from a papule. The patient often has concurrent malaise, fevers, and fatigue. Tender ipsilateral inguinal lymphadenopathy can accompany lymphogranuloma venereum. This is another form of sexually transmitted infection caused by *Chlamydia trachomatis.* **Behçet's syndrome** manifests with multiple painful erosions and ulcers on the vulva. These are recurrent and the company it keeps includes recurrent aphthous erosions and ulcers of the oral mucous membranes and bilateral conjunctivitis. Behçet's syndrome is an autoimmune process. **SCCA of the vulva** manifests with an ulcer that is solitary, erythematous, and often painless, with discrete margins and a relatively clean base. Evidence may be seen of adjacent VIN. This ulcer slowly increases in size. Enlarged ipsilateral inguinal lymph nodes may also be present. Risk factors for SCCA include exposure to UV light, working as a chimney-sweep, and human papilloma virus infection. SCCA is the most common type of vulvar carcinoma.

VAGINAL AND CERVICAL EXAMINATION (Fig. 3.5 and 3.6)

The **vagina** is a hollow muscular canal that lies between the urinary bladder and the rectum. It begins at the vestibule and ends at the cervix of the uterus. The cervix projects into the proximal vagina; a rim of redundant vaginal tissue, termed the fornices, surrounds the cervix. The fornices are divided into quadrants: anterior, posterior, lateral right, and lateral left. The **posterior fornix**, the deepest, is located immediately between the rectum and the distal uterus. This fornix lies immediately anterior to a potential space that is lined with peritoneum, the pouch of Douglas. This space is a potential site of spread of intraabdominal neoplasia, blood, or pus. In addition, in a woman with a uterus that is retroflexed and retroverted, it may be the only site in which it is palpable. The **anterior fornix** lies between the anterior cervix and the urinary bladder, whereas the **lateral fornices** are close to the fallopian tubes.

The **cervix** (Fig. 3.5) is the most inferior aspect of the uterus and the only uterine component that can be visualized by the examiner. The cervix is dome-shaped, usually 2 to 3 cm in diameter and 3 to 5 cm in length; in point of fact, it is approximately one third the total length of the nongravid uterus. The cervical mucosa is divided into the ectocervix and the endocervix. The **ectocervix**, the vast majority of the covering of the cervix, is stratified squamous epithelium; the **endocervix** is an extension of the endometrial lining of simple columnar epithelium. The line of demarcation, also known as the **transformation zone**, which is between these two types of epithelium, is usually visible at or about the cervical os. This transformation zone changes at different times in a woman's life. In a menstruating woman, it is often outside of the os so that the red columnar endocervical mucosa is demonstrable. This is called an **ectropion cervix**. In a premenopausal woman, this line is not demonstrable because it has migrated deeply into the os. The transition zone is the most common site of cervical neoplasia, thus, when sampling for a **Papanicolaou smear**, attempt to sample here. The cervical os, which is the center of the cervix, is round and narrow in a woman who has not had any vaginal deliveries; it is slitlike in any woman who has had one or more vaginal deliveries.

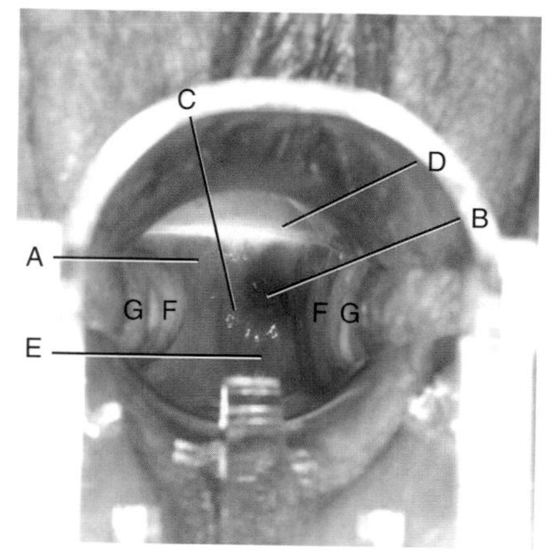

Figure 3.5.

Anatomy of the internal vagina and cervix. **A.** Cervix. **B.** Cervical os. **C.** Transformation zone between ectocervix and endocervix. **D.** Anterior fornix. **E.** Posterior fornix. **F.** Lateral fornices. **G.** Lateral walls: vagina.

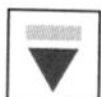

TIPS

- Cervix: inferior protuberance of uterus
- Cervical os: center of cervix, contiguous with the endometrium
- Transformation zone is between ectocervical and endocervical mucosa
- Anterior fornix: between the cervix and urinary bladder
- Posterior fornix: between the cervix and rectum
- Lateral fornices: close approximation with Fallopian tubes

The examination of the vagina and cervix requires specially designed equipment and such examinations are invasive. The first item in performing the examination is patient positioning. The patient must be positioned in a manner to, effectively with the least discomfort, perform the examination required. The two positions that are useful are the traditional dorsal lithotomy position and the lateral decubitus position. The **dorsal lithotomy position** (see page 53 for further description) has been used for centuries and is highly satisfactory for inspection of external genitalia, speculum examination, and bimanual palpation of the uterus and adnexa (Fig. 3.6). An examination table with stirrups should be used for the dorsal lithotomy position. The **lateral decubital position** is one in which the patient is rolled onto one side; an assistant assists the patient and passively forward flexes and holds the superior thigh and leg so as to expose the vulva and genitalia **(Fig. 3.7)**. The examiner then approaches the patient from behind. This is a satisfactory method to perform the entire examination. This position does not require any special examination table. The lateral decubital position is useful in a woman who has severe disability or cannot assume the dorsal lithotomy position. It is important to be deft at performing the pelvic examination using either of these two positions.

Two types of specula can be used to inspect the vagina and cervix: **Graves' speculum**, which is a wide-billed speculum, and the **Pederson speculum**, which is narrow-billed. Other tools required include a spatula and cervical os

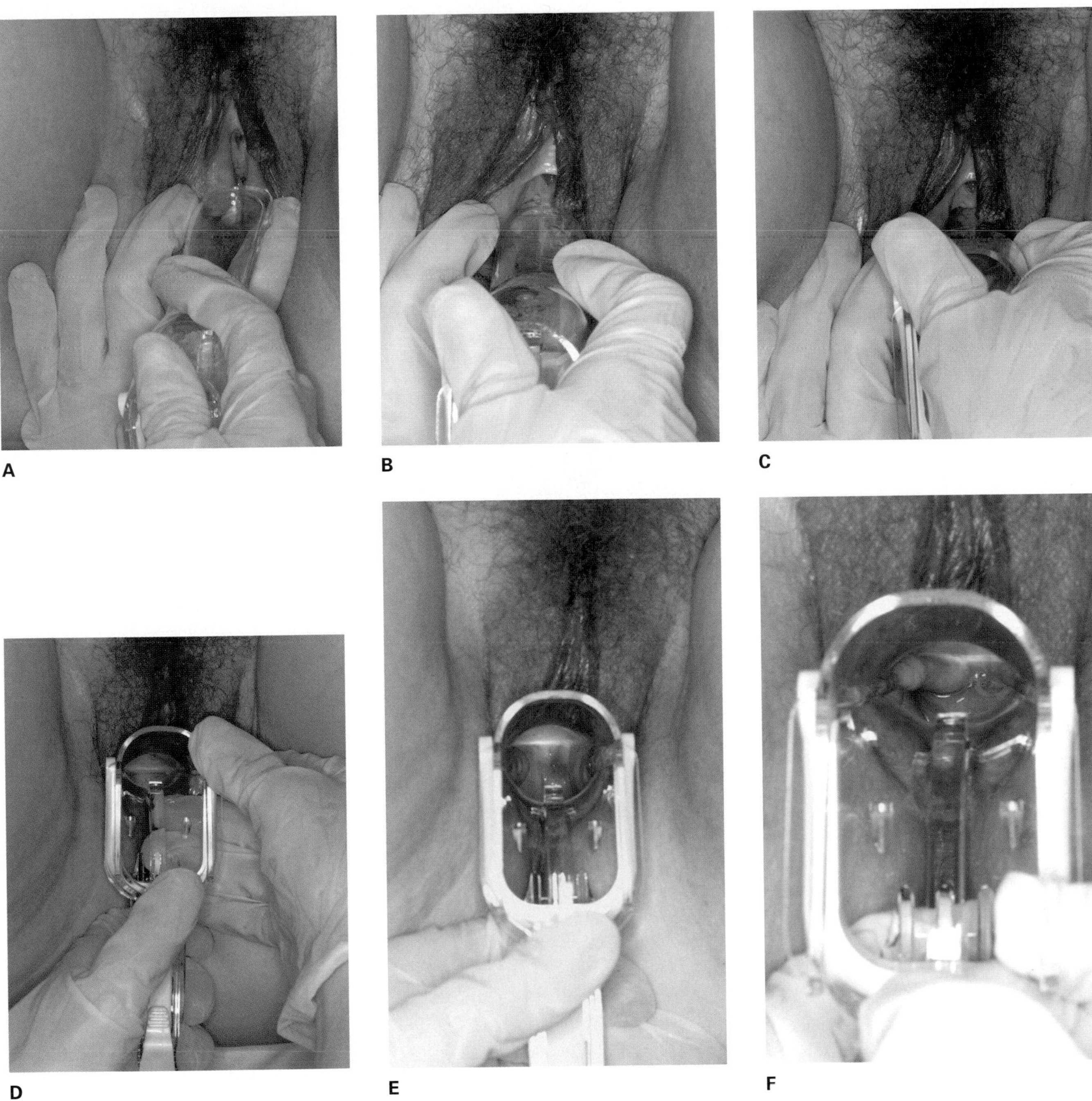

Figure 3.6.

Technique and steps in insertion of a vaginal speculum, with the patient in the dorsal lithotomy position. (**A** through **F**)

TIPS

- **A.** Use fingers 2 and 3 on nondominant hand to gently separate posterior labia
- **B.** With the bill of the speculum closed, gently insert over fingers 2 and 3, through the posterior vaginal introitus. If there is any discomfort or resistance, remove the speculum and start over, turning the bill 90 degrees to facilitate insertion
- **C.** Gently insert speculum with a slight posterior tilt
- **D.** Continue insertion until cervix or posterior vagina (cuff) is reached. If the insertion was with the bill turned 90 degrees, now return to 0 degrees
- **E.** Gently open the bill to expose the cervix. The top portion will be in the anterior fornix, the bottom in the posterior fornix
- **F.** Open the entire speculum to optimize the exposure of the structures

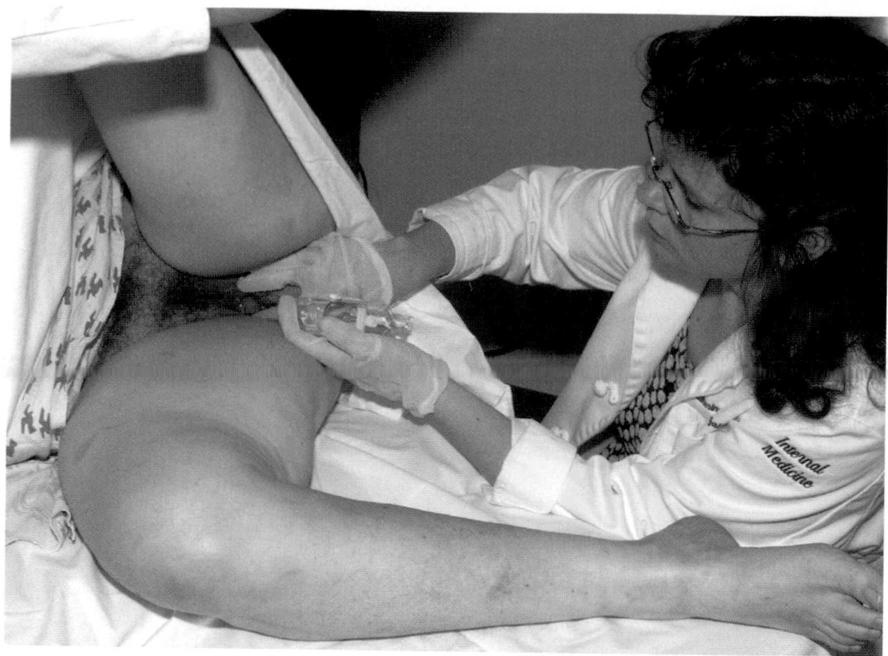

Figure 3.7.

Technique in insertion of a speculum, lateral decubital position.

TIPS

- Use the same procedure as for dorsal lithotomy, except that the speculum handle is directed anteriorly
- Excellent if patient unable to assume dorsal lithotomy position

cytobrush for obtaining a cervical sample. The technique for **speculum insertion** includes warming the speculum with warm water. It is important not to apply any other lubricant than water to the speculum because lubricant may interfere with the Papanicolaou (Pap) smear. The speculum examination component is always performed after inspecting the vulva and after describing to the patient the steps of the procedure. In this technique, the second and third fingers on the nondominant hand are used to separate laterally the labia minora and, thus, open the vaginal introitus. The fingers are then moved posteriorly to press gently on the fourchette. The technique for speculum insertion is with bill closed and parallel to the labia with a slight downward slope. The speculum is inserted completely, turned 90 degrees, and then the bill is gently opened. The bill is adjusted to visualize the cervix. Once positioned, the side screw is tightened to maintain the position of the speculum. The cervix should be between the blades. If on first attempt the cervix cannot be visualized, close the bill and remove it; then, reinsert using same technique only at a different angle. After the cervical examination is complete, loosen the bill and gently remove the speculum. As the speculum is removed, the bill should remain slightly open to inspect the vaginal mucosa.

The technique to obtain a **Papanicolaou (Pap)** smear from the cervical os involves the examiner using a two-pronged spatula or a cytobrush (**Fig. 3.8**). When using the **spatula**, the longer prong of the spatula should be placed into the os of the cervix and the spatula should be rotated the full 360 degrees to obtain a sample from the entire transformation zone. The sample should be placed onto a slide, fixed with the appropriate material, and sent to the laboratory. When using the **cytobrush**, gently place it into the os and rotate one complete 360-degree rotation.

Vaginal Discharge (Table 3.3)

Vaginal discharge is a common problem. Often, the patient will present to the physician with vaginal itching and discharge; she may also have a sensation of urinary hesitancy, dysuria, and pain with intercourse dyspareunia. To further define the vaginal discharge, three tests can be performed: a pH of the vaginal discharge, a wet mount of the discharge, and a KOH preparation of the wet

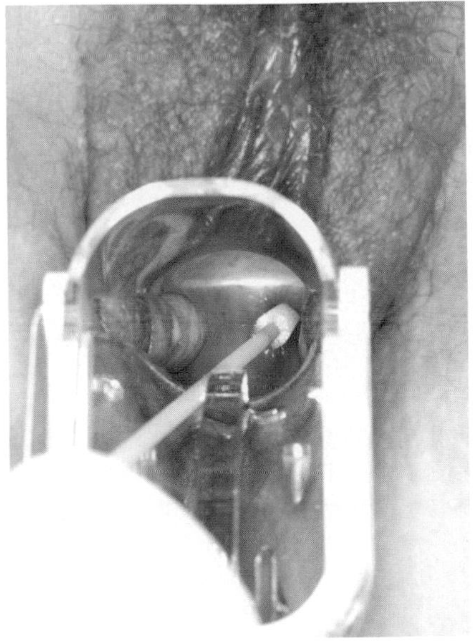

A

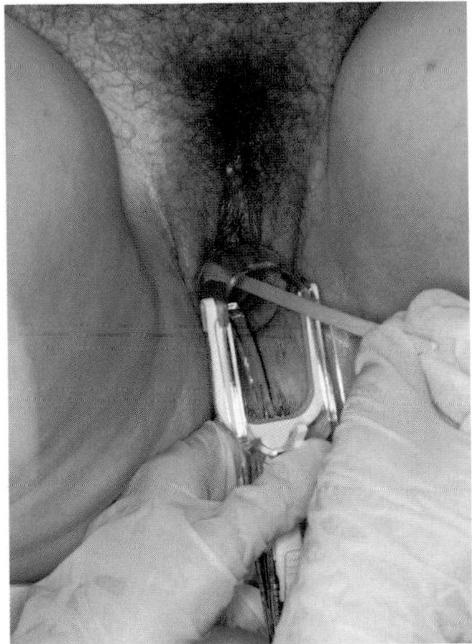

B

Figure 3.8.

Obtaining Pap smear. **A.** Use of cyto-brush. **B.** Use of spatula. In either, the technique involves spatula placed in os and rotated 360 degrees to obtain sample from the entire transformation zone.

TIPS

- Note placement of spatula, longer prong in the cervical os
- Note placement of the cytobrush into the cervical os
- Rotate other device a full turn (360 degrees) and sample entire transformation zone

mount. To perform a **pH test** of the vaginal secretion, place the sterile pH sensitive dipstick against the lateral wall of the vagina, in the lateral fornix, or the area where the discharge appears to be most copious. Note the color of the dipstick and determine the pH. This method has a disadvantage in that an examiner who is color-blind is unable to interpret the strip. Normal pH of vaginal secretions is 3.8 to 4.2. Perform the **wet mount** examination using a sterile cotton-tipped swab to obtain a sample of the discharge from the vagina; then, place the swab in a test tube with 3 mL of normal saline. Then, place a drop of this solution on a glass slide for microscopic analysis. In the normal setting, vaginal epithelial cells and cotton fibers from underpants or pads can be seen. Perform the **KOH preparation** by adding two to three drops of potassium hydroxide 10% solution to the wet mount solution on the slide. Note any odor. The preparation is then again inspected using a microscope. The KOH solution breaks down cellular debris and, thus, makes it easier to observe any fungal elements.

Bacterial vaginosis manifests with the patient complaining of a malodorous whitish-gray, thin, homogeneous liquid discharge that coats the surface of the vagina and vulva. The vaginal walls are diffusely red. The pH of the discharge for bacterial vaginosis is 4.5 to 6; on the wet mount are seen clumps

Table 3.3. Vaginal Discharge

Diagnosis	pH	Discharge	Wet mount	KOH
Normal	3.8–4.2	Minimal	Normal	Nonspecific
Bacterial Vaginosis	4.5–6	Thin white-gray Homogeneous	Clue cells	Odor of fish (amine)
Trichomonas	> 5	Frothy, clear-white	Motile protozoans with antennae	Nonspecific
Atrophic Vaginitis	> 7	Copious, scant, watery	Nonspecific	Nonspecific
Candidiasis	< 4.2	Thick, white Curdled milk	Nonspecific	Yeast

KOH = potassium hydroxide.

of pigment on surfaces of vaginal cells, the clumps being bacteria. These cells are called "clue-cells." The KOH preparation will result in a fishy, amine odor to the wet mount solution. Bacterial vaginosis is caused by an overgrowth of Gardnerella bacteria in the vagina and a loss of the normal lactobacilli flora, which results in lysis and destruction of vaginal epithelial cells. **Cytolytic vaginosis** manifests with the same features as bacterial vaginosis; in point of fact, it is a mild form of the same process. **Trichomonas vaginitis** manifests with a copious quantity of frothy, clear-white discharge with a particular odor. Often, petechiae are present in the walls of the vagina and in the cervix itself. This finding is called "strawberry-cervix." The pH of secretions is >5; the wet mount demonstrates motile protozoan organisms, and the KOH demonstrates the same, nonmotile protozoan organisms. Trichomonas vaginitis is caused by a sexually transmitted infection by *Trichomonas vaginalis.* **Candida vaginitis** manifests with a thick, white, akin to curdled milk-appearing discharge throughout the vulva and vagina. The discharge is often adherent to the vaginal wall and has associated erythema of the vaginal wall and the vulva. The diagnosis is usually made on inspection alone; however, confirmation is with a vaginal pH of 3.8 to 4.2 and a KOH that demonstrates yeast present. This condition is caused by *Candida* infection of the mucosa itself, which can be related to antibiotic use, hormone use, or uncontrolled diabetes mellitus. **Atrophic vaginitis** manifests with overall atrophy of the vagina, vulva, and mucosa. A diffuse loss of vaginal folds and a scanty, watery discharge is present. The pH of secretions is >7; wet mount and KOH are both noncontributory. This process usually occurs in postmenopausal women or in women who have had bilateral oophorectomy and are not receiving hormone replacement.

Vaginal Masses or Nodules

Although vaginal masses or nodules are rare, it is important to recognize these forms and to know and teach of the particular problems that can present with them. A **Gardner's duct cyst** manifests with a discrete, nontender, thin-walled nodule in the anterolateral wall of the vagina. This entity has a yellow hue, is typically 2 to 3 cm in diameter, and rarely, if ever, causes problems for the patient. Often found on routine examination, Gardner's duct cyst is caused by failure of the Wolffian duct (mesonephric duct) to degenerate, which leaves vestigial rests of tissue in the vaginal wall. An **epidermal inclusion cyst** manifests with a nontender, discrete nodule located in the posterior wall of the vagina, almost always in the distal one third adjacent to the fourchette. It often has a yellow hue to it. It most often develops as the result of trauma or surgery, e.g., delivery with a tear or an episiotomy in which a part of vaginal epithelium is included into the submucosal stroma. **Vaginal adenosis** manifests with one or more, usually multiple, red, polyplike, nontender nodules in the wall of the vagina. These are located in the upper one fourth of the vagina or in the vaginal fornices. These structures each have the red color of endocervical columnar epithelium (i.e., the same color as an ectropion cervix). These can change slightly during the different stages of the menstrual cycle. These are rests of columnar epithelium derived from incompletely degenerated müllerian ducts. The most common cause is exposure to diethylstilbestrol (DES) taken by the mother before the eighteenth week of intrauterine gestation. This is important as these individuals are at greater risk for the otherwise exceedingly rare clear cell carcinoma of the vagina. **Endometriosis** of the vagina manifests with one or more red to purple 2- to 5-mm papules in the vagina, especially in the posterior fornix. These entities consist of endometrial tissue that will respond to the hormonal changes of normal menstrual cycles. The company it keeps include other sites of endometrial tissue in the peritoneum that manifest with pain at the time of menstrual flow, often in patients with recurrent, cyclic, and vexing abdominal pain syndromes.

Cervical findings

Examination of the cervix includes visual assessment using the speculum and then obtaining a Pap sample using one or both of the methods described above. **Ectropion cervix** manifests with the transformation zone between the endocervix and ectocervix migrating outward, with a circle or red epithelial tissue surrounding the os, which is caused by a migration of columnar epithelium outside of the os during the reproductive phase of a woman's life. Estrogen is a distinctly powerful factor in its development. If ectropion cervix is present in a postmenopausal woman, further evaluation is mandatory, including, but not limited to, a Pap smear. **Entropion cervix** manifests with the transformation line displaced into the os, thus no red circle of tissue is present about the cervical os itself **(Fig. 3.9)**. This is the normal state in postmenopausal women. **Nabothian cysts** manifest with one or more papules or nodules that range in size from 5 to 25 mm **(Fig. 3.10)**. These are nontender, asymptomatic cysts lined with endocervical columnar epithelium. They are completely benign retention cysts on the cervix, each containing mucus. **Condyloma acuminata** manifests with one or more warty, exophytic papules and nodules on the cervix epithelium. The application of dilute acetic acid solution to the cervix using a cotton-tipped swab, will demonstrate adjacent areas of white and a white color to the specific lesions. This white color is termed "acetowhite staining." Condyloma may be seen in other areas of the vagina and vulva. Condyloma acuminata is caused by infection with human papilloma virus. Because these patients are at increased risk of cervical carcinoma, close follow-up with colposcopic imaging is indicated. **Herpes simplex virus infection** manifests with clusters of indurated erosions and ulcers; rarely are vesicles seen on the cervix. Often, concurrent herpes simplex infection of the vulva is seen, which is caused by the sexually transmitted infection, HSV II. The lesions isolated to the cervix are remarkably asymptomatic, discovered only on speculum examination. **Cervicitis** manifests with the patient complaining of vaginal discharge and lower abdominal pain. On speculum examination, the cervix is mildly swollen, red, and often has purulent discharge from the os. On the bimanual examination, significant tenderness is noted even on gentle palpation of the cervix. There may be concurrent infection and inflammation of the adjacent Fallopian tubes and often marked tenderness in the adnexa. Cervicitis most often results from bacterial infection, including *Neisseria gonorrhea, Chlamydia trachomatis,* or gram-negative rods. In **chlamydia** infection, the erythema and discharge are less prominent. **Cervical polyps** manifest with one or more pedunculated, fragile, red lesions that protrude through the cervical os. These vary in size from 5 mm to several centimeters. The patient often notes spotting of menstrual blood between her periods and often reports postcoital bleeding. These polyps are usually hyperplastic and most often benign but require evaluation. **Endometriosis** manifests with multiple, reddish-blue papules or nodules on the cervix. The company it keeps includes similar lesions on the vagina, especially in the posterior fornix. Often, recurrent abdominal pain occurs that has a cyclic monthly pattern to it. **Cervical hood** manifests with an extra flap of tissue over a portion of the cervix. The company it keeps includes vaginal adenosis and an increased risk of clear cell adenocarcinoma. This is caused by exposure to DES in utero. **Cervical carcinoma** manifests with few specific features until more advanced. Often, early carcinoma is discovered only by routine Pap smear. Thus, screening Pap smears play a markedly important role in the early diagnosis and prevention of cervical carcinoma. More advanced or invasive cervical carcinoma manifests with papules on the cervix, particularly at the transformation zone. Areas of neovascularization may be seen in the papules. In addition, papules are often friable with erosions and ulcers on their surface, and even some adjacent bleeding may occur. Although not discussed in this text the next step in evaluation must be **colposcopic examination** performed by a gynecologist or a

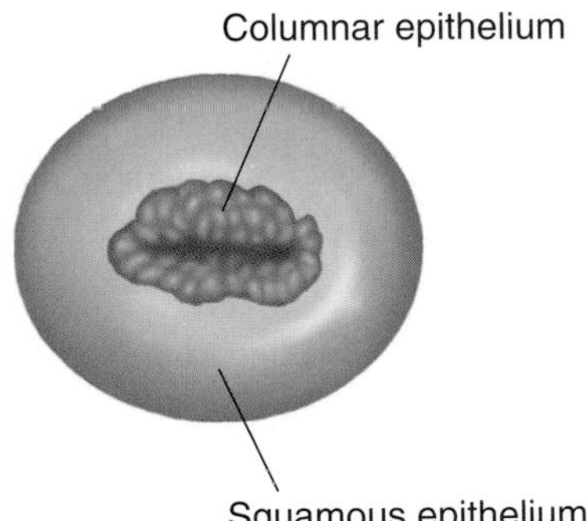

Figure 3.9.

Cervix: marked ectropion. The transformation zone clearly seen.

TIPS

- Ectropion cervix: the squamocolumnar interface is demonstrable outside of the os
- Entropion cervix: no circle or red around the os
- Ectropion in postmenopausal woman, needs evaluation.

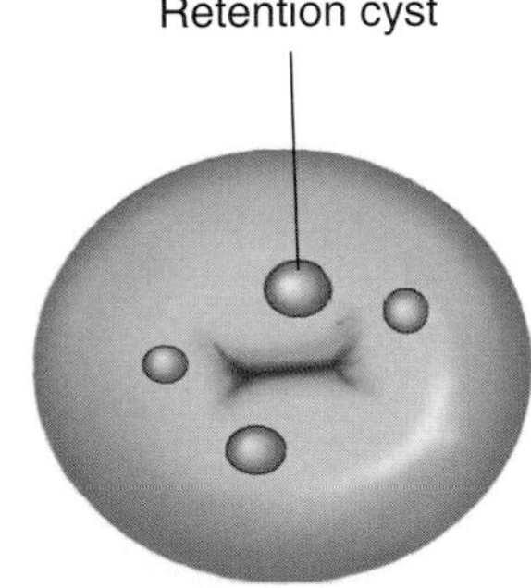

Figure 3.10.

Cervix: Nabothian cysts.

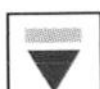

TIPS

- Nabothian cysts: one or more papules or nodules on the cervix, each contains mucus
- Benign

specially trained primary care physician. Cervical carcinoma is closely related to infection with human papilloma virus, especially types 16 and 18. **Pregnancy** manifests with a bluish hue to the cervix (Chadwick's sign) and, late in the third trimester, a softening and thinning of the cervix itself, as it is remodeled for delivery. The company it keeps includes a blue color to the vaginal mucosa and palpably enlarged uterus may be seen in a woman with secondary amenorrhea. In labor, the cervix manifests with softening and thinning and the os beginning to open. The cervical os will dilate to 10 cm during the primary phase of labor. This cervical thinning and os dilation is called the first or primary phase of labor.

Pelvic Relaxation Problems

The speculum examination is the time to inspect and look for features of abnormal relaxation or laxity of the pelvis floor. The patient may complain of urinary incontinence in cases of pelvic relaxation problems or note a bulge, fullness, or "rupture" in the vagina or rectal areas, especially with cough. The most common reason for this is multiple pregnancies with vaginal deliveries. This is a significant quality of life issue that is best diagnosed by physical examination; be cognizant of the evaluation by physical examination. Two specific maneuvers are used to assess the patient for such abnormal laxity, herniations, or bulges. The first is **Valsalva's maneuver** with the patient in a dorsal lithotomy position. This is a nonspecific test that will unmask cystoceles, urethroceles and rectoceles, and prolapses. The next, more invasive, test is the **modified speculum stress maneuver (Fig. 3.11)**. For this, Valsalva's maneuver is repeated with a Graves' speculum, upper blade removed, inserted gently into the vagina. The speculum is then rotated 90 degrees and the Valsalva's maneuver repeated. This is performed so that the four quadrants of the vagina (anterior, lateral left, posterior, and lateral right) have been assessed and stressed. This maneuver is best for the evaluation of the bulges into the vagina—the "celes." **Cystocele** manifests as a soft, bulging mass in the wall of the anterior vagina **(Fig. 3.12)**. The bulge increases with Valsalva's maneuver and, in severe cases, protrudes beyond the introitus. In mild to moderate cases, the modified speculum examination (posterior blade placement) is the only method to demonstrate the bulge, which is an abnormal descent of the urinary bladder into the vagina. **Rectocele** manifests with a soft, bulging mass in the lower two thirds of the posterior rectal wall. The bulge increases with Valsalva's maneuver and, in severe cases, protrudes beyond the introitus. In mild to moderate cases, the modified speculum examination (anterior blade placement) is the method to demonstrate the bulge, which is the abnormal descent of the rectum into the vagina. **Enterocele** manifests with a soft, bulging mass in the wall of the upper one third of the posterior wall of the vagina. The bulge will increase with Valsalva's maneuver and, in severe cases, will protrude beyond the introitus. In mild to moderate cases, the modified

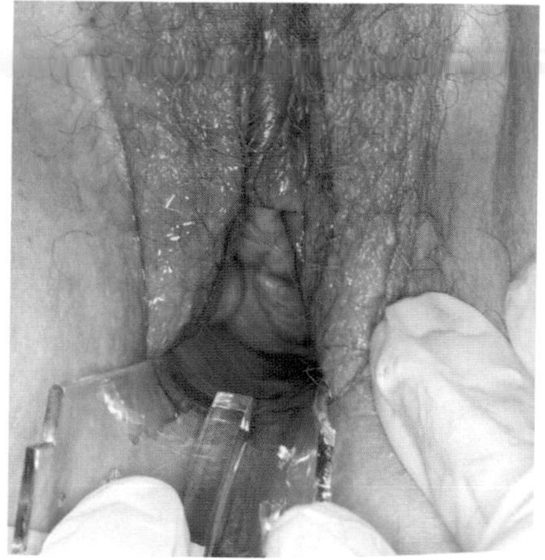

A

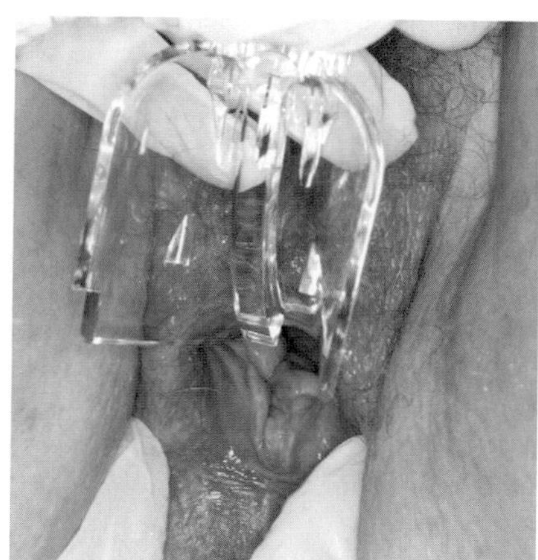

B

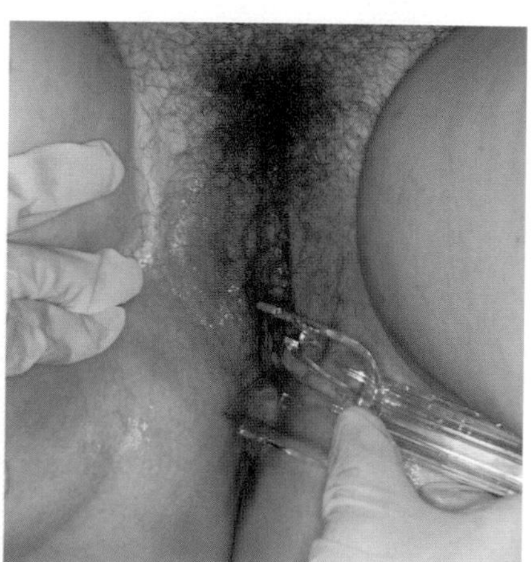

C

Figure 3.11.

Modified speculum pelvic relaxation stress test. **A.** Posterior. **B.** Anterior. **C.** Lateral.

TIPS

- Dorsal lithotomy position is best for this exam component
- Use a Graves' speculum, upper blade removed, inserted gently into vagina
- Patient instructed to perform the Valsalva's maneuver
- The speculum then rotated 90 degrees, and Valsalva's maneuver repeated. This is repeated twice more to stress and assess the four surfaces of the vagina: anterior, lateral left, posterior, and lateral right
- Excellent for diagnosis of laxity

TEACHING POINTS

VAGINAL AND CERVICAL EXAMINATION

1. For incontinence in any patient, the patient must perform the Valsalva's manuever and the clinician a modified speculum examination.
2. Vaginal discharge should be inspected and have a pH, wet-mount, and potassium hydroxide (KOH) analysis performed on it.
3. Vaginal adenosis, cervical hood, and clear cell carcinoma are all associated with diethylstilbestrol (DES) exposure in utero.
4. When performing a Pap smear, always obtain a specimen from the transformation zone.
5. Ectropion is normal in menstruating women, but in postmenopausal women is an ominous finding that requires significant evaluation.

speculum examination (anterior blade placement) will demonstrate the bulge, which is the abnormal descent of the loops of bowel at the pouch of Douglas into the vagina.

Uterine prolapse manifests with the cervix abnormally displaced inferiorly into the vagina. In severe cases, the cervix and the body of the uterus may protrude beyond the introitus **(Fig. 3.13)**. The degree of prolapse is defined by location of the tip of the cervix. In first-degree prolapse, the tip of the cervix is in the proximal one third of the vagina; in second-degree prolapse, the tip of the cervix is to the distal vagina, but not past the introitus; in third-degree prolapse, there is protrusion of the cervix and even the body of the uterus past the vaginal introitus. **Rectal prolapse** manifests with abnormal protrusion of the anus and rectum, such that the rectal mucosa is everted and exposed past the anal verge **(Fig. 3.14)**. This is distinct from, but may be concurrent to, a rectocele. Valsalva's maneuver will increase the size of the prolapse. **Urethral prolapse** manifests with protrusion of the urethra from the urethra meatus; the bulge is increased in size with a simple Valsalva's maneuver.

Uterus and Adnexa

The uterus is a hollow muscular organ that consists of three discrete areas—the cervix, the body, and the fundus—and two appendages—the fallopian tubes.

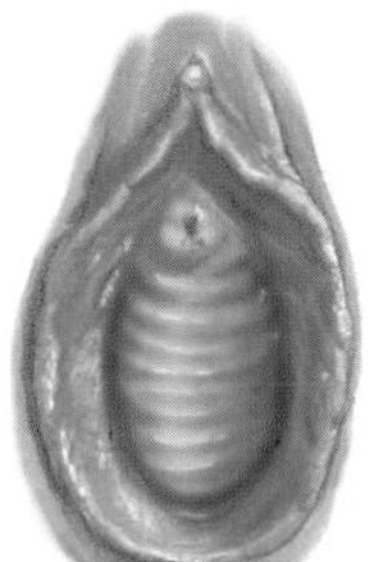

Figure 3.12.

Cystocele: urinary bladder through anterior vaginal wall.

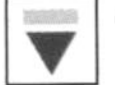 **TIPS**

- Cystocele: note the bulge from the anterior wall of the vagina
- Due to urinary bladder displacement
- Best test: stress test with speculum on posterior vaginal wall

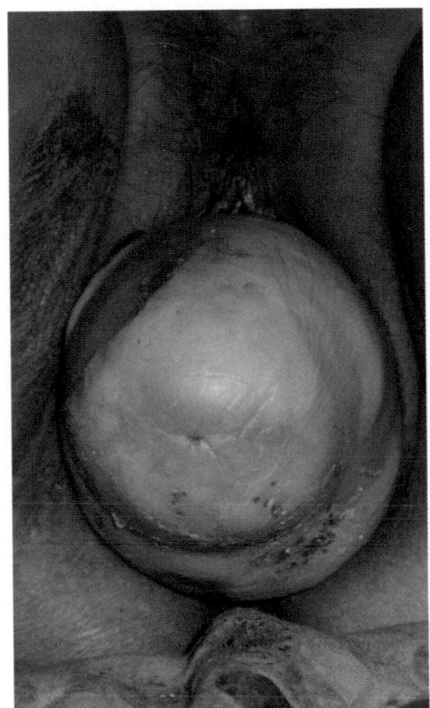

Figure 3.13.

Cervical prolapse—third degree.

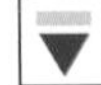 **TIPS**

- Cervical or uterine prolapse: protrusion of the uterus and cervix from the introitus of the vagina

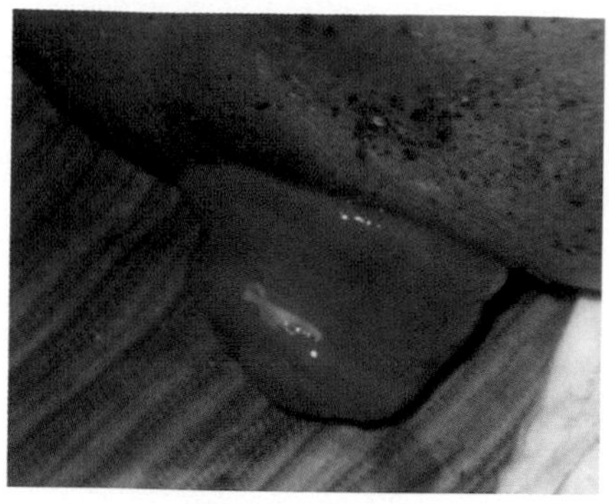

Figure 3.14.

Rectal prolapse.

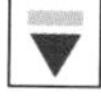 TIPS

- Rectal prolapse: eversion of the anal and rectal tissue, pink ring of rectal mucosa present
- Different from a rectocele

The cervix, the most inferior component, is located in the proximal vagina; the body is the bulk of the uterus; the fundus is the superior aspect between the insertion sites of the Fallopian tubes. The Fallopian tubes are located superior to the uterus; their distal ends are open each with a rim of fimbriae and are adjacent to the ovaries. The Fallopian tubes, with the distal oviducts, fimbriae, and ovaries are collectively called the **adnexa uteri**. The normal size of the uterus is approximately 7 to 9 cm long and 3 to 5 cm in diameter; the normal size of the ovaries is 3 to 4 cm in length. The Fallopian tubes run adjacent to the lateral fornices. The function of this anatomic complex is to provide an environment for fertilization of the ovum with a spermatozoon. The ovum, when extruded from the ovary into the peritoneum, is collected by the fimbriae of the proximal fallopian tube to migrate down to the uterus. If not fertilized, the ovum is passed out with the menstrual flow. Fertilization usually occurs when the ovum is in the proximal tube and, as it is developing into a blastula, will migrate and implant itself into the wall of the uterus. The uterus itself is lined with an endometrium that is simple columnar. The endometrium is responsive to the cyclic hormone changes and thickens at midcycle, i.e., at ovulation and sloughs 2 weeks later if fertilization and implantation have not occurred.

The examination of the uterus and adnexa includes two specific procedures: the bimanual maneuver of palpation and the rectovaginal examination. **Bimanual palpation** is performed in either the dorsal lithotomy or the lateral decubitus position **(Fig. 3.15)**. The bimanual examination is performed after any speculum examination. The specific points and steps in the examination are as follows. Apply water-soluble jelly to the second and third digit on the gloved dominant hand. With the fingers slightly flexed and the thumb in full abduction and extension, gently insert the fingers into the vagina to the level of the cervix. Gently palpate the cervix, the os, the lateral fornices, and the anterior and posterior fornices about the cervix. Then place the nondominant hand, palm to skin, slight flexion of fingers, and directly palpate the suprapubic area. Gently grasp the body and the fundus of the uterus between the hands. The height of the uterine fundus should be assessed and noted; normal height should not be superior to the pubic bones. If indeed it is above the pubic symphysis, further assess and measure, using a tape measure to measure from the top of fundus to the pubis symphysis. As will be described below, a retroflexed, retroverted uterus is difficult to palpate even by experienced examiners.

Once the uterus has been examined, the left and right adnexa must be bimanually palpated **(Fig. 3.16)**. The two digits that are internal are moved to the anterior aspect of the left lateral fornix; with the hand outside, palpate with a hooking maneuver over the left lower quadrant to catch any structure between. The structures between will be the adnexa. Repeat on the right side.

The final step is the **rectovaginal examination**. This is particularly important in a patient in whom you could not easily palpate the uterus or in any patient who has adnexal tenderness. The rectovaginal examination allows the examiner to palpate the anal and rectal lumens and also to feel for any problem in the posterior fornix and adjacent pouch of peritoneum, the pouch of Douglas. Perform this examination by replacing the gloves used in the bimanual examination; apply water-soluble lubricant to the second and third fingers on the dominant hand; insert the second finger into the posterior vagina, and the third digit into the anus and rectum. Palpate the rectovaginal area between the fingers.

The **uterus** itself is positioned in the midline of the pelvis. The two fundamental descriptors of uterine position are first, of the uterus relative to the cervix (i.e., anteflexed versus retroflexed) and, secondly, the tilt between the fundus and the body, anteverted versus retroverted. An **anteflexed** uterus is one in which the body is flexed anteriorly relative to the cervix; whereas,

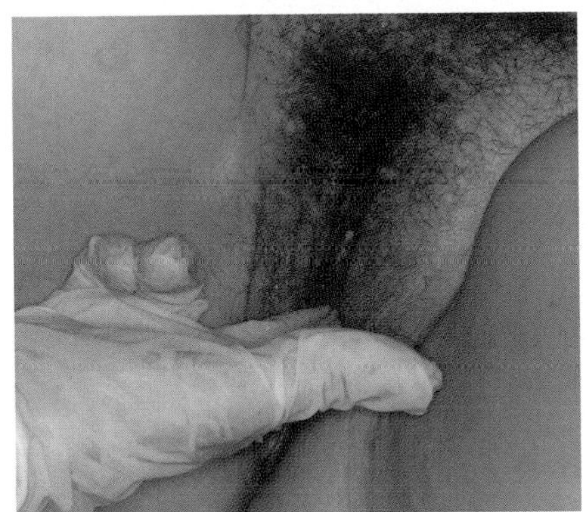
A

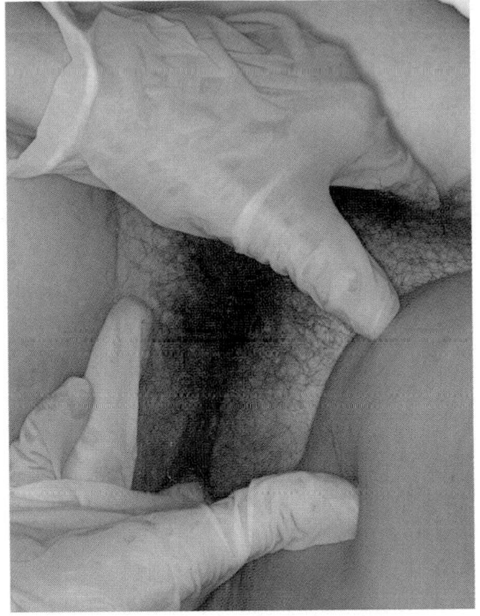
B

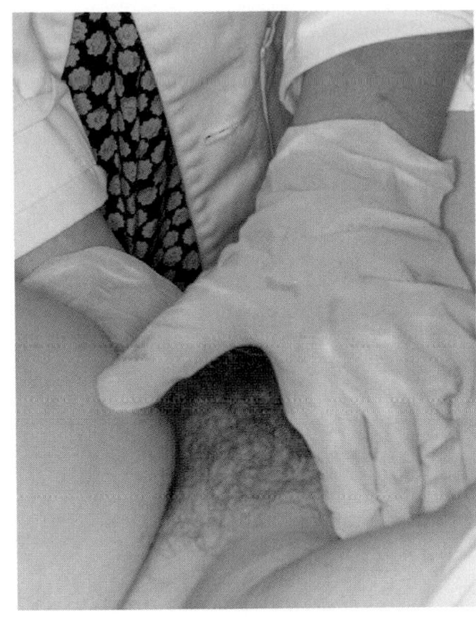
C

Figure 3.15.

Technique for bimanual examination steps-uterus. **A.** Gently insert digits 2 and 3 into posterior vagina to level of cervix and palpate cervix and fornices. **B.** and **C.** Use other hand to palpate using a hooking method.

TIPS

- Examiner applies water soluble jelly to the second and third digit on the gloved dominant hand
- With the fingers slightly flexed and the thumb in full abduction and extension, gently insert the fingers into the vagina to the level of the cervix
- Palpate the cervix, the os, the lateral fornices, and the anterior and posterior fornices about the cervix
- Then place the nondominant hand, palm to skin, slight flexion of fingers and directly palpate the suprapubic area. Attempt to gently grasp the body and the fundus of the uterus between the hands
- Use digits of the hand to gently yet firmly apply pressure with a slight amount of flexion in the fingers (hooking pressure) over the midline area, 2 to 4 cm above the pubis. Assess the presence, size, and characteristics of the uterus by palpating it between two hands

retroflexion is one in which the uterus is flexed posteriorly. Each of these positions is normal. Note the position when describing the uterus itself as a part of the bimanual examination. The **anteflexed and anteverted** uterus is the most common position and the one that makes it the easiest to readily palpate the uterus, in a traditional bimanual approach. A **retroflexed and retroverted** uterus, although completely normal, is one that is more challenging to the examiner. You may not be easily able to feel a normal uterus using a traditional bimanual approach; in point of fact, the uterus may only be palpable when performing a rectovaginal examination as it lies on the pouch of Douglas.

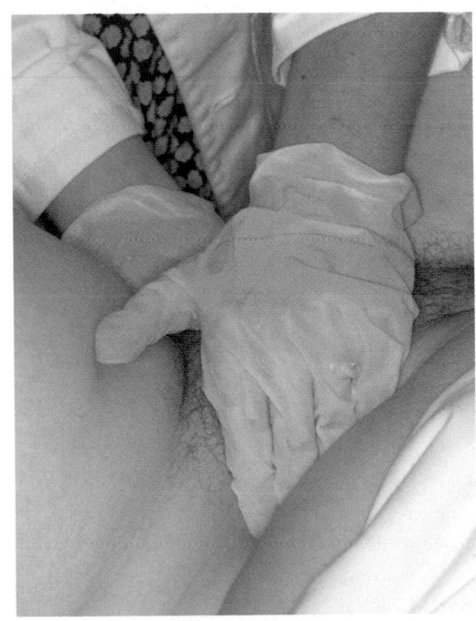

Figure 3.16.

Technique for bimanual examination-adnexa. Palpate the left lower abdomen using the bimanual method to assess presence, size, and characteristics of any adnexal structures or masses. Repeat same on the right (not shown).

TIPS

- The two digits that are internal are moved so that tips are in the anterior aspect of the left lateral fornix
- The hand outside is used to palpate with a hooking maneuver over the left lower quadrant so as to palpate adnexa

Uterus

Bicornuate uterus manifests with two palpably discrete components to the uterus. This is a congenital anomaly that is asymptomatic and discovered on routine first bimanual examination. Bicornuate uterus is caused by a failure of the müllerian ducts to fuse during fetal development and, thus, the patient, in extreme cases, may have two separate vaginas, cervices, and uteri. **Uterine fibroids** manifest with the patient complaining of dysmenorrhea and menorrhagia. They are very common and usually the patient is asymptomatic. On bimanual examination, one or more rubbery, nontender entities may be found in the uterus. Three types of fibroids may be found, which are categorized by location: subserosal, intramural, and submucosa. The **subserosal** type is pedunculated, may twist and thus cause pain. The **intramural** type is associated with excessive menstrual bleeding and pelvic pain; the **submucosal** type is associated with an increased risk of miscarriage. The submucosal is the most unlikely type for an examiner to feel on examination. These fibroids are benign leiomyomata of the uterus, and are extremely common. **Endometrial cancer** manifests with patient reporting irregular vaginal bleeding and the presence of a uterine mass on bimanual examination. Any postmenopausal bleeding should lead to a consideration of endometrial carcinoma and, thus, be aggressively assessed. **Adenomyosis** manifests with a homogenous enlargement of the uterus with minimal to no changes in the patient's menstrual bleeding pattern. This is caused by an abnormal proliferation of the endometrial glands into the myometrium; overall it is a benign process.

Pregnancy manifests with an enlarged uterus. The uterus enlargement is easily found during bimanual palpation during the first trimester and by abdominal examination after the first trimester. At 12 weeks of gestation, the fundus of the uterus is palpable above the pubic symphysis; at 20 weeks, it is at the umbilicus; and, at 34 weeks, it is at the level of the xiphoid process. To measure **fundal height**, use a tape measure to measure the distance between the top of the pubis symphysis to the top of the fundus in the midline of the abdomen. In addition to an enlarged uterus and secondary amenorrhea, a number of signs indicate pregnancy **(Table 3.4)**. On palpation of the cervix, the cervix itself is soft and edematous. It changes from its normal consistency likened to a contracted thenar muscle to that of a flaccid lip. This sign, described by Goodell, occurs at approximately 6 to 8 weeks of gestation. Another sign is the softening of the lower part of the uterine body (Hegar's sign). This is found on bimanual examination, specifically by placing two fingers in the posterior fornix and pressing the lowest part of the body of the uterus. This sign, described by Hegar, occurs in the late third trimester. A bluish color in the mucosa of the vulva, vagina, and cervix indicates pregnancy. (Chadwick or Jacquemier's* sign) The site most

*Chadwick's sign is most appropriately termed Jacquemier's sign.

Table 3.4. Evidence to Support the Diagnosis of Pregnancy

Sign	Author	Sensitivity (%)	Specificity (%)	Positive LR	Negative LR
Chadwick's	Chadwick	51	98	28.7	0.5
Goodell	Goodell et al	18	94	3.17	0.87
Fundus Palpable	Robinson and Barber	9	97	2.77	0.94
Uterine Artery Pulsation	Meeks et al	76	93	10.98	0.26

LR = likelihood ratio.

prominently involved with this bluish-violet hue is the mucosa of the anterior vagina. Described in English literature, first by Chadwick, this occurs at 8 to 12 weeks of pregnancy. Finally, an easily palpable uterine artery is present by the end of the first trimester. This pulse can be easily found by palpating the lateral fornix on bimanual examination.

Adnexa

Ectopic pregnancy manifests with the patient reporting a missed period and the acute onset of unilateral lower right or left quadrant abdominal pain. She may have a purple or blue hue to her vaginal mucosa (positive Chadwick's sign) and a tender mass in one of the adnexa on bimanual examination. If rupture occurs, invariably right or left lower quadrant direct, and rebound tenderness develops, along with flank ecchymosis (Grey Turner sign), hypotension and tachycardia from blood loss. Ectopic pregnancy results from implantation of the fertilized ovum in the Fallopian tube instead of the uterus. **Ovarian cyst** manifests with the presence of a solitary smooth, round mobile mass in the adnexa, indistinguishable from the ovary. The average size of a functional ovarian cyst is 5 cm. These cysts will spontaneously regress in 6 to 8 weeks. These functional cysts comprise 75% of all ovarian masses, and are derived from either a follicle or the corpus luteum. **Corpus luteal cyst** manifests with a mass that is nontender and firm. It is indistinguishable from other neoplastic entities on physical examination and, thus, needs to be evaluated by ultrasound imaging. **Ovarian neoplasia** manifests with few, if any, findings or symptoms until late in the course. One of the first findings may be a firm mass in the adnexa that is fixed to the adjacent tissues. In addition, there is often nodularity present on rectovaginal examination in the pouch of Douglas.

Pelvic inflammatory disease manifests with tenderness in one or both adnexa; sometimes, the tenderness is so severe as to preclude adequate examination. There is often concurrent vaginal discharge and exquisite tenderness on palpation of the cervix. There may be erythema of and discharge from the os of the cervix. This is due to infection with *Neisseria gonorrhea, Chlamydia trachomatis,* or gram-negative rods or anaerobes and is most often a sexually transmitted disease. **Tuboovarian abscess** manifests with an extremely tender mass in one adnexa of a patient who has antecedent or concurrent pelvic inflammatory disease. This is a complication of pelvic inflammatory disease.

Breast Examination

The **surface anatomy** of the breast includes the breast itself, the areola, the nipple, and the nodes that drain the breast, including the supraclavicular, infraclavicular, and axillary sites. Each breast is composed of glandular tissue that is positioned around, and drains into, the nipple via multiple ducts. The areola is the circular area surrounding the nipple. The glandular tissue is supported by connective tissue fibers called Cooper's ligaments. These ligaments not only play a role in the infrastructure of the breast and also contributes to development of a peau d'orange skin associated with a breast cancer. For examination purposes, the breast is geographically divided into **four quadrants**: upper outer, upper inner, lower inner, and right lower outer. The **nipple** is the center point in the lines that form these quadrants. The areola is a unique area that is described separately as the subareolar tissue. The upper outer quadrant extends into the axilla as the tail of Spence. This quadrant is very important in that tumor registry surveys have indicated that 60% of breast cancers are located here. In each of the other quadrants and in the subareolar area, 10% to 12% of all breast cancer occurs. The glandular tissue is

TEACHING POINTS

BIMANUAL EXAMINATION

1. This is best performed with the patient in a dorsal lithotomy position.
2. Palpate cervix and fornices first with dominant hand.
3. Place nondominant hand on suprapubic area to attempt to palpate size and surface of the uterus, most specifically the fundus.
4. Place nondominant hand on left and then right lower areas to palpate the left and right adnexa.
5. The bimanual examination complements the speculum examination.
6. The rectovaginal examination is the best method to palpate a retroflexed and retroverted uterus.

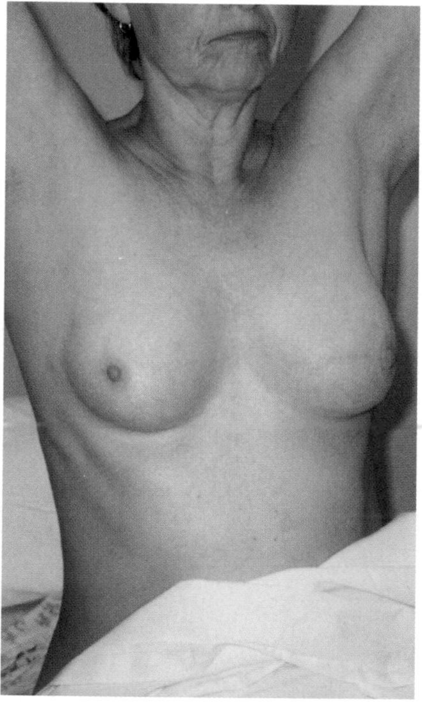

Figure 3.17.

Technique for inspection of the breasts.

TIPS

- Patient sitting
- Inspect the breast, areola, and nipples
- Look for asymmetry, nipple retraction

under the control of multiple hormones and, thus, changes most remarkably at adolescence and during pregnancy and lactation. The breast development during adolescence is described in Tanner stages **(Table 3.5)**. This is a useful staging system to complement the Tanner system for pubic hair distribution (Table 3.1) in the assessment of sexual maturation.

Examination of the breasts must include **inspection of the breasts (Fig. 3.17)** and nipples. On inspection one looks for edema, peau d'orange type thickening of the skin, and discharge from the nipple or nipple retraction. Peau d'orange, a stippled pattern in the skin that looks like the rind of an orange, can indicate an underlying breast carcinoma. The pattern is caused by the Cooper's ligaments maintaining small areas of skin intermixed with edema from the underlying breast carcinoma. Inspection is an important component of the examination that may reveal clues to the underlying diagnosis. **Palpation** is the foundation of the breast examination **(Fig. 3.18)**. To palpate, use the three levels of palpation: soft (Fig. 3.18A), to palpate the subcutaneous structures; medium (Fig. 3.18B), to palpate the intermediate depth structures; and deep (Fig. 3.18C), to palpate the deep structures. Fundamental aspects of the examination include a technique of finger overlap and a specific pattern in order to optimize the examination. The **patterns** are vertical strips (Fig. 3.18F), concentric circles (Fig. 3.18E), or spokes of the wheel. Each of these patterns is useful and appropriate as long as the examiner overlaps the palpation with each step and performs in a reproducible manner. Any nodules or masses discovered are described in terms of tenderness, size, firmness, and surface. Hard, nontender, rough masses are carcinoma until proved otherwise. Furthermore, it is important to describe and note if a mass is fixed to overlying or underlying tissue. The lymph nodes that need to be examined and described are the axillary nodes and the nodes in

Table 3.5. Tanner Staging: Breast Development

Stage	Description
Stage 1:	No breast development—preadolescent girls
Stage 2:	Elevation of the breast and areola—breast bud stage
Stage 3:	Areola and breast enlargement—adolescence, early adult
Stage 4:	Areola elevated to above the breast—adolescence, mid-adult
Stage 5:	Breast enlarged, areola in contour of the breast itself—late adolescence, adult

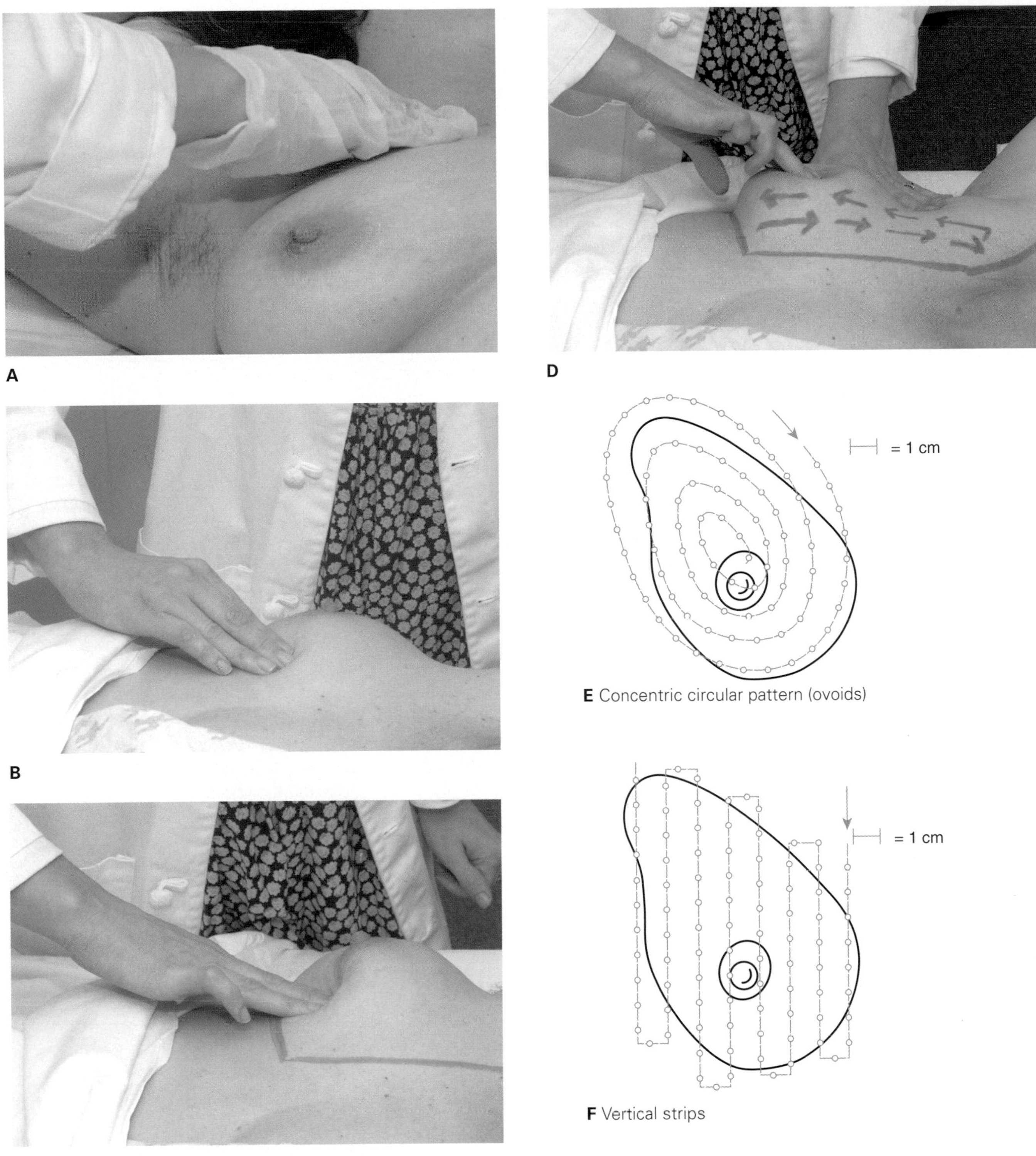

Figure 3.18.

Technique for patterns of palpation of the breasts. Use patterns in **E** or **F** (concentric ovoids or vertical strips) **A.** Light. **B.** Medium. **C.** Deep. **D.** Palpation of subareolar areas. **E.** Concentric ovoid pattern. **F.** Vertical strip pattern.

TIPS

- Patterns for breast palpation, vertical strips and concentric ovoids
- The points of palpation are no more than 1 cm apart
- Include Tail of Spence in pattern

TEACHING POINTS

BREAST EXAMINATION

1. When performing palpation, use a pattern that allows for complete coverage of all breast tissue and overlapping finger technique.
2. Patterns that are excellent include the vertical strips and the concentric circles.
3. Use the index and third fingers on the dominant hand to palpate. Examine each site with light, then moderate, then firm pressure.
4. Remember to drape the patient to optimize comfort and completeness of the examination.
5. Thoroughly examine the tail of Spence, i.e., the breast tissue located in the upper outer quadrant.
6. Palpate for any axillary or supraclavicular lymph nodes present.

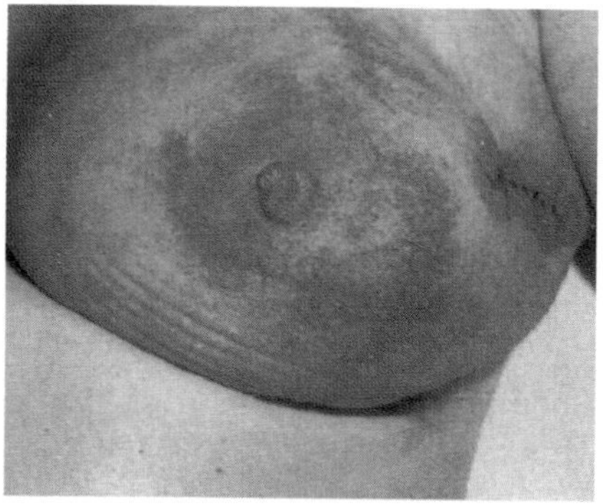

Figure 3.19.

Inflammatory carcinoma. (From Moore KL, Dalley AF. *Clinically Oriented Anatomy,* 4th ed. Philadelphia: Lippincott Williams & Wilkins, 1999:78, with permission).

TIPS

- Inflammatory carcinoma: diffusely erythematous skin with peau d'orange

the infraclavicular and supraclavicular areas. The technique used to examine axillary nodes is described in Chapter 9, Shoulder Examination Fig. 9.6.

Breast carcinoma manifests with a firm, even hard, nodule or mass that, when advanced, is fixed to the underlying pectoralis major muscle or to the overlying skin. Concurrent axillary or supraclavicular nodes may be enlarged, if metastatic disease is present (Fig. 9.24). In very advanced cases, there is a peau d'orange skin edema, acquired retraction of the nipple, bloody nipple discharge, and even inflammation of the skin overlying the cancer—a variant called inflammatory carcinoma of the breast **(Fig. 3.19)**. Risk factors for breast cancer include early menarche, late menopause, nulliparous, and first-degree relative with breast carcinoma. **Breast abscess** manifests with a tender nodule that can erode into the superficial skin to drain pus. The nodule is tender and fluctuant. It is often found in the lactating woman; the tenderness and pain markedly increases with suckling. An abscess may be caused by breast-feeding and if so affects one of the duct systems. **Fibrocystic breast** disease manifests with multiple nodules that often, in the premenstrual period, are modestly tender and increased in size. This is due to a benign condition.

Annotated Bibliography

Apgar BS, Cox JT. Differentiating normal and abnormal findings of the vulva. ***Am Fam Pract*** **1996;53(4):1171–1180.**

Practical overview of normal and abnormal findings in patients who present to primary care physicians; very much written to the primary care provider audience. Entities described include micropapillomas: normal—probable congenital entities on the entire inner labia minora, sebaceous hyperplasia—labia majora (lateral labia) may appear cobblestone when hypertrophy occurs—normal variant. Acetowhite changes (nonspecific) mild postintercourse or yeast or inflammatory process of vulva or if papular with satellites—HPV. Lichen sclerosis—thin atrophic epithelium, labial tissue looks like parchment; white patches coalesce, typical symmetric keyhole appearance about the anus /or the vestibule; can result in atrophy of the labia minora, with decreased size of the introitus and phimosis and paraphimosis of the clitoris glans. Dyspareunia and vaginal pruritus. Squamous cell hyperplasia—surface trauma of recurrent rubbing or scratching; nonspecific—rarely involves the inner labia minora. Red lesions: psoriasis, seborrhea; pigmented, including nevi and melanoma. Finally, a discussion of vulvar intraepithelial neoplasia (VIN). VIN I: mild dysplasia; VIN II: moderate dysplasia; VIN III: carcinoma in situ. Colposcopy should be performed to look for vessel changes and white with application of vinegar papules associated with HPV 16; HPV 16 and 31 highly correlated with VIN in young women. Excellent color illustrations of each of these entities and lesions.

Barton MB, Harris R, Fletcher SW. Does this patient have breast cancer? *JAMA* 1999; 282(13):1270–1280.

An excellent paper demonstrating the technique and importance of clinical breast examination in the diagnosis of early breast carcinoma.

Bastian LA, Piscitelli JT. Is this patient pregnant? Can you reliably rule in or rule out early pregnancy by clinical examination? *JAMA* 1997;278:586–591.

A review of studies to assess, via history and physical examination, and to diagnose pregnancy in the first trimester. Very interesting review; history includes amenorrhea, morning sickness, breast tingling, pain, swelling, patient suspects she is pregnant, sexual activity, and physical examination. Likelihood ratios (LR) are given for breast signs of tenderness and swelling: present positive, LR 2.71, absent 0.55; Chadwick's sign: LR 28.7 and negative LR 0.5, according to Chadwick's study; positive LR 3.17, negative 0.87, and bimanual examination of uterine artery pulsation: positive, LR 10.98, negative LR 0.26.

Cannistra SA, Niloff JM. Cancer of the uterine cervix. *N Engl J Med* 1996;334(16):1030–1036.

A state-of-the-art article in which the epidemiology and risk factors for cervical carcinoma are discussed; the high-risk types of HPV—16, 18, 31, 33, and 35—are associated with cervical intraepithelial neoplasia (CIN). Reviews the performance, interpretation, and recommended follow-up and treatment of various aspects of CIN. The classification specifics are outlined, including the meaning of high-grade squamous intraepithelial lesion (HGSIL) versus low grade (LGSIL) versus atypical squamous cells of undetermined significance (ASCUS). In this class, HG usually reflects CIN II or III, whereas LG suggests CIN I or HPV infection. Colposcopy procedures and evaluation and management of invasive carcinoma are discussed. Excellent images are present in the text, especially of CIN during colposcopy. Indeed, a state-of-the-art paper that all primary care physicians should have.

Chadwick JR. Value of the bluish coloration of the vagina entrance as a sign of pregnancy. *Transactions of the American Gynecologic Society* (1886). 1887;11:399–418.

Chadwick's sign: 8 to 12 weeks the mucous membranes of vulva, vagina, and cervix are congested and bluish-violet in hue. Usually seen in the anterior vagina, rarely if ever before 7 weeks.

Dumesic DA. Pelvic examination. *Consultant* 1996;January:39–46.

A practical overview of the pelvic examination, with emphasis on postmenopausal women. Multiple practical tips for any pelvic examination and some excellent images.

Ferreyra S, Hughes K. *Table Manners: A Guide to the Pelvic Examination for Disabled Women and Health Care Providers.* San Francisco: Planned Parenthood Alameda/San Francisco, 1982.

Very informative, useful, and practical overview of methods to assist the patient and provider in the performance of a pelvic examination in the disabled patient. Includes descriptions and basic illustrations of knee-chest position, diamond-shaped position, M-shaped position, V-shaped position, and tips for hearing and visually impaired patients. Special concerns, including bowel and bladder, or the problem of hyperreflexia or autonomic hyperreflexia in patients with spinal cord injury—common symptoms include increased blood pressure, sweating, botchy skin, nausea, and goosebumps, which may be caused by a reaction to the cold, hard table; the cervical swab; or the bimanual or rectal examination.

Gardner HI, Dukes CD. Haemophilus vaginalis vaginitis. *Am J Ob Gyn* 1955;69:962.

The original description of nonspecific vaginitis.

Germain M, Heaton R, Erickson D, et al. A comparison of the three most common Papanicolaou smear collection techniques. *Obstet Gynecol* 1994;84(2):168.

Using a cotton-tipped applicator, a spatula, and a cytobrush, no difference was found in detecting cervical dysplasia; indeed, an increase in sample of endocervical cells was obtained using the cytobrush.

Hoffman MS, Hill DA, Gordy LW, et al. Comparing the yield of the standard Papanicolaou and endocervical brush smears. *J Reprod Med* 1991;36:267.

Demonstrated that the cytobrush and spatula are superior in collecting endocervical cell samples when compared with cotton-tipped swab and spatula.

Johnson BA. The colposcopic examination. *Am Fam Pract* 1996;53(8):2473–2482.

Nice overview from the point of view of a primary care physician. Reviews indications, tips on the procedure itself, including swabbing the cervix to remove mucus, then imaging the cervix with a green filter on colposcope to image any abnormal vessels or atypical vessels present (green filter makes vessels look darker because of the absorption of red light); 5% acetic acid solution is applied to the cervix (white vinegar is 5%) with three cotton balls in a ring forceps. Acetowhite epithelium has a higher concentration of cellular protein and increased nuclear density thus appears white. Normal and abnormal findings are discussed. Normal: ectocervix: stratified, squamous nonkeratinized; lots of glycogen; endocervix: single layer of mucus-secreting tall columnar cells; beefy red. The squamocolumnar junction (transformation zone) site must be assessed thoroughly. Nabothian cysts (mucus-containing normal branching vessels on surface) caused by occluded epithelial glands-normal. Abnormal: any acetowhite area at transformation zone. Three abnormal vascular patterns on colposcopy: (1) punctuation: dilated, twisted vessels, stippled in appearance; (2) mosaicism: tilelike appearance of vessels; and (3) atypical vessels: corkscrew, spaghetti, commalike—more suggestive of invasion.

Reviews the technique of biopsy, appropriate care of specimen, and postbiopsy management. A practical, well-illustrated article.

Loenzen JR, Gravdal JA. Bloody nipple discharge. ***Am Fam Phys*** **1986:34(1):151–154.**
Good review of the causes and evaluation of bloody nipple discharge.

Majeroni BA. Bacterial vaginosis: an update. ***Am Fam Pract*** **1998;57(6):1285–1289.**
A common cause of vaginal discharge known as nonspecific or Gardnerella vaginalis. Reviews the impact of this disorder on pregnancy which includes increased risk of chorioamnionitis, neonatal sepsis; and increased risk of premature rupture of membranes. Diagnostic criteria are discussed, including homogeneous vaginal discharge; clue cells on vaginal wet mount (often the limit is >20% of cells are "clue," i.e., have stippling of the surface with coccobacilli); the presence of an amine (fishy) smell when 10% solution KOH added to the vaginal secretions(Whiff test) (which is also positive in trichomonas); a pH of vagina >4.5 and no lactobacilli in vagina. Discusses treatment with oral clindamycin or metronidazole or topical metronidazole.

Mayeaux EJ, Harper MB, Barksdale W, Pope JB. Noncervical human papillomavirus genital infections. ***Am Fam Pract*** **1995;52(4):1137–1146.**
Reviews the manifestations of condyloma acuminata—the HPV-related warts that are papular, may be flat and detected only with the application of 1% to 5% acetic acid to the area(s). HPV types 16 and 18 indicate high risk for oncogenic transformation; most of the paper involves various therapeutic modalities and, as such, this is an excellent paper for therapeutic endeavors.

Pennypacker HS, Pilgrim CA. Achieving competence in clinical breast examination. ***Nurse Practice Forum*** **1993;4(2):85–90.**
Tremendously important paper in that it demonstrates a standardized mechanism for performing and teaching clinical breast examination—published in a journal for primary care providers, the very group who needs to master this important technique. Excellent technique discussion.

Reed BD, Eyler A. Vaginal infections: diagnosis and management. ***Am Fam Phys*** **1993;47(8): 1805–1816.**
Very good overview of three specific causes of vaginitis. Bacterial vaginosis: change in the flora of the vagina, etiology not completely clear. There is a decrease in lactobacilli, and an overgrowth of gram-negative findings and anaerobes, specifically Gardnerella vaginalis. Manifestations include increase in pH to >4.5, aromatic amines, fishy odor after intercourse or with the KOH test. Diagnosis is confirmed with a pH>4.5, clue cells (epithelial cells covered with bacteria), positive whiff test, and homogenous white discharge. Trichomonas vaginitis flagellated anaerobic protozoan profuse discharge and vaginal or vulvar irritation with itch, abnormal vaginal odor, dyspareunia. Discharge is white and mild frothy or foamy. Also seen is a strawberry cervix or redness of the vagina, perineum or inner thigh. Other features include elevated pH of>5.0 and >10 white blood cells high power field (Hpf) on wet mount and trichomonads; Candida vaginitis hypha, budding yeast; thick, white discharge, no odor, no clue cells, and Candida on Pap smear. An extensive and excellent discussion of therapy is included; dated but still relevant. A paper that is well illustrated and should be a part of any primary care provider's library.

Robinson ET, Barber JH. Early diagnosis of pregnancy in general practice. ***Journal of the Royal College of General Practice*** **1977;27:335–338.**
Goodell's sign: bimanual palpation of the cervix softens, baseline like a nose tip and pregnant like lips. Hegar sign: a palpable softening of the lowermost portion of the corpus occurs at about 6 weeks . Examiner places two fingers of one hand behind cervix in the posterior vaginal fornix, then compresses the lower part of the corpus anteriorly by suprapubic pressure with other hand. Distinct area of uterine softening is noted.

Scanlon E. A photo checklist for a better breast palpation. ***Primary Care and Cancer*** **1987; Sept:13–20.**
A descriptive paper with multiple images on how to examine the breasts, both by inspection and palpation; ample images included.

Wiese Patel SR, Ohl CA, Estrada CA. A metaanalysis of the papanicolaou smear and wet mount for the diagnosis of vaginal trichomoniasis. ***Am J Med*** **2000;108:301–308.**
Metaanalysis of studies used to detect trichomonas in the vagina: the Pap smear and the wet-mount smear. Used 30 studies (9,501 women) that assessed by wet mount and 7 studies (2,958 women) by the Pap smear. The weighted mean sensitivity, specificity, and positive LR and negative LR for Pap smear were 58%, 97%, 19.3, and 0.4, respectively; whereas for the wet mount they were 68%, 99.9%, 680, and 0.3. Demonstrates the power of either test, but especially the wet mount.

4

Cardiovascular Examination

PRACTICE AND TEACHING

SURFACE ANATOMY

Anterior

The surface anatomy of cardiac structures include the base and the apex of the heart. The **base (Fig. 4.1A** and **B)**, located at the superior aspect of the sternum, is the area overlying the transmission of the aortic (Fig. 4.1A) and pulmonic (Fig. 4.1B) valve sounds. Because blood flows from the left ventricle into the aorta (transmitted in a left to right direction), the **aortic valve** and any problems related to it is best heard over the right side of the base. The **pulmonic valve** and any problems related to it is best heard over the left side of the base. The **apex** of the heart is located 2 cm lateral left to the sternum in the fifth intercostal space **(Fig. 4.1C** and **D)**. The **mitral valve** and any problems related to it is best heard at the apex (Fig. 4.1D); whereas, the **tricuspid valve** and any related problems is best heard to the right of this (Fig. 4.1C). The base is the location where the **second heart sound** is best heard; the apex is the site where the **first heart tone** is best heard. The *left ventricle* is located approximately 2 cm from the left lateral to the sternum; the *right ventricle* is located in the mid-chest and lays on the middle of the diaphragm. The internal

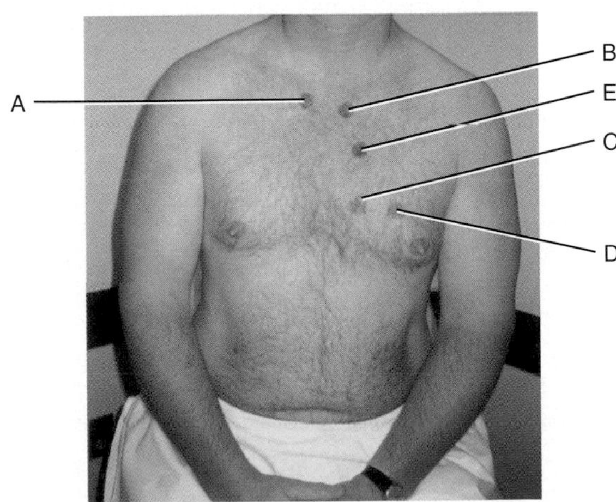

Figure 4.1.

Surface anatomy, anterior chest. **A.** Location where the aortic valve sound is best heard. **B.** Location where the pulmonic valve sound is best heard. **C.** Location where the tricuspid valve sound is best heard **D.** Location where the mitral valve sound is best heard. **E.** Left sternal border of heart.

TIPS

- Base: S_2 is loudest
- Apex: S_1 is loudest
- Base: aortic and pulmonic valve sounds are best heard
- Apex: tricuspid and mitral valve sounds are best heard
- Apex: best site to hear gallops.

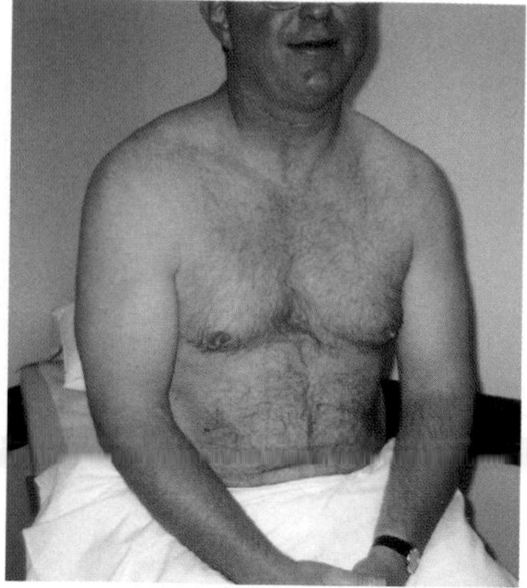

A

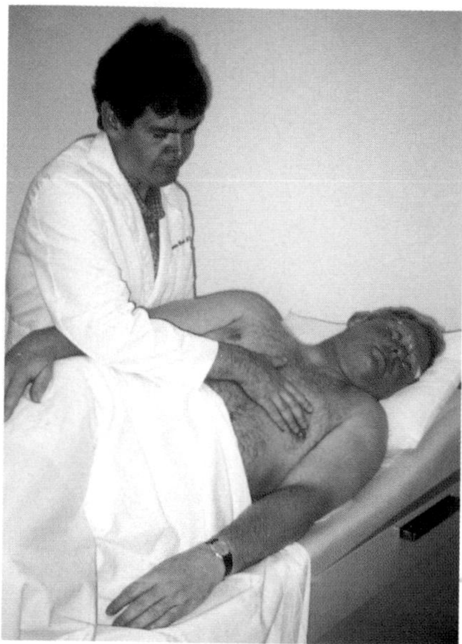

B

Figure 4.2.

Positions for cardiac examination. **A.** Upright best for exam of base. **B.** Left lateral decubital best for exam of apex.

and external jugular veins run with the carotid arteries adjacent to the sternocleidomastoid muscles.

CARDIAC EXAMINATION

Patient position is very important when inspecting, palpating, and ausculting the heart and great vessels. The three different positions are upright, supine, and left lateral decubitus **(Fig. 4.2)**. The **upright position** brings the base of the heart closer to the chest and, thus, facilitates examination of the structures at the base. These structures include the aortic and the pulmonic valve. The **supine position** is a neutral position that is adequate for chest wall inspection, but is *not* the best for any specific site. The **left lateral decubital position** is one in which the patient is rolled onto the left side, approximately 20 degrees. This brings the *apex* of the heart closer to the chest wall and, thus, facilitates examination of structures at the apex. These structures include the left ventricle, the mitral valve, and the tricuspid valve. Also, any gallops are best heard at the apex. A good examination must include both the upright and the left lateral decubital positions. Both positions must be emphasized in practice and teaching.

Chest wall inspection to assess the boney structures of the chest wall is an extremely important first step. This component of the examination, in addition to neck muscle inspection and tracheal location assessment, is often an underutilized component of the physical examination. **Pectus excavatum**, also known as funnel chest, manifests with the inferior sternum displaced posteriorly, i.e., sternal inversion (Fig. 5.3A). This anomaly of the chest wall is associated with mitral valve prolapse (MVP) in up to 15% of cases. It is a potential contributor to restrictive lung disease.

Scars are clues to antecedent trauma or surgical procedures and, as such, provide a rich source of information in the physical examination and history. A **median sternotomy scar** indicates cardiac surgery, either valve or bypass grafting. Furthermore, a scar with a **subcutaneous device** present in the upper chest wall indicates an automatic implantable cardioverter-defibrillator (AICD) or a pacemaker. See Fig. 5.4 for further details.

Pulsations are not uncommonly demonstrated on the chest wall, especially when the patient is in the left lateral decubital position (Fig. 4.2B). The pulsations may be present in the area of the apex, which is the location of the **point of maximal impulse (PMI)**. This pulsation is the transmission of the ventricular contraction across the chest wall itself. It is most prominent in a hyperdynamic setting or in cases of cardiac pathology. The **normal** position of the PMI is in the left midclavicular line, fifth intercostal interspace. The PMI is visible only in minority cases, but, when visible, it makes the examination easier. **Left ventricular hypertrophy** manifests with a laterally and inferiorly displaced point of maximal impulse (PMI), and *left ventricular dilation* manifests with a laterally and inferiorly displaced PMI. **Hyperdynamic state** manifests with a prominent PMI pulsation that is visible, but not laterally or inferiorly displaced. Hyperdynamic states are caused by hyperthyroidism, anemia, fever, and beriberi of thiamine deficiency.

Neck vein inspection is best performed with the patient in a supine position with the trunk elevated 20 degrees **(Fig. 4.3)**. Look at the right lateral neck about the right sternocleidomastoid muscle for any pulsation. Pulsatile areas about the sternocleidomastoid are usually caused by the top of the column of blood in the jugular vein system. The top of the column is called the meniscus. This reflects the volume in and function of the right ventricle.

The **technique of neck vein inspection** includes using a light source, e.g., a penlight or flashlight, directed in an angle that is oblique from the side. This light source adds a dimension of depth to the inspection. Furthermore, if a meniscus is not demonstrable, change the position of the trunk to 0 degrees or 40 degrees and reassess the right neck for pulsations or a meniscus. If one suspects the patient has grossly elevated right neck veins, assess with the patient upright; if no meniscus is present, the veins may be so distended that the meniscus is above the level of the ear or the body habitus prevents adequate examination. Recall, neck vein assessment is difficult even for master examiners. Cook and Simel in their study demonstrated a fair, at best, interrater reliability in neck vein assessment. They report a kappa of 0.65 for students vs attendings, but one of only 0.3 for residents vs attendings. Once the meniscus is found, the vertical drop is measured using a straight-edged ruler from the meniscus to the Angle of Louis*, which is between the body and manubrium of the sternum. This measurement is the jugular venous pressure (JVP). Normally, the JVP measurement is <5 cm; elevated, it is >5 cm. Because the heart is deep to the Angle of Louis, a constant, called the "cardiology constant"—5 cm—is added to the JVP measurement. This sum is the central venous pressure (CVP). Cook and others in their study demonstrated that if indeed the CVP measured is elevated, the likelihood that the CVP is truly elevated is high. (positive LR = 4.1).

A concurrent complementary technique is **arm forward flexion and elevation**, which was first described by von Recklinghausen in the 1870s. This technique uses the principle of raising the right arm above the level of the base of the heart, i.e., the Angle of Louis and thus the base of the heart. The examiner notes the level at which the veins of the skin collapse. Normally, the veins in the arm collapse at the level of the base of the heart; **elevated right-sided pressures** manifest with the veins remaining engorged above the base of the heart. Thus, this may indicate right ventricular failure, superior vena cava syndrome, tricuspid regurgitation, or tricuspid stenosis. Be aware of this subtle, yet important aspect of the physical examination.

The **hepatojugular reflux** (HJR) or **abdominojugular reflux** (AJR) technique is performed with the patient in the supine position, with the trunk elevated to 20–40 degrees, the standard position to assess CVP. The examiner applies pressure with the palm of the hand to the area immediately above the umbilicus for approximately 30 seconds. Inspect the jugular venous meniscus before and during the application of pressure. In the original procedure described by Pasteur, the hand pressure is applied to the liver; as modified by Rondot, the pressure is applied to the area above the umbilicus. **Normal** is an increase of ≤3 cm in the meniscus. **Right ventricular failure** manifests with an increase in this of ≥4 cm. This test, which is complementary to neck vein assessment, is especially useful in assessing borderline cases. The increase is particularly evident in right ventricular failure, tricuspid regurgitation, tricuspid stenosis, constrictive pericarditis, pericardial tamponade, and from left ventricular failure. Thus, it is important to know that the most common reason for elevated JVP to be present is not isolated right-sided heart problems, but actually left ventricular dysfunction or failure.

Once a meniscus and venous pulsations in the right neck are found, look for the discrete individual waveforms at the surface of the meniscus. These were first described at the turn of the last century and includes the *a* wave, the *c* wave, the *v* wave, and the *x* and *y* descents. The ***a* wave**, which is a positive deflection, is the first wave. Produced by the right atrial contraction, it immediately precedes the S_1 and correlates with an S_4. The ***c* wave**, which is a positive deflection, is the second wave, caused by the bulging of the cusps of the tricuspid valve into the right atrium. This correlates with ventricular isovolumetric contraction. This is the hardest wave to see. Of interest, the AC interval is the same as the PR interval on EKG. The ***v* wave**, which is the third and last

*Older texts refer to Angle of Louis as "Angle of Ludwig"

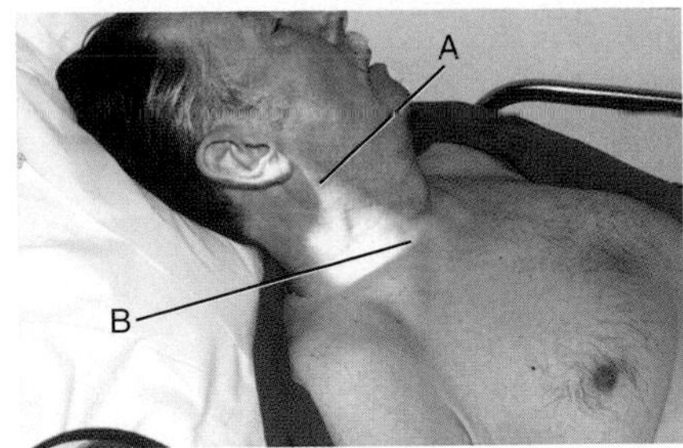

Figure 4.3.

Technique and position for neck vein assessment. **A.** Meniscus. **B.** Angle of Louis

TIPS

- Supine, 20 degrees of trunk elevation
- Angle of Louis: interface between the body and the manubrium of the sternum
- Assess for the meniscus on right neck
- Using a straight edge, that is a ruler, measure the vertical distance between the Angle of Louis and the meniscus; this is the JVP.
- The central venous pressure (CVP) is the jugular venous pressure (JVP) plus 5, 5 being the distance in cm from the Angle of Louis to the right atrium
- Normal JVP: <5 cm
- Normal CVP: <10 cm

Box 4.1.

Increased jugular venous pressure (JVP) with inhalation (positive Kussmaul's sign): evidence basis

Diagnosis	Study	Sensitivity (%)
Right ventricular infarct	Cintron	30
	Dell'Italia	100
Right ventricular failure	Cintron	30
	Dell'Italia	100
Constrictive pericarditis	Shabetai and Spodick	33
Tricuspid stenosis	None	

positive deflection of the contour, correlates with the end of systole of ventricle and early ventricular diastole. The ***x* descent**, which is between the *a* and *c* waves, is a negative deflection. It is produced by right atrial relaxation. The ***y* descent** is a negative deflection. It is produced by ventricular diastole as the tricuspid valve opens. The *y* descent correlates with the S_3 and is accentuated by anything that increases venous return.

Finally, assess the movement of the meniscus of the neck veins when the **patient deeply inhales**. This is the maneuver of Kussmaul. In the normal setting, the jugular vein meniscus decreases with inhalation. In conditions in which there is limited right ventricular filling, a paradoxic increase may occur in the meniscus with inspiration—a positive Kussmaul's sign. **Constrictive pericarditis** manifests with an increase in the meniscus with inhalation, i.e., a positive Kussmaul's sign; whereas, **pericardial effusion** manifests with a decrease in the meniscus with inhalation. Please refer to **Box 4.1** for evidence to support the use of Kussmaul's sign.

Diagnoses in which assessment of JVP and related signs of great importance include **superior vena cava obstruction**, which manifests with increased size of neck and chest wall veins, increased size of arm subcutaneous veins, tongue edema, facial and eyelid edema, and upper extremity edema (Fig. 1.25). The company it keeps is specific to the underlying cause. **Right ventricular failure** manifests with increased JVP; *a* and *v* waves that are both prominent; and increased HJR. **Constrictive pericarditis** manifests with increased JVP, and prominent *x* and *y* descents. The *y* descent is prominent but has a low sensitivity and high specificity. There is an increase in HJR and a positive Kussmaul's sign in one third of patients, but a normal pulsus paradox **(Boxes 4.1 and 4.2)**. **Pericardial effusion** manifests with an increased JVP, a diminished *y* descent, an increase in HJR, a negative Kussmaul's sign, and an

Box 4.2.

Presence of pulsus paradoxus: evidence basis

Exam Findings	Study	Sensitivity (%)
Right ventricular infarct	Lorell	71
Right ventricular failure	Extrapolated from above	71
Pericardial tamponade	Reddy	70 to 100

TEACHING POINTS

INSPECTION OF PRECORDIUM AND NECK

1. One must always inspect the chest wall for pulsations at the apex or in the precordium; this is best performed in left lateral decubital position.
2. One must always inspect the right neck for presence and potential elevation of neck veins; best performed in supine position.
3. Neck vein assessment provides information that further defines and delineates a problem; in and of itself it will not lead to a diagnosis.
4. An elevated jugular venous pressure (JVP) is consistent with right ventricular dysfunction.
5. The *a* wave corresponds to the atrial contraction and an S_4. Atrial fibrillation has no specific *a* waves.
6. The *c* wave is the most difficult to see.
7. The *v* wave is an excellent wave to assess the tricuspid valve.
8. Kussmaul's sign is not specific to constrictive pericarditis. It is caused by right ventricular failure and infarction.
9. Arm forward flexion and hepatojugular reflux are both complementary tests to the standard JVP.
10. Central venous pressure (CVP) = JVP +5. This is a more fastidious measure of neck vein height that effectively means the same as JVP.

elevated pulsus paradox. The sensitivity for pulsus paradox is 70–100% in a study by Reddy. The company a large pericardial effusion keeps includes an area of dullness to percussion over the medial aspect to the left scapula (Ewart's sign) and an associated decrease in tactile fremitus and decreased breath sounds over that area (Fig. 4.14). There have been many other auscultatory and fremitus signs of pericardial effusion but they serve only to confuse the modern clinician educator. **Tricuspid regurgitation** manifests with an elevated JVP, an absent *x* descent, large *c* or *v* waves, and rapid *y* descent, which is also the underlying reason for blinking or bobbing earlobes. Please refer to page 89 for further discussion. **Tricuspid stenosis** manifests with an elevated JVP and a large *a* wave and a slow *y* descent. **Pulmonary hypertension** manifests with an elevated JVP and large *a* waves, caused by an increase in right ventricular end-diastolic pressures. The *a* wave increases with a strong atrial contraction against this increased ventricular pressure. **Atrioventricular (AV) dissociation** manifests with *canon a* waves caused by the atrium contracting against a closed tricuspid valve; this is seen most often in ventricular tachycardia or third-degree AV block. **Atrial fibrillation** manifests with no *a* waves because no effective atrial contractions occur. **Atrial flutter** manifests with flutter *a* waves at a rate of 300 waves/minute.

Palpation of the precordium is important to assess for location of the **point of maximal impulse (PMI),** and any heaves, lifts, or thrills. Inspection of the precordium may give clues to where to place the hands, but it is most likely that palpation will be required to find the specific location of the PMI. Palpation is best performed with the patient in the left lateral decubital position, because it is difficult to assess this with the patient in a supine or upright position. Recall, palpation can be performed with the palmar fingertips or with the palms of the hands (Fig. 4.2B). Use whichever is best for you.

The *PMI* is defined by using the descriptors of size, location, duration, and force. The *size* of the PMI is normally ≤2 cm in diameter; the *location* of the PMI is normally in, or slightly medial to, the left midclavicular line,* fifth intercostal interspace. The duration and force is normally a simple up and down. A concurrent **tap or lift** palpable at the left parasternal border at the third, fourth, and fifth interspace is consistent with hypertrophy of the right ventricle. **Left ventricular enlargement** manifests with a PMI that is >2 cm in diameter, i.e., enlarged and laterally and inferiorly displaced. The left ventricular enlargement may be caused by ventricular hypertrophy or dilatation. The company that hypertrophy keeps includes a strong forceful impulse and a palpable S_4 gallop in late diastole. The company that dilation keeps includes a soft and sluggish impulse with a palpable S_3 gallop.

Tietze's syndrome manifests with discrete tenderness at one or more costochondral joints. This is due to either trauma-related or idiopathic inflammation of the costochondral junctions. **Rib fracture** manifests with severe tenderness and palpable swelling at the site of fracture. There is concurrent splinting to inspiration, ecchymosis, a crunchy sensation palpable over the affected area. The examiner must be aware of the potential for a concurrent pneumothorax. Recall the manifestations of a **severe pneumothorax** include tympany to percussion, diminished breath sounds of the affected side, and deviation of the trachea *to* the side contralateral to the fracture. A **grade 4, 5, or 6 murmur** manifests with a thrill, the vibratory component of a murmur. It is important to palpate the precordium because a **thrill** defines a 4, 5, or 6 murmur and, thus, allows the examiner to auscult and grade **(Table 4.3)** with the fingers. A thrill almost always indicates significant mischief. Finally, the site of the thrill is the location that the murmur is indeed loudest. Some authors, teachers, and students, including Cabot and ourselves, have suggested that an appropriate metaphor for a thrill is the purring of a cat.

Palpation of the pulses, especially the central pulses, is of great clinical and diagnostic importance. Although this is one of the most important aspects of the physical examination in Tibetan and Nepali medicine, it is also of significant importance in the West. Palpation of the pulses should be performed on the carotid, the radial, femoral, dorsalis pedis, and posterior tibialis arteries. The pulses are best palpated by knowing the surface anatomy and placing the palmar aspects of the tips of digits 2 and 3 over the specific site **(Fig. 4.4)**. The sites for each pulse are **carotid**, deep to the sternocleidomastoid muscle in the angle formed by the sternocleidomastoid muscle and the mandible. The **radial artery** is on the radial, palmar side of the wrist, immediately palmar to the first extensor compartment of the wrist (Fig. 10.1). The **femoral artery** is under the inguinal ligament, midway between the anterior superior iliac spine (ASIS) and the pubis symphysis (Fig. 12.1). The **dorsalis pedis pulse** is on the dorsum of the foot, in the interspace between toes 1 and 2, overlying the metatarsals (Fig. 13.2). The **posterior tibialis pulse** is located posterior to the medial malleolus in the ankle (Fig. 13.3).

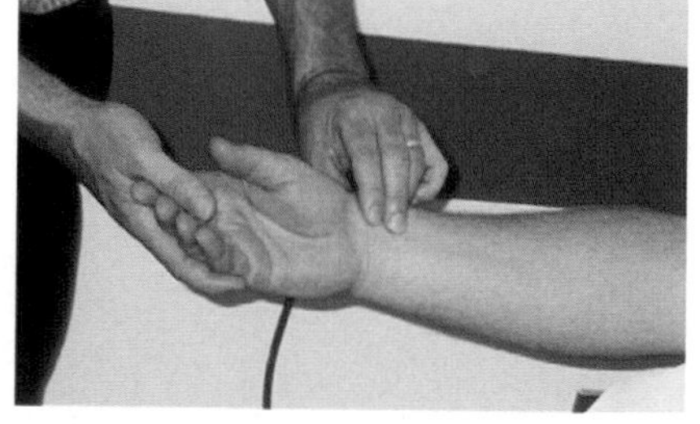

Figure 4.4.

Technique for pulse palpation. Use the palmar fingertips.

TIPS

- Gently apply the palmar sides of digits 2 and 3 to the site
- The most important aspect is knowing the surface anatomy

The pulses are described in terms of intensity and contour. The **scale** used for intensity is 0, not perceptible; 1+, palpable but barely; 2+, easily palpated; 3+, strong; and 4+, hyperdynamic. Contour is the width and height of the waveform as detected by the examiner when feeling the *central* pulse wave. The contour must be measured using a central pulse, i.e., the carotid, femoral, or brachial pulse. The classic arterial pulse wave contours are the ones demonstrated in **Table 4.1**. Normal pulse wave contour is **dicrotic**, i.e., a systolic primary wave and a normally nonpalpable diastolic wave. Only the primary wave is normally palpable. Abnormal pulse contours include bounding

* The left midclavicular line was called the mammillary line by DaCosta in 1909.

TEACHING POINTS

PALPATION OF THE PRECORDIUM AND PULSES

1. Pulsations in the precordium include the point or maximal impulse, a heave, a thrill, and the right ventricular impulse.
2. The rate and rhythm of the pulse is best determined at any site.
3. The contour of the pulse is best palpated and defined at the central sites: carotid, brachial, and femoral arteries.
4. Double pulses include pulsus biferiens, bifid pulse, and pulsus alternans.
5. Bifid pulse is a spike and dome contour in hypertrophic obstructive cardiomyopathy (HOCUM).
6. Pulsus biferiens is a double pulse in aortic insufficiency.
7. Aortic insufficiency has pulsus biferiens and a waterhammer pulse.
8. A tap or lift palpable at the left parasternal border at the third, fourth, and fifth interspace is consistent with hypertrophy of the right ventricle.

pulse, also known as Corrigan's or Waterhammer pulse, pulsus alternans, and pulsus parvus et tardus. **Pulsus bisferiens** manifests with two high-amplitude, quick upstroke and downstroke pulse waves; both beats are in systole. This is usually caused by aortic regurgitation. **Waterhammer pulse**, first described by Corrigan, has a bounding, hyperdynamic pulse contour to all of the pulses palpable. This is especially evident in central sites, i.e., carotid or femoral arteries, but also is easily palpable at the radial pulse site. There is a narrow, staccato-type high-intensity wave that is caused by a markedly increased pulse pressure as the result of aortic insufficiency or profound anemia. **Aortic regurgitation** manifests with an increased pulse pressure—pulsus bisferiens that is a double pulse and a diastolic murmur at the base. The

Table 4.1. Pulse Wave Contours

Diagnosis	Description	Company it Keeps
Aortic insufficiency	Bounding Waterhammer Pulsus biferiens	Increased pulse pressure Diastolic murmur at base
Systolic heart failure	Pulsus alternans	Bradycardia One pulse for every two ausculted beats
Aortic stenosis	Pulsus parvus et tardus	Decreased pulse pressure Systolic murmur at base Dynamic PMI; Brachioradial delay
HOCUM	Bifid pulse	Systolic murmur left upper sternal border
Pulsus biferiens	Two high amplitude Quick upstroke and downstroke	Diastolic murmur at base
Bifid pulse	Spike and dome configuration	HOCUM Systolic murmur loudest at base

HOCUM = hypertrophic obstructive cardiomyopathy; PMI = point of maximal impulse.

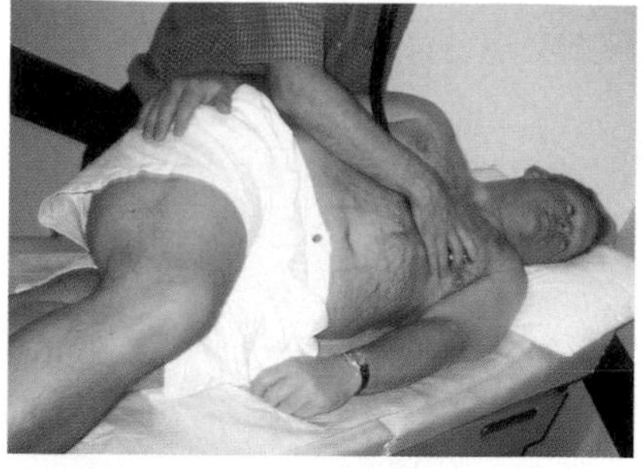

A

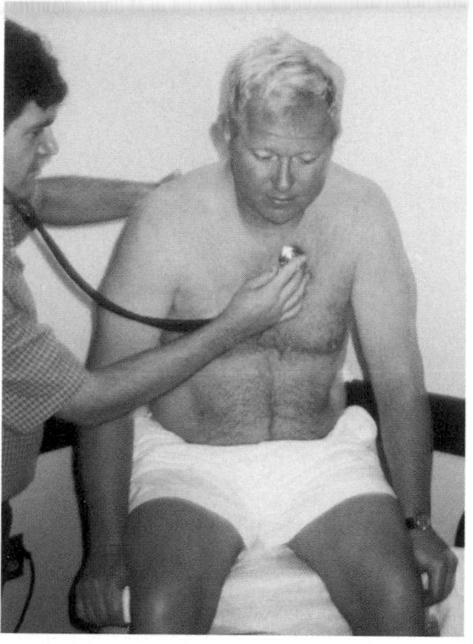

B

Figure 4.5.

Position for auscultation. **A.** Left lateral decubitus. **B.** Upright.

TIPS

- Listen with the diaphragm
- Upright: three sites
- Left lateral decubital: five sites
- Then listen with the bell

pulse wave is a waterhammer type. **Pulsus alternans** is described as a pulse palpable with one beat alternating with an absent pulse with the next beat. This requires the examiner to auscultate the heart and concurrently palpate the pulse. Pulsus alternans is caused by severe systolic heart failure. **Pulsus parvus et tardus** manifests with a low, prolonged, sluggish-type pulse wave. This is caused by decreased systolic blood pressure, with a markedly decreased pulse pressure as the result of aortic stenosis. **Aortic stenosis** manifests with pulsus parvus et tardus, which is a wave that is slow and low. In young healthy individuals, this is an excellent marker for aortic stenosis; in older individuals with significant atherosclerotic disease, this is often falsely negative. The company aortic stenosis keeps includes brachioradial delay. This is a delay in the pulse that occurs between the brachial and the radial site. To perform this procedure, concurrently palpate the brachial and the radial pulse (Fig. 4.8). Normally, the pulses are synchronous; in aortic stenosis, a perceptible delay in the pulse occurs at the radial site relative to the brachial site. **Bifid pulse** manifests with two palpable pulses for each cardiac beat in which there is a spike and dome contour. The spike is rapid early systolic emptying, followed by another slower phase of systolic emptying in a dome pattern of output. This is most often caused by severe **hypertrophic obstructive cardiomyopathy (HOCUM)**. With this there is a concurrent systolic murmur at the left parasternal area. HOCUM manifests with a double or treble apical pulse wave at the apex. According to Sapira in his classic 1990 textbook, 17 of 24 patients with subaortic stenosis (HOCUM) have not only a bifid but even a treble impulse. One of the pulsations is in late diastole, and correlates with an S_4, and the other two are systolic contractions. Bifid pulses also occur in bundle branch block. **Coarctation of the aorta** manifests with delay of the femoral pulse relative to the radial. The company coarctation keeps includes clubbing. Clubbing of the lower extremities and, potentially the left fingers, but not in the right hand.

Auscultation of the Heart (Fig. 4.5)

Recall, the **upright position** brings the base of the heart closer to the chest and, thus, facilitates examination of the structures at the base, which include the aortic and the pulmonic valve. The **supine position** is a neutral position that is adequate for chest wall inspection, but is not the best for any specific site. The **left lateral decubital position** is one in which the patient is rolled

Table 4.2. Cardiac Auscultatory Sounds

Sound	Features	Notes
S_1	Loudest at apex	Mitral and tricuspid
S_2	Loudest at base	Aortic and pulmonic valves Splitting of S_2
Murmur	Turbulent sound	If loud, may have a thrill May be normal In systole, often is normal In diastole, virtually always abnormal
Gallops	Extremely difficult to hear Very low frequency	S_3: mid-diastole S_4: end–diastole
Rub	Creaking, squeaky Three components	Pleuritic-type chest pain relieved with sitting forward

onto the left side, approximately 20 degrees. This brings the apex of the heart closer to the chest wall and, thus, facilitates examination of the apex. While the patient breathes normally, auscult using the diaphragm at least five sites in the left lateral decubital position and at least three sites in the upright position. The five sites include the left apex, the right apex, the left side of base, the right side of base, and the left parasternal area (Fig. 4.1). The three sites in the upright position include the left base, the right base, and the apex. Then, in the left lateral decubitus position, use the bell to auscult at the apex. The bell is not covered with a membrane and is best for low frequency sounds.

Normal findings include the first heart tone also known as S_1, which is loudest at the apex and represents the mitral and the tricuspid valves; the second heart tone, known as S_2, is loudest at the base and represents the aortic and pulmonic valves. The mitral area is at or immediately medial to the apex; the tricuspid area is in the fifth intercostal space on the left parasternal border; the pulmonic area is the second intercostal space at the left sternal border; and the aortic area is the right second intercostal space at the right sternal border (Figs. 4.1 and 4.6). The various findings on auscultation include those listed in **Table 4.2**. **Murmurs** manifest with sounds that represent turbulent flow through or about a valve, which may be caused by valve mischief, hyperdynamic state, or profound anemia. Many, if not most, systolic murmurs are benign whereas most, if not all, diastolic murmurs are caused by an underlying pathology. The grading system for murmurs is on a 1 to 6 scale. This is best described in **Table 4.3**. **Gallops** manifest with sounds that are extremely difficult to hear as they are of very low frequency. Sapira compares them with the "grunt of an old man." They are always in diastole: the S_3 in mid-diastole, the S_4 in late diastole. These are best heard with the patient in the left lateral decubitus position and auscultating with the bell of the stethoscope lightly applied to the chest. S_3 usually results from a systolic ventricular problem, and S_4 from a diastolic ventricular problem. A **rub** manifests with a creaking, squeaky rough noise that often has three components. It is caused by inflammation of the pericardium. Sapira has likened a rub to a rhonchus that is in rhythm with

TEACHING POINTS

CARDIAC EXAMINATION

1. Always examine the heart with the patient positioned in the left lateral decubital position and then in the upright position.
2. There are five sites for the left lateral decubital position; three sites for the upright position.
3. Gallops are always best heard with the stethoscope bell.
4. Atrial fibrillation with a lack of an atrial contraction makes an S_4 impossible, thus any gallop in atrial fibrillation must be an S_3.
5. Auscultation requires role models and practice, practice, practice.
6. Some of the newer standardized teaching models, for example, Harvey, are excellent in reinforcing the techniques and even some of the findings. The true and best method to learn and teach is with a patient at the BEDSIDE.

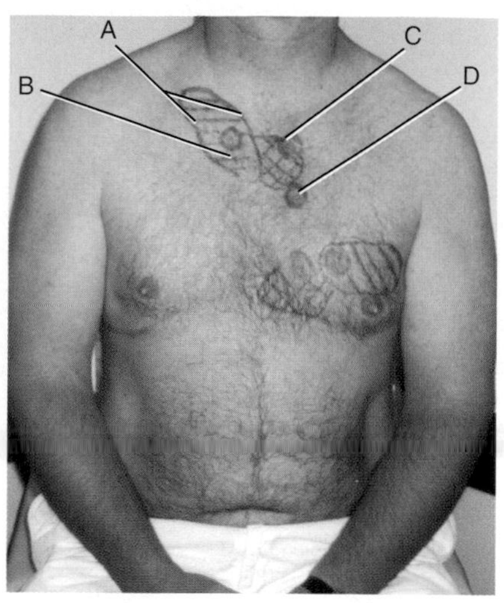

Figure 4.6.

Location (*red*) and radiation (*blue*) of systolic murmurs at base. **A.** Aortic stenosis. **B.** Aortic sclerosis. **C.** Hypertrophic obstructive cardiomyopathy (HOCUM). **D.** Pulmonic stenosis.

TIPS

- Aortic stenosis radiates into the right upper sternal border and neck
- Aortic sclerosis: minimal radiation
- Pulmonic stenosis radiates into the left upper sternal border

Box 4.3.

Entities that cause murmurs at base, systole

1. Aortic stenosis
2. Aortic sclerosis
3. Hypertrophic obstructive cardiomyopathy (HOCUM)
4. Pulmonic stenosis

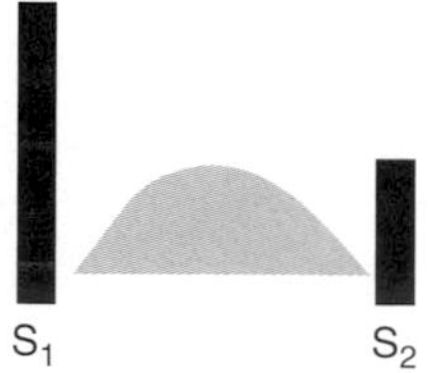

Figure 4.7.

Features of murmur of aortic stenosis. Note diminished S_2.

Table 4.3. Grading System for Murmurs

Grade	Palpation	Auscultation
Grade 1	No finding	Softer than sounds of S_1/S_2
Grade 2	No finding	Same as sounds of S_1/S_2
Grade 3	No finding	Louder than sounds of S_1/S_2
Grade 4	Thrill	Louder than sounds of S_1/S_2
Grade 5	Thrill	Heard with stethoscope Half off area
Grade 6	Thrill	Heard without stethoscope

This is our modification of the system described by Freeman and Levine in 1933 and Levine and Harvey in 1949.

the heart; we think of it as a creaky sensation as when sitting on a rich leather couch. Spodick relates that 85% of rubs are best auscultated over the left sternal border. Rubs can occur in pericarditis or in pleuropericarditis.

CARDIAC EXAMINATION

All murmurs are defined by the ausculatory features and also by related disorders. The **auscultatory features** include descriptions of S_1 and S_2; any concurrent gallops; the timing of the murmur in systole or diastole (or both); the quality of the murmur and where it is loudest; the intensity of the murmur using the 1 to 6 grading system (Table 4.3); and any radiation of the murmur. After this, maneuvers are used to further define and delineate the murmur. In addition other features must be assessed. These include inspection of the chest, assessment of the central and peripheral pulses and their contours, blood pressure and pulse pressure, and jugular venous pulsations, and palpation of the precordium and cardiac apex.

Systolic Murmurs and Sounds (Please see Box 4.3 for entities at base)

Aortic stenosis manifests with the patient having minimal complaints and symptoms, when mild. However, with moderate to severe aortic stenosis, there is exercise-related dyspnea, the onset of syncope, angina, the development of orthopnea, and paroxysmal nocturnal dyspnea (PND) as the result of heart failure.

Table 4.4. Evidence Basis for Maneuvers to Define HOCUM

Manuever	Outcome	Study	Sensitivity (%)	Specificity (%)
Valsalva's	Murmur increased in intensity and duration prolonged	Lembo	65	96
Squat to stand	Murmur increased	Lembo	95	84
Stand to squat	Murmur decreased	Lembo Sapira	95 89	85
Passive leg elevation	Murmur decreased	Lembo	85	91
Active handgrip	Murmur decreased	Lembo	85	75

HOCUM = hypertrophic obstructive cardiomyopathy.

On **auscultation**, S_1 is normal to soft but S_2 is difficult to auscultate, as it often becomes a part of the murmur contour itself. The presence of a gallop is not uncommon: S_4 when left ventricular hypertrophy develops, S_3 when left ventricular dilation develops. The **timing** of the murmur is in midsystole; it is a crescendo–decrescendo, sometimes called a diamond-shaped murmur, that peaks in midsystole **(Fig. 4.7)**. The **location** of the murmur is loudest at the base; however, as demonstrated by Duthie and Tresch, in the older population the murmur may actually be loudest at the left parasternal area or even the apex. In addition, the Gallavardin phenomenon is found in certain cases of aortic stenosis. In this phenomenon, the murmur, which is indeed at the base, can also be auscultated at the apex and sounds are more musical over the apex so as to imitate mitral regurgitation. This was first described by Gallavardin and Ravault in 1925. The **quality** of the murmur is harsh and tearing. The **intensity** of the murmur is any level from grade 1 to grade 6. A murmur that is loud and is now softer usually is a harbinger of malignant outcome. As the stenosis worsens, flow diminishes to the murmur decreased in intensity. This was first written extensively by Cabot at the turn of the last century and remains an important prognostic factor to this day. The murmur often **radiates** into the right neck, especially the right infraclavicular area (Fig. 4.6A).

The company aortic stenosis keeps includes, being on **inspection**, the PMI being often visible and laterally displaced as the left ventricle is hypertrophic and hyperdynamic. The **pulse** in mild aortic stenosis is normal, whereas, when stenosis is moderate to severe, the **pulse contour** becomes low and late. This contour, which is called *pulsus parvus et tardus* (Table 4.1), is best palpated in central arteries, including the carotid, brachial, and femoral. Furthermore, pulse is often delayed when assessed by the **brachioradial delay maneuver (Fig. 4.8)**. In this maneuver, the examiner concurrently palpates the brachial and the radial pulse. In the normal setting, they are synchronous; in severe aortic stenosis, the radial pulse is delayed relative to the brachial. This is a powerful, yet undertaught, feature of severe or critical aortic stenosis. **Blood pressure** is remarkable in that the systolic rarely exceeds 200 mm Hg and there is a decreased pulse pressure. In point of fact the pulse pressure rarely is >40 mm Hg. The **JVP examination** reveals an increase in size, or "giant", ***a*** wave because left ventricular hypertrophy (LVH) is causing the septum to bulge to the right. On **palpation** of the precordium, there is often a left parasternal heave, which is caused by LVH and a palpable thrill over the base. The thrill like the murmur radiates from the mid-heart to the right clavicle, i.e., in the direction of the stenotic flow (Fig. 4.6A). Recall, a thrill indicates the presence of a grade 4, 5, or 6 murmur. The **PMI** in mild stenosis is normal; in moderate to severe disease, it is dynamic, sustained, and laterally displaced. A rule to know, use, and teach is that a combination of weak peripheral pulse with a hyperdynamic apex is consistent with aortic stenosis. Aortic stenosis is caused by rheumatic disease, bicuspid aortic valve, and endocarditis. If the stenosis is caused by a bicuspid aortic valve, one or more ejection sounds will be present in early systole. Please refer to **Table 4.5** for evidence basis for aortic stenosis. Overall, the features of aortic stenosis that are present irrespective of age are the absence of a diminished S_2 and a harsh quality of the murmur.

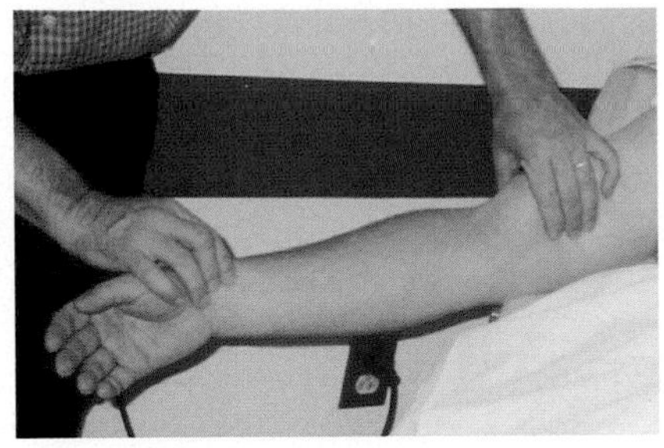

Figure 4.8.

Technique for brachioradial delay for severe aortic stenosis. Concurrent palpation of a central and peripheral pulse.

TIPS

- Concurrently palpate the brachial and the radial pulse
- Normal setting: they are synchronous
- Severe aortic stenosis: radial pulse is delayed relative to the brachial pulse
- This is a powerful, yet *undertaught*, feature of severe or critical aortic stenosis

Box 4.4.

Features of a flow murmur in systole at base—BENIGN features

1. Peaks in early to midsystole
2. Does not involve or diminish S_2
3. Never has thrill, usually grade 2 or 1

Table 4.5. Evidence Basis for Maneuvers for Aortic Stenosis

Manuever	Outcome	Study	Sens	Spec	Pos LR	Neg LR	Kappa
Auscultate at base	Systolic murmur at right upper sternal border	Etchell	100	64	2.6	0	0.45
		Aronow					
		Mild	95				
		Moderate	100				
		Severe	100				
Right infraclavicular	Radiation	Etchell	93	69	3.6	0.10	0.36
Right carotid	Radiation	Etchell	70	91	8.1	0.29	
Carotid volume	Diminished	Etchell	53	93	2.0	0.64	0.24
S_2	Diminished	Etchell	52	93	7.5	0.5	0.54
	Diminished	Aronow					
		Mild	5				
		Moderate	49				
		Severe	74				
Carotid upstroke	Slow	Etchell	47	95	9.2	0.56	0.26
	Slow	Aronow					
		Mild	3				
		Moderate	33				
		Severe	53				

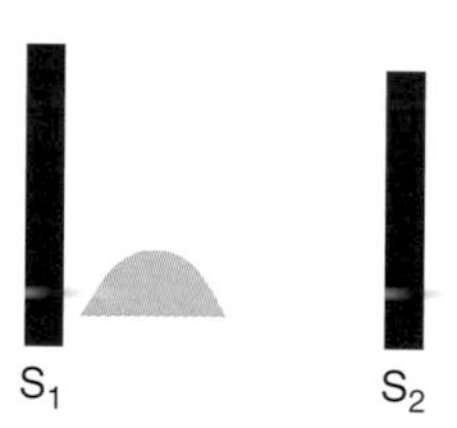

Figure 4.9.

Features of the murmur of aortic sclerosis. Early in cycle, no diminished S_2.

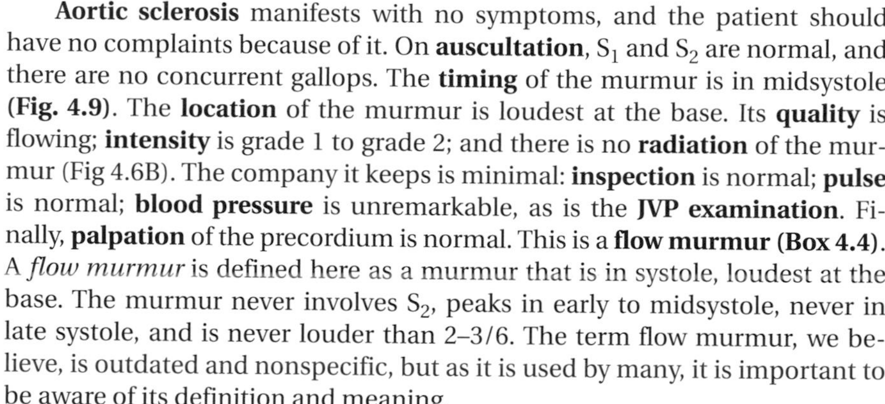

Aortic sclerosis manifests with no symptoms, and the patient should have no complaints because of it. On **auscultation**, S_1 and S_2 are normal, and there are no concurrent gallops. The **timing** of the murmur is in midsystole **(Fig. 4.9)**. The **location** of the murmur is loudest at the base. Its **quality** is flowing; **intensity** is grade 1 to grade 2; and there is no **radiation** of the murmur (Fig 4.6B). The company it keeps is minimal: **inspection** is normal; **pulse** is normal; **blood pressure** is unremarkable, as is the **JVP examination**. Finally, **palpation** of the precordium is normal. This is a **flow murmur (Box 4.4)**. A *flow murmur* is defined here as a murmur that is in systole, loudest at the base. The murmur never involves S_2, peaks in early to midsystole, never in late systole, and is never louder than 2–3/6. The term flow murmur, we believe, is outdated and nonspecific, but as it is used by many, it is important to be aware of its definition and meaning.

Hypertrophic obstructive cardiomyopathy (HOCUM)* manifests with minimal symptoms until advanced or if concurrent problems are present or

*IHSS: Idiopathic hypertrophic subaortic stenosis–old term for HOCUM

Table 4.6. Types of S_2 Splitting

Type	Description	Company it Keeps
Physiologic	With inspiration P_2 is significantly after A_2, i.e., split S_2 With expiration P_2 and A_2 merge into one sound, i.e., not split	Normal
Fixed	Inspiration and expiration P_2 after A_2 with same interval, i.e., split S_2	Right BBB Pulmonary HTN PTE
Paradoxic	A_2 after P_2, i.e., split S_2	Left BBB Aortic stenosis

BBB = bundle branch block; HTN = hypertension; PTE = pulmonary thromboembolism.

Figure 4.10.

Features of the murmur of HOCUM.

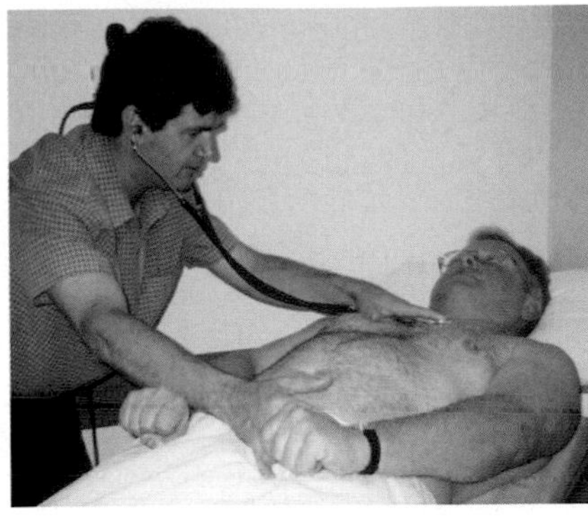

Figure 4.11.

Technique to perform a handgrip maneuver for hypertrophic obstructive cardiomyopathy (HOCUM).

 **TIPS**

- Auscultate over the base, left side, while instructing patient to actively and forcefully clench fists for 30 seconds
- Hypertrophic obstructive cardiomyopathy (HOCUM): the murmur decreases in intensity because of the increase in systemic vascular resistance
- Increases afterload

have developed. When symptomatic, there is dyspnea, which is caused by elevated left ventricular filling pressures; angina pectoris, because of increased demand from increased heart muscle and compression of the arteries from the increased venticular mass; or syncope, which is caused by cerebral hypoperfusion or dysrhythmia.

On **auscultation**, S_1 is normal, S_2 is usually normal but, in severe cases, there may be a fixed or paradoxic split of S_2 **(Table 4.6)**. Often, an S_4 develops in cases of left ventricular hypertrophy and an S_3 may be present even in the setting of normal left ventricular function because of increased inflow of blood into the left ventricle in early diastole. The **timing** of the murmur is in midsystole, but can change over time **(Fig. 4.10)**. The **location** of the murmur is loudest at the base and left upper sternal border (Fig 4.6C). Its **quality** is harsh and **intensity** is any level from grade 1 to grade 6. The murmur can **radiate** into the neck (Fig. 4.6C), but rarely does so with the effect of aortic stenosis. Unlike aortic stenosis, there are never any systolic clicks. **Handgrip maneuver** decreases the intensity of the murmur **(Fig. 4.11)**. For this maneuver, auscultate over the base, left side, while instructing the patient to actively and forcefully clench the fists for 30 seconds. In HOCUM, the murmur decreases in intensity because of the increase in systemic vascular resistance. Furthermore, **Valsalva's maneuver** increases in intensity and lengthens the duration of the HOCUM murmur. For this maneuver, auscultate over the left sternal base while the patient performs a Valsalva's maneuver. An excellent method to make certain the patient is performing this maneuver is to take a sphygnomamometer, inflate it and place it on the abdomen of a patient, and instruct the patient to press his abdomen against it **(Fig. 4.12)**. Please refer to Table 4.4 for the evidence to support these maneuvers.

The company it keeps: on **inspection** the PMI is often visible as the left ventricle is hypertrophic and hyperdynamic; **pulse** is mild in HOCUM and is normal to forceful; when HOCUM is moderate to severe, the **pulse contour** becomes double or bifid (Table 4.1). This bifid pulse is best felt in central arteries and has a spike and dome pattern. The **blood pressure** is unremarkable as is the pulse pressure. The **JVP examination** reveals an increased size ("giant") *a* waves because the LVH is causing the septum to bulge to the right. On **palpation** of the precordium, there is left parasternal heave caused by LVH, and a thrill over the left base because of the murmur. The thrill radiates from the mid heart to the right clavicle, i.e., in the direction of the obstructed flow (Fig. 4.6C). Recall, a thrill indicates a grade 4, 5, or 6 murmur. The **PMI** in mild HOCUM is normal, but in moderate to severe disease, it is dynamic, sustained, laterally displaced, and double or even triple in contour. This triple contour is caused by an S_4 and two different contractions of the ventricle. HOCUM is caused by a hereditary syndrome that is not uncommon and may not manifest until after middle age.

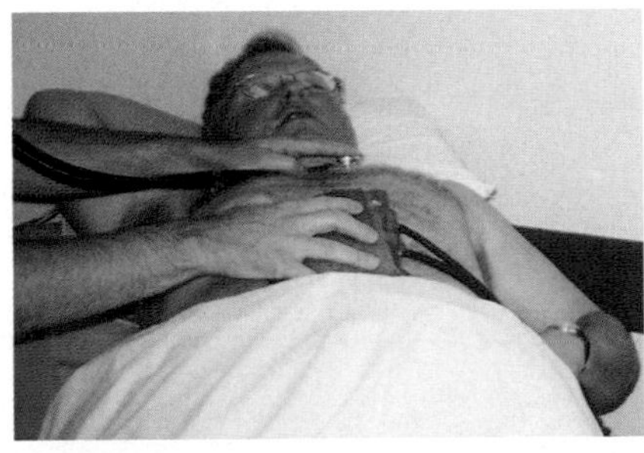

Figure 4.12.

Technique to perform a Valsalva's maneuver for hypertrophic obstructive cardiomyopathy (HOCUM).

 **TIPS**

- Auscultate over the left sternal base while the patient performs Valsalva's maneuver
- An excellent method to make certain patient is performing a Valsalva's maneuver is to take a sphygmotonometer, inflate it, and place it on the abdomen of a patient in left lateral decubital position and instruct the patient to press abdomen against it
- Hypertrophic obstructive cardiomyopathy (HOCUM): increase in intensity and lengthen the duration

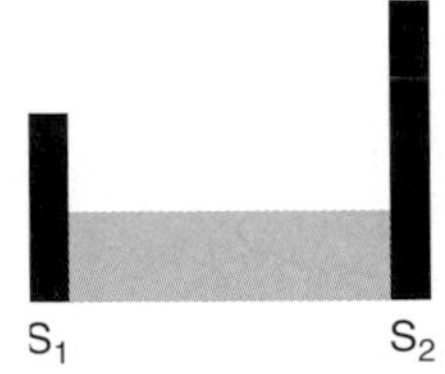

Figure 4.13.

Features of the murmur of mitral regurgitation.

Box 4.5.

Systolic murmurs at apex

1. Mitral regurgitation
2. Mitral valve prolapse
3. Tricuspid regurgitation
4. Ventricular septal defect
5. Aortic stenosis (in the elderly)

Mitral regurgitation manifests with the patient relating complaints only late in the course of disease. Those complaints include dyspnea on exertion, increased fatigue, orthopnea, and PND. Please refer to Box 4.5 for systolic murmur at apex.

On **auscultation**, S_1 is normal to soft, S_2 is normal to soft; P_2 can be accentuated if pulmonary hypertension has developed. An S_3 can develop in severe mitral regurgitation because of increased inflow of blood into the left ventricle in early diastole. No S_4 develops that is specific to mitral regurgitation. The **timing** of the murmur is holosystolic, but can be early, mid, or late systolic **(Fig. 4.13)**. The **location** of the murmur is loudest at the apex **(Box 4.5)**. The **quality** of the murmur is musical, "kazoolike"; its **intensity** is any level from grade 1 to grade 6. It is plateau-shaped and, thus, has no specific peak. The murmur can **radiate** into the left axilla (Fig. 4.16A) and even into the left scapular, rhomboid area **(Fig. 4.14)**. The murmur is not accentuated by any of the maneuvers that accentuate tricuspid regurgitation. Murmur-specific maneuvers include **transient arterial occlusion**, as described by Lembo (see aortic insufficiency, discussed below) in which the murmur increases in intensity. This has a sensitivity of 80%. In addition, **squatting** will also increase the murmur of mitral regurgitation (Fig. 4.17).

The company mitral regurgitation keeps includes: on **inspection** there are few if any remarkable findings. The **pulse** is normal to low, the **rhythm** may become irregularly irregular if atrial fibrillation develops; the **pulse contour** has a pseudocollapsing aspect to it. The **blood pressure** is unremarkable, as is the pulse pressure. The **JVP examination** reveals an increase if right ventricular failure has developed. On **palpation** of the precordium, finding is normal until advanced disease is present, at which time a thrill is heard over the apex that radiates into the axilla. Mitral regurgitation is caused by endocarditis, myocardial infarction, or mitral valve prolapse (MVP) that worsens.

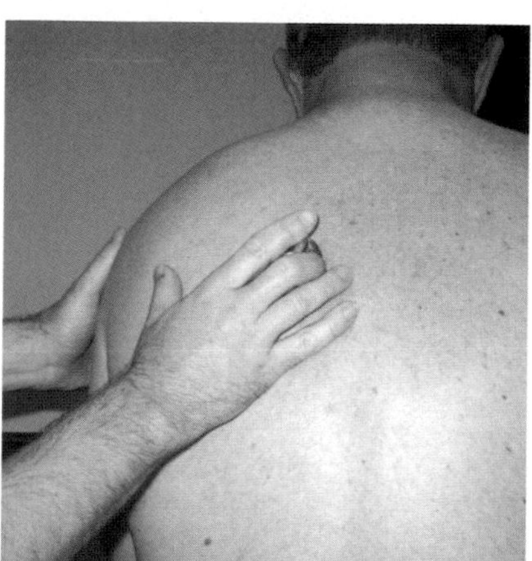

Figure 4.14.

Location for auscultation for mitral regurgitation radiation into the left rhomboid area. This is also location for Ewart's sign of pericardial effusion.

TIPS

- Patient sitting up and leaning forward, auscultate over the left rhomboid
- Mitral regurgitation: may radiate here
- Any other entity: minimal radiation here

Mitral valve prolapse (MVP) manifests with the patient relating few, if any, complaints. The patient may have atypical-type chest pain, but this is a loose association. If MVP progresses to mitral regurgitation, the symptoms of dyspnea on exertion and orthopnea will develop.

On **auscultation**, S_1 is normal to soft, S_2 is normal to soft, and P_2 may be accentuated if pulmonary hypertension is present. An S_3 can develop if mitral regurgitation has developed. The **timing** of the murmur itself is early, mid, or late systolic or, if mitral regurgitation has developed, holosystolic. One or, rarely, more than one midsystolic click is present **(Fig. 4.15)**. High-pitched and loud, these clicks are generated by the prolapse of the mitral valve leaflets into the left atrium. The **location** of the murmur and click are loudest at the apex. Its **intensity** is usually grade 1 to grade 3, but quite variable. It is plateau-shaped and, thus, has no specific peak. The murmur often **radiates** into the left axilla **(Fig. 4.16A)**. **Squatting maneuver** while auscultating over the apex moves the click of MVP closer to P_2 and, in point of fact, decreases the murmur **(Fig. 4.17)**. This is caused by an increase in afterload and preload and, thus, increases the left ventricular diameter and prevents the leaflet from prolapsing. Furthermore, **Valsalva's maneuver** in which the examiner auscultates over the apex while the patient performs the maneuver. See description of technique, page 87. The click is earlier and the murmur is longer and louder during the Valsalva's maneuver. Finally, **standing** increases the intensity of the murmur and according to Sapira accentuates the click in 74% of cases of MVP due to decreased ventricular filling.

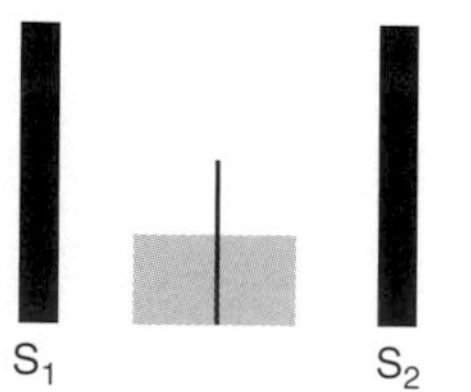

Figure 4.15.

Features of the murmur and midsystolic click of mitral valve *prolapse*.

The company it keeps includes **inspection**, few notable findings. The **pulse wave** is normal, unless mitral regurgitation has developed. The **blood pressure** has no characteristic findings; the **PMI** is normal unless advanced mitral regurgitation has developed, then it is laterally and inferiorly displaced and enlarged. The **JVP** is also unremarkable. The **precordium** is unremarkable, unless mitral regurgitation develops, then there may be a thrill over the apex that radiates into the axilla. Mitral valve prolapse is usually due to congenital degeneration of the posterior mitral valve leaflet.

Tricuspid regurgitation (TR) manifests with the patient stating very few complaints until the lesion is advanced, at which time the features of frank right ventricular failure are noted.

On **auscultation**, S_1 is normal to soft, S_2 is normal, P_2 may be accentuated if and when pulmonary hypertension is present. A right-sided S_3 can develop in severe tricuspid regurgitation because of increased inflow of blood into the right ventricle in early diastole. No S_4 develops related specifically to mitral regurgitation. The **timing** of the murmur itself is holosystolic **Fig. 4.18**. The **location** is in epigastrium or, if the right ventricle is markedly enlarged, it posteriorly displaces the left ventricle and thus tricuspid regurgitation is loudest at the PMI apex. The one best site to auscult for TR is the left sternal border in the fifth intercostal space. The **intensity** of the murmur is usually grade 1 to grade 4. It is plateau-shaped and, thus, has no specific peak. The murmur often **radiates** into the epigastrium (Fig. 4.16B). It is accentuated, that is, made louder with several specific maneuvers; especially useful are the maneuvers described by Rivero Carvallo and Vitum. The **maneuver of Rivero Carvallo** is one in which, with the patient in the left lateral decubital position, the examiner auscultates over the apex and notes the intensity of the apical systolic murmur. The patient is instructed to inhale deeply; examiner continues to auscultate and notes any change in murmur intensity. Tricuspid regurgitation increases in intensity, whereas mitral regurgitation and MVP are unchanged. The sensitivity of this is 61% in a study by Rothman and 100% in a study by Lembo. The **maneuver of Vitum** is one in which the examiner has the patient in left lateral decubital position, auscultates over the apex, and notes intensity of the murmur. The examiner gently presses on the right upper quadrant of the abdomen, and continues to auscultate and notes any change in murmur intensity. Tricuspid regurgitation increases in intensity, whereas mitral regurgitation and MVP are unchanged. This finding has a sensitivity of 56%. A third maneuver is one in which the examiner has the patient in the left lateral decubital position and **passively raises the legs** of the patient, then continues to auscultate and notes any change in murmur intensity. Tricuspid regurgitation increases in intensity, whereas mitral regurgitation and MVP are unchanged. In each of these maneuvers, the underlying physiology is to increase right volume return to increase intensity of any right-sided entity. Of note, especially in the Rivero Carvallo maneuver, emphasize the auscultation

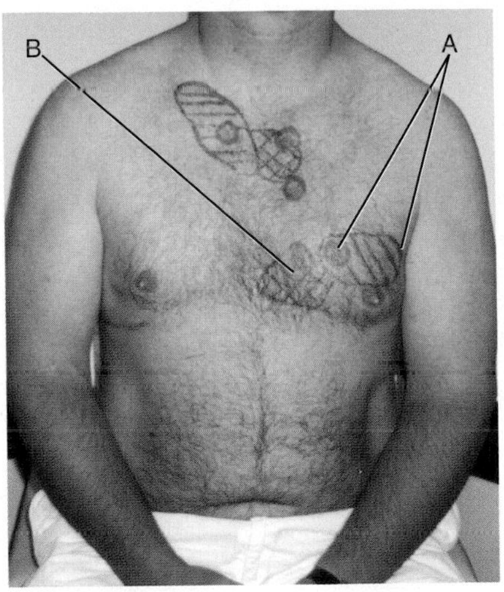

Figure 4.16.

Sites for radiation of systolic murmurs at the apex. **A.** Mitral regurgitation. **B.** Tricuspid regurgitation.

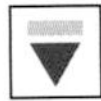

TIPS

- Mitral regurgitation radiates into the axilla
- Tricuspid regurgitation radiates into the epigastrium

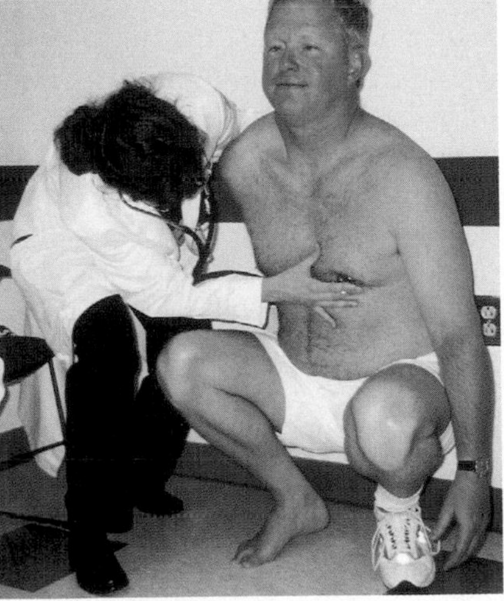

Figure 4.17.

Squatting maneuver to assist in evaluation of mitral valve prolapse (MVP).

TIPS

- Auscultate the apex with the patient squatting
- Mitral valve prolapse: moves the click closer to S_2
- Also useful in aortic regurgitation

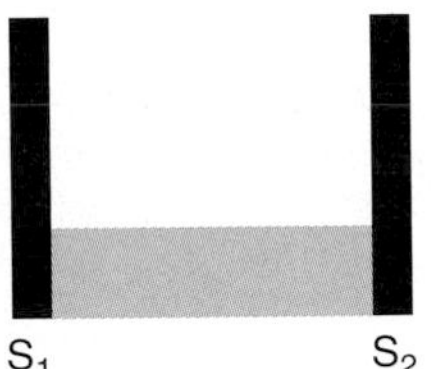

Figure 4.18.

Features of the murmur of tricuspid regurgitation.

Table 4.7. Mitral Versus Tricuspid Regurgitation

Manuever	Mitral regurgitation	Tricuspid regurgitation
Inspiration	Unchanged	Increased
Expiration	Decreased	Unchanged
Elevate legs	Unchanged	Increased
Press on liver	Unchanged	Increased

of the five to eight beats before and during the inhalation, after which, the inhalation will become a Valsalva's maneuver and, when this occurs all bets are off. Because there are several remarkable and positive maneuvers, tricuspid regurgitation is a particularly satisfying diagnosis to teach at the bedside. Please refer to **Table 4.7**.

The company TR keeps includes on **inspection**, few findings except for pitting pedal edema. The **JVP** is elevated with prominent neck veins, elevated to >6 cm, an absent x descent, a pronounced V/CV wave, and a rapid y descent in the neck vein contour. At times, when very advanced, a **winking ear lobe** is noted in which the lobe of the ear wiggles with each heartbeat. Furthermore, there is an abnormal **hepatojugular reflux test**. This test, first described by Pasteur and refined by Rondot, is one in which the patient is in a standard position for inspection of the JVP and neck veins; the examiner applies a hand to the area superior to the umbilicus for >30 seconds. The neck vein meniscus and thus the JVP is observed in the neck. In a healthy individual, there is an increase of <4 cm; in tricuspid regurgitation there is an increase of >4 cm. Maisel and others relate a sensitivity of 66% and a specificity of 100% for this test. The **pulse wave** is normal, **blood pressure** has no characteristic findings, and the PMI is normal. **Palpation** of the precordium is unremarkable early on. In severe tricuspid regurgitation, however, a heave is palpable over the left parasternal or the epigastrium area because of a hyperdynamic and enlarged right ventricle. The enlarged right ventricle pushes the left ventricle posteriorly. It is rare, but in severe tricuspid regurgitation with significant right ventricular hypertrophy, a thrill may be located at the apex. The extracardiac problems that accompany severe tricuspid regurgitation include increased size of the liver, peripheral pitting edema, and ascites. Tricuspid regurgitation is caused by endocarditis, carcinoid syndrome, or ischemic disease.

Other diagnoses with systolic murmurs include **ventricular septal defect**, which manifests with the patient complaining of either mild symptoms or, if it is more significant, dyspnea on exertion, orthopnea, and even PND. There is a direct correlation between the number of symptoms and the flow of blood across the shunt. On auscultation, a systolic murmur is noted at the apex; it radiates throughout the precordium and is often grade 2 to grade 5 in intensity. Murmur-specific maneuvers include **transient arterial occlusion**, as described by Lembo (see aortic insufficiency, discussed below), in which the murmur increases in intensity with a sensitivity of 80% (Lembo). The company VSD keeps includes inspection usually unremarkable unless the patient has developed a shunt that is right to left, i.e., the pressures in the pulmonary bed are so high as to shunt the low O_2 tension blood from the right to the left ventricle. The pulse and blood pressure readings are normal; the PMI is often hyperdynamic, enlarged, and laterally and inferiorly displaced. The precordium has a heave or pulsatile area on the left upper sternal border adjacent to the second intercostal space on the left, which is caused by an enlarged and engorged pulmonary trunk. There is often a thrill from the apex to sternum or sternum to apex, depending on the direction of the shunt. **Pulmonary hypertension** manifests with the patient complaining of no symptoms until moderate to severe pulmonary hypertension occurs. At that point, the patient may develop fatigue and dyspnea on exertion. In severe disease, that is cor pulmonale, there is on inspection, cyanosis and clubbing of the fingernails and toe nails (Figs. 14.3 and 14.4), peripheral pitting edema and ascites. On JVP assessment, large or giant *a* waves are seen. On auscultation, S_1 is normal but S_2 is loud, especially evident in P_2. This accentuation of P_2 is the single best physical finding of this condition. Indeed it may be possible to auscult the splitting of S_2 at the apex; this is a rare finding. Finally, there may be a diastolic murmur at the base due to the secondary formation of pulmonic insufficiency. **Physiologic splitting** of S_2 manifests with no symptoms. A split S_2 is best heard at the base, left upper sternal border, but it is very rare to be heard at the apex. In point of fact, a split S_2 at the apex strongly suggests complications, specifically that of pulmonary hypertension. **Atrial septal defect (ASD)** manifests with the patient complaining of dyspnea and fatigue. Most patients are asymptomatic and ASD is detected only on physical examination or on echocardiogram performed for a different reason. On inspection, there are usually no abnormal findings; however, with a significant right to left shunt, the patient may become cyanotic. The neck veins are usually unremarkable but, if they are elevated, the *a* and the *v* waves are both elevated and equal in height. The pulse contour is usually normal, blood pressure is unremarkable, and the PMI is retracted because the right ventricle is enlarged and, thus, posteriorly displaces the left ventricle. The precordium is hyperdynamic, and there is a prominent left parasternal heave because of the right ventricular hypertrophy. Often, a pulsatile pulmonary trunk is noted in the second intercostal space. The company it keeps is specific to the underlying etiology. **Holt-Oram syndrome** manifests with a hypoplastic or even absent thumb; the arms are underdeveloped; and the patient has a high-arched palate. Other congenital syndromes associated with ASD include Klinefelter's and Ellis-van Creveld syndrome. **Bicuspid aortic valve** manifests with few if any symptoms. Inspection, pulse, blood pressure, PMI, and pericardium are all unremarkable. On auscultation there is a normal S_1 and S_2, with a click at the base early in systole. This entity will often progress to aortic stenosis and/or insufficiency by the patient's fiftieth birthday. Thus, a systolic crescendo–decrescendo murmur with a modified or ablated S_2 should lead to the correct diagnosis of aortic stenosis caused by a congenital bicuspid valve. Bicuspid aortic valve is a common congenital finding. The loss of the early systolic click is a harbinger of stenois development. **Hyperthyroidism** manifests with a systolic sound that Means and Lerman in 1932 described as being between a murmur and a rub. Its timing is in systole, its location is at the base. It is best heard at end expiration. The company it keeps includes tachycardia, tremor, goiter, lid lag, and other classic features of hyperthyroidism. (See Chapter 1, page 29). The sensitivity for this finding is 6% to 12% in the original paper by Means and Lerman. **Mediastinal emphysema** manifests with the patient complaining of an acute onset of left-sided chest pain, which may or may not be pleuritic in nature. This may be spontaneous or after severe vomiting. On auscultation, there is a crackling noise, a crepitus, or rub located in the left chest that is brought on by left lateral decubital position and relieved by assuming a supine or upright position. As the original description was based on seven cases by Dr. Hamman in 1939, the sign is appropriately called "Hamman's crunch." Invariably, crepitus develops in the subcutaneous tissues of the neck. The company it keeps is specific to the underlying cause. If spontaneous, there is shortness of breath; if caused by rupture of the esophagus (Boerhaave's syndrome), antecedent vomiting occurs; or if a recent procedure into the esophagus, tearing chest pain occurs. **Pulmonic stenosis** manifests with a systolic murmur that is virtually identical to aortic stenosis except for location, i.e., at the left second sternal interspace (Fig. 4.6D) and the presence of a

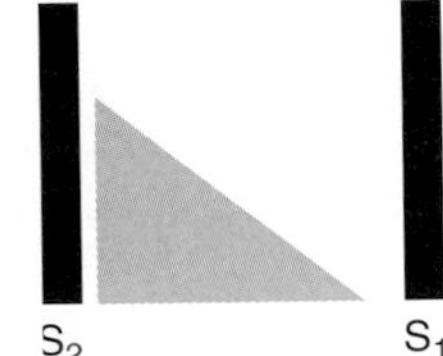

Figure 4.19.

Features of the murmur of aortic insufficiency—a decrescendo, diastolic murmur.

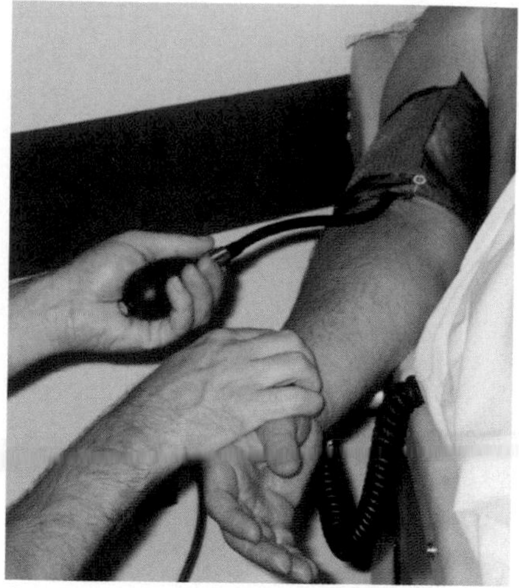

A

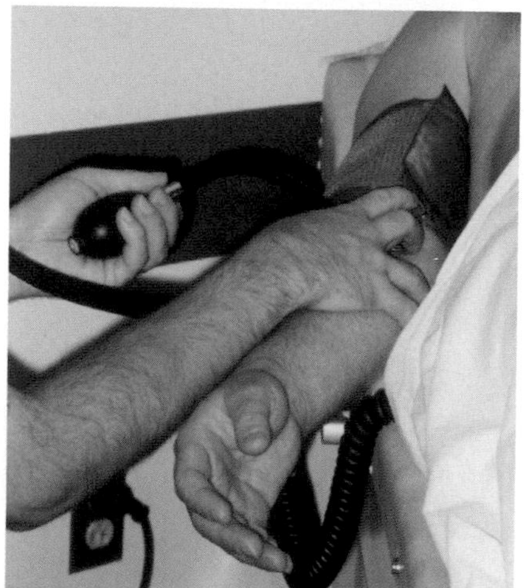

B

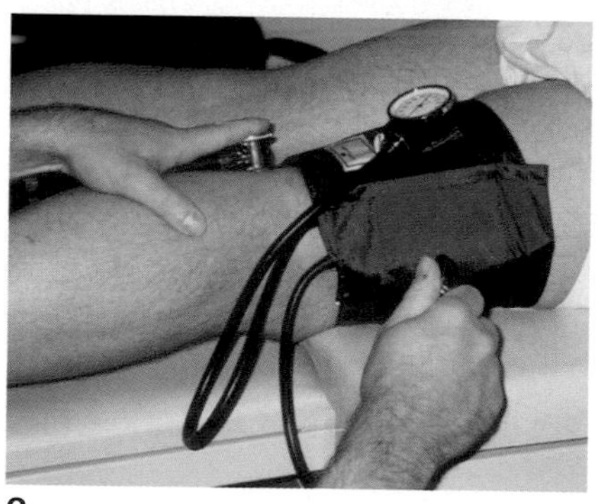

C

Figure 4.20.

Technique to measure arm blood pressure **(A and B)** and thigh blood pressure **(C)**. Here, the right arm and thigh.

TIPS

- Arm blood pressure: sphygnomamometer is placed around the arm
- Auscultate at the antecubital fossa
- Thigh blood pressure: sphygnomamometer is placed around the thigh
- Auscultate at the popliteal fossa

Table 4.8. Evidence Basis for Aortic Insufficiency

Technique	Outcome	Study	Sensitivity (%)
Quincke's	Nail bed pulsation	Tice	90
Hill's	Thigh BP > arm BP		
Durozier's	Diastolic murmur femoral artery	Sapira Tice	58–100 88
Müeller	Pulsation of uvula		
Pulse pressure	Increased		
Corrigan's	Bounding pulse	Tice	95
Transient arterial occlusion	Increases murmur	Lembo	75
Squatting	Increases murmur		

palpable lift at the left parasternal border consistent with a right ventricular enlargement.

Diastolic Murmurs and Sounds (see Table 4.9)

Aortic insufficiency manifests with minimal symptoms early on but, later in the course, there is exertion-related fatigue and dyspnea.

On **auscultation**, there is a normal or soft S_1, a normal to soft S_2; S_3 and S_4 may be present when left ventricular dilation or hypertrophy develops. If the underlying cause is a bicuspid aortic valve, one or more ejection clicks is present in early systole. The **timing** of the murmur itself is early in diastole, beginning immediately after S_2 (**Fig. 4.19**). The **location** is at the base. It is best heard when the patient is sitting upright. In point of fact, a very useful teaching point is that aortic insufficiency may be missed if auscultation is limited to the left lateral decubital position. The **intensity** of the murmur is usually grade 1 to grade 4. The murmur often **radiates** into the left neck. The company aortic insufficiency keeps include that the murmur is accentuated, i.e., is made louder with several specific maneuvers. Especially useful is the maneuver of **transient arterial occlusion** as described by Lembo in 1986. This maneuver consists of placing a sphygmomanometer on each arm and inflating them to exceed the systolic blood pressure by 20 to 40 mm Hg for 20 seconds while auscultating over the base. In aortic insufficiency, the murmur will be increased because of the increase in afterload. This maneuver, according to many authors (including Lembo and Sapira), is the best overall maneuver in the evaluation for aortic insufficiency. Lembo reported a sensitivity of 75% and a positive predictive value of 100% (**Table 4.8**). A further murmur-specific maneuver is **squatting**, which may reveal even a subtle murmur by auscultating the base with the patient squatting (Fig. 4.17). According to Vogelpoel, this is an excellent method to unmask aortic insufficiency and it increases the murmur as the result of an increase in afterload. Finally, often a murmur is best heard at the apex that is in late diastole, and sounds like, but is not, mitral stenosis. This is a specific manifestation of aortic insufficiency caused by a regurgitant jet that keeps the anterior leaflet of the mitral valve modestly closed. This is the "Flint murmur," first described by Dr. Austin Flint.

Table 4.9. Manifestations of Diastolic Extra Sounds

Diagnosis	Diastolic sound description	Company they Keep
Aortic regurgitation	Mid–diastole	Increased pulse pressure Pulsations with Quincke's Bobbing head (deMusset's) Bobbing uvula (Müeller's)
Mitral stenosis	Mid- to late diastole	Rumble plateau fashion Opening snap (OS) Loud S_1 Palpable tapping S_1 at apex ("thumping")
Opening snap	Early diastole	The narrower the distance between P_2 and OS, the more severe the MS (mitral stenosis)
S_3	Early diastole	PMI laterally displaced Orthopnea, PND Bibasilar crackles Systolic heart failure
S_4	Late diastole	PMI laterally displaced Hypertension Basilar crackles Diastolic heart failure
Pericardial rub	Early diastole	Pleuritic type chest pain Pain alleviated by sitting upright
Pericardial knock	Early diastole	Syncope Constrictive pericarditis
Atrial myxoma	Early diastole	Syncope Positional change in plop or in murmur

OS = opening snap; PMI = point of maximal impulse; PND = paroxysmal nocturnal dyspnea.

The company it keeps includes **inspection**, there are bounding visible pulses caused by the high output state. In the setting of severe aortic regurgitation, the head may bob up and down (de Musset's sign) because of the bounding carotid pulses that push the head upward with each systole. The **pulse** is of high volume and has a contour that is rapid ascent and fall of the pulse waveform. The fall is so rapid that it is "collapsing" in contour. The pulse wave is best assessed in the central arteries, e.g., carotid, femoral, and brachial **(Table 4.8)**. This is known as waterhammer pulse contour and was first formally described by the famous Irish professor, Dr. Corrigan, hence the eponym, "Corrigan's pulse." The **blood pressure** (**Fig. 4.20A** and **B**) in severe aortic insufficiency often has a combination of elevated systolic reading, a lowered diastolic reading, and an increase in the pulse pressure. Often, the Korotkoff sounds can be auscultated to 0 in aortic regurgitation. **Blood pressure is measured in the thigh** (Fig. 4.20C), using a thigh cuff and auscultating over the popliteal fossa for Korotkoff sounds. In aortic insufficiency, a difference is seen in systolic blood pressure between that in the arm and thigh that exceeds 20 mm Hg (Hill's sign). The **PMI** is normal early in the course of the disease; later, it is laterally and inferiorly displaced with a forcible and enlarged PMI caused by left ventricular hypertrophy. The precordium is hyperdynamic with a left parasternal heave present. It is rare to feel a diastolic thrill but, if present, it is located at the base and best felt with patient sitting up.

Other findings are almost always related to the increased pulse pressure, including a number of specific maneuvers such as those described by Quincke, Hill, deMusset, Müeller, and Durozier **(Table 4.8)**. **Quincke's maneuver** is performed by placing a sufficiently mild degree of pressure on the distal nail plate on the nailbed to blanch the proximal bed. Normally, the line of demarcation between the pink and white is stable, whereas in aortic insufficiency the line pulsates slightly. This is a highly imperfect finding that, although of clinical diagnostic benefit, may be the least useful classic finding of aortic insufficiency. **Hill's maneuver** is performed by comparing the systolic pressure in the upper extremity (brachial artery) with that in the lower extremity (popliteal artery). Normally, the measured blood pressures are equal; in aortic insufficiency, the blood pressure in the lower extremity is >20 mm Hg. **deMusset's maneuver** is performed by inspecting the patient sitting or standing at baseline. In severe aortic insufficiency, the head bobs with each beat. **Müeller's maneuver** is performed by inspecting the patient's uvula. Normally, the uvula is midline and elevated in midline with AHHHH; in aortic insufficiency, a pulsation occurs with each heartbeat. **Durozier's maneuver** is performed by placing the diaphragm of the stethoscope over the femoral artery. Gradually increase the pressure applied on the artery until the artery is occluded. Early on, a normal systolic murmur occurs; in aortic insufficiency, a diastolic murmur develops two thirds of the way through the application of pressure. Sapira, in 1981, reported that the sensitivity for this maneuver was 58% to 100%. In addition to aortic insufficiency, high-output states, including fever, patent ductus arteriosus (PDA), or hyperthyroidism can cause this finding. Aortic insufficiency is caused by endocarditis, Marfan's syndrome, osteogenesis imperfecta, rheumatoid variants (including Reiter's syndrome), tertiary lues, and a bicuspid aortic valve.

Mitral stenosis manifests with the patient complaining of fatigue and dyspnea on exertion, which over time can become disabling. In addition, the patient often relates palpitations as the result of new onset atrial fibrillation. Finally, the patient may also manifest with orthopnea, PND due to heart failure.

On **auscultation**, the S_1 is very loud, sometimes referred to as "cracking." This is caused by a decrease in diastolic filling due to the stenosis, such that the mitral leaflets do not "float-up" as much as they normally do. Thus, on isometric contraction, the leaflets are further apart and transverse a greater distance in unit time, leading to a louder first sound as the leaflets slam shut. S_2 is normal unless pulmonary hypertension has developed, at which time it is loud because of the marked increase in P_2. An S_3 gallop is present when heart failure develops, it is rare for an S_4 to be present because the patient often develops atrial fibrillation, which precludes an S_4. In addition, there is an **opening snap**, which occurs immediately after P_2. This is as a result of the sudden tensing of the mitral valve leaflets as they initially open rapidly (because of the increased intraarterial pressure) and stop abruptly (because of the stenotic valve). As the valve mobility decreases as the result of worsening stenosis, the opening snap is lost. The shorter the P_2 opening snap interval, the more severe is the stenosis. The **timing** of the murmur itself is in mid-diastole (**Fig. 4.21**). The **location** is loudest at the apex. It is best heard when the patient is in left lateral decubital position. The **intensity** of the murmur is usually grade 1 to grade 3. The murmur often **radiates** into the left chest. The classic description of auscultation in a patient with mitral stenosis is as Duroziez stated, "**Fout ta-ta-rou.**" The loud sharp S_1 is the fout, the S_2 followed by the **opening snap** is the ta-ta, and the rou is the **diastolic murmur** itself. This is most useful when the patient is in sinus rhythm; and much less so when the expected and invariably developed atrial fibrillation occurs.

The company it keeps includes, on **inspection**, nothing specific. The **pulse** is normal until, in advanced disease, an irregular rhythm of atrial fibrillation develops. **Blood pressure** is unremarkable. The **PMI**, in advanced disease, is "tapping", in which the S_1 that is very accentuated becomes palpable; otherwise, the **precordium** is quiet. With the development of pulmonary hypertension, there is a left parasternal heave, which is caused by a hyperdynamic right ventricle. Mitral stenosis, most commonly, is the result of severe rheumatic fever.

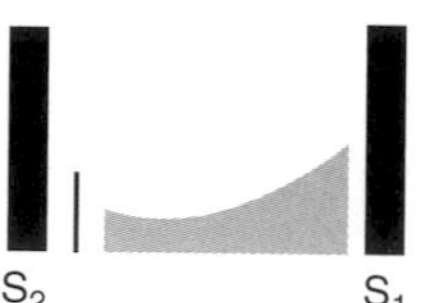

Figure 4.21.

Features of the murmur of mitral stenosis.

The **S_4 gallop** manifests, on auscultation, with a low frequency filling sound in late diastole. This is very difficult to hear, because of a very low frequency (3–60 Hz) of the finding. It is best heard with the bell and with the patient positioned in the left lateral decubital position, listening at the apex; one should listen over mitral area (Fig. 4.1D) if left ventricular; tricuspid area (Fig. 4.1C) if right ventricular. Although the classic teaching is that the term "Ten-nee-seee" is a good cadence for an S_4, we recommend that "Tah-DUP-dah" mimics an S_4. An S_4 is caused by the atrium contracting into a diseased "stiff" left ventricle; thus, if no atrial contraction, e.g., in atrial fibrillation, no S_4 is possible. The wall stiffness is caused by either ischemia or hypertension with hypertrophy. Of interest, this is clinically a marker for diastolic dysfunction.

The **S_3 gallop** manifests, on auscultation, a low frequency filling sound in early diastole. As with an S_4, this is very difficult to hear, because of very low frequency (3–60 Hz). Best heard with the bell at the apex, with the patient in a left lateral decubital position. One should listen over the mitral area if left ventricular; tricuspid area if right ventricular. Although the classic teaching is that the term "Ken-tuck-eee" is a good cadence for an S_3, Ta-ta-dup best mimics an S_3. An S_3 is caused by systolic dysfunction of the ventricle. **Combination gallop** manifests with a combination of S_3 and S_4 that occurs when the patient is tachycardic. This is sometimes called a *quadruple gallop* if the rate is not tachycardic or a *summation gallop* if the rate in tachycardic. **Atrial myxoma** manifests with the patient complaining of near syncope or syncope. On auscultation, an early diastolic plop sound is noted. This sound varies from beat to beat and with specific positions. It is due to a gelatinous tumor derived from the endocardium of the atrium or of one of the valve leaflets. The myxoma may actually cross into the ventricle.

Other diagnoses manifest with diastolic findings. **Pulmonic insufficiency** manifests, on auscultation, with a murmur that is timed in early diastole and is crescendo–decrescendo in nature. It is located at the left second sternal interspace and has company that is specific to the underlying cause. If the etiology is pulmonary hypertension, this murmur is referred to as a Graham-Steell murmur. One of the most common causes today of pulmonic insufficiency is pulmonary hypertension secondary to severe mitral stenosis. **Tricuspid stenosis (TS)** manifests, on auscultation, with a loud S_1, an opening snap, and a mid–diastolic murmur. The company it keeps includes a marked increase in the intensity of the diastolic murmur and its rumble with inspiration. The sensitivity of this application of the Rivero Carvallo maneuver, according to Rothman, is 80%. Finally, a click can be auscultated over the clavicle in TS. The pulse is usually normal; as rarely, does atrial fibrillation develop in TS. The JVP has giant *a* waves and a markedly diminished *y* descent; in addition, it is not uncommon to find Kussmaul's sign, i.e., the paradoxic increase in JVP with inspiration.

Systolic and Diastolic Extra Sounds

Patent ductus arteriosus manifests with the patient being asymptomatic until late in the course of the disease when the patient complains of progressive dyspnea, orthopnea, and PND. On **auscultation**, a continuous murmur across both systole and diastole is noted, loudest over left upper stenal border with patient upright. In other words, it is never really absent **(Fig. 4.22)**. Descriptive metaphors, such as, "machinery like" (obviously a metaphor from the industrial revolution) are not uncommonly used to describe this continuous murmur. On **inspection**, there is clubbing and cyanosis of the toes, but usually sparing of the fingers. Occasionally, the cyanosis will involve the left hand via the left subclavian artery, but the right hand and fingers are always

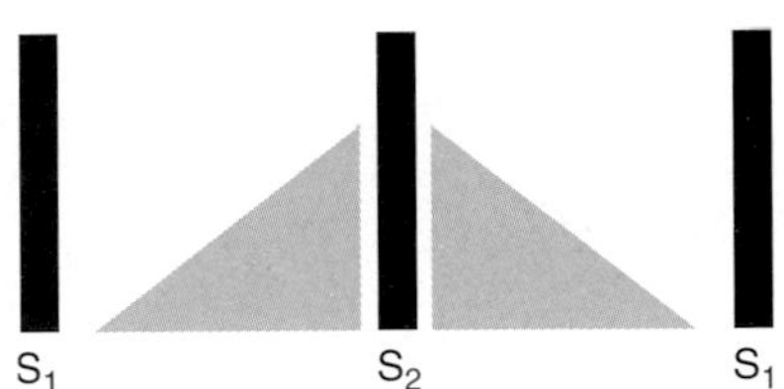

Figure 4.22.

Features of the continuous murmur of patent ductus arteriosus (PDA).

spared clubbing and cyanosis. This differential cyanosis is an important clue in the diagnosis of a PDA with a right to left shunt. At the outset of heart failure, there is an increase in the neck veins with a large *a* wave present. **Pericardial rub** manifests with the patient complaining of a pleuritic-type chest pain that is relieved with sitting up and leaning forward. On **auscultation**, a creaky, squeaky sound is heard in systole, diastole, or both. The rub may have three components: one from the contraction of the ventricle, one from the relaxation of the ventricle, and one with the atrial contraction. The diastolic component of the rub is in early diastole and matches in time within S_3 gallop. Thus, be aware of this overlap. Rubs are best heard on the left lower sternal border. The company pericardial rubs keep includes minimal findings on inspection; the pulse, blood pressure, and apical beat are unremarkable. Occasionally, the rub is palpable in the lower left sternal border. Pericardial rubs are caused by inflammation of the pericardium from autoimmune disease, bacterial infection, uremia, rheumatic fever, or postcardiotomy (Dressler's syndrome). **Calcific or constrictive pericarditis** manifests with a loud, high-pitched, booming sound in early diastole, a sound also known as a knock. It occurs at the same time as an S_3 gallop. **Nicholson's maneuver** is one in which a pericardial knock is unmasked or increased in intensity when the patient squats, which is causes the diastolic filling and, thus, distention of the ventricle against a calcified pericardium. The most common reason for calcific pericarditis is tuberculous pericardial disease. **Hemodialysis fistula** manifests with a palpable fistula in the antecubital fossa in a patient with a history of renal failure. A palpable thrill is noted over the fistula and a grade 5 or grade 6 murmur in systole and diastole located over the fistula. Often, a concurrent murmur is noted in the base of the heart that is transmitted from the fistula. This high output type shunt is a very common site of a continuous murmur and, thus, make certain to look for such a fistula catheter during every physical examination. **Prosthetic valves** manifest with high-pitched sounds in systole, diastole, or both. The sounds from a metallic valve are indeed metallic and loud. These are often the only findings that are truly grade 6/6 in a patient. The **ball-in-cup valve** (Starr-Edwards) has a click in systole and diastole (opening and closing), whereas the more common **disk valves** (Bjork-Shiley and St. Jude) have a single click in systole. Although there may be, and often is, a systolic murmur, any diastolic murmur that develops is abnormal until proved otherwise. **Air embolism** manifests with a gurgling or splashing sound that is rhythmic and continuous. The company it keeps includes hypotension, acute mental status examination changes, and an antecedent history of rapid ascent during a dive (the bends) or air accidentally being infused into a vein or artery. The patient may have sudden death caused by a cerebral embolism.

ORTHOPNEA AND PAROXYSMAL NOCTURNAL DYSPNEA EXAMINATION

Congestive heart failure (CHF) manifests with the patient complaining of shortness of breath. This is often associated with orthopnea, i.e., shortness of breath when supine, alleviated with sitting upright and paroxysmal nocturnal dyspnea, i.e., shortness of breath when supine, dramatically improved with standing bolt upright. Cough is present, which often worsens when the patient is supine and often produces frothy pink sputa. In addition, there is peripheral pitting edema; on auscultation, an S_3 gallop; on palpation of the chest wall, a heave or a laterally and inferiorly displaced PMI. The company CHF keeps includes the presence of red lunula in all fingernails (Terry's heart failure nails) (Fig. 14.6). In addition, an upright sitting position leaning forward with elbows on knees (Fowler's position) is very common. Finally, if severe and chronic, an increased pigment is often seen on the elbows and the anterior thighs (Dahl's sign) (Fig. 5.13). This is due to the chronic need to sit up in order to breathe. If the underlying cause is valvular dysfunction, other features include murmurs of aortic stenosis, mitral stenosis, or of aortic insufficiency; if the underlying cause is myocardial the company may include those of severe longstanding hypertension, i.e., retinal changes, bruits, and diminished peripheral pulses. **Pneumonia—typical consolidative type**—manifests with the patient complaining of a cough, pleuritic-type chest pain, and shortness of breath. The cough is productive of yellow-green sputa. There is dullness to percussion and a marked increase in tactile fremitus over the area. On auscultation the breath sounds are bronchial in nature, with late inspiratory rales, present over the area. Often, there are associated rhonchi or wheezes and concurrent egophony is present over the entire area of dullness. Egophony is performed by auscultating over the area, patient states or sings the sound "EEEEEE". In the normal setting, the term "eeeee" will be heard; in a consolidative process, the sound heard is "AAAAA", like that of a bleating lamb or "A" stated with the patient after inhaling helium. The etiologies of such a consolidative pneumonia include postobstructive pneumonia and the bacterial agents, *Streptococcus pneumoniae* and *Haemophilus influenza*, and, in an immunosuppressed patient, *Pneumocystis carinii.* **Pneumonia—atypical interstitial type** manifests with a nonproductive barking-type cough, normal percussion, and tactile fremitus; but, on auscultation, diffuse rales to all lung fields. The etiologies of this type of acute pneumonia include *Legionella pneumophila, Mycoplasma pneumoniae* and, viral influenza. **Chronic bronchitis** manifests with recurrent or chronic cough that produces white, yellow, or green sputa. On auscultation, diffuse rhonchi and wheezes and in severe cases, inspiratory rales, are noted. **Pleural effusion** manifests with diminished breath sounds. There is dullness to percussion and decreased tactile fremitus, except for a rim of bronchial breath sounds and even hyperresonance at the superior surface of the dullness. Pleural effusion is caused by a collection of fluid in the pleural space. Trepopnea is also present, with the side affected with the pleural effusion being the side that is down when patient sleeps, see Chapter 5.

CHEST PAIN

Pulmonary thromboembolic disease (PTE) manifests with the patient complaining of acute onset of shortness of breath and pleuritic chest pain. There is also mild tachycardia and modest tachypnea. There is often a concurrent or antecedent swollen arm or leg caused by a deep venous thrombosis. In severe PTE, right-sided heart failure develops that manifests with the classic features described by Gorham in 1961. These features include the second sound from pulmonic valve (P_2) being louder than the second sound from the aortic valve (A_2); a pleural rub in the pulmonic area; a systolic murmur at the pulmonic area; an increased area of right-sided cardiac dullness; marked increase in JVP, in which the neck veins are distended even with the patient upright; a right-sided third sound gallop; and hepatomegaly. Hypotension, marked hypoxemia and even sudden death may occur. **Pneumonia** manifests with cough that produces yellow, rusty, or gelatinous sputa. On auscultation there are late inspiratory rales noted over the area; breath sounds are present, bronchial in nature; an associated rhonchi, wheezes, or egophony may be found over the area (see also Chapter 5). **Pneumothorax** manifests with unilateral pleuritic chest pain, diminished breath sounds, and tympany on the affected side, and deviation of trachea to the side opposite. Tracheal deviation indicates that tension pneumothorax is likely (Table 5.3). **Rib fracture** manifests with point tenderness, ecchymosis, swelling, and pleuritic chest pain; pneumothorax or subcutaneous air with crepitus may be an added complication (Table 5.13). **Tietze's syndrome** manifests with tenderness at the costochondral junction(s) adjacent to the sternum. Often in young males, no other rheumatologic findings are present (Table 5.13). **Leukemic infiltration** of the sternum manifests with deep-seated tenderness in the body of the sternum. This is due to acute lymphoblastic leukemia (ALL) or acute myeloid leukemia (AML). **Rib-tip syndrome** of Semble and Wise manifests with pain and tenderness on and around the anterior tenth rib and reproduction of tenderness with the hooking maneuver. The **hooking maneuver** is, with the patient sitting or standing, hook the fingers beneath the margin of the lowest rib (rib 10) anteriorly then gently apply outward traction of the rib. **Acute chest as a sickle-cell crisis** manifests with severe pleuritic chest pain, tachypnea, tachycardia, and features not dissimilar from a PTE. This is in a patient with sickle cell (SS) anemia.

Annotated Bibliography

Aronow WS, Kronzon I. Prevalence and severity of valvular aortic stenosis determined by Doppler echocardiography and its association with echocardiographic and electrocardiographic left ventricular hypertrophy and physical signs of aortic stenosis in elderly patients. *Am J Cardiol* 1991;67:776.

Used echocardiography as a gold standard in elderly patients to assess the sensitivity of signs in detecting mild, moderate, and severe aortic stenosis. Of 142 patients with aortic stenosis, 74 were mild, 49 were moderate, and 19 were severe cases. For mild: systolic murmur at right base; 95%; prolonged duration of the murmur: 3%, late peaking of murmur, 3%, prolonged carotid upstroke 3%, absent A_2: 0%, A_2 decreased or absent: 5%. For moderate: systolic murmur at right base 100%; prolonged duration of the murmur: 63%, late peaking of murmur, 63%, prolonged carotid upstroke 33%, absent A_2: 10%, A_2 decreased or absent: 49%. For severe systolic murmur at right base 100%; prolonged duration of the murmur: 84%, late peaking of murmur, 84%, prolonged carotid upstroke 53%, absent A_2: 16%, A_2 decreased or absent: 74%. Makes the point that, in the elderly, the carotid upstroke may be falsely normal because of decreased compliance and also that the aortic murmur may be loud or even loudest at the apex.

Babu A, Kymes S, Carpenter SM. Eponyms and the diagnosis of aortic regurgitation: what says the evidence? *Ann Int Med* 138(9):736–742, 2003.

The state-of-the-art article.

Badgett RG, Lucey CR, Mulrow CD. Can the clinical examination diagnose left-sided heart failure in adults? *JAMA* 1997;277(21):1712–1719.

An exhaustive review, attempting to stratify by methods how to detect elevated left ventricular filling pressures, decreased ejection fraction, and diastolic from systolic congestive heart failure (CHF). Then, reviews the evidence behind various classic findings of CHF, including vital signs, jugular veins, apical impulse, S_3 gallop, cardiomegaly on radiograph, and pulmonary vascular redistribution. Very densely written paper. Attempted to make overall comments on a topic that is by definition heterogeneous. Perhaps a better method would be to review literature of each specific subset, which would be more useful to the clinician.

Barlow JB, Bosman CK Pocock WA, et al. Late systolic murmurs and non-ejection ("mid-late") systolic clicks. *Br Heart J* 1968;30:203–218.

The original description of this not uncommon syndrome.

Braunwald E, Oldham HN Jr, Ross J Jr, Linhart JW, Mason DT, Fort L III. The circulatory response of patients with IHSS to nitroglycerin and to the Valsalva maneuver. *Circulation* 1964;29:422–431.

Valsalva's maneuver decreases the left ventricular volume by diminishing the venous return, thus increasing the obstruction and the murmur.

Bruns DL, Van Der Hauwert LG. The aortic systolic murmur developing with increased age. *Br Heart J* 1958;20:370.

A descriptive paper of findings and maneuvers to make this diagnosis—the fact that the murmur is decreased during Valsalva's maneuver.

Cintron G, et al. Bedside recognition, incidence and clinical course of right ventricular infarction. ***Am J Cardiol*** **1981;47:224–227.**

Interesting paper that reminded clinicians that a Kussmaul's sign need not indicate pericardial disease, it may also indicate right ventricular dysfunction. Found a sensitivity of 30% for right ventricular infarction with Kussmaul's sign, which is a credible number.

Condos WR, Jr, et al. Hemodynamics of the Mueller maneuver in ma: right ands left micromanometry and Doppler echocardiography. ***Circulation*** **1987;76:1020–1028.**

Defines Müller's maneuver: "With the nares closed, the patient sucks forcibly for 10 seconds on a mouthpiece hooked to a mercury manometer at a negative pressure of 40 to 50 mm Hg. Changes in murmur intensity measured 10 seconds later."

Cook DJ, Simel DL. Does this patient have abnormal central venous pressure? ***JAMA*** **1996;275(8):630–634.**

A thorough overview of the literature and scientific underpinnings of CVP measurement. Reviews the waves pulsations, physiology, and underlying cardiac condition.

Reviews positioning and technique for measuring the CVP; normal is approximately 5 cm H_2O; also relates techniques of abdominojugular reflux (HJR). Furthermore, Kussmaul's sign: the paradoxic increase in CVP with inspiration that occurs in constrictive pericarditis, severe right-sided CHF, amyloidosis, TS, or SVC syndrome. Demonstrates that when the clinical assessment of CVP is high, the positive liklihood ratio (LR) is 4.1, whereas, when the clinical assessment is that the CVP is low, the LR that is indeed low at 3.4. Furthermore, in a study of 62 patients having a right-sided heart catheterization, a student, resident, fellow, and attending physician predicted the CVP low (<0), normal (0–7), or high (>7); sensitivity, 0.33, 0.33, 0.49; sensitivities of 0.73, 0.72, 0.76. The accuracy improved in a low CI, high PCW state and if the patient were not on mechanical ventilation. Reviewed the accuracy of the AJR sign, which was insensitive, but when using strict criteria, a specific method to assess for heart failure (positive LR, 6.4).

Cook DJ. The clinical assessment of central venous pressure. ***Am J Med Sci*** **1990; 299:175–179.**

Reviewed the precision and accuracy of the test for CVP measurement. The precision was measured in 50 patients in the ICU. Blinded to the monitoring results, Cook estimated the patients' CVP to be low (< 5), normal (5–10), high (>10). The kappa was 0 .65 for students (n = 6) and attendings (n =3), but 0.3 between residents (n = 6) and staff. Demonstrated that when the clinical assessment of CVP is high, the positive LR is 4.1, whereas when the clinical assessment is that CVP is low, the LR that it is indeed low is 3.4.

Corrigan DJ: On permanent patency of the mouth of the aorta, or inadequacy of the aortic valves. ***Edinburgh M and SJ.*** **1832;37:225.**

The classic.

Davies-Colley R. Slipping Rib. ***BMJ*** **1922;1:432.**

First description of slipping rib syndrome.

Dell'Italia LJ, et al. Physical examination for exclusion of hemodynamically important right ventricular infarction. ***Ann Intern Med*** **1983;99:608–611.**

Interesting paper that reminds clinicians that a Kussmaul's sign need not mean pericardial disease; it may also mean right ventricular dysfunction. Found a sensitivity of 100% for right ventricular infarction with Kussmaul's sign.

Deluca SA. Coarctation of the aorta. ***AFP*** **1990;Nov:1285–1288.**

Reviews the various types of coarctation and its various manifestations—mainly radiographic—but has some clinical data, specific to the type 1 or preductal type (with upper extremity hypertension and lower extremity claudication); in adult type (II) (collaterals occur anterior or posterior, with rib notching).

Duroziez PI: Du souffle intermittent crural, comme signe de l'insuffisance aortique. ***Arch Gén de Méd*** **1861;17:417,588.**

The classic.

Duthie EH, Gambert SR, Tresch D. Evaluation of the systolic murmur in the elderly. ***J Am Ger Soc*** **1981;Nov:498–502.**

Nice review of the most common entities that manifest with systolic murmurs in the elderly, including aortic stenosis, IHSS, MVP, and mitral regurgitation. A practical and informative review. Makes the point that, with aging, some of the classic manifestations of murmurs described in the young change (e.g., that aortic stenosis often manifests with a murmur loudest at the apex in older patients). This may be because the valve stenosis results from calcifications in the valve in the elderly, with a vibratory component to the murmur in the ventricle as opposed to the tight stricture in youth. Further stated is that the decreased carotid upstroke and pulse parvus et tardus all are less likely found in the elderly. They further make the point that IHSS is similar in manifestations in the elderly versus the young, but it is often overlooked in the elderly.

El-Mofty A, Ismail AA. Detection of gallop rhythm [Letter]. ***Lancet*** **1951;Sept 22:545.**

Described their observation that gallops are diminished with a Valsalva's maneuver (forcibly expiring against a closed glottis) and augmented with a Müeller's maneuver (forcibly inspiring against a closed glottis).

Etchells E, Glenns V, Shadowitz S, Bell C, Siu S. A bedside clinical prediction rule for detecting moderate to severe aortic stenosis. *J Gen Intern Med* 1998;13:699–704.

An excellent study using a gold standard of echocardiography and a definition of moderate to severe aortic stenosis of a valve area of <1.2 cm^2 or a peak instantaneous transvulvar gradient of >25 mm Hg. The study used a standardized physical examination protocol performed by one senior resident and one general medicine faculty member to study the accuracy (using 123 patients on an inpatient ward, 16 of whom had moderate or severe aortic stenosis) and reliability by five residents and one faculty member (using 38 patients) of various findings to diagnose aortic stenosis. Examiners blinded to echocardiographic results. Features included any systolic murmur of >1: sensitivity, 100%; specificity, 64; positive LR, 2.6; negative LR, 0.0; murmur over (radiating to) the right clavicle: sensitivity, 93%; specificity, 69%; positive LR, 3.0; negative LR, 0.10; murmur radiating into right carotid: sensitivity, 73%; specificity, 91%; positive LR, 8.1; negative LR, 0.29; slow carotid upstroke: sensitivity, 47%; specificity, 95%; positive LR, 9.2; negative LR, 0.56; reduced carotid volume: sensitivity, 53%; specificity, 93%; positive LR, 2.0; negative LR, 0.64; diminished second heart sound: sensitivity, 53%; specificity, 93%; positive LR, 7.5; negative LR, 0.5. (values found by resident were similar). They also calculated reliability of specific findings in aortic stenosis: Kappa for diminished S_2, 0.54, for grade II murmur over right second intercostal space, 0.45; for radiation into right clavicle, 0.36; for delayed carotid upstroke, 0.26; for decreased carotid volume, 0.24.

Thus, absence of findings effectively rules out moderate severe aortic stenosis: absence of murmur, absence of radiation into right clavicle findings. When present, the findings that effectively rule in moderate to severe aortic stenosis: include slow upstroke of carotid artery, and murmur radiating into right carotid. History of angina or CHF did not predict either way. The limited number of examiners is a criticism of the study.

Ewart W, Cantab MD. Diagnosis of pericardial effusion. *BMJ* 1896;March:717–721.

Ewart described no less than 12 signs of a pericardial effusion.

Ewy G. The abdominojugular reflux: technique and hemodynamic correlates. *Ann Intern Med* 1988;109:456–460.

An excellent review of a topic that is poorly taught and understood. Brings up a number of excellent points that are of diagnostic importance. Reviews the origins of technique, including Pasteur's original description of liver compression to diagnose tricuspid regurgitation; relates that 10 seconds of upper abdominal compression will result in a marked accentuation of the JVP, followed by an abrupt decrease on release, which is indicative of either right ventricular failure or, more commonly, diastolic left ventricular failure with a wedge of >15 mm Hg.

Ewy GA. Bedside evaluation of precordial pulsations. *Cardiology in Practice* 1984;July/August:127–133.

Excellent overview of the technique and power of this underutilized set of skills. Reviews the site of normal point of maximal impulse (PMI) at the fifth intercostal space in the left midclavicular line. Reviews fact that patient should be examined supine and then in a left lateral decubitus position, at 45 degrees, according to the author. Reviews the sites of palpation, including the aortic, pulmonic, and left parasternal (the site of the normal right ventricular outflow) areas; and the PMI. Stresses the importance of feeling the subxiphoid area for right ventricular findings, especially if the patient has chest wall configuration changes. States that left ventricular findings are most correlated with a prolonged or sustained pulsation over the PMI. Reviews thrills and gallops.

Fink JC, Schmid CH, Selker HP. A decision aid for referring patients with systolic murmurs for echocardiography. *J Gen Intern Med* 1994;9:479–484.

A retrospective case review of 169 asymptomatic patients with systolic murmurs who had concurrent echocardiographic analysis. Found three predictors for increased likelihood of finding abnormalities: increasing age (>35 years), male gender, and murmur intensity of ≥3.

Folland ED, et al. Implications of third sounds in patients with valvular heart disease. *N Engl J Med* 1992;327:458–462.

Excellent paper to assist the clinician in interpreting this finding in specific valve disorders. In mitral regurgitation, third sounds are common but do not necessarily reflect systolic dysfunction; in aortic stenosis, third sounds are common, which usually indicates systolic dysfunction.

Goldblatt A, Harrison DC, Glick G, Braunwald E. Studies on cardiac dimensions in intact, unanesthetized man. II. Effects of respiration. *Circ Res* 1963;13:455–460.

Describes the mechanism for Rivero Carvallo maneuver—inspiration decreases intrathoracic pressure and augments venous return.

Hamman L. Spontaneous mediastinal emphysema. *Bull Johns Hopkins Hosp* 1939;64:1–21.

Describes the crepitant crunching sound, best heard in the left lateral decubital position in seven patients who had mediastinal emphysema. It is interesting to note that several of the original patients were in health care fields. The term "Hamman crunch" has been derived from this paper.

Heberden W. Some account of a disorder of the breast. *Medical Transactions* 1786;2:59–67.

The first description of exercise-related angina pectoris. An incredible description of this very common disorder. "The seat of it and the sense of strangling and anxiety with which it is attended, may make it not improperly called 'angina pectoris'".

Heinz G, Zavala D. Slipping rib syndrome. *JAMA* 1977;237(8):794–795.

Fascinating paper describing an important, but obviously underrecognized cause of chest pain—slipping rib syndrome. Describes the "hooking" maneuver in which the examiner's fingers are curved under the right or left costal margin and pulled upward to unmask the tingling, pain, and dysthesia in the floating ribs 10, 9, and 8.

Howell TH. Cardiac murmurs in old age: a clinico-pathological study. *J Am Geriatrics Soc* 1967;15:509.

Reports that aortic stenosis often manifests with a systolic murmur that, unlike in the younger patient, is loudest at the apex, not the base.

Ishmail AA, Wing S, Ferguson J, et al. Interobserver agreement by auscultation in the presence of a third sound in patients with congestive heart failure. *Chest* 1987;91(6):870–873.

Used 81 patients of whom most had some form of cardiac disease examined by four observers: internist, trainee internist, trainee cardiologist, and a cardiologist. The study was only for agreement, no gold standard was described. The kappa was moderate (0.4–0.5), at best, to poor (0.1–0.3). Makes the point that "gestalt" of sign is important, given the importance of the finding, but relatively moderate to low agreement.

Jeresaty RM. Mitral valve prolapse. *JAMA* 1985;254(6):793–795.

A brief, but satisfactory, review of a not uncommon (prevalence 5%) entity. Discusses pathology, symptoms, signs, diagnosis, and prognosis of this syndrome. The signs include a midsystolic click, which may be associated with a late systolic murmur. The sequalae of or transient ischemic attack (TIA) (40% of TIA in patients <45 years), sudden death, and infectious endocarditis are discussed. Recommends antibiotic prophylaxis in click murmur, but not in silent MVP. If isolated clicks without murmur, prophylaxis may be indicated. Also discusses the indications for beta-blocker treatment.

Jordan MD, Taylor CR, Nyhuis AW, Tavel ME. Audibility of the fourth sound. *Arch Intern Med* 1987;147:721–725.

Used 51 patients (21 normal and 30 abnormal) who were assessed by four cardiologists and five house staff members. Gold standard was phonocardiographic assessment—35/51 had an S_4, 37/51 had splitting of S_1. Interesting but perplexing study that demonstrates that the less-experienced auscultators will diagnose an S_4 more often than those with more experience; also, the less-experienced observers not infrequently misdiagnose a split S_1 as an S_4.

Lembo NJ, Dell'Italia LJ, Crawford MH, O'Rourke RA. Bedside diagnosis of systolic murmurs. *N Eng J Med* 1988;318:1572–1578.

Used 50 patients (ages 6 to 85 years) with systolic murmurs to assess the sensitivity and specificity of physical diagnosis. The underlying diagnoses in these patients included "right-sided murmur" aortic stenosis, IHSS, mitral regurgitation (MR), and ventricle septal defect (VSD). Murmur in the right chambers: increased with inspiration: sensitivity, 100%, specificity, 88%; decreased with expiration: sensitivity, 100%; specificity, 88%; IHSS: increased with the Valsalva's maneuver: sensitivity, 65%; specificity, 96%; increased with squatting to standing: sensitivity, 95%; specificity, 84%; decreased with standing to squatting: sensitivity, 95%; specificity, 85%; decreased with passive leg elevation: sensitivity, 85%; specificity, 91%; decreased with active handgrip: sensitivity, 85%; specificity, 75%. MR and VSD increased with handgrip: sensitivity, 68%; specificity, 92%. Overall, a study that began to assist us in studying the science behind specific tests. Little assistance to the reader in how to differentiate aortic stenosis from MR from VSD; right-sided, very nonspecific. Excellent descriptions of maneuvers including: Müller maneuver: With the nares closed, the patient sucks forcibly for 10 seconds on a mouthpiece hooked to a mercury manometer at a negative pressure of 40 to 50 mm Hg. Changes in murmur intensity measured 10 seconds later.

Transient arterial occlusion: Sphygmomanometer placed around each of the upper limbs, both cuffs simultaneously inflated to 40 mm Hg above systolic blood pressure. Twenty seconds after cuff inflation the murmur changes are recorded.

Lembo NJ, et al. Diagnosis of left-sided regurgitant murmurs by transient arterial occlusion: a maneuver using blood pressure cuffs. *Ann Intern Med* 1986;105:368–370.

Defines the maneuver of transient arterial occlusion: Sphygmomanometer placed around each of the upper limbs, both cuffs simultaneously inflated to 40 mm Hg above systolic blood pressure. Twenty seconds after cuff inflation the murmur changes are recorded.

Lerman J, Means JH. Cardiovascular symptomatology in exophthalmic goiter. *Am Heart J* 1932;8:55–65.

A classic, which describes a cardinal manifestation of profound hyperthyroidism. Although rarely found today, it remains an important concept in the discussion of high output states.

Lind AR, et al. The circulatory effects of sustained voluntary muscle contraction. *Clin Sci* 1964;27:229–244.

Defines the isometric handgrip maneuver: hand dynamometer used changes in murmur recorded 1 minute after maximal contraction.

Lombard JT, Selzer A. Valvular aortic stenosis. *Ann Intern Med* 1987:106:292–298.

A retrospective analysis of 397 patients with aortic stenosis. The study population had a mean age of 61 years and had a valve area of <1.0 cm (i.e., was severe). The study reviewed several physical findings and multiple homodynamic findings of significant aortic stenosis. The physical findings that were studied and found to be of greatest value were the grade of the murmur and the presence of an inaudible S_2. An inaudible S_2 was present in 8.8% of all patients with aortic stenosis; 12.9% with extreme aortic stenosis (<0.045 cm^2); a grade 3 murmur in 65% of all; 65.6% of extreme; a grade 4 to grade 5 murmur in 24 % of all; a grade 4 to grade 5 in 23% of extreme. The remainder of the study reports hemodynamic and right ventricular catheterization parameters for this disorder.

Lorell B, et al. Right ventricular infarction. *Am J Cardiol* 1979;43:465–471.

Interesting paper that reminds clinicians that an elevated pulsus paradox sign need not mean pericardial disease; it may also mean right ventricular dysfunction. Found a sensitivity of 71% for right ventricular infarction with an elevated pulsus paradox.

Lovibond JL. Diagnosis of clubbed fingers. ***Lancet*** **1938;1:363.**
Suggests the use of the profile sign to diagnose clubbing by measuring the angle between the proximal plate and fold and hyponychial—normal angle is 160 degrees; between 160 and 180 degrees early clubbing; >180 degrees gross clubbing. Author notes that in severe clubbing, "the nail can be rocked backward and forward, giving the impression that it is floating on a soft oedematous pad."

Maisel AS, et al. Hepatojugular reflux, useful in the bedside diagnosis of tricuspid regurgitation. ***Ann Intern Med*** **1984;101:781–782.**
A solid overview of the utility of this maneuver to diagnose tricuspid regurgitation. Relates that the sensitivity for elevated HJR is 66% and specificity is 100%.

Marantz PR, Kaplan MC, Alderman MH. Clinical diagnosis of CHF in patients with acute dyspnea. ***Chest*** **1990;97:776–781.**
Nicely designed study based on a patient problem and the clinical assessment by a primary care (emergency [ER]) physician using the abdominojugular reflux examination. Using ER physicians, the sensitivity for the test was 0.33, specificity was 94; positive LR: 6.0, negative LR 0.7, similar to numbers if strict criteria are used to measure. Excellent evidence that the test is insensitive but specific for the diagnosis of CHF.

Nellen M, Gotsman MS, Vogelpoel L, Beck W, Schrire V. Effects of prompt squatting on the systolic murmur in IH cardiomyopathy. ***BMJ*** **1967;3:140–143.**
The murmur intensity is decreased because of increased venous return and increase in left ventricular volume by decreasing the obstruction.

Nicholson WJ, et al. Early diastolic sound of constrictive pericarditis. ***Am J Cardiol*** **1980;45:378–382.**
The description of method to accentuate a pericardial knock.

Nishimura RA, Tajik J. The valsalva maneuver and response revisited. ***Mayo Clin Proc*** **1986; 61:211–217.**
Reviews the four phases of Valsalva's maneuver: I; 61: Straining onset: increased intrathoracic pressure at outset of straining, slight increase in systemic blood pressure. II: Active phase of straining: decrease in pulse pressure and stroke volume, with reflex tachycardia. III: Release of straining: blood pressure further decreases due to pooling of blood in pulmonary bed due to abrupt decrease in intrathoracic pressure. IV: Continued release of strain; overshoot of the systemic blood pressure with modest bradycardia. Reviews the clinical applications, including those in patients with autonomic dysfunction and CHF; heart murmurs and coronary artery disease (CAD). Reviews the side effects, including those in patients with autonomic dysfunction. In scenario of heart murmurs: During phase II, the intensity of most murmurs decreases because of decreased stroke volume and cardiac output, except for IHSS and MVP, both of which increase. A good and useful review of a maneuver that is frankly difficult to use for diagnostic purposes.

Pretre R, Von Segesser LK. Aortic dissection. ***Lancet*** **1997;349:1461–1464.**
Nice overview of the pathogenesis, classification (De Bakey). Type I dissection extends distally to the aortic arch. Type II is confined to the ascending aorta. Type III originates in descending aorta. Stanford type A involves the ascending aorta; type B is distal to the left subclavian artery. Manifestations are described: acute, severe retrosternal interscapular pain, with migration down the back—90% sensitivity; concurrent findings of diastolic murmur of AI and pericardial effusion are not uncommon. Reviews the imaging and outlines acute and chronic follow-up for ultrafast computed tomography (CT) of the aorta (sensitivity, 80% to 100%; specificity, 95% to 100%) echocardiogram (TT and TE: sensitivity, 95% to 100%; specificity 85 to 90) and aortic valve assessment with echocardiogram.

Quincke HI: Ueber capillar puls und centripetal venenpuls, Berl-Klin-Wchnsch 1890; 27:265.
The classic.

Rivero Carvallo JM. Signo para el diagnostico de las insuficiencia tricupidideas. ***Arch Inst Cardiol Mex*** **1946;16:531–540.**
Original description of this classic and useful test to diagnose tricuspid regurgitation.

Ronan JA, Gordon MS. Jugular venous pulse. ***Cardiology*** **1984;July:103–112.**
A splendid overview of the methods behind, and utility of, the measurement of the jugular venous pulse. Describes the method, the normal measurement, and then the various waves and their abnormalities. Description and illustrations of the a, c, and v waves and the x and y descents.

Rondot E. Le reflux hepato-jugulare. ***Gaz Hebdomadaire Sci Med Bordeaux*** **1898;19:567–571, 579–582, 590–592.**
The paper on the performance of abdominojugular reflux is a variant of Pasteur's original description that has better bedside characteristics and utility. This is the standard for teaching today.

Rothman, Goldberger. ***Ann Intern Med*** **1983;Sept:346.**
A review of the sensitivities and specificities of maneuvers used to diagnose systolic murmurs. Data from various studies were combined to determine values. In tricuspid regurgitation, the increase of murmur with inspiration has a sensitivity of 61% (102/167); in IHSS, squatting decreased the murmur in 10/11 (sensitivity of 92%), but did not decrease intensity in systolic murmurs of other etiology (0/16 had a decrease in intensity—100% specificity). Amyl nitrate inhalation increased intensity of murmur in 24/27 patients with IHSS.

Sapira JD. Quincke, de Mussets Duroziez, Hill,: Some aortic regurgitations. ***Southern Med J*** **1981:74(4): 459–67.**
A joy to read. Written by a (the) master.

Schamroth L. Personal experience. *South African Med J* 1976;50:297.

Loss of the rhomboid window when the dorsal surfaces of the plates are apposed. Reported this when he received his care during bouts of endocarditis in a South African hospital.

Shabeti R, et al. The hemodynamics of cardiac tamponade and constrictive pericarditis. *Am J Cardiol* 1970;26:480–490.

Reviews the clinical features of these entities, with nice discussion of technique described by Kussmaul useful in the diagnosis of constrictive pericarditis.

Sharpey-Schafer EP. The effects of squatting on the normal and failing circulation. *BMJ* 1956;1:1072–1074.

The procedure for squatting is as described in paper. Patient instructed to breathe normally and not to perform Valsalva's maneuver during the squatting. Changes in murmur intensity were recorded immediately after squatting.

Squatting to standing: patient squatted for >30 seconds, then rapidly assumed a standing position. Changes in the murmur intensity recorded during the first 15 to 20 seconds after standing.

Spodick DH. The normal and diseased pericardium: current concepts of pericardial physiology, diagnosis and treatment. *J Am Coll Cardiol* 1983;1:240–251.

An excellent paper that describes the physical examination of patients with pericardial disease, including constrictive pericarditis. Reviews Kussmaul's sign; 33% sensitivity for constrictive pericarditis.

Still GF. *Common Disorders and Diseases of Childhood.* London: Oxford University Press, 1915.

In this text is described a specific type of innocent or physiologic murmur (Still's murmur) in children aged 2 to 6 years. This is a systolic murmur at the apex; has a "twang sound, very like that made by a piece of tense string." Also, a significant variability in intensity is noted between various beats.

Terry R. Red half-moons in cardiac failure. *Lancet* 1954;2:842–844.

Of 23 patients with this finding of red lunale, 14 had cardiac failure, the remaining had systemic disease such as Hodgkin's, malnutrition, or cirrhosis. Interesting finding that is, at best, the company with which the problem keeps.

Tice F: The clinical determination and significance of some peripheral signs of aortic insufficiency. Illinois MJ 1911;20:271.

A series of 124 cases; one of first papers on evidence to support exam in aortic insufficiency.

Traube L. Uber den doppleton in der cruralis bei insufficienze der aortenklappen (on the femoral doubletone of aortic insufficiency). *Berl Klin Wochenchr* 1872;9:573–574.

The classic paper in the diagnosis of aortic insufficiency—a must for any zealot in physical diagnosis or medical history.

Trousseau A. Clinique medicale de l'Hotel Dieu de Paris. *Editiones Baillere*:707.

This was probably the first time the term "clubbing" was used. Trousseau was lecturing to students in 1865 and stated, "there is not one among us who does not recognize the significance of finger clubbing or Hippocratic fingers."

Voelpoel L, et al. The value of squatting in the diagnosis of mild aortic insufficiency. *Am Heart J* 1969;77:709–710.

In this overview, it is stated that squatting is indeed an excellent method to unmask the diastolic murmur of aortic insufficiency in that it increases the intensity of the murmur as the result of increased afterload.

Vongpatanasin W, Hillis LD, Lange RA. Prosthetic heart valves. *N Engl J Med* 1996; 335(6):407–415.

An excellent, state-of-the-art paper on the types of heart valves used for replacement, including manifestations and complications. An excellent paper to be included in any primary care physician's library.

Wang K, Hodges M. The premature ventricular complex as a diagnostic aid. *Ann Intern Med* 1992;117:766–770.

Review that demonstrates the usefulness of a premature ventricular complex (PVC). Emphasizes the utility of a PVC to diagnose specific electrocardiographic (ECG) findings; it also relates one physical examination finding—that a PVC may assist in differentiating an S_3 from an S_4; S_4 is ablated during a PVC, S_3 is not.

Weitzman D. The mechanism and significance of the auricular sound. *Br Heart J* 1955; 17:70–78.

Very good study, demonstrating 100 consecutive healthy individuals without the presence of an S_4.

Wood P. Aortic stenosis. *Am J Cardiol* 1958;1:553.

Seminal work on the physical examination and features of aortic stenosis. This is a wealth of information for the clinician and the teacher.

5

Lung and Chest Examination

PRACTICE AND TEACHING

SURFACE ANATOMY

Posterior

The left lung structures include the **lingula**, which is lateral; the **left lower lobe**, which is from the diaphragm to the midscapula; and the **left upper lobe**, which is from midscapula to the apex **(Fig. 5.1)**. The heart is distant from the posterior chest wall and, thus, cannot be examined from the back. The right lung structures include the **right middle lobe**, which is lateral; the **right lower lobe**, which is from diaphragm to midscapula; and the **right upper lobe**, which is from midscapula to the apex. The structures in the chest wall and overlying tissue include the **scapula**; its vertebral surface is medial, the inferior angle at T7, the scapular spine at T3, and the superior angle at T2. The rhomboid muscle attaches from the medial lower scapula to the vertebral spinous processes. The vertebral spinous processes of **C7** is called "vertebra prominens;" it is the most prominent of the spinous processes and the end of the cervical lordosis. Spin-

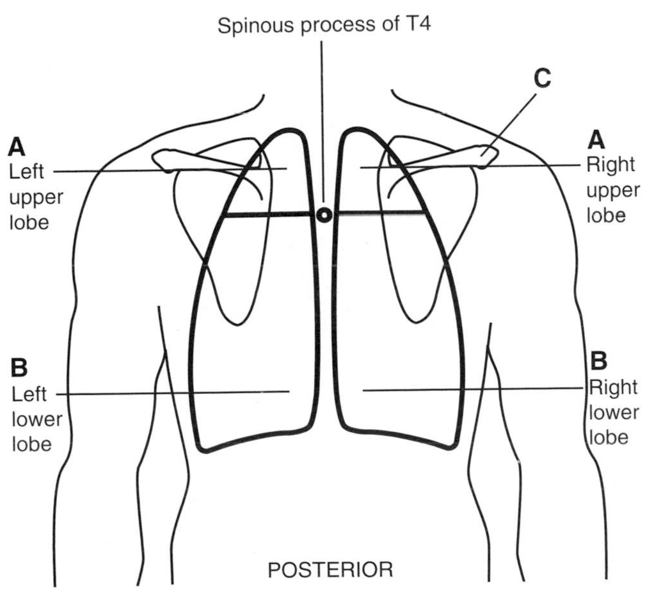

Figure 5.1.

Schematic of surface anatomy: posterior chest. **A.** Upper lobes, small areas in superior chest. **B.** Lower lobes, large areas in lower chest. **C.** Spines of scapula approximately at T3; patient should be positioned with arms at sides. (Adapted from Bates, p. 236).

TIPS

- Left lingula: extreme lateral and inferior; upper lobe; small area superiorly; and lower lobe, largest posterior component
- Right middle lobe: lateral, upper lobe—small area superiorly and lower lobe most of posterior
- Posterior midclavicular line
- Vertebral surface of scapula with spine of scapula at level of T3 and superior and inferior angle of scapula at T2 and T7, respectively
- Thoracic spinous processes 1—12 with paired ribs
- Ribs are all bone posteriorly

ous processes **T1 through T12** each have a pair of ribs that comprise the posterior chest wall. Ribs 1 through 7 are **complete**; ribs 8 through 10 are **incomplete** (i.e., they are attached to the bottom of rib 7 via cartilage); and ribs 11 and 12 are **floating**, i.e., unattached laterally. The **posterior midclavicular** line is an excellent reference on both the left and right sides. The **diaphragm** is located on the **right**, approximately level T10, with a range of T7 on full expiration and T12 on full inspiration; on the **left**, approximately level T9, with a range of T6 on full expiration and T12 with full inspiration.

Anterior

The left lung structures include the **lingula**, which is lateral to the heart, below rib 5; the **left upper lobe**, which is from the area above the clavicle to the heart, at approximately rib 2 medially and rib 4 laterally; the **left lower lobe** is posterior to the heart, i.e., "retrocardiac," and not represented anteriorly **(Fig. 5.2)**. The **heart** is close to the left chest wall and is easily palpated, auscultated, and visualized here. The right lung structures include the **right middle lobe**, which is lateral and inferior; and the **right upper lobe**, which is from the diaphragm and edge of the liver to the area above the clavicle (i.e., the apex). The **right lower lobe** is not represented anteriorly. The overlying structures include the **sternum** (Fig. 5.2C) to which the **complete ribs** (1–7) directly attach; the **manubrium**, which is superior, and to which the clavicles attach via the sternoclavicular joints; and the **xiphoid** process, in lowest point in the midline. The **incomplete ribs** (8–10) are attached by cartilage to rib 7. The **clavicles** extend from the sternum to the acromion. All lung tissue above the clavicles is termed "apical tissue;" it is effectively the upper lobes. The medial aspect of the apical tissue is a site often overlooked and undertaught in the physical examination—**Koenig's isthmus** (Fig. 5.2D). The **pectoralis major** is the major muscle of the upper chest, over which the breast lies. The **anterior midclavicular line** (Fig. 5.2G) is an excellent line for reference on both the left and right sides. The **diaphragm** is located on the right, approximately at T6 with a range of T5 with full expiration and T8 with full inspiration and on the left, approximately at T7 with a range of T5 with full expiration and T8 with full inspiration. The **anterior axillary line** (Fig. 5.2F), which starts at the left acromioclavicular joint, is important for geographic definition in both chest and abdomen examinations.

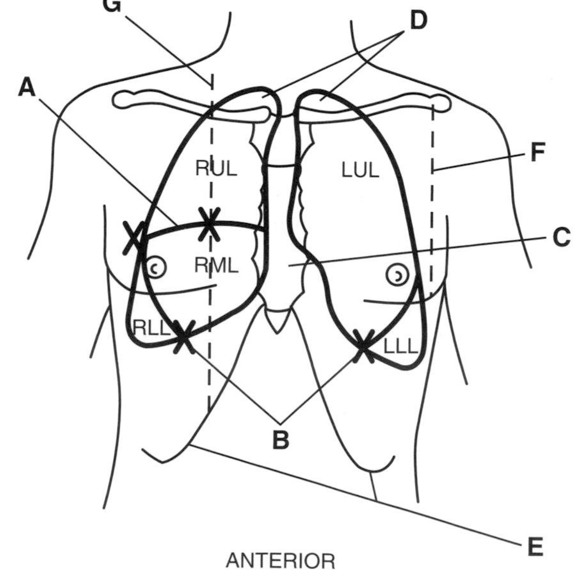

Figure 5.2.

Schematic of surface anatomy, anterior chest. **A.** Minor fissure located between right middle and upper lobes approximately at the fourth rib. **B.** Lower borders of lungs, approximately sixth rib bilaterally at midclavicular line. **C.** Sternum. **D.** Apices; note upper lobes extend superior to clavicles. **E.** Rib 10. **F.** Anterior axillary line. **G.** Midclavicular line. (Adapted from Bates, p. 237).

TIPS

- Left lingula is lateral and inferior; left upper lobe, large area including apex, above the clavicle
- Right middle lobe is lateral and inferior; right upper lobe, large area including apex, above the clavicle
- Anterior midclavicular line, right and left
- Clavicles, define the lower edge of apices
- Sternum, manubrium, and xiphoid, all boney
- Ribs 1–7: cartilaginous attachments to sternum; 8–10 cartilage to the ribs
- Anterior axillary line, especially on the left

PULMONARY EXAMINATION

Chest wall inspection to assess the boney structures of the chest wall is an extremely important first step in the pulmonary examination. Chest wall inspection, neck muscle inspection, and tracheal location assessment are often underutilized in the physical examination. Abnormal deviations of the chest configuration can lead to significant **restrictive-type disease**. Some of these deviations and other chest wall findings are described in **Table 5.1**. **Pectus excavatum**, also known as "funnel chest," manifests with the inferior sternum displaced posteriorly (i.e., sternal inversion) **(Fig. 5.3A)**. This anomaly of the chest wall has concurrent mitral valve prolapse (MVP); with a prevalence of 15% in pectus excavatum. **Pectus carinatum**, also known as "pigeon chest,"

Table 5.1. Chest Wall and Skin Changes

Diagnosis	Chest Wall Findings	Company it Keeps
Pectus excavatum (funnel chest)	Inferior sternum is displaced posteriorly (inverted)	Mitral valve prolapse Restrictive lung disease
Pectus carinatum (pigeon chest)	Narrow thorax, sternum protrudes anteriorly (everted)	Marfan's syndrome Rickets
Barrel chest	Increased anteroposterior diameter	Emphysema COPD
Harrison's sulcus	Outward flare of anterior lower ribs (the incomplete ribs)	Old healed rickets
Scoliosis	Lateral deviation of the thoracic spine to right or left Deviation worsened by forward bend	Restrictive disease
Dowager's hump	Accentuated kyphosis in upper thoracic vertebrae (T1 to T6)	Restrictive disease
Thoracic ankylosis	Straight thoracic spine, loss of kyphosis Straight lumbar spine, loss of lordosis	Decreased Schober's maneuver Decreased chest wall expansion SI tenderness Erythema nodosum FABERE with tenderness over the SI joints Achilles tendinitis Aortic insufficiency Restrictive lung disease
Superior vena cava syndrome	Marked increase in size of chest wall veins	Right apical dullness Tongue edema Facial edema Right brachial plexus problems Right apical dullness and wheezes, if tumor Pemberton's sign, if caused by a retrosternal goiter
Empyema necessitatis	Subcutaneous fluctuant nodule or mass Warm and overlying redness	Underlying empyema that dissected peripherally
Actinomycosis	Orifice of a fistula in chest wall Drains pus and mucus Yellow granules, akin to sulfur, in the material	Underlying pleural based pneumonia Upper lobes Poor dentition with gingivitis
Rib fracture	Focal tenderness, ecchymosis Specifically over rib(s) Boney step-off on affected rib(s)	Splinting on affected side

COPD = chronic obstructive pulmonary disease; SI = sacroiliac joint.

Table 5.2. Intercostal Movements with Respiration

Diagnosis	Local or Diffuse	Bulging or Retracted
Normal	Diffuse	Inhalation: retract Exhalation: bulge
COPD/asthma	Diffuse	Inhalation: retract, accentuated Exhalation: bulging, accentuated
Restrictive	Diffuse	Inhalation: retract, accentuated
Tension pneumothorax	Local	Exhalation: accentuated, bulging
Flail chest	Local	Inhalation: retract, accentuated Exhalation: bulge, accentuated
Pleural effusion	Local	Inhalation: bulge Exhalation: bulge, accentuated
Constrictive pericarditis	Local, left	Focal retractions with each ventricular systole (Broadbent's sign)

COPD = chronic obstructive pulmonary disease.

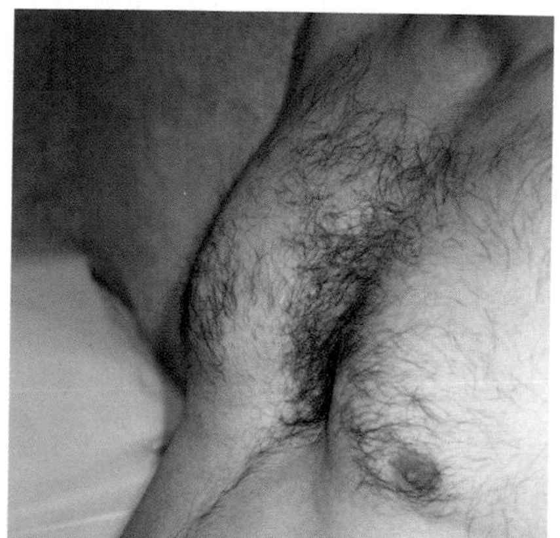

A

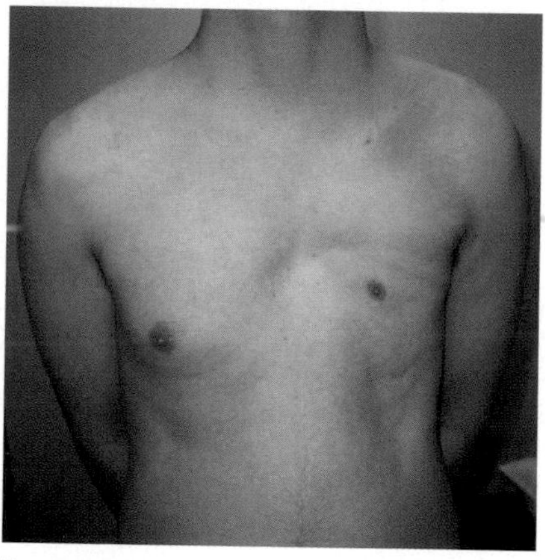

B

Figure 5.3.

A. Pectus excavatum. **B.** Pectus carinatum.

TIPS

- Chest wall anomaly in which there is an inverted (posteriorly displaced) sternum
- Concurrent restrictive lung disease may be present
- Mitral valve prolapse present in 15%
- Also known as "funnel chest"

manifests with a narrow thorax, with the sternum protruding anteriorly, i.e., sternal eversion **(Fig. 5.3B)**. It is associated with Marfan's syndrome and with severe rickets. **Harrison's sulcus**, which manifests with the lower ribs being flared outward, is associated with old, healed rickets. **Rickets** manifests with chest wall variants or anomalies of pectus excavatum, Harrison's sulcus, and valgus deformity of the tibia, bilaterally. Rickets is uncommon today in the United States, but the manifestations may be present in older patients who grew up during the Depression when these disorders of malnutrition were not uncommon.

Scoliosis manifests with lateral deviation of the spine to left or right. This finding is often accentuated when the patient forward bends at the waist. Often significant restrictive disease is present, as measured by both the qualitative and quantitative chest expansion tests. This is most often developmental in nature; it is uncommon in the United States today because of a very successful screening and intervention program in the elementary school system. It is, however, not uncommon in older individuals and in patients from the Third World (See Chapter 12). **Barrel chest** manifests with a marked increase in the anteroposterior (AP) diameter of the chest as assessed at the angle of Louis. This is a relatively advanced manifestation of emphysema. The presence of a barrel chest configuration should prompt the examiner to look for emphysema. **Dowager's hump** manifests with an accentuated kyphosis in the upper thoracic vertebrae, i.e., T1–T6. The patient has a forward displaced head at the neck such that she/he must significantly backward flex the neck to look forward. Overall, in kyphosis there is a decrease in height and qualitative and quantitative decrease in chest expansion. This is most often caused by osteoporotic-related vertebral body compression fractures.

Thoracic ankylosis of ankylosing spondylitis manifests with the patient complaining of significant overall back stiffness and discomfort in the upper and lower back. On examination, a "straight as a poker" gait is seen, as are a

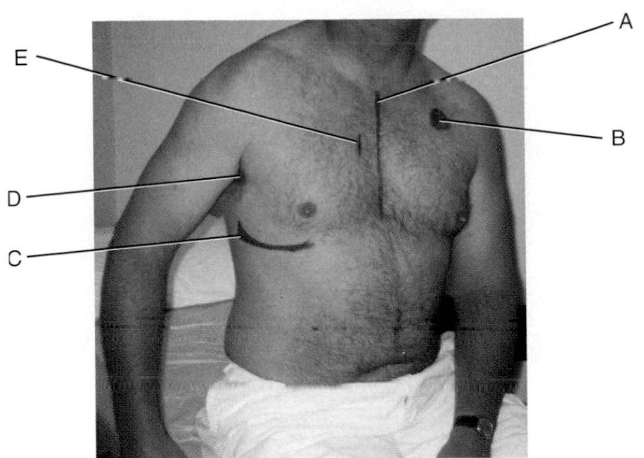

Figure 5.4.

Scar sites for various procedures. **A.** Median thoracotomy. **B.** Placement of pacemaker. **C.** Lobectomy. **D.** Chest tube placement. **E.** Right parasternal (Chamberlain) scar.

 **TIPS**

- Various sites of scars for various procedures
- Excellent information gleaned from simple visual inspection

thoracic spine that has minimal kyphosis and a lumbar spine that has minimal lordosis. Recall, ankylosis means straightening and fusion. The straight thoracic and lumbar spines remain straight with forward bend at the waist. In fact, on forward bend, there is no reversal of the lumbar spine to kyphosis, no curve, and, thus, no increase in length when performing Schober's maneuver (Fig. 12.13). The **qualitative chest wall expansion** demonstrates significant symmetric restriction; the **quantitative** is limited, i.e., an increase in circumference that is <2.5 cm. This is an important finding, as described by Fries. The company ankylosing spondylitis keeps includes tenderness at the sacroiliac joints with iliac compression and with the FABER* test, erythema nodosum, polyarticular arthritis, the diastolic murmur of aortic insufficiency, and tenderness discrete to the insertion of the Achilles tendon to the calcaneus, i.e., Achilles tendinitis.

Scars are clues to antecedent trauma or surgical procedures and, as such, provide a rich source of clues in the physical examination and history **(Fig. 5.4)**. A **median sternotomy scar** (Fig. 5.4A) indicates cardiac, either valve or bypass, grafting surgery. Furthermore, a scar with a **subcutaneous device** present in the upper chest wall (Fig. 5.4B) indicates an automatic implantable cardioverter-defibrillator (AICD) or a pacemaker. In addition, a **unilateral arc-shaped costal** scar (Fig. 5.4C) indicates lobectomy or pneumonectomy. A scar that is on the **right sternal border**, rib level 4 to 5, indicates a limited thoracectomy and surgical exploration of the mediastinum (Fig. 5.4E) (Chamberlain incision). A scar at **midaxillary line in intercostal space of 6 or 7** indicates an old chest tube placement (Fig. 5.4D) for the treatment of a pneumothorax or drainage of a pleural effusion.

Assessment of active chest wall expansion is an important complementary technique in the chest examination, in general, and restrictive lung disease, specifically. Two tests are used to assess the chest wall function: one is qualitative and performed first; the second is quantitative. In any patient, the qualitative test should be performed; in any patient in whom the clinician suspects restrictive disease, both the qualitative and quantitative tests should be performed. For the **qualitative chest expansion** test **(Fig. 5.5)**, stand behind the patient and place the hands, in a horizontal position, parallel to floor, thumbs perpendicular to floor, pointing upward over the medial chest wall; and instruct the patient to actively deeply inhale. Repeat this procedure on both the lower and upper chest walls. In the normal setting, a symmetric outward movement is noted with the thumbs tilted medially; in **restrictive disease**, there is decreased movement of hands; and, in **pleural disease**, there is decreased movement on the affected side. The **quantitative chest expansion**

*FABER: Passive forward flexion, abduction, external rotation of hip.

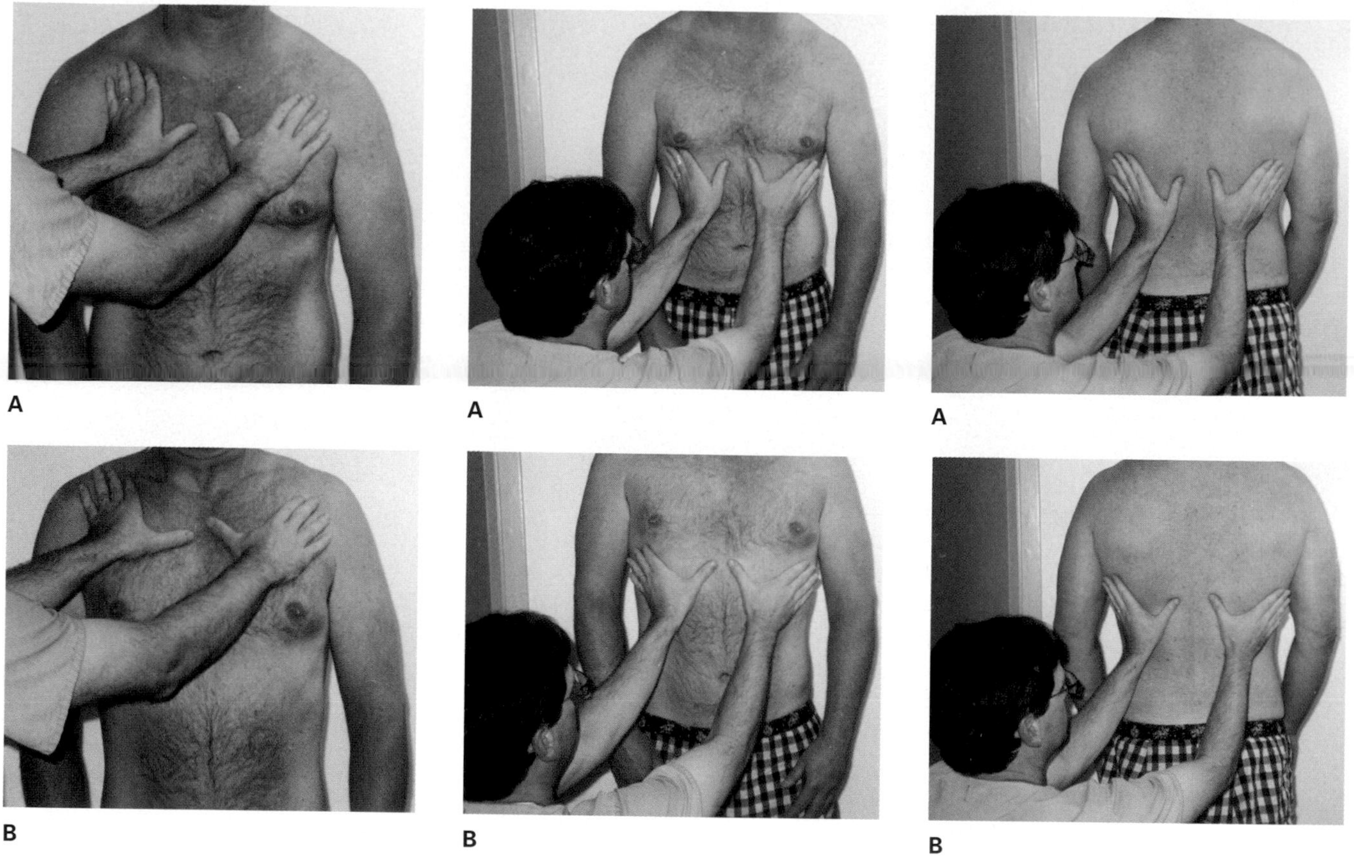

A A A

B B B

Figure 5.5.

Technique for qualitative assessment of chest wall expansion, here normal symmetric expansion. **A.** Baseline, full exhalation. **B.** Full inspiration. Note the placement of hands and thumbs.

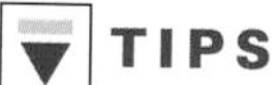

TIPS

- With patient standing, stand behind the patient and place hands, horizontal to floor, thumbs on or off the skin on lower lateral rib cage, and instruct patient to take an active deep inhalation
- Watch movement of hands
- Repeat this from the front-lower anterior and upper anterior chest wall
- Normal: symmetric outward movement
- Pleural disease: no movement on affected side
- Restrictive disease: decreased movement of hands

examination involves measuring the circumference of the chest at the fourth rib in full exhalation and inhalation with a tape measure. Normally, an increase of >5 cm is noted in the circumference of the chest with inhalation. In restrictive disease, an increase of <2.5 cm in chest circumference is noted.

Other diagnoses include **superior vena cava obstruction (SVC)**, which manifests with increased size of neck and chest wall veins; increased size of arm subcutaneous veins; and tongue, facial, eyelid, and upper extremity edema. The company it keeps is specific to the underlying cause. If SVC is caused by a **right apical tumor**, there usually is a malignant bronchogenic neoplasm, like that first described by Pancoast more than 100 years ago, manifestations include dullness to percussion in the right apex and, on auscultation, wheezing or bronchial breath sounds in the right anterior chest. In addition, there may be neuropathy involving the brachial plexus; the development of miosis, ptosis, and anhidrosis on the right side caused by Horner's syndrome; and the development of hard right-sided supraclavicular nodes. If

TEACHING POINTS

CHEST WALL ANOMALIES AND FINDINGS

1. Chest wall complications, restrictive disease.
2. Pectus excavatum (funnel chest): associated with mitral valve prolapse.
3. Pectus carinatum (pigeon chest): inverse of excavatum, associated with Marfan's syndrome.
4. Three levels of restrictive disease assessment: inspection of the chest, qualitative inspection with hands on chest, and quantitative inspection with a tape measure.
5. A straight thoracic spine: strongly consider for ankylosing spondylitis.
6. Dowager's hump (i.e., upper thoracic kyphosis): assess for osteoporosis.
7. Scars: provide a wealth of historical data for the examintion.
8. Localized bulging of the intercostal spaces: indicates fluid in the pleural space.
9. Diffuse intercostal retractions: consistent with moderate to severe asthma.
10. Diffuse mild retractions with inspiration: normal, only marked ones indicate a complication.

SVC is caused by a **retrosternal goiter**, manifestations of hypothyroidism may be seen. In addition, marked facial suffusion and exacerbation of symptoms may be noted on passive forward flexion of the arms above the horizontal (i.e., a positive Pemberton's sign) (see Fig. 1.65). **Metastatic carcinoma** to the chest wall manifests with a hard nodule or mass that is fixed to the underlying rib. This is usually seen in a patient who has weight loss and in whom the diagnosis of metastatic carcinoma is already known. **Empyema necessitans** manifests with a fluctuant subcutaneous nodule or mass, located specifically in an intercostal space. Often erythema and warmth are noted in the overlying skin. Invariably present are dullness to percussion, diminished tactile fremitus, and diminished breath sounds in an area adjacent to the empyema necessitatis, reflective of the underlying pleural-based empyema. **Actinomycosis** manifests with a specific form of empyema necessitatis in that it will open and drain as a fistula. Often, the drainage is mucopurulent and has yellow sulfurlike granules in it. Again, there is dullness to percussion, decreased tactile fremitus, and decreased breath sounds in the area adjacent. This indicates the location of the underlying pleura-based pneumonia. A **rib fracture** manifests with point tenderness and even gross deformity over a rib, ecchymosis, swelling, and severe pleuritic chest pain. The patient often has marked restriction to inspiration as assessed qualitatively. This inspiratory embarrassment is called **splinting**. Quantitative assessment is painful and unnecessary in such a case. Rib fracture(s) is often caused by blunt trauma to the chest; for instance, a helmeted head of a football player thrust into the side of a quarterback. The company it keeps is specific to the complications, including a **pneumothorax**, which can manifest with tympany to percussion; decreased tactile fremitus; and diminished breath sounds over the affected area. In addition, if severe, the trachea may be pushed to the other side, indicating the emergent life-threatening condition of a **tension pneumothorax**.

Intercostal retractions (Table 5.2) manifest with passive invaginations of the skin and tissue in the intercostal spaces, either local or diffuse. These are normal in inspiration. Diffusely present and accentuated retractions, however, may be consistent with moderate to severe asthma. In point of fact, if

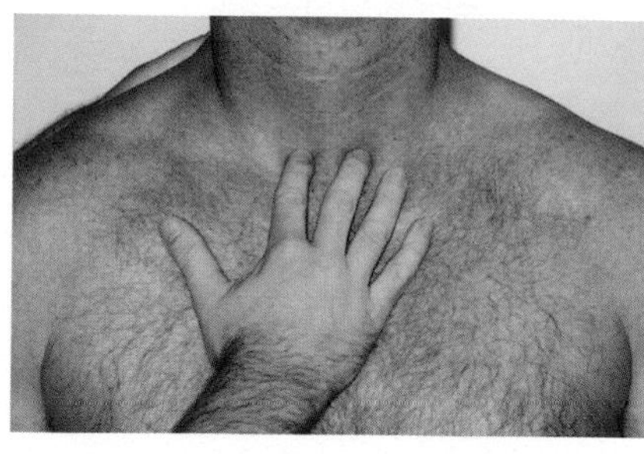

Figure 5.6.

Technique to assess tracheal location.

TIPS

- With patient standing or sitting, inspect the position of the trachea in the anterior neck and as it passes deep to the manubrium sternum
- Normal: midline
- Tension pneumothorax: pushed away
- Pleural effusion: pushed away
- Lung collapse: pulled toward

Table 5.3. Tracheal Location Inspection

Diagnosis	Tracheal Deviation	Related Symptoms	Intervention
Tension pneumothorax	Toward side away from pain Pushed away	Tympany and decreased breath sounds, side away	STAT
Massive pleural effusion	Toward side away from pain Pushed away	Dullness and decreased breath sounds, side away	Emergent
Obstructed bronchus with atelectasis	Toward side of pain Pulled toward	Dullness and decreased breath sounds	Urgent/emergent

asthma is severe such that air movement is minimal, this may be more prominent, important, and diagnostic than the traditionally taught finding of wheezes. **Intercostal bulges** (Table 5.2) manifest with evaginations of the skin and tissue in the intercostal spaces. These can be either local or diffuse. In normal expiration, there is a mild diffuse bulging of the spaces. Usually, local areas of bulging indicate underlying large collections of fluid in the pleural or pericardial spaces. See **Table 5.2** for specifics on interpretation and utility of these. These findings comprise the company and become more important in patients with potentially confounding problems. These are not primary items introduced in second year curricula, but as company on rounds.

Inspection of neck muscles is important in the pulmonary examination. The examination includes baseline inspection of the size of the sternocleidomastoid, trapezius, and scalene muscles and whether the muscles are used during inspiration or any phase of respiration except during vigorous exercise. Normally, these muscles are not used during respiration. **Severe chronic obstructive pulmonary disease (COPD)** manifests with hypertrophy of these muscles. In point of fact, McFadden and colleagues have related that hypertrophy correlates with a forced expiratory volume in 1 second (FEV_1) of 1.0 to 1.5 L. In addition, **inspect the trachea (Table 5.3)** with the patient standing or sitting upward; observe the trachea relative to the midline of the anterior neck, the midline being the midaxis of the jugular notch **(Fig. 5.6)**. Normally, minimal to no deviation, i.e., <4 mm from midaxis, is noted. In **tension pneumothorax**, the trachea is deviated (i.e., pushed away from the side of complications). With a **large pleural effusion**, the trachea is deviated, i.e., pushed away from the side of complications. With a **bronchus obstruction** with atelectasis, the trachea is deviated, i.e., pulled toward the side of complications (Table 5.3). The obstruction is usually caused by a bronchogenic carcinoma.

Palpation of the chest wall is important to assess for nodules and points of tenderness in the muscles or bones of the chest wall. **Tietze's syndrome**, which manifests with discrete tenderness at one or more costochondral joints, is either trauma related or idiopathic inflammation of the costochondral junctions. **Rib fracture** manifests with severe tenderness and palpable swelling at the site of fracture. There is concurrent splinting to inspiration, ecchymosis, a crunchy sensation palpable over the affected area, and, potentially, a pneumothorax. Recall, the features of a **severe pneumothorax** because this should be sought in any rib fracture. The company it keeps includes tympany to percussion, diminished breath sounds of the affected side and deviation of the trachea to the contralateral side.

Assess the **respiratory pattern** when counting the respiratory rate. The pattern should be observed for at least 30 seconds and, if any abnormality is suspected, a minimum of 2 minutes **(Table 5.4)**. Normal is a pattern of

Table 5.4. Respiratory Patterns

Pattern	Features	Company it Keeps	Causes
Normal	Regular, rate of 12–14/minute	Normal	Normal
Kussmaul	Rapid, deep respirations	Ketones on breath	Metabolic acidosis Diabetic ketoacidosis Ethanol ketoacidosis
Biot	Periodic apnea intermixed with rapid deep breathing	Decreased level of consciousness	Brainstem damage
Cheyne-Stokes	Periodic, repetitive apnea Periods of breathing, the depth increases with each breath	Third sound Decreased level of consciousness Increased age	Congestive heart failure
Sleep apnea	Intermittent period of apnea to 20 seconds while asleep	Morning headaches Snoring Increased size of neck	Obesity Retrosternal goiter

regular rhythm with a rate of 12 to 14/minute. **Kussmaul's respiration**, which manifests with rapid deep breathing, is highly correlated with marked metabolic acidosis. A classic example of this is diabetic ketoacidosis. **Biot's breathing** manifests with periods of rapid, deep breathing interspersed with periods of apnea. It is correlated with a brainstem infarct or damage. **Cheyne-Stokes** pattern manifests with periodic breathing in which there is apnea followed by a period of low, then increasing in depth breathing. This is consistent with severe heart failure.

Table 5.5. Descriptors of Percussion

Diagnosis	Percussion Note
Normal	Normal percussive notes, especially tympanic in apices
Consolidation, not obstructed (i.e., bronchus open)	Dullness throughout
Consolidation, obstructed (i.e., bronchus closed)	Dullness throughout
Pleural effusion	Dullness, with a rim of tympany at top
Lobectomy	Dullness throughout
Pneumonectomy	Dullness throughout
Pneumothorax, severe	Tympanic over area
Tuberculosis	Bilateral apical dullness, especially about Kronig's isthmus
Massive pericardial effusion	Dullness to percussion at the posterior left lower chest, adjacent to the tip of left scapula (Ewart's sign)

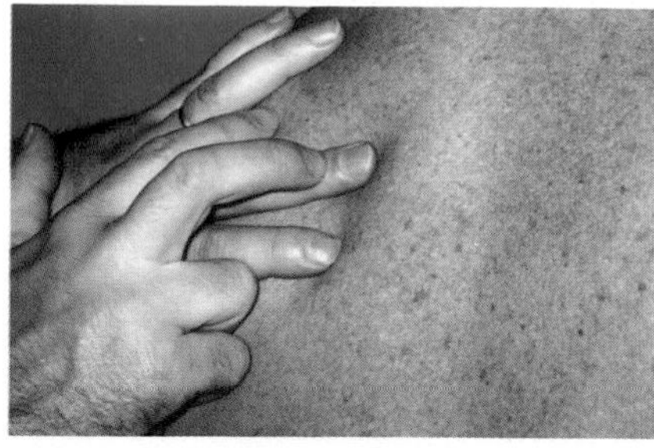

Figure 5.7.

Technique for chest percussion.

TIPS

- Place third digit of nondominant hand on skin of chest wall (pleximeter), strike with tip of dominant hand as a mallet (plexor)
- Feel and listen to the percussion note

Table 5.6. Fine Points of Tactile Fremitus

Diagnosis	Fremitus Features
Normal	Tactile fremitus present and symmetric; left chest, the heart site: no tactile fremitus
Consolidation, not obstructed (i.e., with bronchus still open)	Increased tactile fremitus over area
Consolidation, obstructed (i.e., with bronchus closed)	Decreased or absent tactile fremitus over the area
Pleural effusion	Decreased tactile fremitus at inferior part, with a thin rim of increased tactile fremitus at superior rim
Lobectomy	Absent tactile fremitus
Pneumonectomy	Absent tactile fremitus

Percussion of the chest is one of the fundamental techniques of medicine **(Table 5.5)**. Every teacher should be a master of this set of techniques and be able to deftly teach them. Once a student has learned this, it marks a passage from preclinical to clinical years of learning medicine. With the patient standing or sitting, arms crossed in front, slightly leaning forward **(Fig. 5.7)**, place the third digit of the nondominant hand on the skin of chest wall (pleximeter), strike with tip of dominant hand as a mallet (plexor) **(Fig. 5.8)**. Feel and listen to the percussion note; use Pacinian corpuscles to hear also. Chest percussion is a systematic method in which three sites are percussed in the anterior chest, two sites in the lateral chest, and four sites in the posterior chest. Compare and contrast the sides by percussing from the superior to inferior aspect, side to side. Normally, the notes are resonant, approaching tympany at the anterior apices above the clavicles, including the medial anterior apices, i.e., Koenig's isthmus. This resonance results from the fact that, in the upright position, ventilation is highest relative to perfusion in the upper zones, thus, normally more gas, more tympanic. Furthermore, in the left

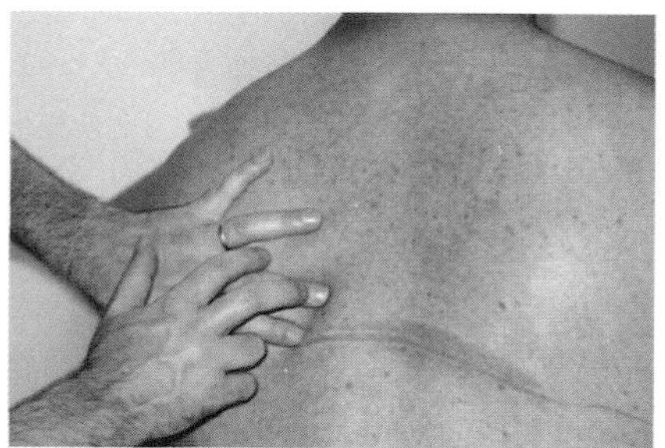
A

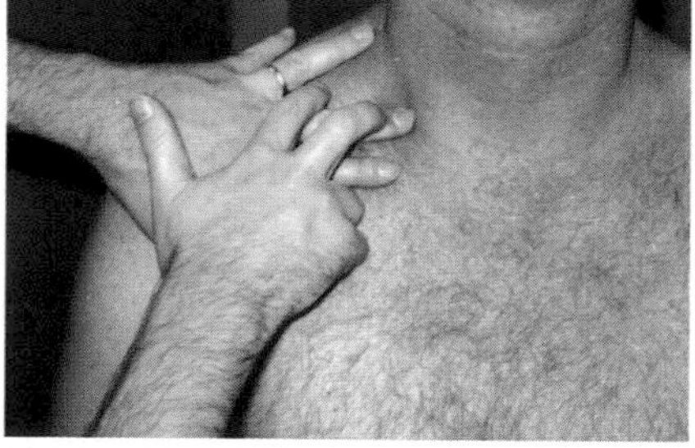
B

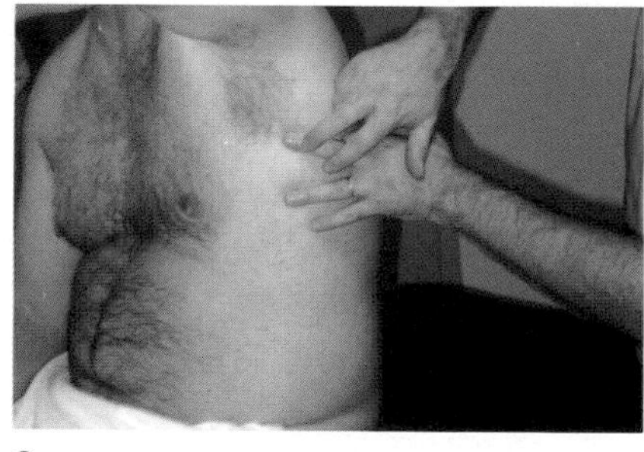
C

Figure 5.8.

Sites for percussion. **A.** Posterior. **B.** Anterior and apices. **C.** Lateral.

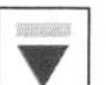
TIPS

- With patient standing or sitting, crossing arms in front, leaning slightly forward; compare and contrast the sides
- May start from top and go down or from bottom and go upward
- Percuss the anterior, lateral, and the posterior sites
- The apices, the most tympanic areas of the lungs, are a great reference site

anterior chest, there is dullness to percussion because the heart is in the left anterior chest. **Consolidation** of, or in, the lung tissue manifests with dullness throughout the area, which is caused by fluid, pus, or blood in the alveoli of the affected lung area. **Lobectomy** or pneumonectomy manifests with dullness to percussion in the affected area. **Pleural effusion** manifests with dullness to percussion in the area affected with a rim of hyperresonance on the superior aspect—also called Skodiac resonance, which was first described by the famous Czech clinician educator Skoda. The dullness is caused by fluid in the pleural space. **Reactive tuberculosis** manifests with bilateral apical dullness if typical mycobacterial disease; in atypical disease, the dullness may be unilateral. **Pericardial effusion** manifests with dullness on the medial aspect of the tip of the medial left scapula, which is also known as Ewart's sign (Fig. 4.14).

Tactile fremitus of chest is another fundamental technique in the chest and pulmonary examination **(Table 5.6) (Fig. 5.9)**. The technique consists of the patient standing or sitting, leaning slightly forward, with arms crossed in front. Place hands, palms on the skin of chest wall, and instruct the patient to say "ninety-nine" or "o-ing," e.g., as in boy or toy or coin. According to some, including Dock and Sapira, o-ing is superior to the standard ninety-nine, but it is recommended to use both. Use the part of hand that is most receptive to the fremitus: palm, palmar fingertips, or the ulnar aspect. To gain experience, place the hands on your own lower chest and state ninety-nine or o-ing, feeling normal fremitus and experiment to determine if o-ing or ninety-nine is better and whether the palms, fingertips, or ulnar aspect of the hands are the best tools to sense the fremitus.

Be systematic in approach. Assess the anterior, lateral, and posterior chest at sites marked on the chest wall. In the procedure, compare and

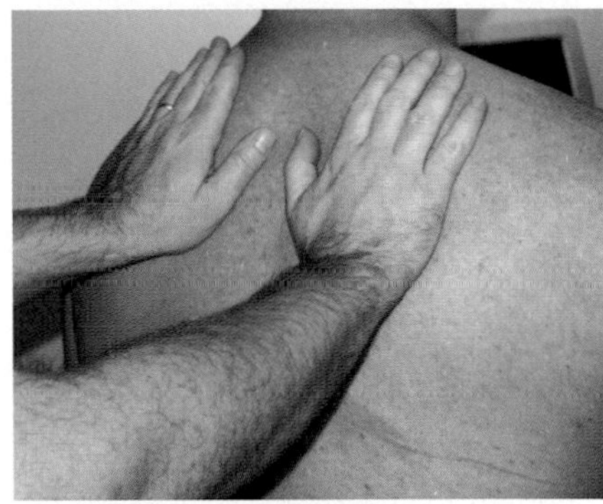

A

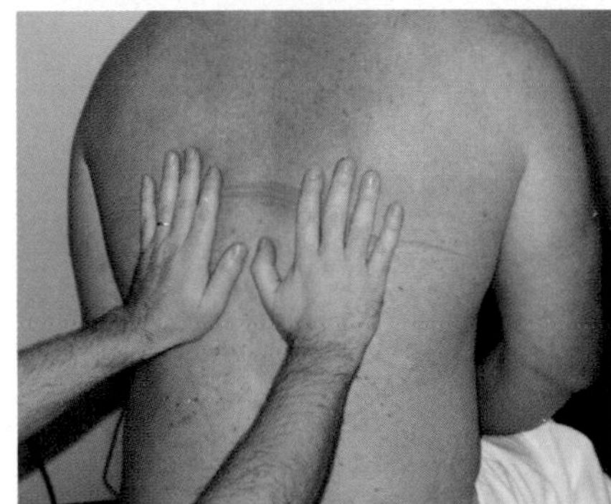

B

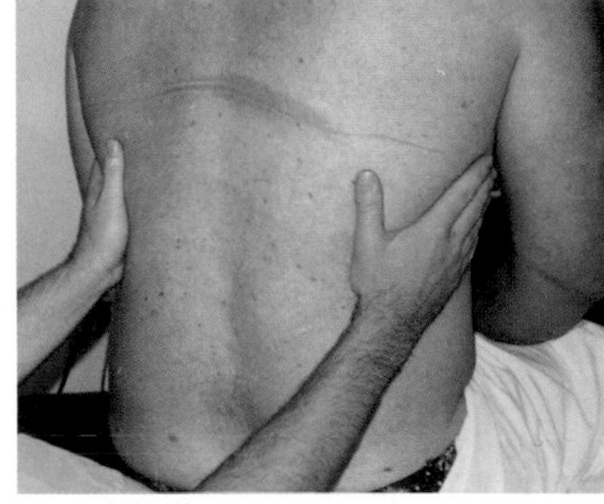

C

Figure 5.9.

Technique for performing tactile fremitus. **A.** Upper. **B.** Lower. **C.** Lateral.

Table 5.7. American Thoracic Society (ATS) Classification of Adventitious Sounds

Sound	ATS Features	Metaphor	Laennec Description
Coarse crackle	Discontinuous, interrupted explosive sounds Loud, low in pitch	Like hairs being rubbed together	Rale muquex ou gargouillement
Fine crackle	Discontinuous, interrupted explosive sounds Loud, higher in pitch		Rale humide ou crepitation
Wheeze	Continuous, high-pitched, hissing		Rale sibilant sec ou sifflement
Rhonchus	Continuous low-pitched, snoring quality	Phlegmatic sounding	Rale sec sonore ou ronflement
In addition:			
Rubs	Leathery, creaky sound Inspiratory and expiratory phase	Sit on leather couch	
Stridor	High-pitched Always inspiratory Upper airway angioedema Ludwig's angina Superior vena cava syndrome Epiglottitis		

TIPS

- With patient standing or sitting, cross arms before the patient, slightly leaning forward
- Place hands on chest wall, in pairs, side-to-side
- Patient states term "99" or "oingg," e.g., booyyy, tooyyy, coin

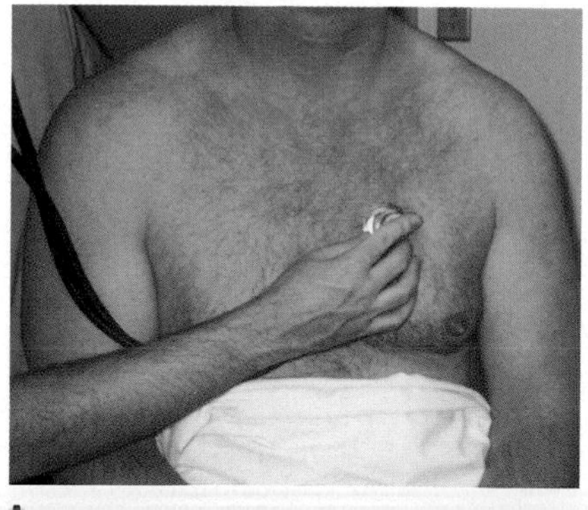

A

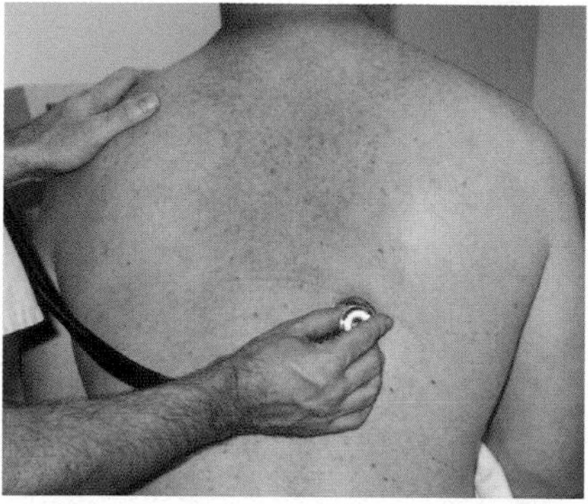

B

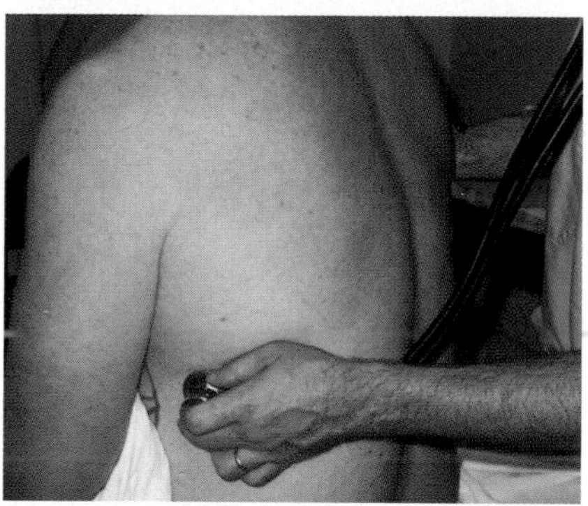

C

Figure 5.10.

Technique for auscultation. **A.** Anterior in midclavicular line. **B.** Posterior in midclavicular line. **C.** Lateral in midaxillary line.

TIPS

- With patient standing or sitting, cross arms before the patient, slightly leaning forward
- Place the diaphragm of the stethoscope on bared skin—not through clothes

contrast the sites by placing the hands in pairs, side-to-side from the superior to inferior aspect: three times anteriorly, two times laterally, and four times posteriorly. **Normal** manifests with tactile, symmetric fremitus present throughout. Little, if any, tactile fremitus is noted over the left chest as this is the heart site. **Consolidation with filled airways** manifests with decreased tactile fremitus throughout; the radiographic correlate of this is the complete absence of air bronchograms because the airways are filled with pus, blood, fluid, or other material. **Lobectomy** or **pneumonectomy** manifests with decreased tactile fremitus throughout. **Consolidation with open airways** manifests with increased tactile fremitus throughout the area. The radiographic correlate of this is consolidation with air bronchograms. A **pleural effusion** manifests with decreased tactile fremitus throughout, which is caused by fluid in the pleural space. **Reactive tuberculosis** manifests with bilateral apical decreased tactile fremitus, caused by pleural thickening and cavitary lesions. **Pericardial effusion** manifests with mildly increased tactile fremitus on the medial aspect of the tip of the medial left scapula, which is caused by a rim of adjacent atelectasis. All of these will have dullness to percussion.

Auscultation of the chest involves the patient standing or sitting, slightly leaning forward, with arms crossed in front (**Fig. 5.10**). Auscultation is one of the classic items that both the physician and the patient think of when they define physical examination. Place the diaphragm of stethoscope on the skin of the chest wall. In many ways, the use of a stethoscope adds credibility to the patient–physician encounter. NEVER listen through cloth or linen. The examination must be performed on bare skin with appropriate draping. Instruct the patient to inhale and exhale, then auscultate the sites using the diaphragm of the stethoscope. The auscultation must be performed in a systematic manner: four pairs posteriorly, two pairs laterally in the midaxillary lines, and three pairs anteriorly in the midclavicular lines. On auscultation, you should be able to describe, define, and delineate the breath sounds using the features of intensity, type, inspiratory:expiratory ratio, adventitious sounds and where in the cycle the adventitious sounds are located. The **intensity** of breath sounds should be described: are they present, diminished, or absent? The **type** of breath sounds: are they vesicular or bronchial? **Vesicular breath sounds** are those that are normally present over the periphery; tubular or bronchial breath sounds are those that are normally located over the trachea. **Describe** the inspiratory:expiratory ratio of the breath sounds. Finally, it is important to describe the presence of any **adventitious sounds,** e.g., wheezes, crackles, rubs, rhonchi, and, if present, determine if they are inspiratory or expiratory. One of the best methods to reproducibly categorize adventitious breath sounds is the classification developed by the American Thoracic Society (**Table 5.7**). This classification is almost universally used and, as such, should be the paradigm used to teach and describe findings. This nomenclature is fascinating in that it is different from that used by the father of stethoscopy, Rene Laennec. Please refer to **Table 5.8** for clinical and teaching data on ausculatory findings. **Wheezes** are described as continuous, high-pitched, and almost hissing in quality. Wheezes are caused by airway obstruction, but are often nonspecific and may be present in the normal setting. **Coarse crackles or rales** are described as discontinuous, interrupted, explosive sounds—loud, low in pitch. **Fine crackles or rales** are described as discontinuous, interrupted explosive sounds—loud, slightly higher in pitch than coarse crackles. Crackles are caused by interstitial processes, including fibrosis and edema. **Rhonchi** are described as continuous, low-pitched, snoring quality. Rhonchi are caused by fluid, mucus, foreign material, pus, or blood in the airway itself. Other adventitious sounds include rubs, whoop, and stridor. **Rubs** are described as leathery, creaky sounds that occur in both inspiration and expiration. The company it keeps includes pleuritic chest pain and even

Table 5.8. Fine Ausculatory Descriptors of Common Lung Diagnoses

Diagnosis	Findings on Auscultation	Company it Keeps
Normal	Breath sounds symmetric Vesicular throughout Bronchial central Minimal adventitious sounds May have wheezes with forced expiration	Nonspecific Mild retraction inhalation Mild bulge exhalation
Consolidation	Crackles over area	Cough productive of yellow-green, often rust streaked, sputa
Open airways	Rhonchus or wheeze Late inspiratory crackles	Breath sounds present, bronchial in nature Dullness Increased tactile fremitus
Consolidation, obstructed	Diminished breath sounds Crackles present Breath sounds are bronchial	Dullness Decreased to absent tactile fremitus
Pleural effusion	Diminished breath sounds Bronchial breath sounds at superior rim	Dullness Decreased tactile fremitus Focal intercostal bulge inhalation and exhalation
Lobectomy or pneumonectomy	Complete absence of breath sounds	Scar over area Dullness No tactile fremitus Loss of intercostal movements
Asthma/reactive airways	Diffusely diminished breath sounds Vesicular breath sounds Prolonged expiratory phase Expiratory wheezes In moderately severe, expiratory and inspiratory wheezes Expiratory stridor-type sounds	Eczema Accentuated retraction with inspiration
Severe asthma	Paucity of wheezes Wheezes may become inspiratory and expiratory Diffusely diminished breath sounds Early inspiratory crackles	Somnolence because of CO_2 narcosis Use of sternocleidomastoid muscles Use of scalene anterior muscles
Upper airway compromise	Diffusely diminished breath sounds Vesicular breath sounds Prolonged expiratory phase Inspiratory (usually holoinspiratory) stridor	Position of "sniffing the flowers" Accentuated retraction with inspiration
Pneumothorax	Locally diminished breath sounds Rub adjacent may be present	Tympany over area If tension, trachea deviated to (pushed toward) other side If tension, hypotension, sudden cardiac collapse
Emphysema	A few wheezes Diffusely diminished breath sounds Early inspiratory crackles if severe	Tympany throughout Increase anteroposterior diameter Lowered and flattened hemidiaphragms
Chronic bronchitis	Normal intensity breath sounds Diffuse wheezes and rhonchi Early inspiratory crackles if severe	Chronic cough Productive cough If cor pulmonale, clubbing, right S_3
Bronchiectasis	Midinspiratory crackles over area Bronchial breath sounds over area	Dullness over area Increased tactile fremitus Chronic cough produces yellow-green sputa
Interstitial lung disease	Diffuse, dry, fine crackles	Clubbing Often concurrent Pleural disease

(continued)

Table 5.8. **(continued)**

Diagnosis	Findings on Auscultation	Company it Keeps
Pulmonary edema	Lower zones, late coarse crackles A few wheezes, diffuse	Peripheral edema Gallop—S_3 or S_4 Cardiomegaly Laterally displaced, PMI, lift or heave Increased JVP
Situs inversus	Decreased breath sounds right Anterior	Decreased tactile fremitus, right anterior Dullness to percussion, right anterior Liver scratched and palpated in left midclavicular line If Kartengener's, recurrent pneumonias

JVP = jugular venous pressure; PMI = point of maximal impulse.

a pericardial rub. Rubs are caused by areas of pleural inflammation. **Whoops** are described as high-pitched sounds, heard without a stethoscope and associated with a cough. Whoops are caused by the relatively uncommon disease of pertussis, caused by *Bordetella pertussis.* **Stridor** is described as a high-pitched, loud, always inspiratory, finding that is often noted with or without auscultating the chest. Stridor is caused by upper airway obstruction, angioedema, epiglottitis, or foreign body.

Normal auscultatory findings include vesicular breath sounds in all areas except the center, where they become bronchial; breath sounds are present throughout and symmetric; no adventitious sounds are noted. An exception to this is the presence of wheezes when the patient is instructed to exhale forcefully and maximally. **Consolidation** with **airways open** manifests with breath sounds that are present and bronchial in nature; associated rhonchus or wheeze is present. Often, crackles are present late in inspiration. The company it keeps includes dullness to percussion, increased tactile fremitus, and a productive cough. This is caused by infection with bacteria, most often *Streptococcus pneumoniae* or *Haemophilus influenzae.* **Consolidation** with **airways filled** with fluid manifests with diminished breath sounds; any sounds present are bronchial. There are crackles present. The company it keeps includes dullness to percussion, and decreased to absent tactile fremitus. This is caused by a severe pneumonia in which fluid is in alveoli and the airways or one in which there is concurrent blockage of the bronchus itself. **Pleural effusion** manifests with diminished breath sounds. Dullness to percussion and decreased tactile fremitus are noted, except for a rim of bronchial breath sounds and even hyperresonance at the superior surface of the dullness, which is caused by a collection of fluid in the pleural space. **Lobectomy or pneumonectomy** manifests with a complete absence of breath sounds. Dullness to percussion and an absence of tactile fremitus are noted over the area. The company it keeps includes a scar and complete loss of intercostal movements. **Upper airway obstruction** manifests with diffusely diminished breath sounds to all lung fields, and breath sounds are vesicular in nature. A prolonged expiratory phase and inspiratory stridor are noted. The head position is one of "sniffing the flowers." The stridor, which is not only present on auscultation, usually is present throughout inspiration. Accentuated intercostal retractions may be noted with inspiration. This is caused by angioedema, epiglottitis, Ludwig's angina, or an inhaled foreign body. **Asthma or reactive airways** manifests with diffusely diminished breath sounds to all areas. The breath sounds are vesicular in nature. A prolonged expiratory phase, expiratory wheezes, and, at times, expiratory stridor sounds are noted. The company it keeps includes eczema and an accentuation of intercostal retractions with inspiration. Asthma is caused by increased reactivity to the bronchial smooth muscle. **Severe asthma** manifests with diffusely diminished breath sounds that are vesicular in nature. Noted is a remarkable paucity of wheezes and a prolonged expiratory phase. The wheezes may become inspiratory and expiratory, and early inspiratory crackles may be heard. The patient may be somnolent because of elevated carbon dioxide in blood. Often, the use of accessory muscles of respiration is noted. **Pneumothorax** manifests with locally diminished breath sounds, and a rub may be noted over the area. There is tympany over the area and decreased tactile fremitus. If a severe pneumothorax, the trachea is deviated toward, i.e., pushed to, the other side; hypotension and sudden cardiac death may occur. A pneumothorax is caused by the entry of air into the pleural space because of trauma. The air can emanate from the bronchi or the skin. A tension pneumothorax is progressive and, without intervention, a mortal event. **Emphysema** manifests with diffusely diminished breath sounds, a few diffuse wheezes, and if severe, some diffuse early inspiratory crackles. Tympany is noted throughout the chest, as are decreased tactile fremitus throughout the chest, an increase in the anteroposterior (AP) diameter of the chest, and the diaphragms being located lower in both inspiration and expiration. This is a specific type of chronic obstructive lung disease in which there is general loss of lung tissue. **Chronic bronchitis** manifests with normal intensity breath sounds, diffuse rhonchi, a few scattered wheezes, and, if severe, early inspiratory crackles. The patient relates a cough that is chronic and produces mucoid or purulent sputa. The company it keeps includes, if cor pulmonale, diffuse clubbing, a loud P_2 and a right-sided S_3. **Bronchiectasis** manifests with a discrete area of bronchial breath sounds and concurrent midinspiratory rales, with breath sounds that are very loud. Dullness to percussion and marked increase in tactile fremitus over the area are noted. The patient complains of a chronic cough productive of yellow-green purulent sputa, which is caused by a chronic infection, with chronic dilation of the area involved. **Interstitial lung disease** manifests with diffuse, late inspiratory crackles. Often, concurrent dullness and decreased tactile fremitus are noted, as are concurrent pleural disease and clubbing. Interstitial lung disease is caused by fibrosis or infiltration of the interstitial tissue with various substances, including iron or asbestos, or is autoimmune. **Pulmonary edema** manifests with coarse crackles in the lower lung zones, which are late in inspiration. Often, a few wheezes are present. It is important to recognize that the differential diagnosis of wheezes include asthma, or normal or pulmonary edema. Pulmonary edema is caused by fluid in the interstitial lung from left-sided to backward heart failure.

A final component of the physical examination must include an assessment of the digits of all four extremities for **clubbing**. The specific criteria for clubbing include a flattening of the angle formed between the nail plate and the proximal nail fold (Lovibond's angle) so that it is >170 degrees and, second, a sponginess of the nail plate on the underlying nailbed (Fig. 14.3 and 14.4). Both criteria need to be met to diagnose clubbing. Perform the **Schamroth procedure** to confirm a flattened or normal angle. In this procedure, instruct the patient to place the dorsal aspects of digits 2 or 3 together or the dorsal tips of the thumbs together, and observe the apposition of the nail plates when viewed from the side. The presence of a diamond-shaped area of light rules out flattening and, thus, rules out clubbing; its absence makes the angle indeed flat and fulfills one criterion for clubbing. (Refer to skin and fingernails for further discussion and images). Both criteria need to be met to diagnose clubbing and, once diagnosed, the pattern of involvement of extremities must be outlined. See **Table 5.9** for specific causes of clubbing. Advanced clubbing is relatively easy to diagnose—the tips of the digits appear as "lollipops."

TEACHING POINTS

PULMONARY EXAMINATION

1. Inspection of chest, inspection of trachea, tactile fremitus, chest percussion, and auscultation of chest should be performed on all patients; they are the five pillars of chest examination.
2. Examine the patient without any overlying clothes or bedlinens, i.e., to the bare skin; but drape to maintain privacy.
3. Restrictive disease always trumps obstructive disease, thus inspect the chest wall and assess the patient's ability to inhale first.
4. A finding by auscultation in restrictive disease more suggestive of significant pathology.
5. Wide differential for adventitious sounds, especially for wheezing. Wheezing can be normal or caused by reactive airways; if local, it is caused by partial obstruction of lower airways (e.g., a peanut) or results from pulmonary edema.
6. The seminal component of chest examination is percussion; use this to establish a pretest assessment with the other techniques; it should and must be mastered.
7. The examination must be performed in a systematic manner on anterior, lateral, and posterior chest.
8. The acquired absence of wheezes in a patient with asthma indicates either improvement or, if airways have become very tight, a harbinger of imminent demise.
9. Diagnoses are not made by auscultation or percussion alone, but by the constellation of manifestations together.

Table 5.9. Diseases Associated with Clubbing of Digits

Diagnosis	Extremities Involved	Company it Keeps
Rheumatoid arthritis	All four	Synovitis, swan necking
Inflammatory bowel disease	All four	Bloody diarrhea
Emphysema	All four	Increased anteroposterior diameter Signs of right ventricular failure
Hypertrophic pulmonary osteoarthropathy	All four	Pulmonary mass, postobstructive pneumonia
Coarctation of aorta	All extremities, except right hand	Diminished pulses and decreased blood pressure In left arm, both legs recurrent paresthesia and cyanosis in affected limb
Thoracic outlet	The hand on side involved	Diminished pulse with Adson's maneuver
Atrial septal defect	Toes, not fingers	Systolic murmur

Table 5.10. Sputa Characteristics of Various Disorders

Diagnosis	Color	Consistency	Odor
Abscess	Nonspecific	Thin to thick	Fetid, putrid
Pneumococcal	Yellow-green with rusty red streaks	Thick	Nonspecific
Acute bronchitis	Red-streaked yellow sputa	Thick	Nonspecific
Tuberculosis	Frank hemoptysis	Thin	Nonspecific
Chronic bronchitis	White to yellow	Thick	Nonspecific
Asthma	Yellow-green	Thick	Nonspecific

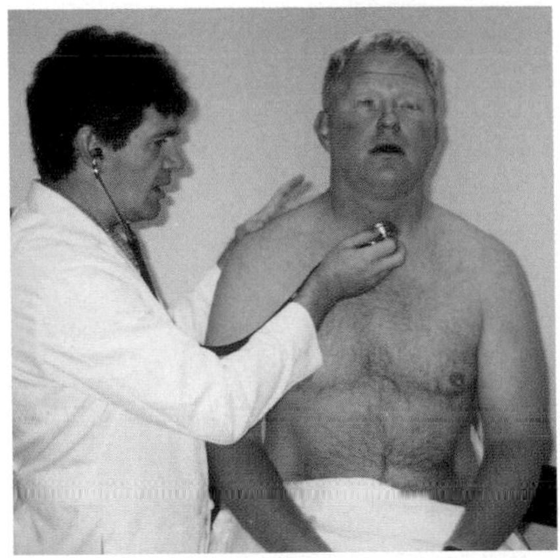

Figure 5.11.

Technique for performing the forced maximal expiration. Note auscultation is performed over the trachea.

 **TIPS**

- Place stethoscope over the midanterior trachea
- Instruct patient to inhale maximally and then fully exhale maximally
- Normal: <3 seconds
- Airway disease, nonspecific: >6 seconds

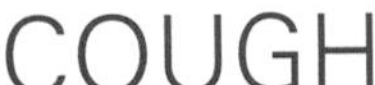

COUGH

Asthma manifests with mild shortness of breath and a recurrent paroxysmal cough, which may produce yellow-green sputa **(Table 5.10)**. On auscultation, breath sounds are diffusely diminished, vesicular in nature, with a prolonged expiratory phase and with diffuse expiratory wheezes. In addition, the forced expiratory respiration is prolonged (i.e., >6 seconds). This forced expiratory volume is measured by placing the stethoscope over the midanterior trachea, instructing the patient to inhale maximally and then maximally, and then fully exhale. Normal finding is <3 seconds **(Fig. 5.11)**. Shapira relates a sensitivity of 74% and specificity of 75%. **Severe asthma** manifests with shortness of breath and a cough that is usually nonproductive. On auscultation are noted diffuse inspiratory and expiratory wheezes and midinspiratory crackles. When very severe, there is a remarkable paucity of wheezes because of the marked decrease in air movement. The company it keeps is specific to the underlying cause. If indeed **atopic**, eczema; if **gastroesophageal reflux disease (GERD)**, a nonproductive cough that often occurs on assuming a supine position, a few diffuse wheezes, significant pyrosis, halitosis, and erosions on the lingual side of teeth. **Pneumonia—typical, consolidative type**—manifests with the patient complaining of a cough, pleuritic-type chest pain, and shortness of breath. The cough produces yellow-green sputa **(Fig. 5.12)**. Noted are dullness to percussion over the area and a marked increase in tactile fremitus; on auscultation, breath sounds present, bronchial in nature, with late inspiratory rales over the area. Often, also noted are an associated rhonchus or wheeze and concurrent egophony over the entire area of dullness. Egophony is performed by auscultating over the area while the patient states or sings the sound eeeeee **(Table 5.11)**. In the normal setting, the term eeeee is heard; in a consolidative process, the sound heard is "AAAAA", like that of a bleating lamb or A stated with the patient

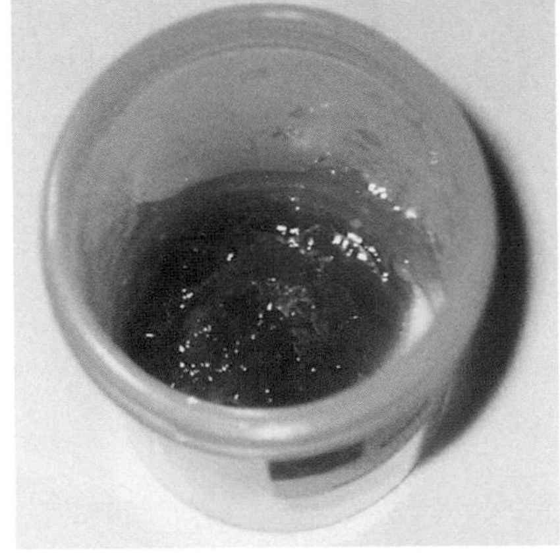

Figure 5.12.

Inspection of the sputa. This is the thick, rusty sputa of a patient with a pneumococcal pneumonia.

 **TIPS**

- Visually inspect and indirectly smell the sputa that the patient is producing
- This is, indeed, a part of the physical examination
- Note color, consistency, and any odor
- See Table 5.10

Table 5.11. Egophony Findings

Diagnosis	Patient States	Examiner Hears
Normal	eeee	eeeee
Consolidation, open airways	eeee	AAAAA
Consolidation, closed airways	eeee	Nothing
Effusion	eeee	Nothing, except aaaa upper rim

Table 5.12. **Evidence to Support the Physical Examination—Pneumonia**

Test	Study	Positive LR	Negative LR
Tachycardia >120/min	Hackerling, et al Gennis, et al	2.3 1.9	0.49 0.89
Fever, >37.8 C	Hackerling, et al Gennis, et al	2.4 1.4	0.58 0.63
Decreased breath sounds	Hackerling, et al Gennis, et al	2.5 2.3	0.64 0.78
Dullness	Hackerling, et al Gennis, et al	4.3 2.2	0.79 0.93
Egophony	Hackerling, et al Gennis, et al	5.3 2.0	0.76 0.96

on helium. Causes of such a consolidative pneumonia include postobstructive pneumonia and the bacterial agents of *Streptococcus pneumoniae* and *Haemophilus influenzae.* Evidence to support exam is in **Table 5.12.** **Pneumonia—atypical, interstitial type**—manifests with a nonproductive barking cough, normal percussion, and tactile fremitus, but on auscultation, diffuse rales to all fields. Causes of this type of acute pneumonia include *Legionella pneumophila, Mycoplasma pneumoniae* and *viral influenza.* **Acute bronchitis** manifests with an acute onset of cough that produces yellow-green, sometimes red-streaked sputa. On auscultation are noted diffuse rhonchi and occasional wheezes, normal fremitus, and percussion. **Chronic bronchitis** manifests with recurrent or chronic cough that produces white, yellow, or green sputa. Often, on auscultation are noted diffuse rhonchi and wheezes; in severe cases, early inspiratory rales. **Tuberculosis** manifests with a cough that is chronic and nonproductive to productive of frank hemoptysis, unintentional weight loss, night sweats, and fevers. On percussion is noted bilateral, atypical dullness to percussion; on auscultation, amphoric or cavernous breath sounds—akin to listening to a shell for the sounds of the ocean. A pulmonary **abscess** manifests with fetid or putrid sputa, low-grade fever, dullness to percussion, and bronchial breath sounds at one apex. Poor dentition with gingivitis are related features (Fig. 1.37).

ORTHOPNEA AND PAROXYSMAL NOCTURNAL DYSPNEA EXAMINATION

Congestive heart failure (CHF) manifests with the patient complaining of shortness of breath. This is often associated with **orthopnea**, i.e., shortness of breath when supine, alleviated with sitting upright, and **paroxysmal nocturnal dyspnea**, i.e., shortness of breath when supine, dramatically improved with standing bolt upright. There is cough that is often worse when supine and often produces frothy pink sputa. Also noted are peripheral pitting edema; on auscultation, an S_3 gallop; and, on palpation of the chest wall, a heave or a laterally and inferiorly displaced point of maximal impulse (PMI). The company CHF keeps includes the presence of red lunula in all

TEACHING POINTS

ORTHOPNEA AND PAROXYSMAL NOCTURNAL DYSPNEA (PND)

1. Orthopnea can be caused by COPD, bilateral lower pneumonia, bilateral pleural effusions, or pulmonary edema from heart failure.
2. COPD and heart failure often are present in the same patient and, as such, it can be vexing to differentiate which is the primary condition. It is necessary to know the related symptoms to learn how to best differentiate between the two.
3. Most of the causes have a cough, often productive, except for pleural effusions.
4. The fundamental aspects of the examination—inspection, percussion, tactile fremitus, and auscultation allow the physician to best differentiate one from another.

fingernails, i.e., Terry's heart failure nails (Fig. 14.6). In addition, an upright sitting position, leaning forward with elbows on knees (Fowler's position), is very common. Finally, if this is severe or chronic, increased pigment is seen on the elbows and the anterior thighs (Dahl's sign) **(Fig. 5.13)**. If the underlying cause is valvular dysfunction, the company it keeps includes murmurs of aortic stenosis, mitral stenosis, aortic insufficiency; if the underlying cause is myocardial dysfunction, evidence is seen of severe long-standing hypertension, i.e., retinal changes, bruits, and diminished peripheral pulses. **Pneumonia—typical, consolidative-type**—manifests with the patient complaining of a cough, pleuritic-type chest pain, and shortness of breath. The cough is productive of yellow-green sputa. There is dullness to percussion over the area, and a marked increase in tactile fremitus over the area; on auscultation, breath sounds present, bronchial in nature, with late inspiratory rales over area. There often is an associated rhonchus or wheeze and concurrent egophony over the entire area of dullness. Egophony is performed (Table 5.11) by auscultating over the area, patient states or sings the sound eeeeee. In the normal setting, the examiner hears the term eeeee; in a consolidative process the sound heard is AAAAA, like that of a bleating lamb or A stated with the patient on helium. Etiologies of such a consolidative pneumonia include postobstructive and the bacterial agents of *Streptococcus pneumoniae* and *Haemophilus influenza*. **Pneumonia—atypical, interstitial type**—manifests with a nonproductive barking cough, normal percussion, and tactile fremitus, but on auscultation, diffuse rales to all fields. Etiologies of this type of acute pneumonia include *Legionella pneumophilia, Mycoplasma pneumoniae,* and *viral influenza.* **Chronic bronchitis** manifests with recurrent or chronic cough productive of white, yellow, or green sputa. There is often, upon auscultation, diffuse rhonchi and wheezes, and in severe cases, early inspiratory rales. **Pleural effusion** manifests with diminished breath sounds. There is dullness to percussion and decreased tactile fremitus, except for a rim of bronchial breath sounds and even hyperresonance at the superior surface of the dullness, which is caused by a collection of fluid into the pleural space. There is also trepopnea, with the side affected with the pleural effusion being the side that is down when patient sleeps.

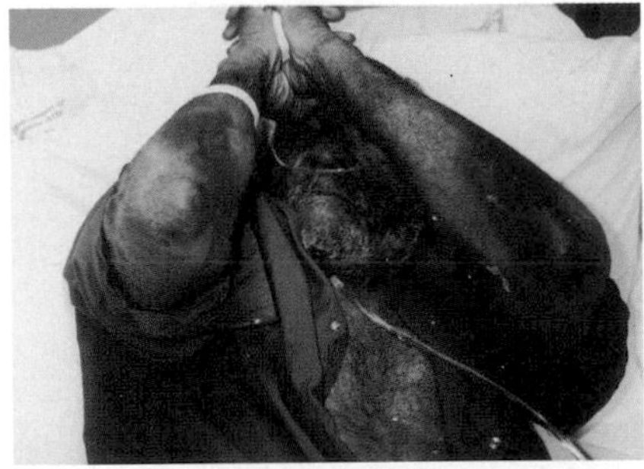

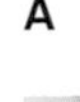

A

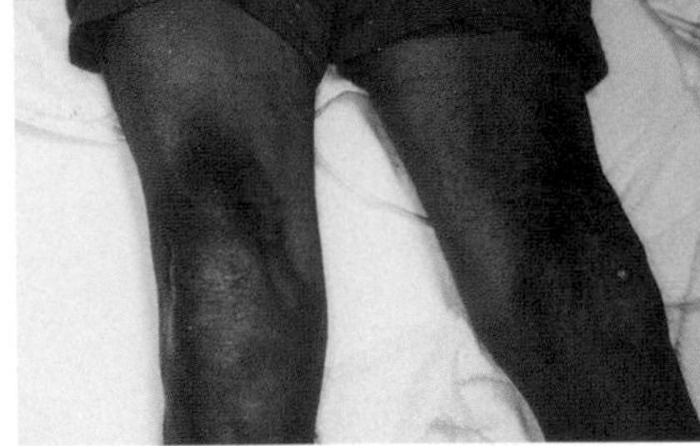

B

Figure 5.13.

Dahl's sign of chronic need to position oneself in Fowler's position. **A.** Elbows. **B.** Anterior thighs.

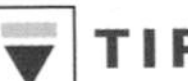

TIPS

- Inspect the skin of the elbows and thighs in a patient who has orthopnea
- Severe long-standing chronic heart failure (CHF) or chronic obstructive pulmonary disease (COPD): increased pigment on the elbows and the anterior thighs (Dahl's sign), which indicates chronicity

TEACHING POINTS

PLEURITIC CHEST PAIN PHYSICAL EXAMINATION

1. Always include chest wall examination as a component of pleuritic chest pain.
2. The company thromboembolic disease keeps is lower or rarer, upper extremity proximal deep venous thrombosis.
3. There are few physical findings of PTE, unless it is severe.
4. Pneumothorax has few easily detected physical findings until significant.
5. The findings of tracheal deviation and tympany to percussion throughout the opposite lung field are consistent, if not diagnostic, of a severe pneumothorax.

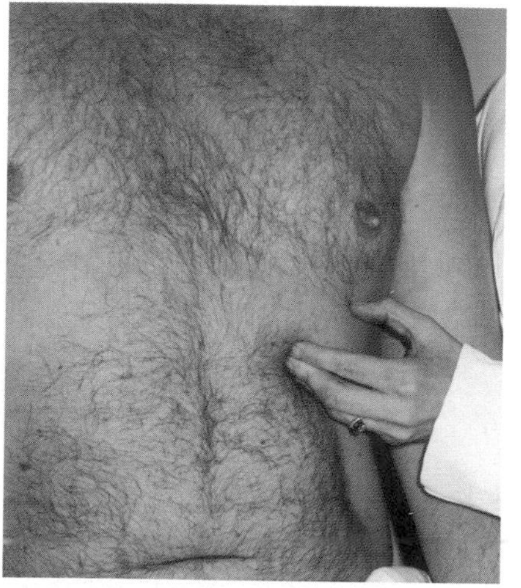

Figure 5.14.

Technique for hooking maneuver for rib-tip syndrome.

TIPS

- With patient sitting or standing, hook fingers beneath the lower margins of rib 10 anteriorly
- Apply gentle pulling force on the rib
- Described by Semble and Wise
- Rib-tip syndrome: reproducible or exacerbation of the pain and tenderness

PLEURITIC CHEST PAIN (Table 5.13)

Pulmonary thromboembolic disease (PTE) manifests with mild tachycardia and modest tachypnea; the company it keeps is a concurrent or antecedent swollen arm or leg caused by deep venous thrombosis. In severe disease, right-sided heart failure occurs, which manifests with the classic features described by Gorham in 1961: the second sound from pulmonic valve (P_2) is louder than the second sound from the aortic valve (A_2); a pleural rub in the pulmonic area; a systolic murmur at the pulmonic area; an increased area of right-sided cardiac dullness; a marked increase in JVP, in which the neck veins are distended, even with the patient upright; a right-sided third sound gallop; and hepatomegaly. Often, hypotension and marked hypoxemia are present when disease is this severe. **Pneumonia** manifests with cough productive of yellow, rusty, or gelatinous sputa; on auscultation, late inspiratory rales are heard over the area; breath sounds are present, bronchial in nature, and may have an associated rhonchus or wheeze, and egophony over the area. **Pneumothorax** manifests with unilateral pleuritic chest pain, diminished breath sounds, and tympany on the affected side, and deviation of the trachea to the opposite side. A tracheal deviation makes tension pneumothorax a likely diagnosis. **Rib fracture** manifests with point tenderness, ecchymosis, swelling,

Table 5.13. Chest Wall Problems

Diagnosis	Site of Tenderness	Company it Keeps
Leukemic infiltration	Sternum itself	Leukocytosis Fatigue, pale mucous membranes and nailbeds
Costal chondritis (Tietze's syndrome)	Costosternal junctions	
Xiphoiditis	Xiphoid process	
Rib fracture	Specific rib site	Ecchymosis Pneumothorax Crepitus
Rib-tip syndrome	Anterior medial tenth rib	Pain with hooking maneuver

TEACHING POINTS

IMPENDING RESPIRATORY FAILURE PHYSICAL EXAMINATION

1. Always remember ABCs of basic and advanced life support.
2. Always assess for tracheal deviation, which is a very important clue.
3. Inspiratory sounds suggest stridor, which is an upper airway complication.
4. Expiratory sounds suggest wheezes, which is a lower airway complication.
5. Assess position of patient; orthopnea is helpful in diagnosis.

and pleuritic chest pain; the complication of pneumothorax or subcutaneous emphysema with crepitus may be present. **Tietze's syndrome** manifests with tenderness in the costochondral junction(s) adjacent to the sternum. Due to inflammation of costochondral joints. **Leukemic infiltration** of the sternum manifests with deep-seated tenderness in the body of the sternum. The company it keeps includes acute lymphoblastic leukemia (ALL) or acute myeloid leukemia (AML). **Rib-tip syndrome**, as described by Semble and Wise, manifests with a positive hooking maneuver and tenderness on anterior tenth rib **(Fig. 5.14)**. For this examination, with the patient sitting or standing, hook the fingers beneath the margin of the lowest rib (10) anteriorly. Gently apply outward traction of the rib. Due to abnormal mobilization of the false ribs. **Acute chest, as a sickle-cell crisis**, manifests with severe pleuritic chest pain, tachypnea, tachycardia, and features not dissimilar from a PTE. This is seen in a patient with sickle cell (SS) anemia.

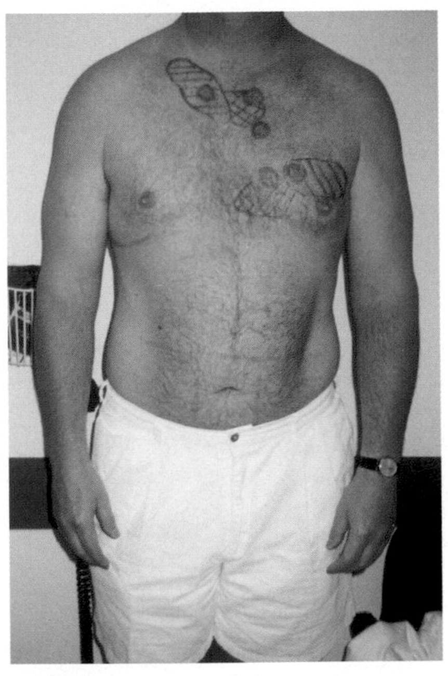

Figure 5.15.

Technique to assess abdominal muscles in respiration.

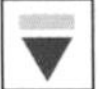

TIPS

- Examine with patient erect; note the movement of the abdomen with normal respiratory efforts
- *Normal:* abdominal wall outward during inspiration, inward during expiration
- *Severe COPD or abdomen*: abdomen retracts during inspiration as it is needed to inhale (Macklem respiratory paradox).
- *Diaphragmatic weakness*: normal pattern in the morning; abdomen retracts in the afternoon during inspiration (Macklem respiratory alternans)

IMPENDING RESPIRATORY FAILURE

Nonspecific markers for impending respiratory failure include cyanosis of the fingernails and mucous membranes, which are caused by an increase in deoxyhemoglobin. There is also a marked decreased in level of consciousness or a confusional state, i.e., delirium. These are caused by an increase in the CO_2 in the blood (i.e., also called CO_2 narcosis). As the symptoms worsen, there is less shortness of breath and a decrease in respiratory effort, with fatigue of the diaphragm, also called "respiratory alternans"; and periods of apnea. To assess for **respiratory alternans**, Macklem and colleagues recommend the following procedure **(Fig. 5.15)**. With the patient standing erect, if possible, but may perform sitting or supine, and breathing normally, inspect the abdomen for movements with respiration. In the normal setting, the abdomen moves outward with expiration, inward with expiration. In severe COPD, the opposite occurs: it retracts during inspiration, which Macklem calls a "**respiratory paradox**." In weakness to the diaphragm because of phrenic nerve problem or proximal muscle weakness, the pattern is normal during the morning, but by afternoon, the muscles have tired to retract during inspiration; this, too, Macklem calls respiratory alternans. This was a manifestation of poliomyelitis that indicated potential respiratory com-

Table 5.14. Overall Description of Pulmonary Problems with Fremitus, Percussion, and Auscultation

Mischief	Percussion	Fremitus	Auscultation	Company it Keeps
Consolidation, with open airways	Dull	Increased	Increased	Productive cough Egophony throughout area of dullness
Consolidation, with closed airways	Dull	Decreased	Decreased	Nonproductive cough Minimal egophony
Pneumonectomy	Dull	Decreased to absent	Decreased to absent	Surgical scar No egophony
Pleural effusion	Dull	Decreased	Decreased	Trepopnea Egophony of superior surface of dullness
Asthma, mild	Nonspecific	Nonspecific	Diffuse wheezes	
Asthma, severe	Nonspecific	Nonspecific Remarkable absence of breath sounds	Diminished Minimal wheezes, little airflow Cyanosis	Intercostal retractions Decreased mentation due to CO_2 narcosis Use of sternocleidomastoid muscles
Bronchiectasis	Dull	Marked increase	Marked increase	Chronic productive cough
Bronchitis	Nonspecific	Nonspecific	Rhonchi Wheezes Both diffuse	Productive cough
Chronic bronchitis	Nonspecific	Nonspecific	Rhonchi Wheezes Both diffuse	Chronic productive cough If cor pulmonale: S_3 gallop Cyanosis Clubbing Peripheral edema
Pneumothorax	Tympany	Decreased	Decreased	Small, minimal findings Large, classic unilateral findings Tension, deviation of trachea away from side of pneumothorax
Emphysema	Tympany, diffuse	Decreased, diffuse	Decreased, diffuse	Decreased sensitivity for other adventitious sound findings Inferior placed diaphragms, minimal excuration Increased anteroposterior diameter of chest
Interstitial lung disease	Nonspecific	Nonspecific	Diffuse crackles	Clubbing Nonproductive cough Restrictive disease, if chronic
Restrictive lung disease	Nonspecific	Nonspecific	Nonspecific	Markedly decreases sensitivity of findings As restriction always trumps obstruction Thus, if wheezes, rhonchi or crackles, very meaningful and probably bespeak pathology
Pulmonary edema	Nonspecific	Nonspecific	Bilateral lower zone Crackles	May have findings of concurrent pleural effusion
Situs inversus	Dullness right, anterior	Decreased right, anterior	Decreased right, anterior	Recurrent pneumonias
Cardiomegaly	Dullness left, anterior	Decreased left, anterior	Decreased left, anterior	Gallop, S_3/S_4 Peripheral edema Increased JVP

JVP = jugular venous pressure.

promise. Finally, Macklem and colleagues have demonstrated that the use of accessory muscles for breathing is a marker for severe COPD with an FEV_1 of <1 to 1.5 L.

Severe asthma manifests with shortness of breath and a cough that is usually nonproductive. On auscultation, is noted diffuse inspiratory and expiratory wheezes and midinspiratory crackles. When very severe, there is a remarkable paucity of wheezes because of the marked decrease in air movement. **Severe congestive heart failure** manifests with dyspnea, orthopnea in Fowler's position, paroxysmal nocturnal dyspnea (PND), diffuse crackles at the bases more than upper fields, a third sound gallop, neck vein distension, and Cheyne-Stokes pattern. **Upper airway obstruction** manifests with diffusely diminished breath sounds in all lung fields; breath sounds are vesicular in nature. A prolonged expiratory phase and inspiratory stridor are noted. The head position is one of "sniffing the flowers." The stridor, which is not only present on auscultation, usually presents throughout inspiration. There may be accentuated intercostal retractions with inspiration, which are caused by angioedema, epiglottitis, Ludwig's angina, or an inhaled foreign body. **Pneumothorax** manifests with locally diminished breath sounds; there may be a rub over the area. Tympany is noted over the area as is decreased tactile fremitus. Company it keeps includes, if a tension pneumothorax, the trachea is deviated toward and pushed to the other side. Also, there may be hypotension and sudden cardiac death. This is caused by the entry of air into the pleural space because of trauma. The air can be from the bronchi or the skin. A tension pneumothorax is progressive and, without intervention, a mortal event. **Massive pleural effusion** manifests with tracheal deviation to the opposite side, orthopnea and trepopnea, dullness to percussion with diminished breath sounds and decreased tactile fremitus, focal expiratory bulging, and inspiratory retraction **(Table 5.14)**.

Annotated Bibliography

American Thoracic Society ad hoc Committee on Pulmonary Nomenclature. Updated nomenclature for membership reaction. *ATS News* 1977;Fall:3:5–6.

A report of the new definitions discussed in the Loudon and Murphy paper cited below.

Bradding P, Cookson JB. The dos and don'ts of examining the respiratory system: a survey of British Thoracic Society members. *JR Soc Med* 1999;92:632–634.

A survey of 403 senior members of the British Thoracic Society was used to query them on how they teach the respiratory examination. Of these, 95% taught tracheal deviation, 98% taught chest expansion; only 26% routinely taught tactile fremitus.

Cohen MH. Signs and symptoms of bronchogenic carcinoma. *Semin Oncol* 1974;1(3): 183–188.

An excellent review of the clinical manifestations of non–small-cell and small-cell carcinoma of the lung. The local, metastatic, and paraneoplastic manifestations are covered, including postobstructive pneumonia, Horner's syndrome, superior vena cava syndrome, migratory thrombophlebitis, hypertrophic osteoarthropathy (12% of adenocarcinoma), peripheral neuropathies, encephalopathy, and carcinomatous meningitis. Designed as an overview for the primary care provider.

Crump HW. Pectus excavatum. *Am Fam Phys* 1992;46(1):173–179.

A robust review of the manifestations, associated conditions, and surgical management of this not uncommon congenital chest anomaly.

Dock W. Examination of the chest: advantages of conducting and reporting it in English. *Bull NY Acad Med* 1973;49:575–582.

Discusses the etymology of the statement "99" for tactile fremitus—a derivative of the German 99, which has the "ooing" diphthong. The 99 was Americanized in late nineteenth and early twentieth centuries. Overall, "oing" is better than saying 99 for the test.

Fletcher CM. The clinical diagnosis of pulmonary emphysema-an experimental study. *Proc R Soc Med* 1952;45:577–584.

Restriction is present if chest wall expansion is <1.5 inches.

Forgacs P. Lung sounds. ***Br J Dis Chest*** **1969;63:1–12.**

Tremendous wealth of auscultatory findings and some theories on their pathophysiologic underpinnings. Discusses findings in upper airway compromise: breath sounds that are diffusely diminished, vesicular, prolonged expiratory phase, and inspiratory (usually holoinspiratory) stridor. Also states that rales that migrate downward when patient sits up are caused by congestive heart failure (CHF).

Fries JF. The reactive enthesopathies. ***Dis Mon DM*** **1985;31:1–46.**

Reports on the importance of measuring chest wall expansion. If <2.5 cm difference, consistent with restriction; normal is approximately 5 cm. This should be performed in all patients with ankylosis spondylitis.

Gennis P, Gallagher J, Falvo C, et al. Clinical criteria for the detection of pneumonia in adults: guidelines for ordering chest radiographs in the emergency room. ***J Emerg Med*** **1989;7:263–268.**

Determined the likelihood ratios for various physical examination findings: heart rate (HR) >120; positive LR, 1.9; negative LR, 0.89; temperature >37.8; positive LR, 1.4; negative LR, 0.63; dullness to percussion: positive LR, 2.2; negative LR, 0.93; decreased breath sounds: positive LR, 2.3; negative LR, 0.78; egophony: positive LR, 2.0; negative LR, 0.96.

Gorham LW. A study of pulmonary embolism. Part 1. A clinicopathological investigation of 100 cases of massive embolism of the pulmonary artery: Diagnosis by physical signs and differentiation from acute myocardial infarction. ***Arch Intern Med*** **1961;108:8–22.**

Relates the physical diagnosis features of very severe, in these cases, lethal pulmonary emboli. Study performed when no effective therapy was available for this devastating disorder. Relates the classic findings taught today, include P_2 louder than A_2, a pleural rub in the pulmonic area, a systolic murmur at the pulmonic area, an increased area of right-sided cardiac dullness, distended neck veins with the patient upright, a right-sided third sound gallop, and hepatomegaly.

Hackerling PS, Tape TG, Wigton RS, et al. Clinical prediction rules for pulmonary infiltrates. ***Ann Intern Med*** **1990;113:664–670.**

Determined likelihood ratios of various physical examination findings: HR, >100; positive LR, 2.3; negative LR, 0.49; temperature >37.8; positive LR, 2.4; negative LR, 0.58; dullness to percussion: positive LR, 4.3; negative LR, 0.79; decreased breath sounds: positive LR, 2; negative LR, 0.64; egophony: positive LR, 5.3; negative LR, 0.76.

Hamman L. Spontaneous mediastinal emphysema. ***Bull Johns Hopkins Hosp*** **1939;64:1–21.**

A classic description of the mediastinal crunch.

Laennec RTH. Treatise on the diseases of the chest. Translated by JT Forbes and C Underwood, London, 1821. Republished under the auspices of the Library of the New York Academy of Medicine. New York: Hafner Publishing Co., 1962.

The classic by the father of auscultation, but, alas, a difficult paper to read.

Loudon R, Murphy RLH. Lung sounds. ***American Review of Respiratory Diseases*** **1984; 130:663–673.**

A tremendous resource and reference. This paper makes sense of a confusing topic—describing breath sounds. They used data from the American Thoracic Society, the Committee of the International Lung Sounds Association, and Laennec himself. Reviews the history of these and fact that crackles replaced rales as a term recently.

Reviews the pathophysiology and mechanism of each of theses sounds in addition to vesicular and bronchial breath sounds. The references are a veritable gold mine of data for research and to include in teaching. A must for all students and teachers of clinical skills.

Macklem PT. The diaphragm in health and disease. ***J Lab Clin Med*** **1982;99:601–610.**

Excellent paper regarding function and exam of the diaphragm.

Macklem PT. Respiratory muscle dysfunction. ***Hosp Practice*** **1986;21:83–95.**

Nice overview of neuromuscular cause of respiratory failure.

McFadden ER Jr, Kiser R, de Groot WJ. Acute bronchial asthma: relations between clinical and physiologic manifestations. ***N Engl J Med*** **1973;288:221–225.**

In severe COPD, the use of the sternocleidomastoids and their hypertrophy; correlates with a severely embarrassed FEV_1 of 1.0 to 1.5 L.

McGee SR. Percussion and physical diagnosis: separating myth from science. ***Disease a Month*** **1995;41(10):641–692.**

Very robust and scholarly review of percussion. Uses extant data to develop a set of recommendations on which components of percussion are clinically useful. Dr. McGee concludes that percussion is useful in diagnosing pleural effusions and ascites, but only of limited utility in percussing the size of solid organs (heart, liver). He comes out strongly in opposition to auscultatory percussion. Reviews that the interobserver variation is high to percussion interpretation to dull, normal, and tympany.

Metlay JP, Kapoor WN, Fine MJ. Does this patient have community-acquired pneumonia? ***JAMA*** **1997;278(17):1440–1445.**

Reviews the papers to date regarding the diagnosis of pneumonia; based on this review, no significant conclusions were made regarding the physical examination. Nice review of the papers, although the interobserver variation is so poor and the physical examination is of less than robust utility to make this common diagnosis. My bias is that we need to train and make the diagnosticians better at these techniques.

Morgan WC, Hodge HL. Diagnostic evaluation of dyspnea. *Am Fam Phys* 1998;57(4): 711–716.

Basic overview paper for the primary care provider. A fair description of the associated symptoms and concurrent signs. A good overview of the causes and primary care evaluation of a patient with dyspnea.

Nath AR, Capel LH. Inspiratory crackles-early and late. *Thorax* 1974;29:223–227.

Early inspiratory rales occur in asthma or COPD when the FEV_1/FVC is <44%.

Philip EB. Chronic cough. *Am Fam Phys* 1997;56:1395–1402.

Primary care overview of common and rare causes of chronic cough and a well thought-out evaluation paradigm is included. Historic questions are robust, including history of smoking, postnasal drip, asthma, GERD, and use of medications like angiotensin-converting enzyme (ACE) inhibitors. Highly satisfactory paper, even with its limited physical examination discussion.

Ravitch MM. The operative treatment of pectus excavatum. *Ann Surg* 1949;129:429–436.

The five findings of pectus excavatum: depressed sternum, rounded shoulders, dorsal kyphosis, prominent potbelly, and retraction of sternum with deep inspiration.

Sapira JD. *The Art and Science of Bedside Diagnosis.* Baltimore: Williams & Wilkins, 1990.

The pulmonary chapter contains a nice discussion on egophony (E to a changes).

Schapira RM, Reinke LF. The outpatient diagnosis and management of chronic obstructive pulmonary disease. *J Gen Intern Med* 1995;10:40–45.

Nice review of the pathophysiology, manifestations, and therapy of this common disease process. Reports the forced expiratory time as measured over the trachea is a good clinical marker of COPD: a forced expiratory time (FET) of >6 seconds has a sensitivity of 74% and specificity of 75%.

Schapira RM, Schapira MM, Funahashi A, et al. The value of the forced expiratory time in the physical diagnosis of obstructive airways disease. *JAMA* 1993;270:731–736.

Reports the forced expiratory time, as measured over the trachea, is a good clinical marker of COPD; a FET of >6 seconds has a sensitivity of 74% and specificity of 75%.

Semble EL, Wise CM. Chest pain: a rheumatologists perspective. *South Med J* 1988;81: 64–68.

Nice description of the rib-tip syndrome as a cause of anterior musculoskeletal chest pain.

Shim CS, Williams H Jr. Relationship of wheezing to the severity of obstruction in asthma. *Arch Intern Med* 1982;143:890–892.

Excellent discussion of the physical examination findings of asthma and reactive airways: presence of diffusely diminished, vesicular, prolonged expiratory phase, expiratory wheezes, and, at times, expiratory stridor sounds. Also makes the points that, as the airway disease increases in severity, the wheezes become inspiratory and expiratory, and is associated with early inspiratory rales. In severe asthma are noted diffusely diminished breath sounds, and then a paucity of wheezes—a particularly ominous sign.

Skoda J. Treatise on percussion and auscultation. Vienna: JG Ritter, 1839.

This great Czech physician has described a classic, but paradoxic, feature of a pleural effusion: dullness throughout, but, with a rim of hyperresonance at top (Skodaic resonance).

Spiteri MA, Cook DG, Clarke SW. Reliability of eliciting physical signs in examination of the chest. *Lancet* 1988;1:873–875.

Reliability of various physical examination findings of the chest, using 24 physicians and 24 patients. Kappa for the techniques included wheezes: 0.51; dullness to percussion, 0.52; crackles: 0.41; decreased breath sounds: 0.43; and bronchial breath sounds: 0.32.

Stein PD. Prospective Investigation of Pulmonary embolism diagnosis (PIOPED).

Signs of PTE: tachypnea: 73%; rales: 55%; tachycardia: 30%; dyspnea: 78%; pleuritic pain: 59%; and cough: 43%. Further delineates that this can be a vexing problem to diagnose on physical examination alone.

Wynder EL, Graham EA. Tobacco smoking as a possible etiologic factor in bronchogenic carcinoma. *JAMA* 1950;143:329–336.

One of the first studies in the United States that conclusively linked smoking with a disease, which was (and is) epidemic—lung cancer. Fascinating, in that categories of smoking included the terms moderate, heavy, excessive, and the highest category—chain. Also concluded from their data that adenocarcinoma was found in nonsmokers. Study included only men, barely commenting on the disease in women.

6

Abdominal Examination

PRACTICE AND TEACHING

ANATOMY

To define and describe the abdominal examination, it is important to review and utilize paradigms for the surface anatomy of the abdomen **(Fig. 6.1)**. These paradigms allow the clinician to optimize the examination and teaching and, by applying knowledge of anatomy, find a reasonable differential diagnosis for problems at various sites. Specific lines used in the examination of the abdomen include the **midclavicular lines.** Each is a longitudinal line through the midclavicle. This is particularly important on the right (Fig. 6.1B) as a marker for the liver and gallbladder. In addition, the **anterior axillary lines**, each of which is a longitudinal line through the acromioclavicular joint, is particularly important on the left (Fig. 6.1A) as a marker for the spleen. Further lines include the **subcostal** margins, which are the inferior arcs over the lower ribs, these are useful in gallbladder and spleen examination. **Murphy's point** is the intersection of the right midclavicular line and the right subcostal margin. This is the site of the gallbladder. The **inguinal ligaments** extend from the anterior superior iliac spine to the pubis symphysis. In addition, **McBurney's point** and **McBurney's line** (Fig. 6.1D) are very important markers. The point is 1.5 to 2 inches or three finger breadths medial to the anterior superior iliac spine (ASIS) on a straight line between the umbilicus and the ASIS. This very specific point, according to McBurney, is useful in the diagnosis of acute appendicitis. Finally, **Hesselbach's triangle** (Fig. 6.1E) is formed by, at its base: inguinal ligament; medial border: linea alba; and, superior border: the inferior epigastric artery. This is the site of direct inguinal hernias.

In addition, a grid is useful in mapping the surface of the abdomen **(Fig. 6.2)**. A grid that is mapped using ones mind's eye complements the lines and points described above. The grid can be of the four quadrants or of nine squares on the abdominal surface or a combination of the two. Either grid pattern is useful and each has advantages and disadvantages. As neither grid system is vastly superior to the other, we choose to use and teach a combination of the two grids, the four quadrants, and the three midline squares: epigastric area, periumbilical area, and suprapubic area; we call this the "**4 plus 3" grid** system (see **Table 6.1**). The four quadrants are the **left upper**, which contains the spleen, part of the transverse colon, left kidney, and pancreas; the **right upper**, which contains the liver, gallbladder, right kidney, and part

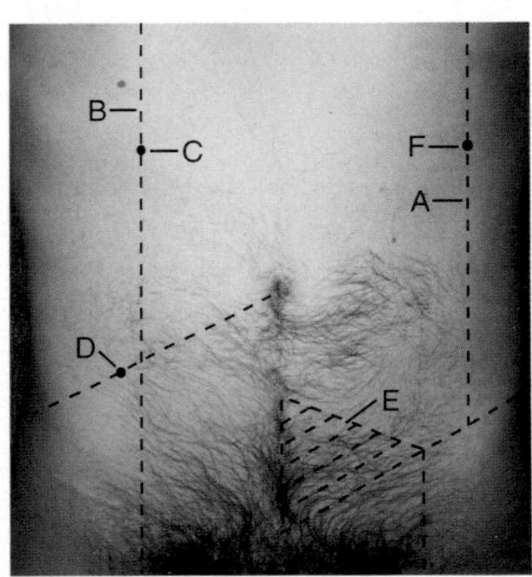

Figure 6.1.

Surface anatomy-abdomen. **A.** Left anterior axillary line. **B.** Right midclavicular line. **C.** Murphy's point. **D.** McBurney's line and point. **E.** Hesselbach's triangle. **F.** Castell's point.

TIPS

- Left anterior axillary line: important in the assessment of the spleen
- Right midclavicular line: important in the assessment of the liver and the gallbladder
- McBurney's line and McBurney's point: important in assessment of appendicitis
- Murphy's point: important in assessment of gallbladder
- Hesselbach's triangle: site of direct inguinal hernias

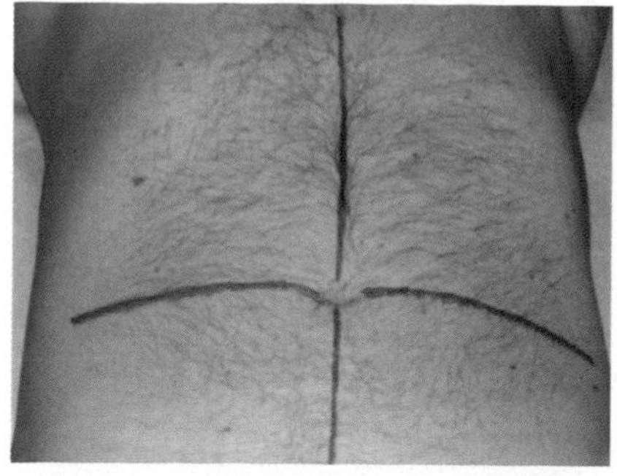

A

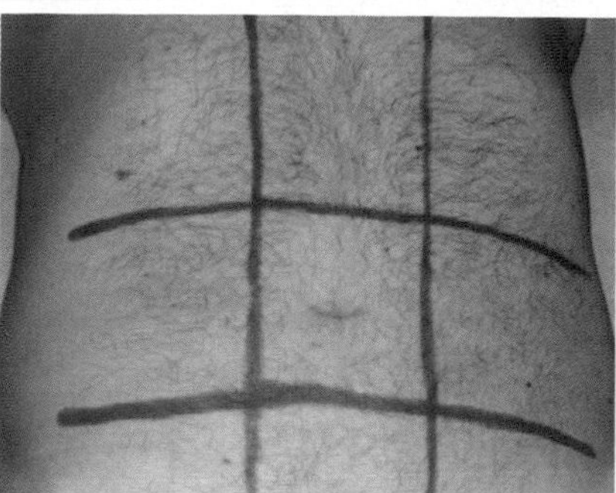

B

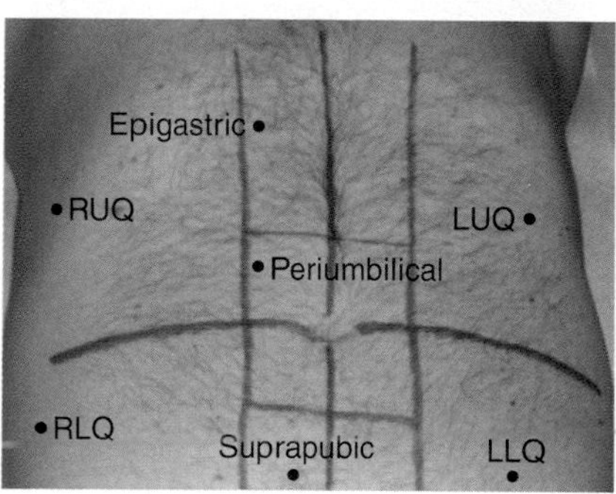

C

Figure 6.2.

Surface anatomy grids. **A.** Four quadrants. **B.** Nine squares. **C.** The 4 plus 3 pattern.

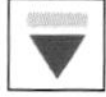

TIPS

- Grid patterns are useful to define, describe, and begin to diagnose abdominal complications
- Four quadrants: right upper, left upper, right lower, left lower
- Nine squares
- "4 plus 3" grid: the four quadrants and three squares in midline (epigastric, periumbilical, and suprapubic)

Table 6.1. Abdominal Structures in the "4 Plus 3" Grid

Grid	Abdominal structures	Potential diagnoses
Right upper	Gallbladder	Cholecystitis
	Liver	Hepatomegaly
		Hepatitis
	Kidney	Pyelonephritis
Epigastric	Stomach	Gastritis
		Peptic ulcer disease
	Pancreas	Pancreatitis
	Esophagus	Esophagitis
Left upper	Spleen	Splenic rupture
		Splenomegaly
	Kidney	Pyelonephritis
Periumbilical	Small intestine	First site for acute appendicitis
Right lower	Appendix	Second site for appendicitis
	Ascending colon	Diverticulitis
	Ureter	Nephrolithiasis
		Pyelonephritis
	Fallopian tube	PID
		Ectopic pregnancy
Suprapubic	Urinary bladder	Cystitis
		Bladder distention
	Uterus	Pregnancy
Left lower	Descending colon	Diverticulitis
	Ureter	Nephrolithiasis
		Pyelonephritis
	Fallopian tube	PIP
		Ectopic pregnancy

PID = Pelvic Inflammatory Disease.

of the transverse colon; the **right lower**, which contains the appendix, the ascending colon, the right ureter, and the right Fallopian tube; and the **left lower** quadrant, which contains the descending colon, left ureter, and left fallopian tube. The **epigastric** area contains the distal esophagus, and the stomach. The **periumbilical area**, which contains the small intestine, is a

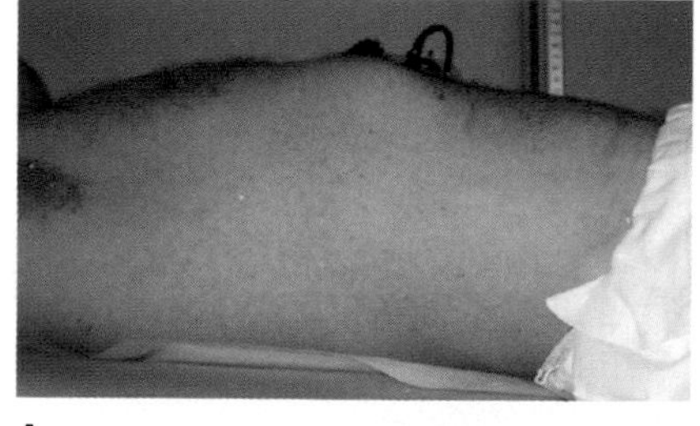

A

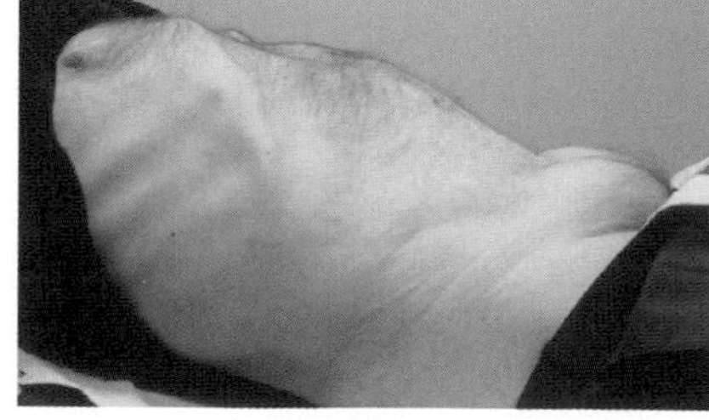

B

Figure 6.3.

Technique to inspect the abdomen. **A.** Normal. **B.** Patient with a distended urinary bladder.

TIPS

- Patient supine, relaxed: visually inspect entire abdomen, make note of skin, umbilicus, overall configuration
- Hips forward flexed to 45 degrees, knees flexed to 90 degrees; assist the patient in relaxing the abdominal wall
- Scaphoid abdomen: sunken in relative to the chest
- Enlarged abdomen: nonspecific increase in size

TEACHING POINTS

SURFACE ANATOMY

1. The lines and grid patterns are useful to define, delineate, and describe the site of complications.
2. The grid pattern provides a paradigm complementary to the classic lines and points in the examination.
3. This is a great application of anatomy applied to clinical medicine.
4. It is useful to know the potential problems associated with each of the quadrants and squares.

site where the pain associated with appendicitis commences. The **suprapubic area** contains the urinary bladder and the uterus.

ABDOMEN EXAMINATION

For the overall examination of the abdomen, with the patient supine, inspect the **abdomen** and assess it from the side and front **(Fig. 6.3)**. Obviously, the patient's abdomen must not be covered with clothing or linen. Assess the size of the abdomen, and the presence of any discernible ecchymoses, masses, or any abnormal venous pattern **(Table 6.2)**. Normal veins in the abdominal wall are often not visible and, if visible, not prominent in the skin.

Table 6.2. Diagnoses Found in the Abdominal Wall

Diagnosis	Abdominal wall finding	Company it Keeps
IVC obstruction	Distended venous collaterals Lateral to umbilicus Upward flow for all	Lower extremity edema Scrotal or vulvar edema
Portal hypertension	Distended venous collaterals Flow radiates from the umbilicus Flow above umbilicus: upward Flow below umbilicus: downward	Ascites Internal hemorrhoids Small liver ESLD
Retroperitoneal bleed	Grey Turner's sign Cullen's sign Back pain	Hypotension Anemia Hypocoagulable state Pelvic or hip trauma
Subcutaneous heparin use	Sites of ecchymosis No skin atrophy	Indication for heparin
Subcutaneous insulin use	Sites of ecchymosis Sites of skin atrophy	Diabetes mellitus
Sister Mary Joseph's	Nodule in umbilicus Secondary ulceration of nodule	Weight loss Early satiety Painless jaundice Hard node of Troisier/enlarged node of Virchow
Rectus Sheath hematoma	Tender mass in rectus Ecchymosis Cullen's sign	Trauma Tender increases with active forward flexion Tender increases with passive backward flexion

ESLD = End Stage Liver Disease; IVC = inferior vena cava.

Collateral veins from portal hypertension manifest with one or more dilated, often serpiginous-appearing veins above and below the umbilicus (Fig. 6.28B). Of interest, but of little clinical importance, is that when compressing a segment of these veins, those located above the umbilicus flow upward and those located below the umbilicus flow downward. The specific pattern of veins can appear to be radiating and, in fact, flowing from the umbilicus, analogous to the mythologic head of Medusa from which snakes radiated. Hence, the term, **Caput medusae** is an apt descriptor. The company it keeps includes manifestations of end-stage liver disease (see discussion later). **Collateral veins from inferior vena cava (IVC) obstruction** manifest with dilated veins that are predominantly in the lateral abdominal wall. On vessel compression, flow is almost always in the upward direction. The company it keeps includes bilateral lower extremity edema and significant scrotal, penile, or vulvar edema. IVC obstruction is most commonly caused by tumor or massive lymphadenopathy in the abdomen or pelvis or from the placement of an IVC filter. **Retroperitoneal bleed** manifests with the patient complaining of significant low back discomfort. Often, a history of trauma or use of an anticoagulant, e.g., warfarin is reported. Often, an ecchymosis is present on the flank (Grey Turner sign), (Fig. 14.19), either unilateral or bilateral, or on or near the umbilicus (Cullen's sign). The company it keeps is specific to the sequela. This includes manifestations specific to blood loss, which includes pale nail beds and mucous membranes, syncope, hypotension, and tachycardia. **Sister Mary Joseph's sign** manifests with a nodule that may secondarily ulcerate in or near the umbilicus. The company it keeps includes significant unintentional weight loss, early satiety, and a palpable hard, fixed node in the left supraclavicular fossa, that is the node of Troisier (Fig. 9.24). This usually results from metastases from a pancreatic or gastric carcinoma. Use of **subcutaneous heparin** in the abdominal skin manifests with multiple small sites of ecchymosis, each with a small puncture site; subcutaneous **insulin** use manifests with multiple small sites of ecchymosis and skin adipose atrophy at each site of injection. **Rectus Sheath hematoma** manifests with acute onset of tender mass in abdominus rectus muscle. The company it keeps includes an increase in pain with active forward flexion of trunk and with passive backward flexion of trunk. This is due to blunt trauma or severe trunk-stretching.

Incisional scars manifest as healed suture sites for specific procedures (**Table 6.3** and **Fig. 6.4**). These are powerful clues to confirm or complement the history given by the patient. A **Pfannenstiel** incisional scar (Fig. 6.4A) manifests in the suprapubic area, parallel to the pubis. It indicates a cesarean section or abdominal hysterectomy. A **subcostal** incisional scar manifests beneath the costal margin on the left or right (Fig. 6.4B and C). One on the left is consistent with a splenectomy; if on the right, it is consistent with a cholecys-

Table 6.3. Scars and Their Meaning

Scar	Site	Potential meaning
Pfannenstiel	Suprapubic	Abdominal hysterectomy Cesarean section
Right subcostal	Subcostal	Cholecystectomy
Left subcostal	Subcostal	Splenectomy
Midline	Linea alba	Vascular procedure Bowel resection Gastric resection
Right lower quadrant	Right lower quadrant	Appendectomy
Inguinal	Above and parallel to inguinal ligament	Inguinal herniorrhaphy
Periumbilical	Small, about umbilicus	Laparoscopy

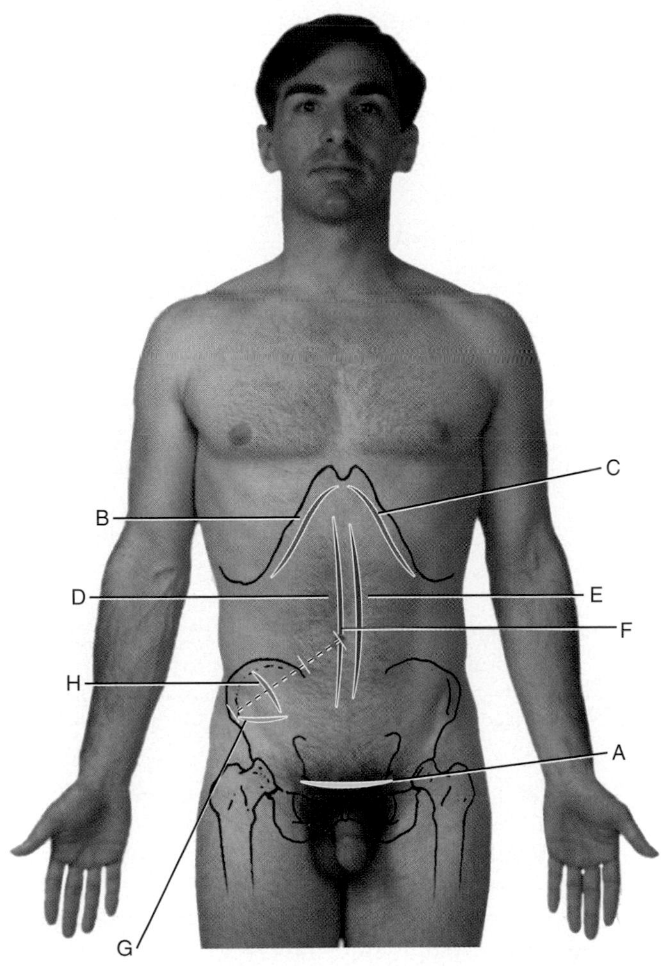

Figure 6.4.

Types and locations of various incisional surgical scars. **A.** Pfannenstiel. **B.** Right subcostal. **C.** Left subcostal. **D.** Midline abdominal. **E.** Left paramedian. **F.** Periumbilical. **G.** Inguinal, **H.** Appendix (From Moore KL, Dalley AF. *Clinically Oriented Anatomy*, 4th ed. Philadelphia: Lippincott Williams & Wilkins, 1999:190, with permission.)

TIPS

- Patient supine or erect: visually inspect the skin for scars and their location
- Excellent data derived

tectomy. A **midline** incisional scar is consistent with colon, gastric, or small bowel resection, or with a vascular surgical procedure. A **right** lower quadrant incisional scar, over McBurney's line is consistent with an appendectomy. Furthermore, a left or right **inguinal** scar (Fig. 6.4G), parallel to the inguinal ligament, is consistent with a herniorrhaphy. A small **periumbilical** incisional scar is consistent with an umbilical herniorrhaphy or today, more commonly, laparoscopic surgery.

These scars give significant clues and provide a foundation for the patient's history. In addition, these are sites of potential **incisional hernia**, which manifests with a palpable and even visible mass (Fig. 6.12) or nodule associated with the scar. This is often a palpable defect in the fascia underlying the scar, and the mass increases in size or develops with cough or Valsalva's maneuver. Furthermore, if a mass or nodule is seen adjacent to the scar, consider and teach that incisional hernia is in the differential diagnosis. Finally, look for the rashes of pigment changes affiliated with the scars themselves. Recall,

Table 6.4. **Findings on Auscultation**

Diagnosis	Findings	Company it Keeps
AAA	Epigastric bruit	Epigastric pulsatile mass Popliteal aneurysm Bruits in femoral and carotid arteries
Small bowel obstruction	High pitched (high C) Tinkling Rushes admixed with silence	Distention Tympany Diffuse tenderness
Ileus	Absent bowel sounds	Nonspecific Nonfocal Postsurgical
Renal arterial stenosis	Flank bruit	Hypertension Hypokalemia
Mesenteric angina	Epigastric bruit	Bruits over other arteries Postprandial pain
Third trimester pregnancy	Epigastric bruit (21%)	Gravid uterus Fetal heart tones
Hepatocellular carcinoma	Right upper quadrant bruit	Hepatomegaly Nodules

AAA = Abdominal Aortic Aneurysm.

rashes of **psoriasis** (Fig. 14.69) and **lichen planus** (Fig. 14.18) often develop in areas of scar, the process called Koebner's phenomenon. The loss of pigment in **vitiligo** also can manifest at a scar (Fig. 14.53) and **Addison's disease** can manifest with increased pigment at scars.

Auscultate the abdomen, with the patient in the same supine position, using the diaphragm of the stethoscope **(Table 6.4)**. Auscultate for a minimum of 30 seconds involving at least two of the four quadrants. Auscultation should precede palpation. This statement, however, has little scientific basis and, in our opinion, is more tradition than foundation. As there is no harm in teaching that auscultation should be performed first we follow the dictum of Thomas Jefferson (paraphrased here), "in matters of style go, with the flow." Note bowel sounds and, if bowel sounds are present and of normal quality, note and report as such. **Ileus** manifests with a marked decrease in quantity of bowel sounds. The abdomen is nonspecific in size and tenderness. The patient often reports a decrease in bowel movements, significant anorexia, nausea, and a marked decrease in flatus. This can be caused by complications involving the abdomen, including the postoperative period after virtually any abdominal surgery. Normal **hyperactive bowel sounds** manifest with a marked increase in bowel sounds, which may be so loud that they can be heard without a stethoscope; they are called **Borborygmi. Small bowel obstruction** manifests with a high-pitched bowel sound that is defined as higher than high C (the sound from a 512 Hz tuning fork). In addition to their distinct pitch, the sounds are tinkling in quality, have rushes i.e., the bowel sounds are accelerated to a rate three times normal, admixed with periods of silence for 10 to 20 minutes. During these silent periods, the patient has a marked increase in a cramp-type of abdominal discomfort. Furthermore, the abdomen is often tender and diffusely distended, with tympany to percussion throughout. **Renal arterial stenosis** manifests with a systolic or continuous bruit in the left or right upper quadrant. To auscultate the renal arteries, place the diaphragm of the stethoscope over the left and then right flank of the patient. Duration of auscultation, at minimum, should be 20 seconds on each side. Often, the company it keeps includes significant hypertension and concurrent hypokalemia are present. **Aortic artery atherosclerotic disease**, including aortic abdominal aneurysm and celiac arterial disease, manifests with epigastric bruit. **Aortic abdominal aneurysm** manifests with a bruit in the epigastric area and, potentially, a pulsatile mass palpable superior to the umbilicus. Lederle confirmed that the physical exam for AAA is of very limited clinical utility. **Mesenteric angina** manifests with postprandial cramping, periumbilical discomfort and a bruit over the epigastric area. This is caused by celiac artery atherosclerosis with resultant small intestine or large intestine ischemia. **Pregnancy—third trimester**—manifests with an epigastric bruit in addition to the obvious findings of an enlarged gravid uterus and fetal heart tones. McSherry relates a 21% prevalence of the finding in the third trimester. **Hepatocellular carcinoma** or metastatic carcinoma to liver manifests with a rub (with or without a bruit) in a nodular enlarged liver, which has been described by Sherman. Such a rub has a high specificity but low sensitivity.

Palpate the abdomen with the patient supine, relaxed, and with knees and hips flexed in an orderly manner in the "4 plus 3" specific sites. If the patient reports any subjective pain, start at the side and site opposite this pain. In **deep palpation**, use the fingers to probe, palpate, and feel the abdominal structures. The techniques include the **hooking technique (Fig. 6.5A)** in which the fingers are slightly flexed or the **pressing–mashing** technique **(Fig. 6.5B)** in which the fingers are fully and rigidly extended. For either technique, use a gentle, rotatory component to palpate to three levels: superficial, intermediate, and deep **(Fig. 6.5)**. We prefer the hooking maneuver because it is easier to teach and perform, and easier on the patient. In any site of direct tenderness, assess for rebound tenderness. For this technique, rapidly release from the deepest palpation position. On release, the presence of tenderness at the site is called "rebound tenderness" or Blumberg's sign. Rebound tenderness indicates irritation of the peritoneum in the tender area. **Involuntary guarding** manifests with a rigidity of the abdominal wall muscles, such that the abdomen is hard as a marble table. Although it is a rare finding in the United States today, it is virtually diagnostic of diffuse advanced peritonitis and defines an acute or surgical abdomen. Recall, a surgical abdomen is one that any delay in surgical intervention can lead to morbid or mortal outcome for the patient. It is a true emergency. If during palpation an undefined structure is localized, describe its presence, location, tenderness, and size. A **mass** is >4 cm in diameter; whereas, a **nodule** is <4 cm in diameter. **Appendicitis** manifests with pain in the periumbilical area with nausea and anorexia, followed by resolution for 6 hours, only to return with great intensity at McBurney's point for 24 to 36 hours. The pain then disseminates throughout the abdomen. Please see Table 6.9 and extensive description of appendicitis on page 149.

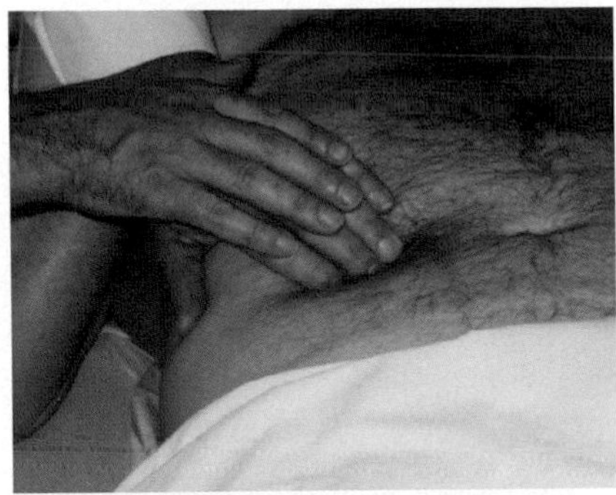

A

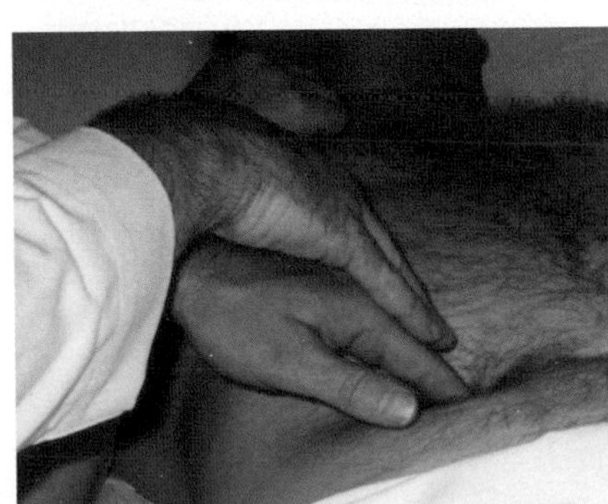

B

Figure 6.5.

Technique to palpate the abdomen. **A.** Hooking. **B.** Pressing. (We prefer the hooking technique.)

TIPS

- Patient supine, relaxed, knees and hips flexed: palpate the abdomen in an orderly manner involving nine specific sites; deep palpation using flexed fingers, the hooking technique **(A)**, or extended fingers; and the pressing technique **(B)** at three levels
- Perform rebound from the deepest direct palpation position
- If any subjective pain from outset, start at side opposite of pain site

Liver

Examination of the liver includes determining its size in the right midclavicular line via the **scratch test (Fig. 6.6)**. Perform the scratch test with the patient supine, relaxed, and with knees and hips flexed. Place the diaphragm of the stethoscope over the epigastrium, then use the index or third finger to gently scratch the skin. Perform the scratching in a reproducible manner by flicking the index or third finger, from a flexed to an extended position, as though flicking a grain of sand off the skin. Perform the scratch test procedure in the right midclavicular line from midchest into the lower abdomen. On auscultation, the scratch sound is much louder over the liver than above and below it. Normally, the sound is loudest in a span of 8 to 12 cm in the right midclavicular line. A *small liver* manifests with a scratch test in which no discernible difference in the scratch findings is noted; in *hepatomegaly*, the increased scratch is usually >14 cm and can actually extend into the pelvis in massive liver enlargement. The scratch test is an excellent first-line test for assessment

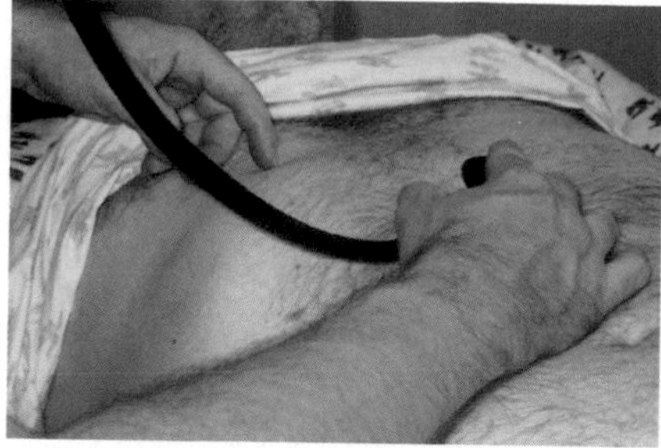

A

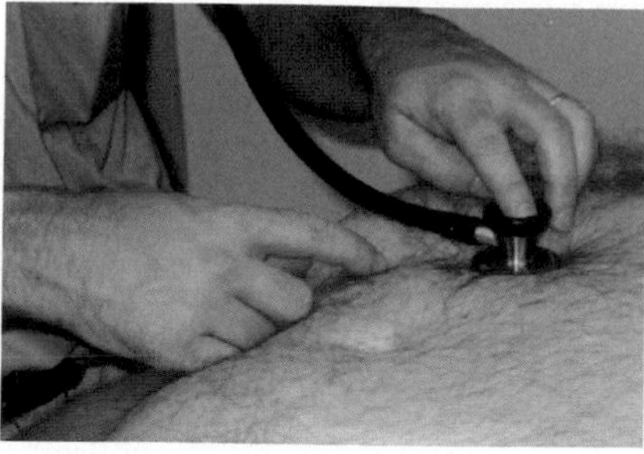

B

Figure 6.6.

Technique to scratch out the span of the liver in the right midclavicular line.

TIPS

- Patient supine, relaxed, knees and hips flexed: place the diaphragm of stethoscope over the epigastrium
- Use index finger to scratch skin; perform in a reproducible manner by flexing the digit
- Scratch in the midclavicular line from midchest into lower abdomen
- Patient breathing normally
- Normal: increased intensity of scratch sound over liver, 8 to 12 cm in the right midclavicular line
- Technique is best used to screen out upper and lower borders to further define upper border by percussion and lower border by palpation

of liver size and span because it sets the overall parameters and causes little if any discomfort to the patient. Indeed, in a patient who has significant abdominal pain, it may be the only method that can be used to assess liver size. The scratch test is complemented and refined by both percussion of the upper edge and palpation of the lower edge of the liver.

Percussion of the upper edge of the liver and palpation of the lower edge confirm the location of the upper and lower liver borders. For **percussion**, with the patient supine, stand on right side of the patient; place the nondominant hand on the lower right chest wall, fingers in the lower rib interspaces; use the third digit of the other hand as a plexor on digits 2, 3, 4, 5 and percuss in the right midclavicular line. Feel and listen for normal (lung) to dull (liver) sounds and note the level of demarcation. This should confirm the upper level of the scratch test **(Fig. 6.7)**. For **palpation** of the lower edge, with the patient supine, stand on right side of the patient and place the hands, palms toward patient, fingers pointing toward patient's feet **(Fig. 6.8)**. Place the fingertips 2 to 3 cm inferior to the lower border found at scratch test, with the middle finger in the right midclavicular line. Gently flex the digits (hooking maneuver) and instruct the patient to inhale in order to feel the liver hit fingers. You do not feel for the liver, the liver is pushed down to hit your fingertips. Be passive in the examination. If no edge is felt, repeat the procedure with fingers placed 1 cm cephalad; repeat this until the edge is felt or the costal margin is reached. **Hepatomegaly** is a liver span >14 cm in size, a **small liver** is a span <6 cm in width. The company a large or small liver keeps are discussed in Table 6.7. **Hepatocellular carcinoma** manifests with an enlarged liver with nodules and a bruit or rub over one of those nodules or masses. The company it keeps includes jaundice and cachexia.

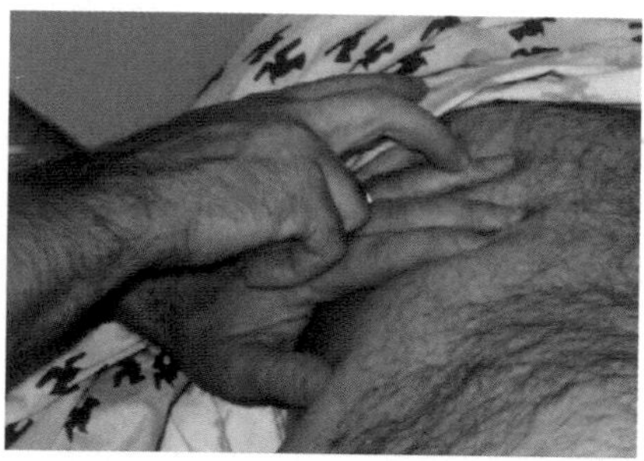

Figure 6.7.

Technique to percuss the upper edge of the liver.

TIPS

- Patient supine, relaxed, knees and hips flexed: stand on right side of patient, place nondominant hand on lower right chest wall, fingers in the lower rib interspaces; use third digit of other hand as plexor on digits 2–5; percuss in the right midclavicular line
- Feel and listen for normal (lung) to dull (liver): note level of demarcation
- Normal: able to detect and confirm the upper edge of the liver as detected by scratch

Anorectum

An **anorectal examination** is indicated in most, if not all, cases related to the abdomen **(Fig. 6.9). Inspection** alone often indicates the diagnosis of certain processes. The **digital rectal examination** (DRE) then is performed to examine the structures deep to the junction between the external anus and the internal anus i.e., the dentate line and palpation of the distal rectum, the prostate in men, and the uterus* in women. See **Box 6.1** for techniques to assist in the performance of this inherently challenging examination technique. Any stool sample obtained, including a small quantity on the gloved finger, should be inspected for color. **Red or mahagony-colored stool** has frank blood in it; **white stool** or classically "clay-colored" stool may indicate disease in the common bile duct, whereas **black stool** can be caused by inorganic iron e.g., the use of $FeSO_4$ as a mineral supplement, or by organic iron, e.g., hemoglobin from a gastrointestinal bleed, or by a nosebleed or from eating poorly cooked (raw) meat. In addition, black stool may be from oral ingestion

*Especially a uterus that is retroflexed and retroverted.

Table 6.5. Anorectal Disorders

Diagnosis	Anal findings	Company it Keeps
External hemorrhoid	Dilated, blue veins External to dentate line	Nonspecific Anal pruritus Soiling of underpants Constipation
Thrombosed external hemorrhoid	Thrombosed vein Firm, tender Easily bleeds	Antecedent external hemorrhoids
Internal hemorrhoid	Dilated, blue veins Internal to the dentate line Painless Bleeding	Portal hypertension Liver disease
Anal fissure	Severe pain Midline longitudinal fissure usually in posterior anus	Constipation Anal intercourse is risk factor
Fistula-in-ano	Painful orifice with swelling in external anus Orifice adjacent to a crypt of Morgagni at dentate line	Crohn's disease Diabetes mellitus
Perirectal abscess	Painful, tender mass in perineum, lateral to anus, medial to ischial Tuberosity	Fistula-in-ano Diabetes mellitus
Rectal prolapse	Eversion of pink, soft, velvetlike mucosa through the anus	Constipation, rare by itself Pelvic laxity Uterine prolapse Urinary and fecal incontinence
Pinworm	Anal pruritus White 1- to 2-mm thin worms in the perianal area	Family members with similar symptoms

of bismuth or of charcoal. Any stool sample should have a guaiac test performed on it. In this test, stool sample is applied to a guaiac card and a reagent is added. Organified iron e.g., hemoglobin turns the sample blue; inorganic iron does not (see **Table 6.6** for specifics on stool and guaiac results). Although not discussed in detail here, visual inspection using an **anoscope** will complement these two examinations. Please see Table 6.5.

Box 6.1.

Points to Remember When Performing a Rectal Examination

1. Use index finger of dominant hand, apply water soluble lubricant to gloved finger, place the palmar tip of finger on anal midline, finger pointed posteriorly, with slight flexion of finger
2. Patient attempts to relax
3. Index finger gently inserted into anus and rectum via direct pressure and mild finger flexion; insert finger to base of the proximal phalanx
4. Palpate with the palmar tip the posterior rectum, turn finger 90 degrees to left, turn finger 180 degrees to right then 90 more degrees to assess the anterior

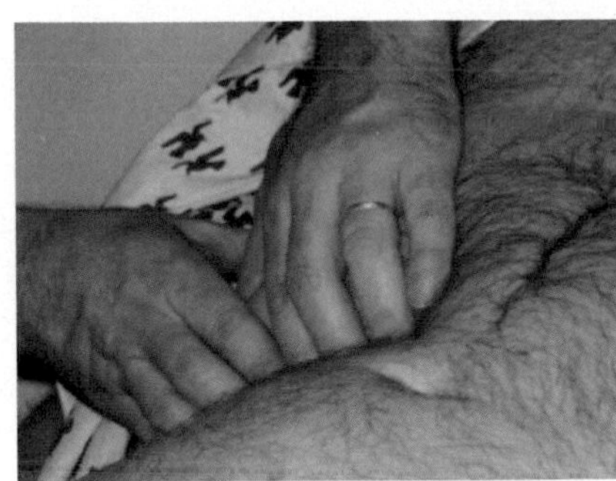

Figure 6.8.

Technique to palpate the lower edge of the liver.

TIPS

- Patient supine, relaxed, knees and hips flexed: stand on right side of patient and place hands palms toward patient, fingers pointing toward patient's feet, finger tips 2 to 3 cm inferior to the lower border found at scratch test; place index fingers near the right midclavicular line; gently flex digits to feel any edge; instruct patient to inhale; feel the liver hit fingers
- If no edge felt, repeat procedure 1 cm cephalad; repeat this until edge felt or costal margin reached
- Hooking procedure: better than mashing
- Normal: usually can find the edge, smooth, nontender; make note of lower edge

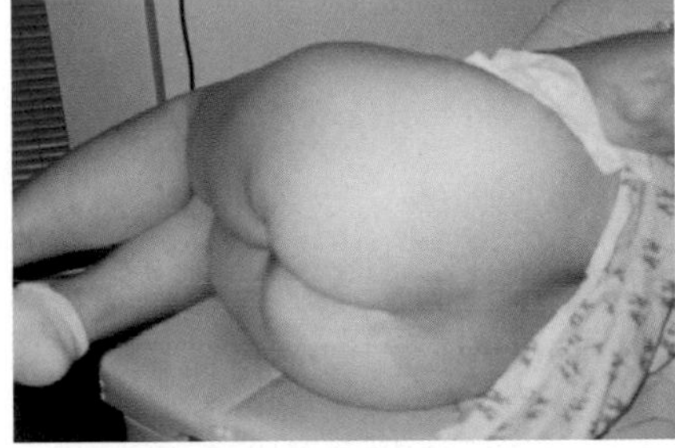

Figure 6.9.

Technique and decubital position for anorectal examination.

TIPS

- Patient in decubital position, left or right, knees and hips flexed
- With gloved hands, lift one buttock to reveal the gluteal cleft, perineum, and anus
- Inspect the skin of the area
- Remember to drape

TEACHING POINTS

OVERALL ABDOMINAL EXAMINATION

1. Always must include the male and female genitourinary examination when performing an abdominal examination.
2. Always examine the sites of discomfort last.
3. Inspection of the wall itself is important for scars.
4. Divide the abdomen into either four quadrants or nine areas, or the "4 plus 3" grid, which is probably the best model for localizing, defining, describing, and even diagnosing the problem.
5. Repeated examinations on a serial basis is important to follow and diagnose a finding.
6. Digital rectal examination is very important in the evaluation.

External hemorrhoids manifest with one or more palpable and visible venous structures (**Fig. 6.10**). The entities, which are painful and tender, are located distal to the dentate line. These are caused by straining, Valsalva's maneuver, and irritation. **Thrombosed external hemorrhoids** manifest with one palpable, visible, and extremely painful dilated vein that is firm and tender and often easily bleeds. There are often antecedent and concurrent external hemorrhoids. **Internal hemorrhoids** manifest with one or more dilated, palpable veins in the area proximal to the dentate line. The company it keeps includes those of hepatic portal venous system hypertension. These include abdominal venous collaterals, small liver, and ascites. The most common reason for internal hemorrhoids is indeed portal hypertension. **Rectal prolapse** manifests with an eversion of the rectal and anal mucosa (Fig. 3.14). It is a soft pink, velvetlike doughnut of tissue that protrudes past the anal verge. The company it keeps includes stool incontinence, uterine prolapse, and past history of multiple pregnancies with vaginal deliveries. **Anal fissure** manifests with an exquisitely tender and painful longitudinal fissure in the posterior midline anus, often accompanied by bleeding. This is usually caused by mild trauma to the anus or to constipation. **Fistula-in-ano** manifests with a visible orifice in the external anus. There may be a palpable nodule adjacent to the orifice. The other end of the fistula is located proximal to the dentate line. This may be caused by Crohn's disease or proctitis. **Perirectal abscess** manifests with a tender even fluctuant swelling in the area lateral to the anus (Fig. 2.14). This swelling is limited anatomically by the ischial tuberosity. In severe cases or in immunocompromised patients, Fournier's gangrene (Fig. 2.13)

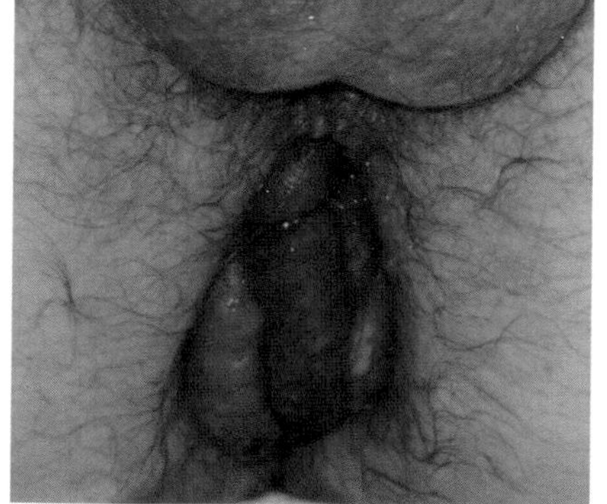

Figure 6.10.

External hemorrhoids.

TIPS

- External hemorrhoids: one or more venous structures that are palpable and visible distal to the dentate line
- May secondarily thrombose

Table 6.6. Stool Sample Tests

Diagnosis	Gross assessment	Guaiac
Charcoal	Black	Negative
Bismuth	Black	Negative
Iron sulfate	Black	Negative
Occult blood	Brown	Positive
Blood	Black	Positive
Frank blood	Red or mohagoney	Positive
Biliary obstruction	White or clay-colored	Negative

may develop, which manifests with crepitus and necrosis. **Pinworm infestation** manifests with the patient complaining of anal pruritus. Multiple, thread-sized (1–3 mm in length) worms are found in the perianal area. Often, other members of the family, especially children in daycare, will have similar symptoms. See **Table 6.5** for specific anorectal and perianal disorders.

ABDOMINAL MASSES

Inguinal hernia manifests with a palpable and even visible mass in the lower medial abdomen **(Fig. 6.11)**, through the floor of Hesselbach's triangle. The hernia is usually not tender and, on application of gentle pressure, usually is reducible. Incarcerated or strangulated hernias are tender and not reducible.

Incisional hernia manifests with a palpable and even visible mass in the site of a healed surgical scar in the abdomen **(Fig. 6.12)**. The hernia is usually not tender and, on application of pressure, reducible. Incarcerated or strangulated hernias, however, are tender and not reducible. An increased risk for incisional hernia is found in patients who have surgery when their diabetes mellitus is out of control or in patients who are taking high dose steroids.

Umbilical hernia manifests with a palpable and visible nodule or mass from, and often effectively replacing, the umbilicus **(Fig. 6.13)**. This is usually not tender and, on application of pressure, reducible. Again, it can be incarcerated or strangulated, but rarely so. The company it keeps includes either ascites or pregnancy. Tanyol observed that the hernia caused by pregnancy points upward, whereas one from ascites points downward—an interesting observation, but rarely of clinically relevance.

Aortic abdominal aneurysm manifests with a palpable, pulsatile mass in the midline epigastric area of the abdomen; a concurrent epigastric bruit may be present. The company it keeps includes long-standing hypertension, diminished pulses in the lower extremities, and often a pulsatile mass in one or both popliteal fossa (popliteal aneurysm). See discussion page 137.

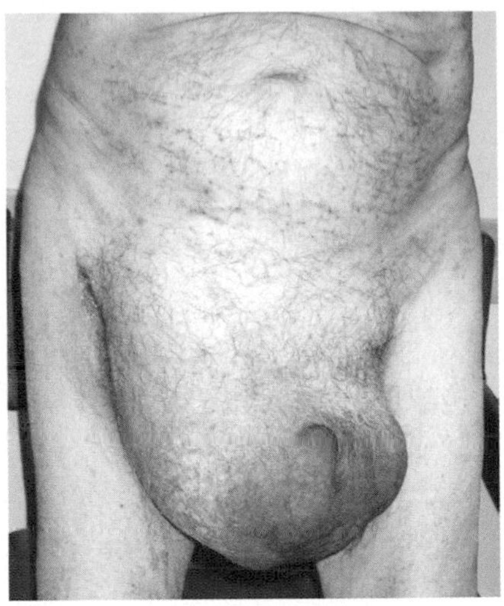

Figure 6.11.

Inguinal hernia, direct.

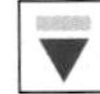

TIPS

- Direct inguinal hernia: mass through the floor of Hesselbach's triangle and often into the scrotum or labia majora
- Can become massive
- Relatively low risk of incarceration

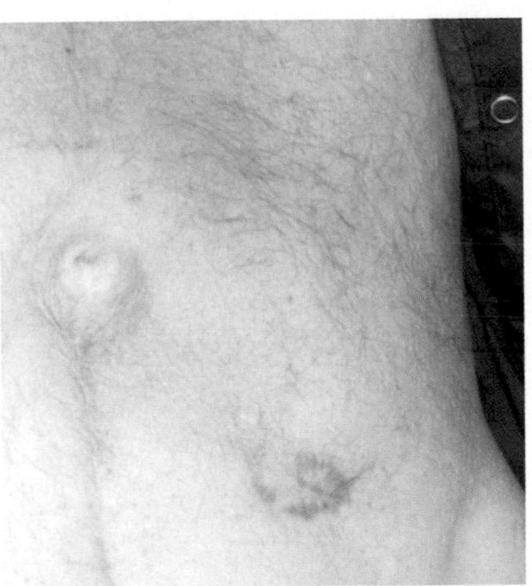

A

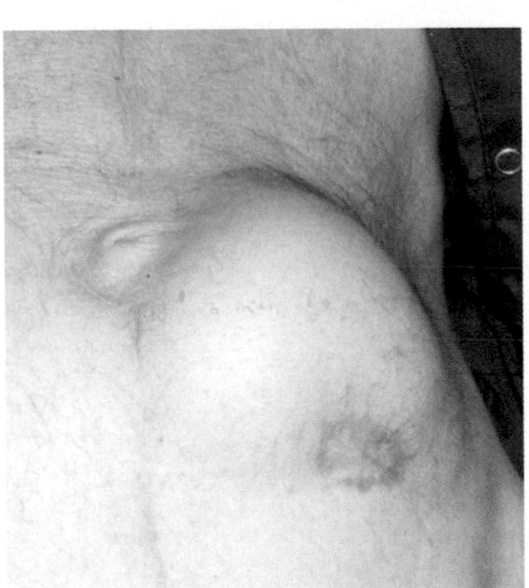

B

Figure 6.12.

Incisional hernia.

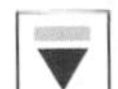

TIPS

- Incisional hernia: palpable and even visible mass through an incisional site i.e., scar
- Can be massive; usually a low risk of incarceration

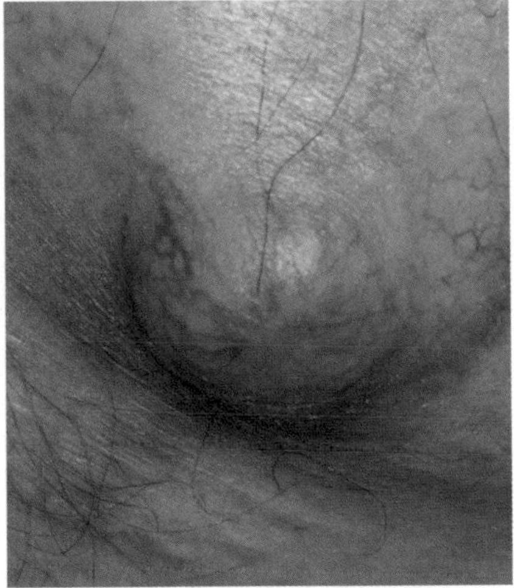

Figure 6.13.

Umbilical hernia.

TIPS

- Umbilical hernia: bulge at the umbilicus, usually easily reduced
- Must assess patient for increased intraabdominal pressure, e.g., pregnancy versus ascites

TEACHING POINTS

ABDOMINAL MASSES

1. Carnett's maneuver is a method useful in differentiating wall from intraabdominal processes. It may be even more appropriate to use in pain syndromes.
2. By convention, any unknown structure >4 cm is a mass, <4 cm is a nodule.
3. Incarcerated hernia: nontender, nonreducible is a surgical urgency.
4. Strangulated hernia: tender, nonreducible is a surgical emergency.
5. A mass in an area adjacent to a surgical scar is likely to be an incisional hernia.
6. Suprapubic masses are often either a distended urinary bladder, a uterine fibroid, or a gravid uterus.
7. Very rare to find a palpable gallbladder; when discovered, strongly consider periampullary carcinoma.
8. Lipomas are one of the most common causes of nodules found in abdominal examination.
9. The physical examination for an abdominal aortic aneurysm is unsatisfactory and, thus, requires imaging techniques to evaluate.

Periampullary carcinoma manifests with a palpable, nontender mass in the right upper abdomen (Courvoisier's sign), which is located near Murphy's point immediately inferior to the right costal margin. The company it keeps includes significant jaundice, clay-colored stool, and darkened urine. **Lipomas** manifest with one or more subcutaneous fleshy, nontender to tender nodules that remain present and palpable with contraction of the abdominal muscles (Carnett's sign) (Fig. 6.26). Lipomas are very common. Their symptoms can wax and wane and may be tender if irritated, twisted, or traumatized. **Hepatomegaly** manifests with a liver that is >14 cm in the right midclavicular line as demonstrated by the scratch test (Fig. 6.6) and confirmed by percussion (Fig. 6.7) and palpation (Fig. 6.8). The liver may cross over midline. A **distended urinary bladder** manifests with fullness in the suprapubic area, best seen by inspecting the abdomen from the side (Fig. 6.3B). Dullness to percussion is noted over the area and, in men, usually an enlarged prostate is noted on digital rectal examination. This is usually due to bladder outlet obstruction, e.g., from benign prostatic hypertrophy. **Splenomegaly** manifests with dullness to percussion at Castell's point and in Traube's space (Fig. 6.14B); often, a palpable spleen is noted in the left upper quadrant (Fig. 6.16) (see discussion below).

LIVER EXAMINATION

End-stage liver disease usually manifests with a **small liver** by the scratch test, confirmed by percussion of the upper edge and palpation of the lower edge. The company it keeps includes **ascites** which manifests with bulging flanks (Fig. 6.28 and 31), fluid wave, and a percussible meniscus with shifting dullness are noted. Furthermore, **peripheral dependent edema** that is most often pitting and bilateral is noted (Fig. 6.32). It often involves the vulva or the scrotum and penis. In addition, there is **abdominal venous dilation.** In this, the venous blood flow is upward above the umbilicus and downward when below the umbilicus. This is so prominent that it may cause the rare pattern of caput medusae. Furthermore, there is **decreased mental status**, with lethargy and **asterixis**, as assessed by instructing the patient to actively dorsiflex hands, spread fingers in a full position of abduction, and maintain that position for 60 seconds (Fig. 7.48); this can also be assessed with the feet in full dorsiflexion for 60 seconds. The inability to maintain the position, i.e., an irregularly irregular flap of extension, then voluntary dorsiflexion indicates asterixis. **Icterus** of the sublingual mucosa, conjunctiva, and skin may be seen. This is manifested by a yellow discoloration to the conjunctiva (not the sclera) at which level the bilirubin is usually is >4. Of interest, several agents, e.g., rifampin, can cause tears and in fact, all body secretion to become orange-colored and be mistaken for icterus. **Gynecomastia**, which manifests with enlargement of breast tissue itself, and **small testes** are also not uncommon findings. One or more **spider angiomata** (Fig. 14.13) in the distribution of the superior vena cava are common, along with multiple purpura and ecchymosis. Finally, bilateral palmar and plantar erythema are seen, which appears mottled, as if sitting on one's hands. The physical examination plays a significant role, both in diagnosis and in staging the severity of liver disease. Many of the **Child-Pugh-Turcotte** classification features involve the physical examination **(Table 6.7)**. These include pitting edema and Meurcke's lines of *decreased albumin*, asterixis and changes in **mental status exam** (MSE) of *encephalopathy*, examination features for *ascites*, evidence of *poor nutrition*, and the presence of icterus in the sublingual and conjunctival areas for *elevated bilirubin*. **Hepatomegaly** manifests with a liver that is >14 cm in the right midclavicular line, as demonstrated by scratch test, percussion of the upper edge and palpation of the lower edge. Always palpate the lower edge so as not to miss any crossover to the left side or any nodules or masses in the liver.

Hepatitis manifests with a tender liver, which can be normal size or enlarged; tenderness brought out by palpation of the lower edge of the liver; and from the **fist percussion test** in which the examiner places the palm of one hand over the lower right chest wall (over the liver) and strikes with the ulnar surface of other hand to unmask the tenderness. The company it keeps includes **icterus** of sublingual and conjunctival areas and skin; orange to brown urine; and, usually, normal stool color. In addition, the patient has a marked increase in fatigue and malaise, new onset of nausea and vomiting, and, in many cases, a recent history of significant polyarticular small joint arthritis.

Table 6.7. Child-Pugh-Turcotte Classification of End-Stage Liver Disease: Correlates to Physical Examination

Feature-physical examination	A	B	C
Albumin assessment	*> 3 g* Minimal edema	*2–3 g* Pitting edema dependent Tiger-striping	*< 2 g* Meurcke's lines Diffuse pitting edema
Total bilirubin	*< 2 mg%* No findings	*2–3 mg%* Minimal findings May be able to note sublingual icterus	*> 3 mg%* Sublingual Conjunctival icterus
Ascites	*Minimal* to none	*Present*, but not tense, easily controlled	*Poorly controlled*, often tense
Asterixis	*Minimal* to none	*Present*, but easily controlled	Decreased level of consciousness, poor control
Nutritional status	*Good* Normal tongue surface Normal lips No purpura	*Fair* Atrophic Glossitis Angular chelosis Ecchymosis Purpura	*Poor* Atrophic Glossitis Cheilosis Ecchymosis Purpura Petechiae (perifollicular of scurvy)

TEACHING POINTS

LIVER EXAMINATION

1. Perform scratch test first, then confirm the upper edge with percussion, the lower edge with palpation.
2. Normal liver span in right midclavicular line: approximately 8 to 14 cm.
3. Firm nodules with a bruit or rub are likely neoplastic.
4. Fist percussion is good to assess for inflammation in a normal sized liver.
5. ESLD manifestations include spider angiomas, gynecomastia, small testes, small or large liver, icterus, ascites, and asterixis.
6. The physical examination plays a significant role both in the *diagnosis* and in *staging* the severity of liver disease.

SPLEEN EXAMINATION (Table 6.8)

The spleen is located in the extreme upper lateral left abdomen; in fact, it is in the lower chest beneath ribs 6 and 7. Palpation of this structure is one of the most challenging aspects of the physical examination. Several reasons exist why this is so challenging, including that today in the United States splenomegaly is relatively uncommon and mild to moderate splenomegaly is best first ruled out by inspection and percussion. Thus, if percussion rules out any splenomegaly, palpation becomes less important **(Fig. 6.14)**. Most important to percussion is the **point of Castell**, which is the intersection of the left subcostal margin and the anterior axillary line. In addition, the **triangle of Traube**, which is bordered laterally by the anterior axillary line, superiorly by the sixth rib, and inferiorly by the subcostal margin, is important because this is a common site for moderate splenomegaly. To optimize detection rates, with the patient having fasted, both tests should be performed with the patient in full expiration and then in full inspiration (empty stomach is filled with gas, thus tympanic). A *normal spleen* in expiration or inspiration will remain proximal to this point and to this triangle.

Splenectomy manifests with tympany to percussion at Castell's point and in Traube's space. Furthermore, a scar is present in the left subcostal area or midline abdomen.

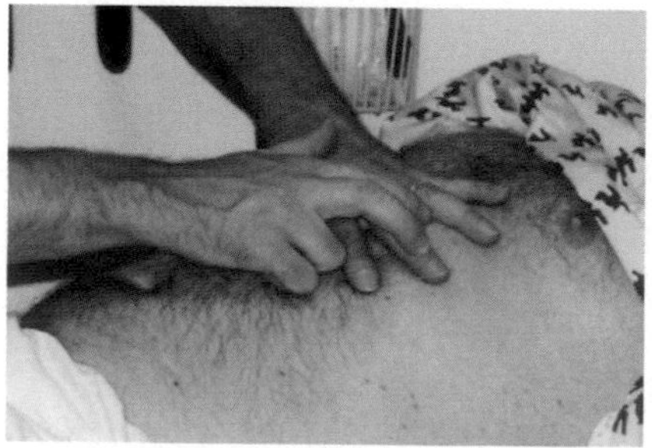

A

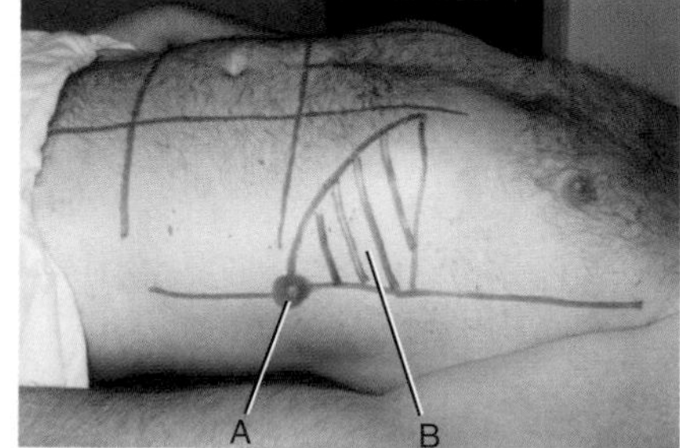

B

Figure 6.14.

Technique for percussion for splenomegaly. **A**. Castell's point. **B**. Traube's space.

 **TIPS**

- Patient supine, percuss at Castell's point **(A)**: left anterior axillary line, costal margin
- Patient supine, percuss over Traube's space **(B)**: sixth rib, anterior axillary line, costal margin
- Repeat with the patient in full inspiration
- Best to perform in early morning or when patient has an empty stomach
- Normal: tympanic or resonant note
- If tympany present, highly unlikely that spleen is enlarged
- Mild splenomegaly: dull to full inspiration, not in expiration
- Moderate or large splenomegaly: dull to both inspiration and expiration

TEACHING POINTS

SPLEEN EXAMINATION

1. Always check first for a left subcostal scar and query patient if spleen has been removed.
2. Percussion is first best examination technique.
3. If tympany at Castell's point, unlikely to have splenomegaly.
4. Examination of the spleen should proceed in the following order: percuss at Castell's point, percuss over Traube's space, palpate left upper quadrant in the right decubital position, palpate with the patient in the supine position.
5. The biggest spleens are the ones that are missed, remember to start palpation low in the left lower quadrant and palpate in a step-wise cephalad direction, 1 to 2 cm.

Moderate splenomegaly manifests with dullness to percussion at Castell's point, with both expiration and full inspiration, and dullness to percussion in Traube's space. Dullness to percussion at either site does not necessarily mean splenomegaly because dullness can also be caused by a large pleural effusion or cardiomegaly; tympany however, makes an enlarged spleen decidedly unlikely. For palpation, place the patient in the **right lateral decubital** position. The examiner places one hand on flank and back **(Fig. 6.15)**, and the other on the left subcostal margin, while the patient inhales deeply; in moderate splenomegaly palpable spleen should be noted in the left upper quadrant only. Furthermore, in moderate splenomegaly the spleen is not palpable in the supine position when the examiner hooks (hook of Middleton) the palmar aspects of the flexed fingers beneath the left subcostal margin and instructs the patient to inspire **(Fig. 6.16). Marked to massive splenomegaly** manifests with the patient complaining of early satiety and nausea and even postprandial

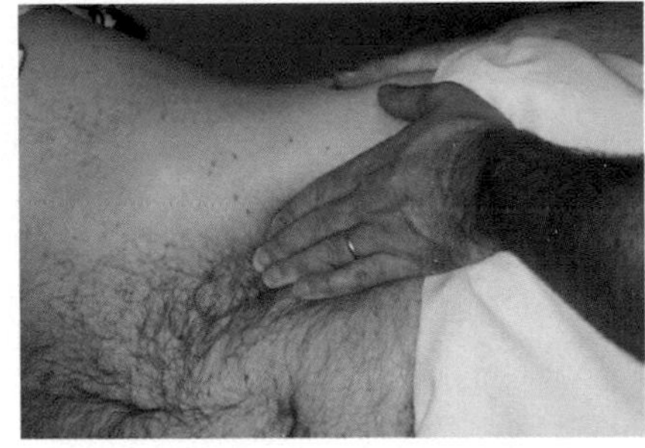

Figure 6.15.

Technique and position to palpate enlarged spleen in the right decubital position.

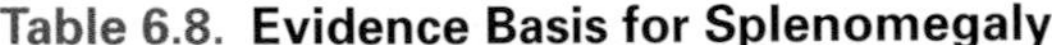

Table 6.8. Evidence Basis for Splenomegaly

Procedure	Paper	Sensitivity	Specificity	Notes
Percussion Castell's point	Barkum (1991)	79%	46%	
	Grover	82%	83%	
	Castell	82%	83%	
	Tamayo			LR 1.97
Percussion Traube's space	Barkum (1989)	78%	82%	
	Barkum (1991)	62%	72%	
	Grover	78%	82%	
Palpation (overall)	Barkum (1991)	39%	97%	
	Grover	58%	92%	
	Tamayo			LR 1.69
Palpation-Hooking Manuever	Grover	56%	93%	
	Shaw	56%	93%	
	Tamayo			LR 2.66

TIPS

- Palpation of little benefit if tympany at Castell's point
- Patient in right lateral decubital position
- Place one hand on flank and back, other hand hooking under the left subcostal margin, patient inspire maximally
- Splenomegaly: spleen edge palpable

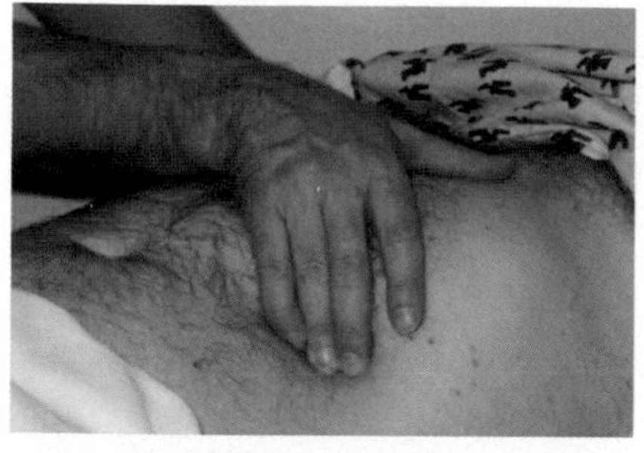

A

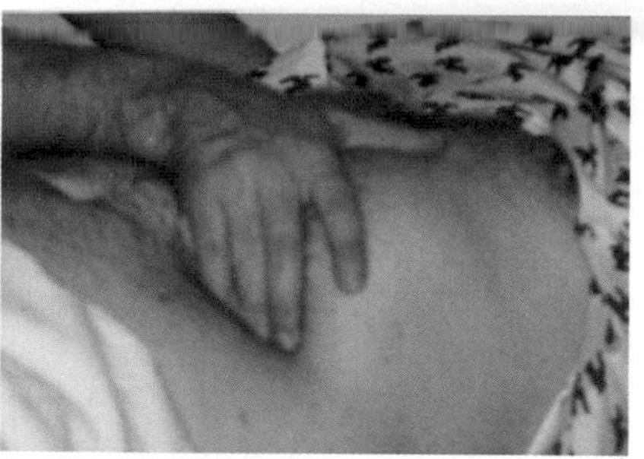

B

Figure 6.16.

Position and technique to palpate enlarged spleen in supine position.

 **TIPS**

- Palpation of little benefit if tympany at Castell's point
- Hook fingers beneath the left subcostal area, instruct patient to inhale
- Mild or moderate splenomegaly: no spleen palpable
- Marked to massive splenomegaly: spleen palpable, may extend into the pelvis

vomiting. Dullness to percussion is noted at Castell's point, with both expiration and inspiration; dullness to percussion in Traube's space; and a palpable spleen in the left upper quadrant in the right decubital or supine position. In marked to massive splenomegaly, the spleen can extend into the pelvis; in such cases, palpation should be begun in the left lower quadrant and progressively repeated each 1 to 2 cm cephalad. Please refer to Table 6.8 for evidence basis.

ABDOMINAL PAIN (Table. 6.10)

A thorough examination must emphasize **palpation**, both **direct** and **rebound**. It is incumbent for the examiner and teacher to stress two points: first, what is involved in an appropriate examination for a patient with an acute abdomen and, second, localize, to define, delineate, and describe the tenderness in order to optimize the potential to diagnose the problem. Rebound tenderness and guarding are related signs that make the constellation more troubling and can indicate peritoneal irritation. Localize the seat of maximal pain and geographically place it on the abdominal "grid of nine" or quadrants or the **4 plus 3 grid**. A patient with an **acute abdomen** manifests with anorexia, diffuse abdominal pain, diffuse deep and rebound tenderness, and, most troubling and noticeable, involuntary guarding. This is also called a "surgical abdomen" for it always requires emergent intervention by a surgeon.

Pancreatitis manifests with an acute onset of epigastric and left upper quadrant pain with associated nausea and often vomiting. The pain is worsened by any oral intake and relieved with fasting. Local direct and often rebound tenderness is noted in the left upper quadrant and the epigastrium. This tenderness is reproduced and increased on placing the patient in a right lateral decubitus position with the knee to the chest and then palpating in the left upper quadrant (Guy-Mallet sign) **(Fig. 6.17)**. The pain and tenderness often will radiate into the left shoulder (Kehr's sign). The company it keeps is specific to any complications of pancreatitis. **Retroperitoneal hemorrhage** manifests with flank ecchymosis (Grey Turner's sign) and in the periumbilical skin (Cullen's sign). **Noncardiogenic pulmonary edema** manifests with diffuse crackles on chest auscultation and desaturation of oxygen from the blood. Pancreatitis is most commonly caused by ethanol ingestion or by a stone in the biliary tree.

Cholecystitis manifests with nausea, vomiting, and right upper quadrant pain. There is right upper quadrant tenderness, both to direct and rebound, and the pain worsens with oral intake. In addition, splinting is noted when performing **Murphy's sign (Fig. 6.18)**. To test for this sign, have the patient sit and lean slightly forward. Stand behind the patient, place an arm around and hook under the right subcostal margin in the right midclavicular line (Fig. 6.18A); or, with the patient supine, stands adjacent to the patient's head and place the hands in a

Figure 6.17.

Technique and positioning for Guy-Mallet sign.

 **TIPS**

- Patient in right lateral decubitus, knee to chest position: press deeply into the left upper quadrant
- Pancreatitis: marked increase in tenderness in left upper quadrant

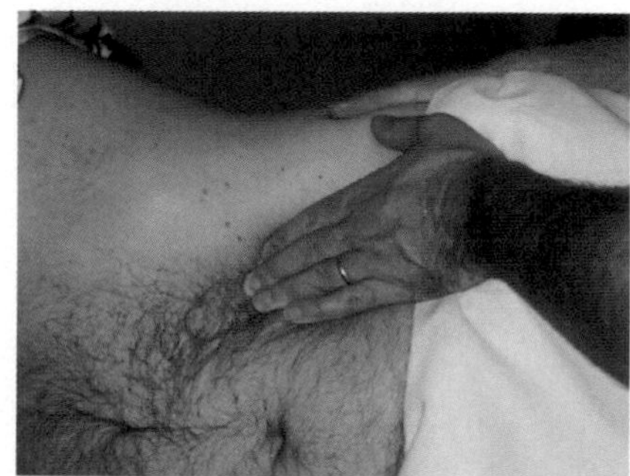

hooking position over the subcostal area in right midclavicular line (Fig. 6.18B). Either position is good, the supine position being the conventional one. Murphy, however, used the upright position and the clinician may find that in certain patients, e.g., those who cannot assume a supine position this position is indeed best. In both positions, instruct the patient to inhale deeply. In acute cholecystitis, the patient splints i.e., stops inhalation. The test for Murphy's sign is complementary to direct and rebound tenderness; in Murphy's test the patient controls the pain, the examiner is static and passive. The sensitivity for this has been reported to be 27% by Gunn, but, in our view, this is a low number.

In acute cholecystitis, there is also right **flank hyperesthesia** (Boas' sign). Hyperesthesia is assessed by lightly stroking the skin with fingertips or cotton-tipped swab or by the technique described by Cope in which the examiner gently pinches the skin between the thumb and index finger **(Fig. 6.19)**. The stroking or pinching is repeated several times in the same general area. The sensitivity of hyperesthesia, as reported by Gunn and colleagues, is 7%. The pain often radiates into the right shoulder (Kehr's sign). This pain may be precipitated by Valsalva's maneuver, cough, or palpation of the right upper quadrant. The company it keeps is specific to the underlying cause. If biliary obstruction, icterus, dark urine, and clay-colored stools are often noted. If ascending cholangitis, there are fevers and more generalized abdominal tenderness. Ascending cholangitis is very close to an acute abdomen.

Peptic ulcer disease manifests with subacute or even progressively worsening nausea and epigastric pain, with vomiting possibly occurring later in the course. The epigastric discomfort is decreased with oral intake and increased with fasting. Often noted is tenderness to direct palpation but rarely any significant rebound tenderness. When severe, there may be concurrent emesis that appears like old coffee grounds, which is also known as hematemesis; and jet black stools, also known as melena; or even frank red blood in stool, also known as hematochezia. When mild, the stool is brown, but it may be guaiac positive for occult blood **(Fig. 6.20)**.

Pyelonephritis manifests with pain in the right or left flank that radiates into the ipsilateral groin. There is antecedent dysuria, urgency, hesitancy, when urinating increased urinary frequency, and even frank pyuria. Tenderness is reproduced by a tap over the ipsilateral costophrenic angle **(Murphy's "punch" maneuver) (Fig. 6.21)**. This tenderness often radiates into the ipsilateral groin. The company it keeps includes nausea, vomiting, and fevers. **Nephrolithiasis** manifests with severe pain, intermittent and spasmodic, with nausea and vomiting. The pain often radiates into the ipsilateral groin. Although gross hematuria may be present, most often the hematuria is occult, i.e., detected only via microscopic or dipstick analysis. Thus, be aware of the importance of a dipstick and microscopic urinalysis.

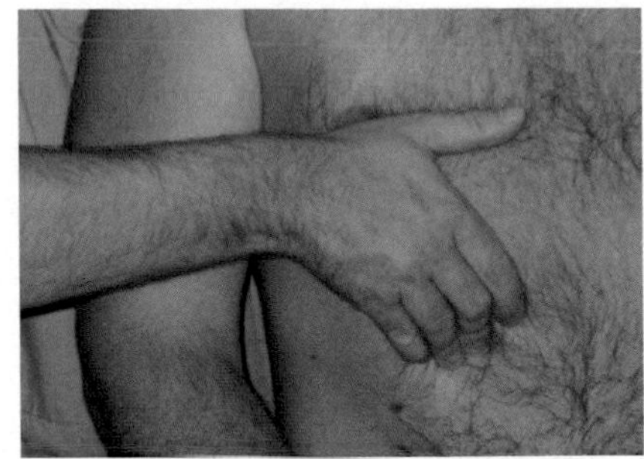

A

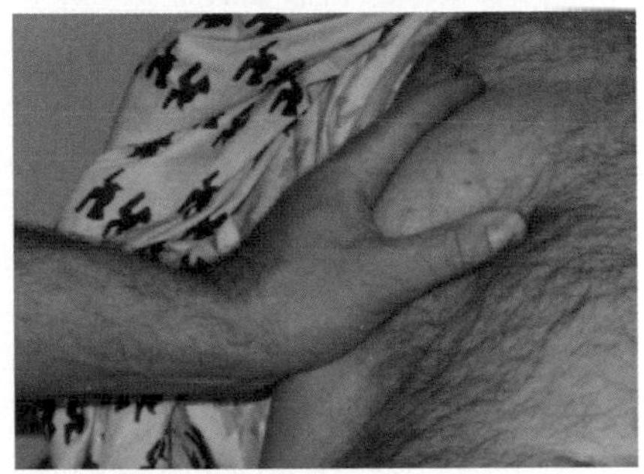

B

Figure 6.18.

Techniques and positions for Murphy's sign. **A.** Sitting up technique. **B.** Supine technique.

TIPS

- Patient sitting and leaning forward: stand behind patient, place arm around and hook under the right subcostal margin in right midclavicular line **(A) or**
- Patient supine: stand at head of patient and place hands in a hooking position over subcostal area in right midclavicular line **(B)**
- Patient instructed to inhale deeply
- This is complementary to direct and rebound tenderness; the patient controls the pain, the examiner is static and passive
- When the patient splints (i.e., stops inhalation), the test is positive—no need to actively palpate
- Cholecystitis: inspiration stopped (splinted) because of the palpation
- Sensitivity: 27%

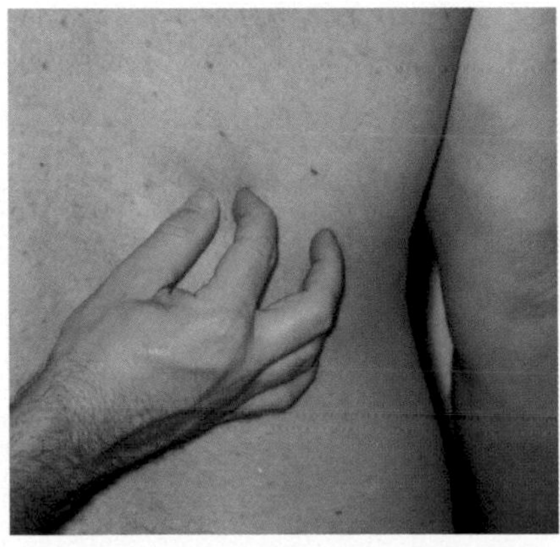

Figure 6.19.

Technique for Copes' pinch. Excellent to assess hyperesthesia.

TIPS

- Patient sitting or supine: gently pinch skin between thumb and index finger, perform in two to three sites in each area of examination
- Cholecystitis: right flank hyperesthesia (Boas' sign)
- Gunn and colleagues found 7% sensitivity

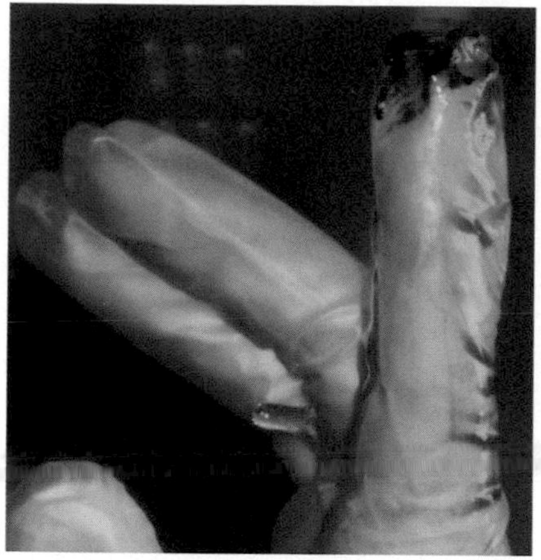

A

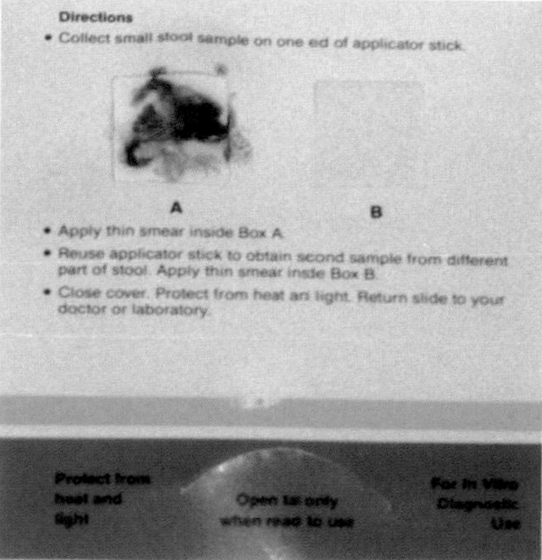

B

Figure 6.20.

A. Jet black (melena) stool with some frank blood (hematochezia). **B**. Guaiac positive stool sample (blue color indicates hemoglobin. Patient was having a massive gastrointestinal bleed.

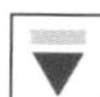

TIPS

- Frank blood in stool: black (melena) that is guaiac positive
- Occult blood in stool: brown stool that is guaiac positive

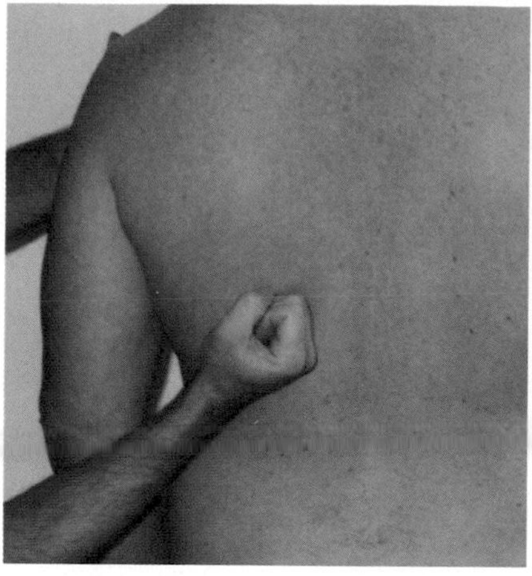

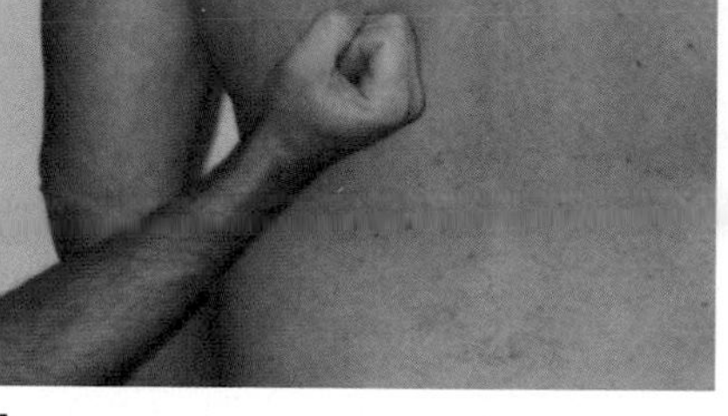

A

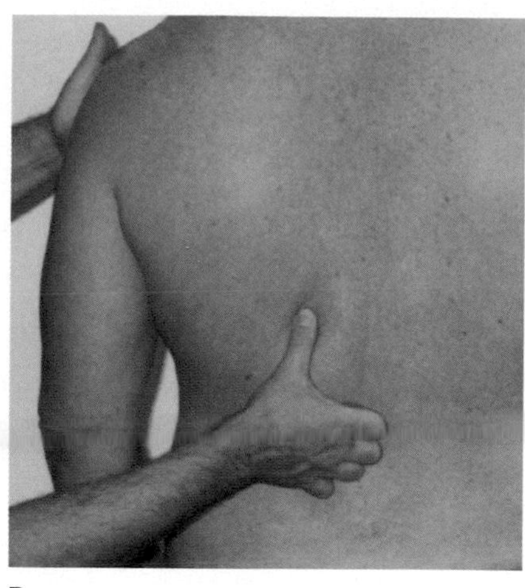

B

Figure 6.21.

Technique to perform Murphy's "punch" maneuver. **A.** Punch technique. **B.** The finger tap technique.

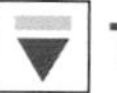

TIPS

- Patient sitting upright or standing
- Use the ulnar aspect of hand to gently punch the right and then left costovertebral angle
- Normal: no tenderness
- Pyelonephritis or nephrolithiasis: left or right tenderness that radiates into the ipsilateral groin

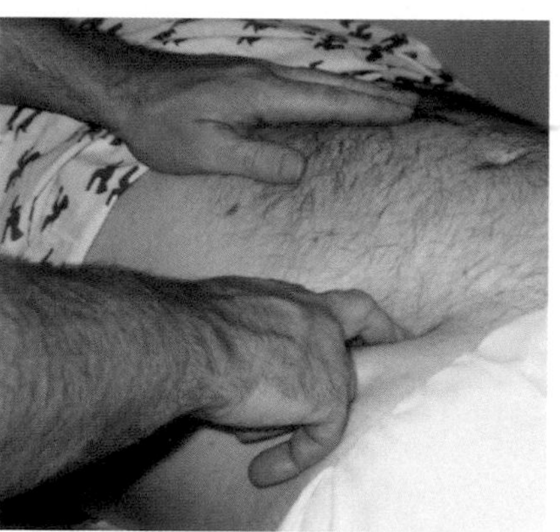

Figure 6.22.

Technique for McBurney's point palpation maneuver in the assessment of acute appendicitis.

TIPS

- Patient supine: pressure over the point 2 inches medial to the ASIS on a line from the ASIS to the umbilicus (McBurney's line)
- Appendicitis: tenderness in right lower quadrant pain, specifically at McBurney's point

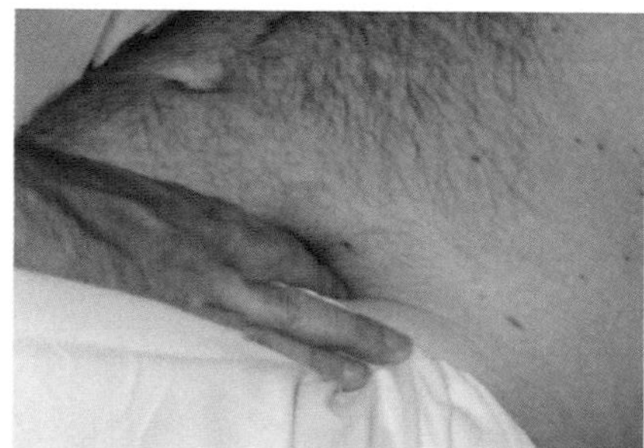

Figure 6.23.

Technique for Rovsing's (Owen's) maneuver in the assessment of acute appendicitis.

TIPS

- Patient supine: firm pressure over left iliac fossa—causes gas to retrograde into the right colon
- Appendicitis: tenderness in right lower quadrant pain, specifically at McBurney's point

Table 6.9. Evidence Basis for Appendicitis

Procedure	Paper	n	Sensitivity	Specificity	Notes
Pain periumbilical, Radiates to Right Lower quadrant	Alvarado	305	69%	84%	PPV .95
Anorexia	Alvarado	305	61%	72%	PPV .91
Right lower Quadrant Tenderness	Berry		96%		
	Izbicki	686	96%		
McBurney's Point Tender	Alvardo	305	100%	12%	PPV 1.0
Right lower Quadrant Hyperesthesia	Cope	185	59%		
Rebound Tenderness	Alvarado	305	55%	78%	PPV 0.92
	Berry		70%	39%	LR 1.1
	Colledge	100	82%	89%	
	Izbicki	686	76%	56%	
Psoas Sign	Berry		13%	91%	
	Izbicki	686	15%	97%	LR 5.0
Rovsing's Sign	Izbicki	686	22%	96%	LR 5.5

LR = Likelihood Ratio; PPV = positive predictive value, n = number of patients.

Appendicitis manifests with a reproducible natural course: manifestations of pain in the periumbilical area that then resolve, only to return 6–8 hours later with intensity to the right lower quadrant often specific to McBurney's point; if untreated, the tenderness then becomes generalized because of the development of generalized peritonitis. Tenderness in the right lower quadrant is specific to McBurney's point. See **Table 6.9** for evidence. **McBurney's point** is 2 inches medial to the ASIS on a line from the ASIS to the umbilicus (McBurney's line) **(Fig. 6.22** and Fig. 6.1). Tenderness is noted to direct and rebound palpation, is reproducible on performance of Rovsing's maneuver, Psoas maneuver, and the Obturator maneuver. **Rovsing's (Owen's) maneuver** is performed with the patient supine, place firm pressure over the left lower abdominal quadrant. Tenderness over McBurney's point indicates appendicitis. High specificity see Table 6.9. It has been postulated that the retrograde movement of gas results in the tenderness **(Fig. 6.23). Psoas maneuver** is performed with the patient supine: apply resistance to the distal thigh while the patient actively forward flexes the thigh at hip **(Fig. 6.24)** see Table 6.9. Finally, the **obturator maneuver** is performed with patient supine: with the patient passively forward flex the hip and knee and then passively internally then externally rotates the hip **(Fig. 6.25)**. This passively stretches the obturator muscle, and causes right lower quadrant pain in appendicitis. Furthermore, with gentle stroking or skin pinch, hyperesthesia is noted over the right lower quadrant skin (Cope's sign). Finally, the patient often has nausea, anorexia, and constipation but very little, if any, vomiting. See Table 6.9 for evidence.

Splenic rupture manifests with an acute onset discomfort in the left upper part of the mid area. Often, the patient reports a history of antecedent trauma to left flank or left lower chest wall or a syndrome of infectious mononucleosis. The discomfort starts sharp and over hours becomes dull. Tenderness is noted in direct and rebound palpation and there is ecchymosis of the flank, left side more commonly than the right side (Grey Turner's sign)

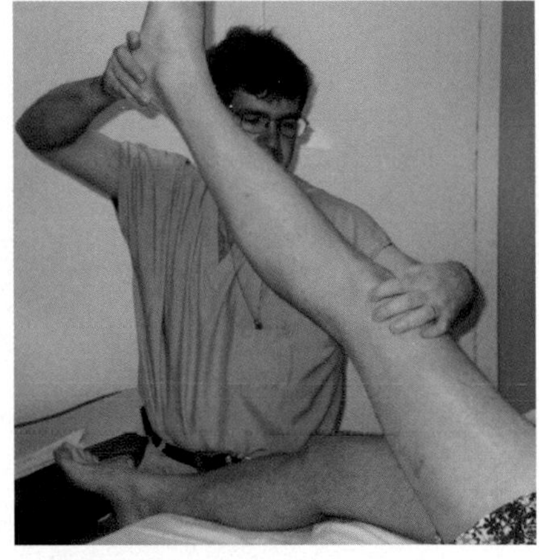

Figure 6.24.

Technique for Psoas maneuver in assessment of acute appendicitis.

TIPS

- Patient supine: place hand over mid-distal thigh; patient actively flexes thigh at hip against resistance
- Appendicitis: right lower quadrant pain, at McBurney's point

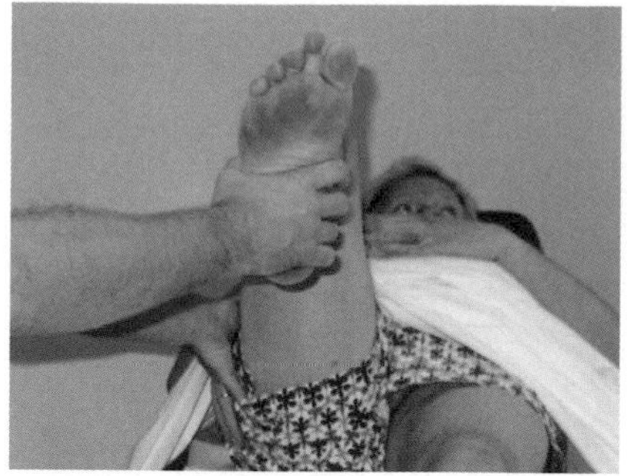
A

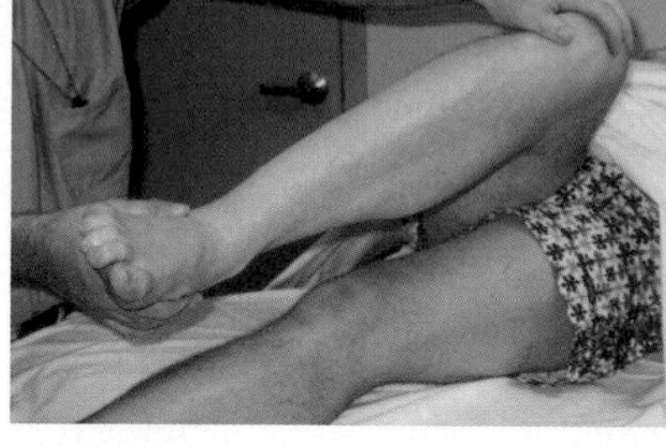
B

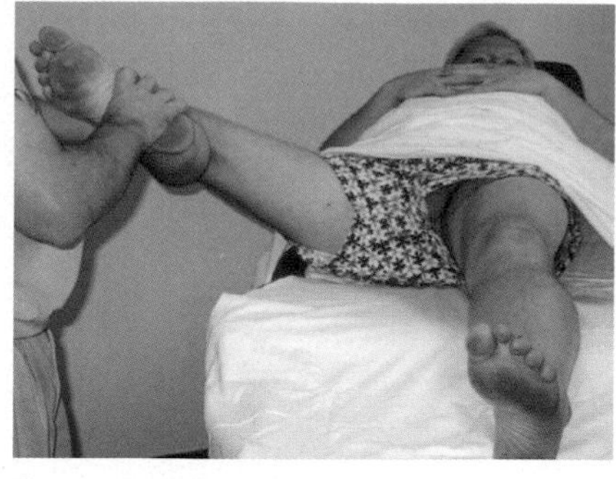
C

Figure 6.25.

Technique for obturator maneuver in the assessment of acute appendicitis.

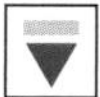 **TIPS**

- Patient supine: passively flex hip and knee; passively internally then externally rotate hip maximally. This passively stretches the obturator muscle
- Appendicitis or any pelvic inflammation: pain especially in right lower quadrant

because of retroperitoneal bleeding. The pain often radiates into the left shoulder (Kehr's sign). In addition, the discomfort is increased on **passive elevation of the legs** when the patient is supine (Ballance sign). Hypotension and even shock may develop up to several days after acute event.

Abdominal wall pain manifests with a discrete area of tenderness in the abdominal wall. The pain or any complication remains unchanged or even increases when the examiner places a finger over the tender site and instructs the patient to contract abdominal muscles by performing an active sit-up **(Carnett's maneuver) (Fig. 6.26)**. An intraabdominal site of mischief will manifest with a decrease in discomfort with this maneuver. Carnett originally described this test with the reasoning that an overlooked cause of abdominal pain may be specific peripheral nerves in the abdominal wall that are irritated or entrapped. The causes of abdominal wall pain include lipomas that become irritated, superficial sensory nerves that become irritated or entrapped, small, trauma-related contusions or rectus hematoma (page 134). The company it keeps includes a discrete area of tenderness with slight fullness or nodule, or, in entrapment, paresthesia or dysesthesia in a specific area or site.

Hepatitis manifests with right upper quadrant tenderness; the liver may be of normal size or enlarged; tenderness is exacerbated or precipitated by palpation of the lower edge of the liver or by the fist percussion test. For the fist percussion test, place one hand on the lower rib cage and gently punch using ulnar side of hand over the other hand. This tenderness can radiate into the right shoulder. This is particularly useful when the patient's liver is not enlarged. The company it keeps includes icterus of sublingual and conjunctival areas and the skin; orange to brown urine, but normal stool color. Often, the patient complains of a marked increase in fatigue and malaise, new onset of nausea and vomiting, and, in many cases, a recent history of significant polyarticular small joint arthritis; all of which are antecedent to icterus. **Diverticulitis** manifests with mild nausea and mild diarrhea, which can be bloody. Often, left or right

Figure 6.26.

Technique for Carnett's procedure to differentiate an abdominal wall from an intraabdominal site. **A**. Relaxed, **B**. Sit-up position.

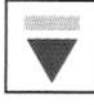 **TIPS**

- Place fingers over the tender site, instruct patient to contract abdominal muscles by sitting up slightly or lifting head
- Note if pain changes or if nodule or mass becomes less or more prominent
- Intraabdominal site of complications: decreased tenderness when muscles contracted, any nodule becomes less apparent
- Abdominal wall site of complications: same or increased pain with or without contraction of muscle—nodule or mass approximately the same

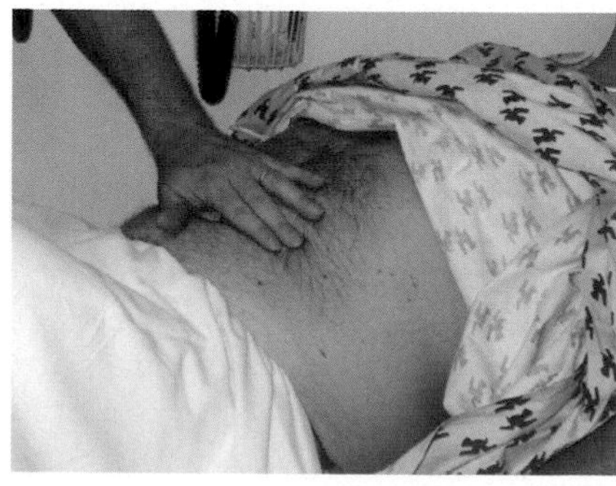
A

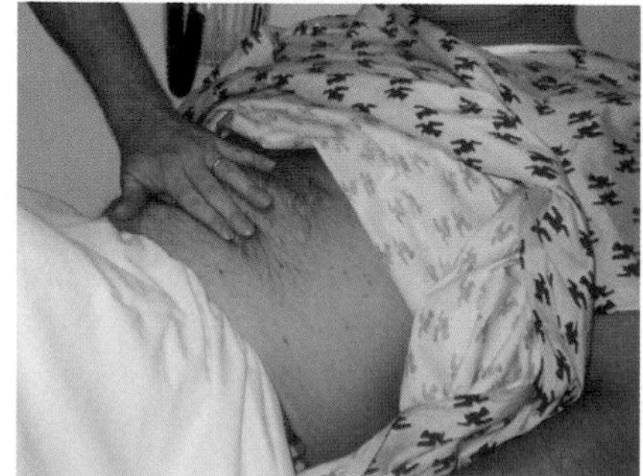
B

mid- or lower abdominal pain and tenderness are noted to direct and even rebound palpation. **Pelvic inflammatory disease** manifests with nausea and pain and tenderness in the left or right mid- to lower abdominal area. In addition, there is often vaginal discharge and severe tenderness on ipsilateral side, with fullness on pelvic bimanual examination. **Ruptured ectopic pregnancy** manifests with an acute onset of pain and tenderness in the left or right side. This is in a woman who has missed one, two, or three periods. She may even know that she is pregnant but has not yet had an ultrasound. There is often a blue color to the vaginal and cervical (Chadwick's sign) mucosa (see Chapter 3, Table 3.4.) If the complication of retroperitoneal hemorrhage is present, there is a flank ecchymosis (Grey Turner's sign) (Fig 14.19).

Table 6.10. Abdominal Pain: Physical Examination

Diagnosis	Abdominal grid site	Company it Keeps
Pancreatitis	Left upper	Exacerbated by oral intake Radiates into back Nausea, vomiting Decreased with fasting Radiates into left shoulder (Kehr's sign) Ethanol use or history of gallstones common Severe: crackles with dyspnea of noncardiogenic pulmonary edema; Grey Turner's sign Positive Guy-Mallet sign
Cholecystitis	Right upper Often specific to Murphy's point	Murphy's sign Hyperesthesia (Boas' sign) Exacerbated with oral intake Nausea and vomiting Decreased with fasting Radiates into right shoulder (Kehr's sign) If stone in common duct: dark urine and conjunctival icterus
Hepatitis	Right upper	Fist-percussion tenderness Normal to slightly enlarged Icterus not uncommon Ethanol binge, use of acetaminophen or exposure to viral agent or IVDA
Peptic ulcer disease	Epigastric	Decreased with oral intake Increased with fasting If bleeding, melena and guaiac positive stool
Pyelonephritis	Right or left flank	Dysuria Pyuria Hematuria Murphy's punch sign
Diverticulitis	Right or left mid to lower	Localized rebound Mild diarrhea or irregular bowel habits Rare in true diverticulitis to have hematochezia or melena; may have occult blood in stool
Appendicitis	Early: periumbilical Intermediate: right lower, specifically, McBurney's point Late: diffuse	Nausea and anorexia Rarely, vomiting Late: fever
Pelvic inflammatory disease	Right or left mid to lower	Nausea Sexually active Discrete reproduction of tenderness with pelvic examination, specifically palpation of adnexa or cervix Purulent discharge from cervical os

(*continued*)

Table 6.10. **(continued)**

Diagnosis	Abdominal grid site	Company it Keeps
Ruptured ectopic pregnancy	Right or left mid to lower	Secondary amenorrhea Chadwick's sign Grey Turner's or Cullen's signs Tenderness of adnexa on affected side
Acute abdomen	Generalized	Involuntary guarding-rigid Rebound tenderness hemodynamically unstable
Splenic rupture	Left upper	Grey Turner develops relatively fast Hiccups due to diaphragmatic irritation Marked increase in pain in left shoulder on elevating both legs, with patient supine Antecedent infectious mononucleosis or blunt trauma Hemodynamically unstable
Abdominal wall	Nonspecific	Soft fleshy nodules: lipomas Positive Carnett's sign for wall, e.g., nerve entrapment, versus intra-abdominal etiology Paresthesia or dysesthesia in specific area for any nerve entrapment

IVDA = intravenous drug abuse.

TEACHING POINTS

ABDOMINAL PAIN

1. Need to find McBurney's line to find McBurney's point.
2. Always perform gynecologic or genitourinary examination in any patient with abdominal pain.
3. Hyperesthesia using the pinch maneuver of Cope is an adjunct to the standard examination that may be of help to the clinician.
4. Repeated, reproducible serial examinations over time will be of great importance to the diagnosis.
5. Carnett's maneuver helps differentiate abdominal wall from intraabdominal process.
6. Left upper quadrant pain after trauma, think of and evaluate for spleen rupture.
7. Murphy's sign complements direct and rebound palpation in evaluation of cholecystitis.

ABDOMINAL DISTENTION

The patient with an enlarged abdomen presents a diagnostic and teaching challenge to the clinician. It is important to emphasize the differential diagnosis and the methods best to define, describe, delineate and thus diagnose the problem **(Table 6.11)**. The most common causes of an enlarged abdomen are adipose tissue (obesity) and pregnancy. Other causes include bowel obstruction, ascites, and an enlarged urinary bladder.

Table 6.11. Physical Examination of the Patient with a Distended Abdomen

Technique	Ascites	Bowel obstruction	Adipose	Pregnancy
Bulging flanks	Mild: present Tense: present	Absent	Absent	Absent
Percussion	Mild: meniscus of Dull (fluid), dome of gas (tympany) Tense: dull throughout	Tympany If marked, like a snare drum	Nonspecific	Nonspecific
Meniscus	Mild: present Tense: absent	Absent	Absent	Absent
Shifting dullness	Mild: shifts Tense: no shift	Absent	Absent	Absent
Fluid wave	Mild: present Tense: present	Absent	Absent	Absent
Dependent edema	Mild: present Tense: present Absence of pitting edema makes ascites unlikely	Absent	Nonspecific	Often present
Inspection	Venous collaterals	Tense skin	Nonspecific striae	Linea nigra
Auscultation	Nonspecific	High-pitched Tinkling	Nonspecific	Fetal heart tones
Tenderness	Nontender, unless associated peritonitis	Diffuse tenderness	Nonspecific	Nonspecific
Hernia	Umbilical pointed down	May be present, especially if incarcerated	None	Umbilical pointed up (Tanyol's sign)
Company it keeps	Conjunctival Icterus New use of suspenders Tiger-striping of skin Spider angioma Palmar erythema	Decreased flatus	Other areas of adipose	Amenorrhea Linea nigra Palpable fetus Epigastric bruit Fetal heart tones

Bowel obstruction manifests with the patient complaining of mild to moderate cramp-type abdominal discomfort and notes a decreased to absent flatus. In addition, there is associated nausea and then vomiting. On **inspection**, there are no bulging flanks. On **percussion** of the abdomen, diffuse tympany is noted **(Fig. 6.27)**. If the obstruction is severe and tense, it may be so taut as to sound like a snare drum. On **auscultation**, the classic features of bowel obstruction are noted. These include periods of absent bowel sounds admixed with rushes, high-pitched* tinkling-type bowel sounds. It is important to examine for any **hernias** in inguinal, femoral, and umbilical sites as an incarcerated hernia may cause obstruction.

Ascites manifests with the patient complaining of increasing size of abdomen **(Tables 6.11** and **6.12)**. The patient often reports the new need to use suspenders to keep trousers up and lower extremity edema. On **inspection**, bulging flanks are noted **(Fig. 6.28)**. On **percussion** performed with patient supine and from the highest point of the abdomen posteriorly, repeated in four to five different lines. Note any pattern of tympany and dullness. Tense ascites is dull throughout; bowel obstruction is tympanic; modest ascites has

*High-pitched = higher than a 512 Hz tuning fork (High C).

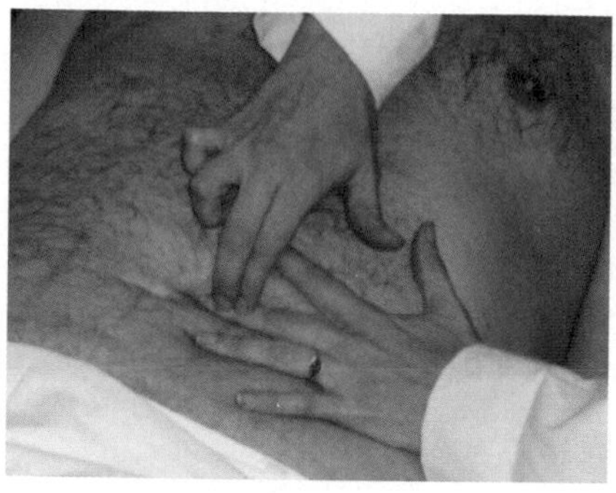

Figure 6.27.

Technique to percuss the abdomen.

 **TIPS**

- Patient supine
- Find the highest point of the abdomen, place palmar side of third digit there
- Use third finger of dominant hand to percuss
- Percuss on a line from highest point, posteriorly
- Note any change in percussion note from normal or tympanic to dull
- Make note of this point of change
- Repeat the procedure in four to five different lines from the center, again noting any change from normal or tympany to dull
- Normal or adipose: nonspecific
- Ascites: pattern of a circle of dullness (a meniscus) on rim, radius is same from center point
- Tense ascites: dullness throughout, often with pitting edema in abdominal skin
- Bowel obstruction: tympany throughout

Table 6.12. Evidence to Support the Physical Examination: Ascites

Test	Study	Sensitivity (%)	Specificity (%)	LR	LR
Flank dullness	Simel, et al	80	69	2.6	0.3
	Cattau, et al	94	29	1.3	0.2
Bulging flanks	Simel, et al	93	54	2.0	0.1
	Cattau, et al	78	44	1.4	0.5
	Cummings, et al	72	70	2.4	0.4
Shifting dullness	Simel, et al	60	90	5.8	0.5
	Cattau, et al	83	56	1.9	0.4
	Cummings, et al	88	56	2.0	0.2
Fluid wave	Simel, et al	80	92	9.6	0.2
	Cattau, et al	50	82	2.8	0.6
	Cummings, et al	53	90	5.3	0.5

distinct meniscus. If a **meniscus** is present, it can be confirmed by performing the *shifting dullness maneuver.* This maneuver is performed with the patient supine: note the meniscus line between the normal or tympany and the dull area, then roll the patient over onto a decubitus position, and percuss the interface again. A shift in this interface (meniscus) makes ascites likely. If no meniscus is present, there is no need to perform the shifting dullness examination; instead, a *fluid wave maneuver* should be performed to confirm fluid. The **fluid wave maneuver** is performed with the patient supine. The examiner places one hand, palm side to skin, on the lowest side of one flank, then use the second or third digit as a plexor on the mid to lower part of the contralateral side and briskly taps once **(Fig. 6.30)**. Feel for a bump, thump, or thud transmitted across the fluid as a result of the tap. A ripple in the skin is perfectly normal and, if distracting to the examiner, the hand of a colleague can be placed in the midline abdomen to tamp it out. This third hand technique is of minimal diagnostic help. In addition, there is often **pitting peripheral edema**, scrotal and penile or labia majora and minor edema and abdominal wall edema (Fig. 6.28B) **(Figs. 6.31 and 6.32)**. The absence of pitting peripheral edema is an excellent marker to decrease the likelihood that the abdominal enlargement is a result of ascites. Finally, if the underlying cause of ascites is end-stage liver disease, liver-related manifestations are not uncommon. The company it keeps includes a small liver, gynecomastia, small testes, collateral venous distension in the abdomen above and below the umbilicus (Fig. 6.28A), palmar erythema, spider angiomas, asterixis, and white transverse bands in the nail beds (Muercke's lines) of profound (albumin of <2.2) hypoalbuminemia **(Fig. 6.33)**.

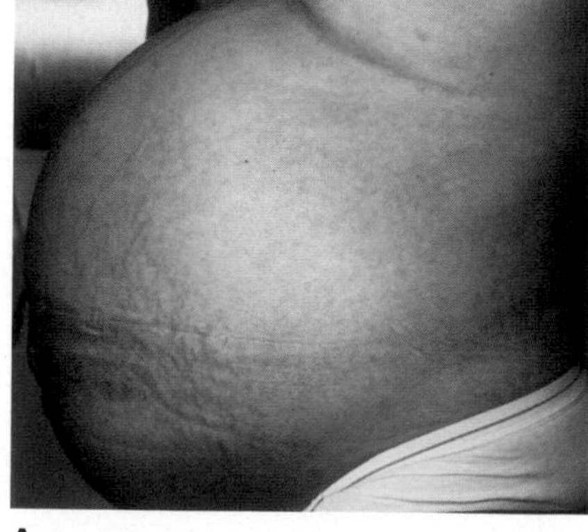

A

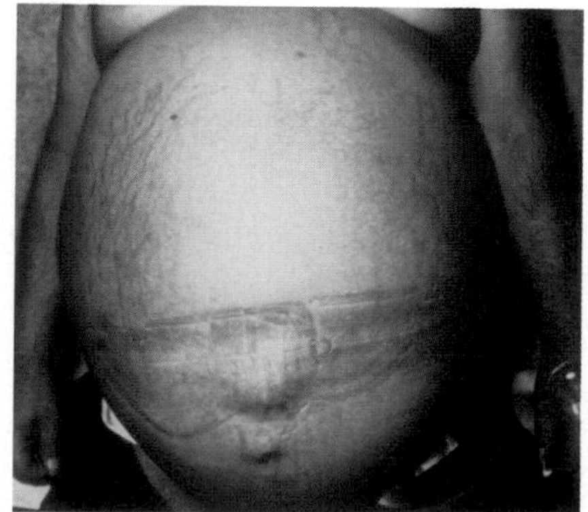

B

Figure 6.28.

Ascites. **A**. Side view. Massive ascites with "tiger-striping" edema. **B**. Front view. Bulging flanks, collateral veins.

 **TIPS**

- Ascites: distention; when tense, dull throughout, no shifting dullness; fluid wave present however

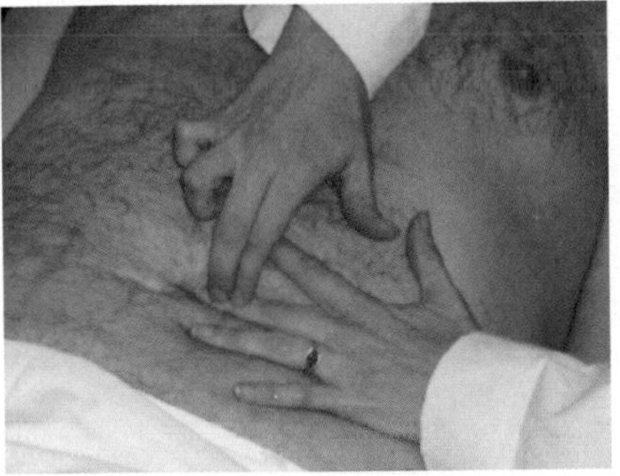

A

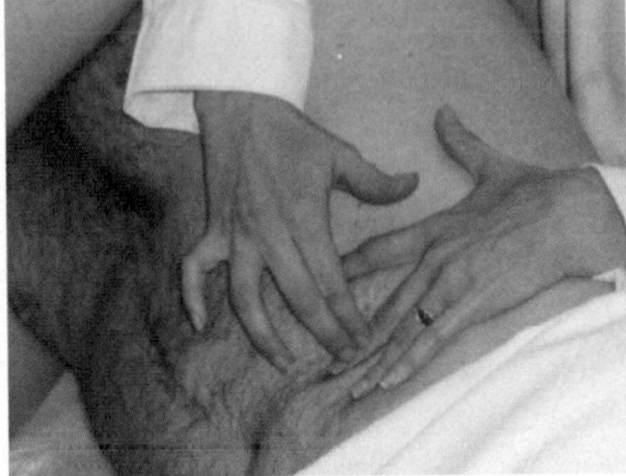

B

Figure 6.29.

Technique to perform shifting dullness. **A**. Supine, **B**. Right decubital position.

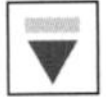

TIPS

- Note line of meniscus of tympany to dull: if no such meniscus, no need to perform
- Have patient roll over into lateral decubitus position: repeat the percussion procedure, make note of point of change between normal or tympany to dull
- Mild to moderate ascites: clear shift or movement of the line or point, i.e., the fluid moves

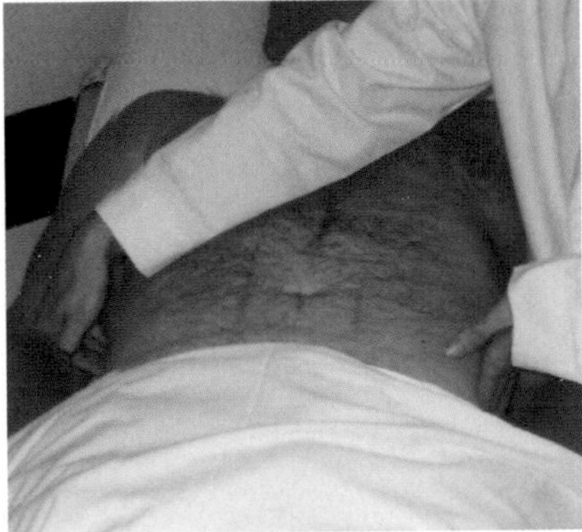

Figure 6.30.

Technique for fluid wave.

TIPS

- Patient supine
- Place one hand, palm to skin, on the lowest site of one flank
- Use the second or third digit as a plexor on the mid to low flank on contralateral side
- Tap once
- Note ripple in skin and subcutaneous tissue; note any slurp or thud wave felt in other hand
- If the skin ripple is distracting, have an associate place a hand, ulnar side to midline of abdomen, to tamp this out
- Normal or adipose: ripple wave present, no thud wave
- Mild or tense ascites: ripple wave present, thud or bump wave felt with other hand

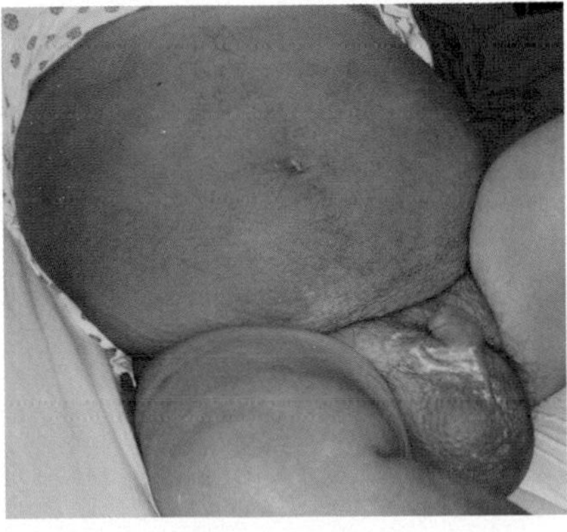

Figure 6.31.

Ascites due to right heart failure. Scrotal edema, and pitting edema.

TIPS

- Ascites: Often concurrent dependent pitting edema and scrotal or vulvar edema

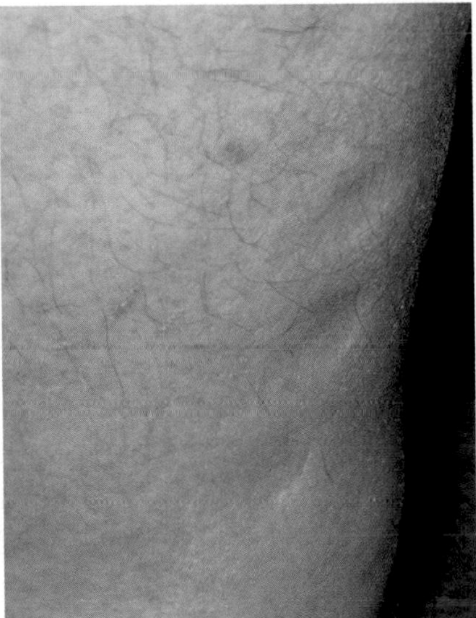

Figure 6.32.

Peripheral pitting edema; here is left ankle.

TIPS

- Ascites: often there is concurrent dependent pitting edema and scrotal or vulvar edema

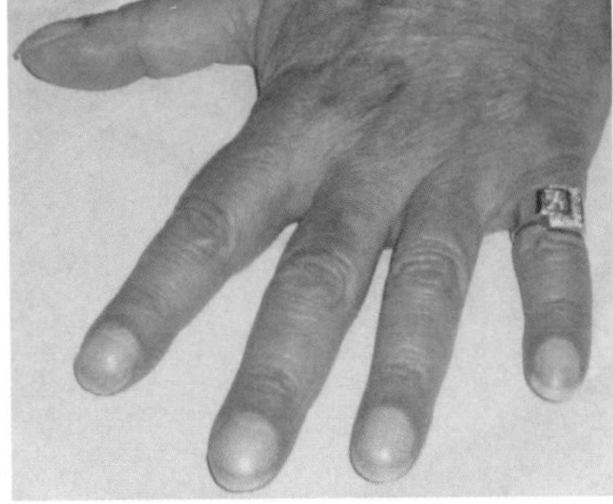

Figure 6.33.

Ascites: white nails and Muercke's lines of liver disease.

TIPS

- Ascites: often concurrent white nails or transverse white bands in the nail beds
- Highly correlated with profound hypoalbuminemia

TEACHING POINTS

ABDOMINAL DISTENSION

1. Distension may be caused by gas (bowel obstruction), fluid (ascites), fat, mass (gravid uterus), or distended urinary bladder.
2. Gas is easiest to differentiate: tympany throughout.
3. Massive ascites is dull throughout; only classic findings in such a case are peripheral edema, bulging flanks, and fluid wave.
4. Remember to include a massively distended urinary bladder in the differential diagnosis.
5. Must assess for a large prostate in males with distended urinary bladder.

Adipose obesity manifests with no specific complaints from the patient. On **inspection**, there are no bulging flanks. On **percussion**, there is no specific pattern of tympany or dullness and no shifting dullness. **Auscultation** is nonspecific and normal. Often, adipose tissue is noted in other areas and multiple lipomas may be found in the abdomen and chest.

Pregnancy manifests with secondary amenorrhea and lower abdominal distension. On **inspection**, distention is seen in the lower anterior abdomen. On **palpation**, a palpable uterus is noted, which is symmetrically enlarged, up to the level of the umbilicus at 20 weeks and to the xiphoid process at 38 weeks. The uterus has a smooth surface (see Chapter 3; Table 3.4.) **Leopold maneuver**—a bimanual examination of the fetus—is performed during the third trimester to assess the position of the baby's head, rump, and back. Furthermore, on auscultation, fetal heart tones at a rate of 135 to 140 beats/minute are distinctly heard over the uterus. The company pregnancy keeps includes cervical mucosal purple coloration (Chadwick's sign), line of pigment in the midline of the abdomen (linea nigra), tingling in the anterior-lateral thighs bilaterally (meralgia paresthetica), thickening of the interdental papillae, systolic epigastric bruits (prevalence of 21%, Sherrin), mild tachycardia, and dependent bilateral lower extremity pitting edema.

Massively enlarged urinary bladder manifests with the patient complaining of fullness in the suprapubic area, often with urinary hesitancy, burning with urination (dysuria), dribbling of urine, and the sensation of incomplete urinary evacuation (tenesmus). On inspection, a diffuse bulge is noted in the lower abdomen (best seen from the side) (Fig. 2.15 and 6.3B); on percussion, dullness is noted over the suprapubic area. In addition, in men, a symmetrically enlarged prostate is often noted on digital rectal examination.

Annotated Bibliography

Overall

Julius S, Steward BH. Diagnostic significance of abdominal murmurs. ***N Engl J Med*** **1967; 276:1175–1178.**

Found a small, but finite, number of healthy individuals have a systolic bruit in epigastrium—probably in a high-output state.

McSherry JA. The prevalence of epigastric bruit. *Journal of the Royal College of General Practice* 1979;29:10–172.

Epigastric bruits can be associated with high output states, e.g., fever or pregnancy; prevalence of 21%.

Rob C. Surgical diseases of the celiac and mesenteric arteries. *Arch Surg* 1966;93:21–32.

Epigastric bruit: 90% sensitive for celiac or mesenteric artery obstruction, but not very specific.

Anorectal Disorders

Metcalf A. Anorectal disorders. *Postgrad Med* 1995:98(5):81–94.

Practical and problem-oriented description of these common problems. Includes discussion of findings of internal hemorrhoids, external hemorrhoids, anal fissure, anal fistula, pruritus ani, and condyloma acuminatum. Some good color images of several of these entities.

Raymond PL. The ubiquitous umbilicus. *Postgrad Med* 1990;87(2):175–181.

Practical and primary care-based discussion of periumbilical problems, including Sister Mary Joseph's nodule, caput medusae, fistula, and umbilical hernia. Mentions Tanyol's sign in which an umbilical hernia is pointed upward in pregnancy, downward in ascites.

Liver Examination

Castell DO, O'Brien KD, Muench H, Chamlmers TC. Estimation of liver size by percussion in normal individuals. *Ann Intern Med* 1969;70:1183–1189.

Percussed liver size and developed a nomogram using weight, height, and sex to determine normal (in 116 individuals).

Fenster LF, Klatskin G. Manifestations of metastatic tumors of the liver. *Am J Med* 1961; 31:238–248.

Of patients with tumor metastatic to liver, 10% have a rub.

Fuller GN Hargreaves MR, King DM. Scratch test in clinical examination of liver [Letter]. *Lancet* 1988;1:181.

Scratch test has merit in physical examination.

Meidel EJ, Ende J. Evaluation of liver size by physical examination. *J Gen Intern Med* 1993; 8:635–637.

Solid review of this topic.

Naylor CD. Physical examination of the liver. *JAMA* 1994;271(23):1859–1865.

Overview of the techniques and interpretation of physical examination of the liver.

Sherman HI, Hardison JE. The importance of a coexistent hepatic rub and bruit: a clue to the diagnosis of cancer in the liver. *JAMA* 1979;241:1495.

Hepatic rub and bruit, together, markedly increase the likelihood of metastatic disease.

Sullivan S, Krasner N, Williams R. The clinical estimation of liver size: a comparison of techniques and an analysis of the source for error. *BMJ* 1976;2:1042–1043.

Demonstrates the problems in reproducibly assessing liver span using the scratch test, percussion, and even scintiscan imaging.

Abdominal Pain

Alvarado A. A practical score for the early diagnosis of acute appendicitis. *Ann Emerg Med* 1986;15:557–564.

Retrospective analysis of 305 patients hospitalized with abdominal pain (epigastric, periumbilical, or right lower quadrant). Of these, 254 (83%) had an appendectomy, 27 (11%) did not have appendicitis. Symptoms and signs included migration of pain—periumbilical or epigastric into the right lower quadrant sensitivity, 69%; specificity, 84%; positive predictive value (PPV), 0.95; anorexia: sensitivity, 61%; specificity, 72%; PPV, 0.91; nausea or vomiting: sensitivity, 0.74; specificity, 0.36; PPV, 0.84; tenderness at McBurney's point: sensitivity, 100%; specificity, 12%; PPV, 1.0; rebound pain: sensitivity, 55%; specificity, 78%; PPV, 0.92; fever: sensitivity, 0.73; specificity, 0.5; PPV, 0.87. Also leukocytosis: sensitivity, 93%; specificity, 38%; PPV, 0.87; left shift: sensitivity, 71%; PPV, 0.91. Based on these, came up with a scoring system to assess appendicitis. This is a retrospective analysis with problems inherent to such a design.

Berry J, Malt RA. Appendicitis near its centenary. *Ann Surg* 1984;200(5):567–575.

Manifestations of appendicitis, including right lower quadrant tenderness: sensitivity, 96%; likelihood ratio (LR), 1.0; rebound tenderness: sensitivity, 70%; specificity, 39%; LR, 1.1; and psoas sign: sensitivity, 13%; specificity, 91%; LR, 1.6.

Carnettt JB. Intercostal neuralgia as a cause of abdominal pain and tenderness. *Surgery Gynecology and Obstetrics* 1926;42:625–632.

Fascinating paper that describes the procedure to assist a clinician in differentiating abdominal wall problems from intraabdominal problems.

Cope Z. Cutaneous hyperesthesia in acute abdominal disease. *Lancet* 1924;(Jan):121–125.

An elegant and practical review of this relatively useful, yet underutilized, test for intraabdominal pathology. Describes two different methods: pin-stroke (we do not recommend this, but instead the use of a cotton-tipped swab) and the light pinch. The pinch test: "corresponding portions of skin on each side of the middle line are gently pinched between the finger and thumb and patient is asked if there is any difference in sensation." Dr. Cope found the pinch test to be slightly superior to the pin-stroke. Definitions of hyperalgesia (pain over area) and hyperesthesia (increased sensitivity but not necessarily pain). Used the outcome of hyperesthesia—sensitivity of 59% (110/185 cases) for acute appendicitis in right lower quadrant; 47% for acute abdomen. States that other writers report sensitivities of 32% (Sherren) and 21% (Robinson) for hyperalgesia in appendicitis. He found the test to be most useful in appendicitis, less so in cholecystitis (6/16 cases had hyperesthesia). Also used the test for perforated ulcers, inflamed ovarian cysts, and abscesses of the spermatic cord as case series of two to three cases. Made a point of examining on skin with" clothes or bedclothes well out of the way".

Dowdall GG. Five diagnostic methods of John B. Murphy. *Archives of Diagnosis* 1910;(Jan): 459–466.

Describes five physical examination techniques invented by Murphy, as reported by one of his staff members, Dr. Dowdall. Murphy constantly referred to these as "five diagnostic methods." Two of these are used today: "fist percussion of kidney...the patient, with clothing removed above the waist, is seated in an upright position on a stool, and is then instructed to bend forward as far as possible. One hand placed flat over site one kidney or the other, the clenched fist of examiner is brought down with considerable force upon the dorsum of flexed hand. If acute congestion ...the patient will cry out with the pain of the blow." A control test is advised by first striking the sound side and then the suspected side. The second is the classic Murphy's sign used today, which he called "deep-grip palpation" in suspected gallbladder disease. "Standing directly behind the patient, provided that the patient is well enough to assume an upright position, if not the examiner reaches over the recumbent patient from the head, the right hand of the examiner curls up under the costal arch at the tip of the ninth cartilage, the patient is requested to take a deep breath and at the end of expiration, the examining fingers seek the gallbladder area and fix it from beneath. The diaphragm, descending from above with the beginning of inspiration, brings down the liver and gallbladder and if cholecystitis or cholelithic obstruction present, the descent is checked suddenly with an accompanying groan from the patient. Other tests, including piano percussion for small quantities of ascites, comparative bimanual examination of iliac fossa for acute appendicitis, and "hammer stroke percussion" for cholecystitis are fascinating. Excellent images, but no data on predictive values.

Fitz Reginald H. Perforating inflammation of the vermiform appendix. *Am J Med Sci* 1886; 321–345.

A classic, although ponderous and light on the descriptions of physical findings, it is one of the original descriptions of appendicitis. Classic description of sudden severe abdominal pain, resolving on day 2, followed by fever to 103°F, then peritoneal signs and even swelling in right iliac fossa. No diarrhea, but often constipation.

Golledge J, Tom AP, Franklin IJ, Scriven MW, Galland RB. Assessment of peritonism in appendicitis. *Ann R Coll Surg* 1996;78(1):11–14.

Excellent overview of the signs of appendicitis. Prospectively assessed 100 patients with right iliac fossa pain. Of the 100 patients, 58 had surgery, 44 had appendicitis on pathology. Cat's eye symptom: sensitivity, 80%; specificity, 52%; PPV, 57; cough sign: sensitivity, 82%; specificity, 50%; PPV, 0.56; percussion tenderness: sensitivity, 57%; specificity, 86%; rebound tenderness: sensitivity, 82%; specificity, 89%; PPV, 0.86. Noted that the most false-positive diagnostic findings were in young woman (11/14 normal appendices removed from young women).

Gunn A, Kedie N. Some clinical observations in patients with gallstones. *Lancet* 1972; 2:230–241.

Boas' sign: sensitivity, 7%; Murphy's sign: sensitivity, 27%.

Izbicki JR, Wolfram TK, Dietmar KW, et al. Accurate diagnosis of acute appendicitis: a retrospective and prospective analysis of 686 patients. *Eur J Surg* 1992;158:227–231.

Used 686 patients to assess the physical examination of patients with potential acute appendicitis. Manifestations of appendicitis included right lower quadrant tenderness: sensitivity, 96%; LR, 0.96; rebound tenderness: sensitivity, 76%; specificity, 56%; LR, 1.7; Rovsing's sign: sensitivity, 0.22; specificity, 0.96; LR, 5.5; psoas sign: sensitivity, 15%; specificity, 97%; LR, 5.0.

Abdominal Mass

Courvoisier LG. *Casuistisch-Statistische Beitrage zur pathologie und Chirugie der Gallenwege.* Leipzig: Verlag von FCW Vogel, 1890.

A classic. In patients with jaundice, a palpable gallbladder indicates neoplastic process in ducts; nonpalpable gallbladder, an inflammatory process.

Fortner G, Johansen K. Abdominal aortic aneurysms *West J Med* 1984;140:50–59.

A diameter of>3.5 cm of the infrarenal aorta indicates aneurysm.

Lederle FA. Selective screening for abdominal aortic aneurysm with physical examination and ultrasound. *Arch Intern Med* 1988;148:1753–1756.

A solid paper that demonstrates the significant limits and uses of physical examination in the diagnosis of aortic abdominal aneurysm.

Abdominal Distension (Except for Ascites)

Guarino JR. Auscultatory percussion of the urinary bladder. *Arch Intern Med* 1985;145: 1823–1825.

Interesting application of this technique in which 170 men were examined. The upper extent of the urinary bladder was noted in reference to the symphysis pubis and then correlated with urinary bladder volume. Technique was with patient supine, diaphragm placed superior to the symphysis *pubis, scratch test applied in midline using palmar fingertip. Fluid loud, gas soft, if border at 0 cm; empty bladder, if at >2 cm full; or distended bladder. Found that mean urinary volumes at the 3-cm level (and above) were significantly >250 mL or that of a full bladder (P < .01). Interesting use of this technique.*

Ascites

Cattau EL, Benjamin SB, Knuff TE, et al. The accuracy of the physical examination in the diagnosis of suspected ascites. *JAMA* 1982;247:1164–1166.
Used gastroenterologists to assess the accuracy of the history and physical examination for ascites in 21 patients referred to a gastroenterologist to assist the primary physician in the diagnosis. Flank dullness: sensitivity, 94%; specificity, 29%; positive LR, 1.3; negative LR, 0.2; bulging flanks: sensitivity, 78%; specificity, 44%; positive LR, 1.4; negative LR, 0.5; shifting dullness: sensitivity, 83%; specificity, 56%; positive LR, 1.9; negative LR, 0.4; fluid wave: sensitivity, 50%; specificity, 82%; positive LR, 2.8; negative LR, 0.6.

Cummings S, Papadakis M, Melnick J, et al. The predictive value of physical examination for ascites. *West J Med* 1985;142:633–636.
Used board-certified general internists to assess the accuracy of the history and physical examination for ascites in 90 patients with chronic liver disease. Bulging flanks: sensitivity, 72%; specificity, 70%; positive LR, 2.4; negative LR, 0.4; shifting dullness: sensitivity, 88%; specificity, 56%; positive LR, 2.0; negative LR, 0.2; fluid wave: sensitivity, 53%; specificity, 90%; positive LR, 5.3; negative LR, 0.5.

Lawson JD, Weissbein CA. The puddle sign—an aid in the diagnosis of minimal ascites. *N Engl J Med* 1959;260:652–654.
Describes a test that, at best, is minimally beneficial in diagnosis and, in all cases, difficult for the patient, in that it requires the patient to lie prone, then go onto all four extremities to be examined. It is especially difficult if the patient is ill. Not discussed or recommended by us.

Simel DL, Halvorsen RA, Feussner JR. Clinical evaluation of ascites. *J Gen Intern Med* 1988; 3:423–428.
Used internal medicine house staff to assess the accuracy of the history and physical examination for ascites (ultrasound documented). Flank dullness: sensitivity, 80%; specificity, 69%; positive LR, 2.6; negative LR, 0.3; bulging flanks: sensitivity, 93%; specificity, 54%; positive LR, 2.0; negative LR, 0.12; shifting dullness: sensitivity, 60%; specificity, 90%; positive LR, 5.8; negative LR, 0.5; fluid wave: sensitivity, 80%; specificity, 92%; positive LR, 9.6; negative LR, 0.2. One of the best papers on this topic, it also set the standard for evidence-based physical examination. Also demonstrates that the patient's subjective assessment of no ankle swelling was an excellent marker for no ascites (negative LR, 0.10), and the objective absence of peripheral edema has a great negative LR of 0.17.

Williams JW, Simel DL. Does this patient have ascites? *JAMA* 1992;267(19):2645–2648.
Nice review of the pathophysiology and clinical manifestations of ascites based on several papers, including data from Cummings, Simel, and Cattau. Includes a history of increased girth: positive LR, 4.6; negative LR, 0.17; sensitivity, 87%; specificity, 77%; ankle swelling: positive LR, 2.8; negative LR, 0.10; sensitivity, 93%; specificity, 66%. Focused physical examination, including inspection of bulging flanks, pooled data: positive LR, 2.0; negative LR, 0.3; sensitivity, 0.81; specificity, 0.59; percussion for flank dullness: positive LR, 2.0; negative LR, 0.3; sensitivity, 84%; specificity, 59%; with an inference of a circle of differentiation between dullness and the tympany, testing for shifting dullness: positive LR, 2.7; negative LR, 0.4; sensitivity, 77%; specificity, 72%; and test for fluid wave: positive LR, 6.0; negative LR, 0.4; sensitivity, 62%; specificity, 90%. They did not recommend the puddle sign: positive LR, 1.6; negative LR, 0.8; sensitivity, 45%; specificity, 73%; or auscultatory percussion as useful tests at the bedside to assess patient for ascites.

Abdominal Wall

Bailey H. *Demonstrations of Physical Signs in Clinical Surgery*, 11th ed. Baltimore: Williams & Wilkins, 1949:227.
Hamilton Bailey first credited Sister (Mary) Joseph with the eponym for this finding (10 years after her death).

Cullen TS. A new sign in ruptured extrauterine pregnancy. *Am J Obstet* 1918;(3):78.
Terse description of one case of a 38-year-old woman with the finding and diagnosis of ruptured extrauterine pregnancy.

Issa M, Feeley M, Kerin M, Tanner A, Keane F. Umbilical deposits from internal malignancy: Sister Mary Joseph's nodule. *Ir Med J* 1987;80:152–153.
Excellent review of this rare, but diagnostically and prognostically important, finding.

Schwartz I. Sister (Mary?) Joseph's nodule. *N Eng J Med* 1987;316:1348–1349.
Fascinating discussion of the evolution of this eponym—Mary Joseph or Joseph. (Actually, her birth name was Julia Dempsy).

Turner GG. Local discoloration of the abdominal wall as a sign of acute pancreatitis *Br J Surg* 1920;7:394–7395.
The original by Dr. Grey Turner.

LR = Likelihood Ratio.

Splenomegaly

Barkun AN, Camus M, Meager T. Splenic enlargement and Traube's space: how useful is percussion? ***Am J Med*** **1989;87:562–566.**

Percussion of Traube's space: supine, arm slightly abducted, percuss space defined by rib 6, midaxillary line, left costal margin, patient breathing normally; dull abnormal, normal note-normal: sensitivity, 62%; specificity, 72%; if in a fasting, nonobese patient: sensitivity, 78%; specificity, 82%.

Barkun AN, Camus M, Green L, Meagher T, Coupal L, De Stempel J, Grover SA. The bedside assessment of splenic enlargement. ***Am J Med*** **1991;91(5):512–518.**

Prospective assessment of 118 patients using various techniques to diagnose splenomegaly; the gold standard is ultrasound. Traube's space percussion: sensitivity, 62%; specificity, 72%; splenic percussion sign: sensitivity, 79%; specificity,46%. Palpation was useful in those with dullness to percussion, but was poor if no percussion dullness. Palpation characteristics: sensitivity, 39%; specificity, 97%; positive LR, 13.

Grover SA, Barkun AN, Sackett DL. Does this patient have splenomegaly? ***JAMA*** **1993;270 (18):1218–1221.**

An excellent review of the physical examination techniques to detect an enlarged spleen. Reviewed most of the papers written to study this issue. Percussion by Nixon's maneuver, Sullivan and William's modification, right lateral decubitus position: percuss from left arc in a line perpendicular to the margin, dullness <8 cm from margin—splenomegaly, patient breathing normal: sensitivity, 59%; specificity, 94%. Percussion by Castell's method: patient supine, percuss in lowest intercostal space in left anterior axillary line, in both expiration and full inspiration—normal; normal note, any dullness-splenomegaly: sensitivity, 82%; specificity, 83%. Percussion of Traube's space: supine, arm slightly abducted, percuss space defined by rib 6, midaxillary line, left costal margin, patient breathing normally—dull abnormal, normal note-normal: sensitivity, 62%; specificity, 72%. If in a fasting, nonobese patient: sensitivity, 78%; specificity, 82%. Two-handed palpation: patient in right lateral decubitus position, examiner's left hand is on posterior flank lifting anteriorly, the right hand under the left costal margin; patient takes a large inhalation; repeat with right hand moved inferiorly 2 cm for four cycles. One-handed palpation: patient supine, the right hand under the left costal margin, patient takes a large inhalation; repeat with right hand moved inferiorly 2 cm for four cycles. The Hooking palpation procedure of Middleton: patient supine with fist beneath left costal area, examiner on left side of patient, facing feet, examiner's fingers under left costal margin, patient takes a long deep inhalation: sensitivity, 56%; specificity, 93%. Overall palpation for splenomegaly, pooled study data: sensitivity, 58%; specificity, 92%. All procedures described in detail. Kappa findings for Traube's space percussion were 0.19 to 0.41 and for studies using palpation were 0.56 to 0.7. The recommendation was to percuss first and then, if dullness present, to palpate.

Castell DO. The spleen percussion sign: a useful diagnostic technique. ***Ann Intern Med*** **1967;67:1265–1267.**

Percussion by Castell's method: patient supine, percuss in lowest intercostal space in left anterior axillary line, in both expiration and full inspiration—normal; normal note, any dullness-splenomegaly: sensitivity, 82%; specificity, 83%.

Shaw MT, Dvorak V. Palpation of minimally enlarged spleens. ***Lancet*** **1973;1:317.**

Hooking palpation procedure of Middleton: patient supine with fist beneath left costal area, examiner on left side of patient, facing feet, examiner's fingers under left costal margin, patient takes a long deep inhalation: sensitivity, 56%; specificity, 93%; overall palpation for splenomegaly.

Sullivan S, Williams R. Reliability of clinical techniques for detecting splenic enlargement. ***BMJ*** **1976;2:1043–1044.**

Percussion by Nixon's maneuver, Sullivan and William's modification: right lateral decubitus position, percuss from left arc in a line perpendicular to the margin, dullness <8 cm from margin—splenomegaly, patient breathing normal: sensitivity, 59%; specificity, 94%.

Tamayo SG, Richman LS, Mathews WC, et al. Examiner dependence on physical diagnostic tests for the detection of splenomegaly: a prospective study with multiple observers. ***J Gen Intern Med*** **1994;8:69–75.**

Small study of 27 patients to assess for splenomegaly. Percussion using Nixon's maneuver: positive likelihood ratio (LR), 1.74; Castell's: positive LR, 1.97; palpation bimanual: positive LR, 1.69; Middleton's: positive LR, 2.66.

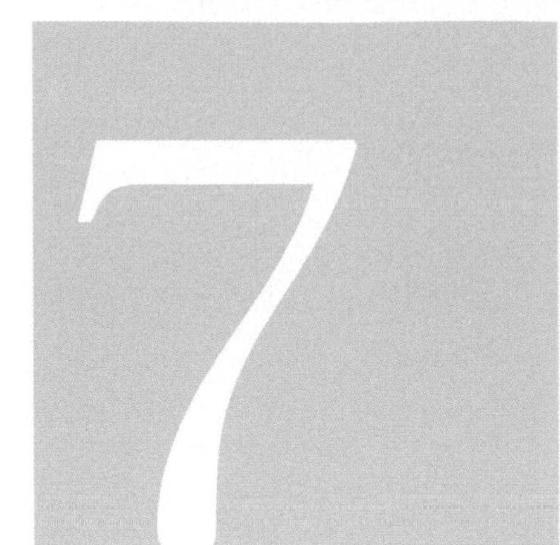

Neurologic Examination

PRACTICE AND TEACHING

OVERALL EXAMINATION

Overall neurologic examination includes the thorough assessment of power, tone, reflexes, cranial nerves, and function of the sensory structures.

Power Assessment

The **neurologic examination** includes the assessment of the **power**, also known as strength of various muscle groups. Two muscle groups from the proximal upper and lower extremities should be examined. **Shoulder elevation or shrugging** against resistance is assessed for proximal muscle strength, trapezius muscle function, and cranial nerve (CN) XI function **(Fig. 7.1)**. For this assessment, the patient actively elevates the shoulders, i.e., shrugs, while the examiner applies resistance; feel the trapezius muscle. **Arm extension** is assessed for triceps function, radial nerve, and root C7 **(Fig. 7.2)**. For this, the patient's arm is passively abducted to horizontal (90 degrees), forearm dangling down at the elbow; the patient then actively extends the forearm at the

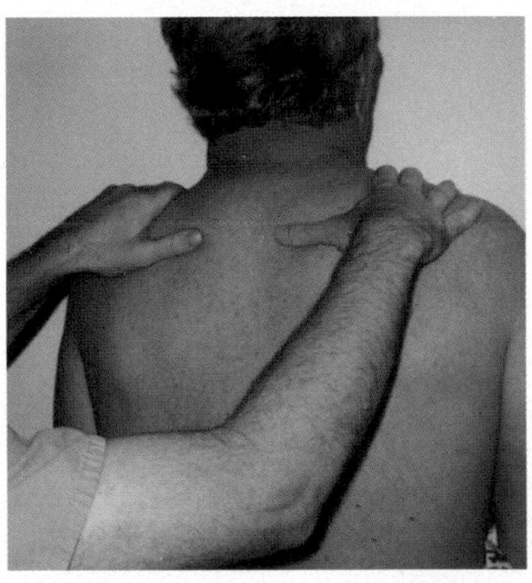

Figure 7.1.

Technique for power assessment of proximal upper extremities: elevation of shoulders.

 **TIPS**

- Active shoulder elevation or shrugging: apply resistance to tops of the scapula
- Trapezius contraction
- Proximal muscle problems: bilateral weakness

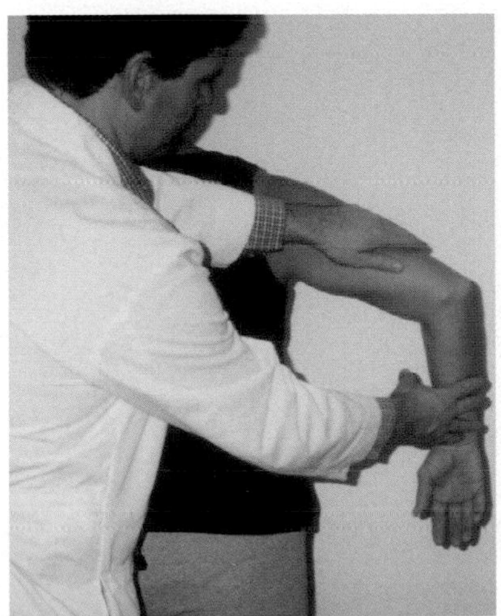

Figure 7.2.

Technique for power assessment of triceps and proximal arm: extension of elbows.

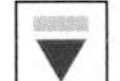 **TIPS**

- With patient's arm abducted to 90 degrees, forearm dangling at the side, actively extended at elbow: apply resistance to the distal forearm
- Triceps muscle contraction
- Radial nerve or root of C7 problem: unilateral paresis, fasciculations, and even atrophy of the triceps muscle
- Proximal muscle weakness: bilateral paresis

Figure 7.3.

Technique for power assessment of proximal hip. **A.** Forward flexion of hip with patient standing. **B.** Patient supine.

TIPS

- Patient standing **(A)**, or supine **(B)**, or sitting (see Hip Examination chapter)
- Start from about 10 to 20 degrees, leg supported by the examiner at this baseline; apply resistance on the distal anterior thigh
- Iliopsoas muscle damage or nerve roots L2 and 3: unilateral paresis
- Proximal muscle problem: bilateral paresis

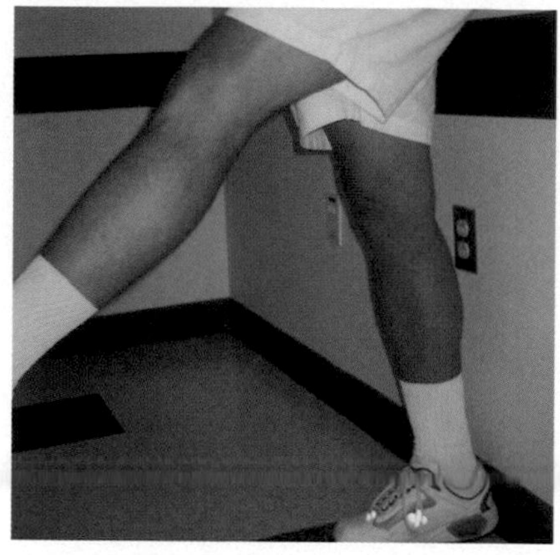

A

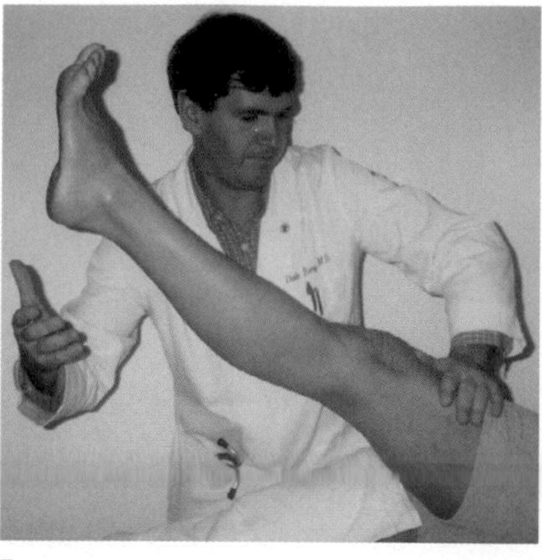

B

elbow against resistance applied by the examiner; feel the triceps muscle. **Hip forward flexion** is assessed for proximal muscle strength, upper lumbar roots (L1, 2, 3), and iliopsoas muscle function **(Fig. 7.3)**. Assessment is either from a baseline position of standing, supine, or sitting. The standing position (Fig. 7.3A) or with the patient supine with leg suppported by examiner at 10 degrees of forward flexion (Fig. 7.3B) or, sitting with knees flexed are all acceptable. The patient then actively forward flexes the leg while the examiner applies resistance to the distal anterior thigh. From the seated position, the patient is instructed to raise the knee straight upward. **Hip backward flexion** is assessed for proximal muscle strength, gluteal muscle function, and lower lumbar and upper sacral root function (L4, 5 and S1, 2) **(Fig. 7.4)**. Assessment is with the patient either standing and leaning onto a wall supported by hands placed on wall (Fig. 7.4A) or in the prone position with the leg assessed slightly off the side of the table (Fig. 7.4B). The patient actively backward flexes the leg against resistance applied to the posterior distal thigh. **Extension at knee** is assessed for proximal muscle weakness, midlumbar root function (L3, 4), femoral nerve and quadriceps muscle function **(Fig. 7.5)**. Assessment is one in which the patient is either supine or sitting with knees flexed and supported in 40 degrees of flexion. The patient actively extends the leg at the knee while the examiner applies resistance at the middistal anterior leg.

The **grading of power** uses the classic 5 to 0 numerical system. In this system, 5 is normal, 0 is completely absent; 3 is able to perform against gravity alone **(Table 7.1)**. The **pattern** of weakness (paresis) or paralysis (plegia) is of greatest diagnostic use. See **Table 7.2** for specific details. The various patterns

Figure 7.4.

Technique for power assessment of proximal hip. **A.** Backward flexion of hip, patient standing. **B.** Patient prone.

TIPS

- Note patient standing, stabilized by examiner or wall **(A)** or supine **(B)**; active backward flexion of hip: apply resistance on the distal posterior thigh
- Gluteus maximus muscle damage: unilateral paresis
- L5 or S1 or S2 roots or gluteal nerve damage: unilateral paresis
- Proximal muscle weakness: bilateral paresis

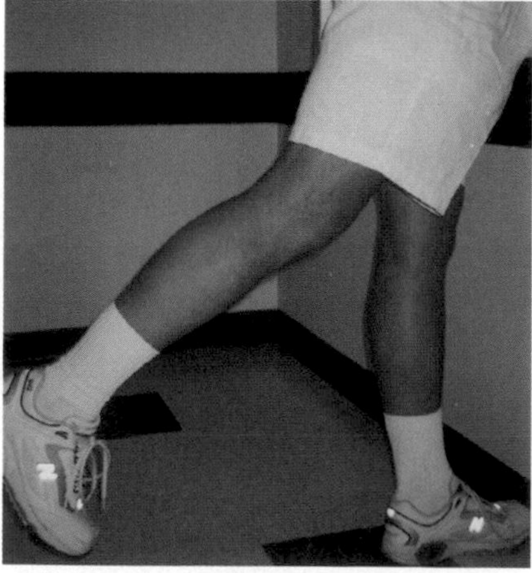

A

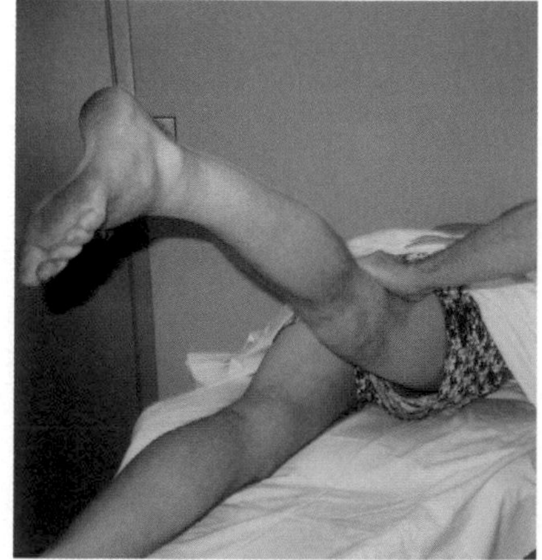

B

Table 7.1. Grading of Power

Proximal muscle groups		
0 Absent	Plegia	Paralysis
1 Twitch	Paresis	Weakness
2 Move, but not to gravity	Paresis	Weakness
3 Gravity	Paresis	Weakness
4 Gravity with two fingers of resistance	Paresis	Weakness
5 Gravity with full hand of resistance	Normal	
Distal muscle groups		
0 Absent	Plegia	
1 Weakness	Paresis	
2 Normal		

Often excellent to repeat this set of tests for follow-up because incremental improvement or decremental deterioration of strength indicates specific diagnoses.

include paraparesis, paraplegia, tetraparesis, tetraplegia, hemiparesis, hemiplegia, and proximal muscle weakness (see Table 7.1). Although useful, the grading system of power itself has several problems inherent to it. First, there is a significant amount of interobserver variation: 5 (normal) that may be markedly different for different examiners. Second, the grading system is best used on proximal muscle groups like the pectoralis and pelvic, and is not easily used on distal muscle groups. The distal muscle groups are best graded as normal, weak, or absent. Finally, the effectiveness of the examination is diminished when concurrent joint swelling or pain is present.

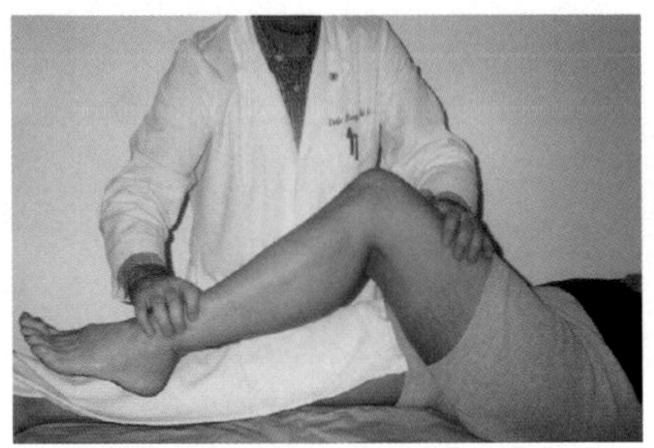

Figure 7.5.

Technique for power assessment of the proximal lower extremity, quadriceps muscle. Extension at the knee, patient supine.

TIPS

- Patient sitting or supine
- Note knee held in 30 to 40 degrees flexion; patient told to actively straighten the leg
- Apply resistance on the middistal leg
- Quadriceps muscle or femoral nerve (L4) problem: unilateral paresis
- Proximal muscle problem: bilateral paresis

Table 7.2. Definitions of Weakness and Paralysis

Type	Pattern	Company it Keeps
Paraparesis	Bilateral Usually lower extremity weakness	Trauma to thoracic or lumbar spine Decreased anal wink Sacral sparing if a thoracic lesion Incomplete transection
Paraplegia	Bilateral Usually lower extremity paralysis	Trauma to thoracic or lumbar spine Absent anal wink Complete transection
Tetraparesis	All four extremities Weakness Also called quadriparesis	Trauma to cervical spine Incomplete transection
Tetraplegia	All four extremities paralyzed Also called quadriplegia	Trauma to cervical spine Complete transection High risk of respiratory defect
Hemiparesis	Unilateral, upper and lower weakness	Contralateral CVA Spastic hemiparetic gait Positive Hoffman or Tromner maneuver Positive Babinski sign Clonus
Hemiplegia	Unilateral, upper and lower paralysis	Contralateral CVA Usually unable to ambulate Positive Hoffman maneuver Positive Babinski sign Clonus

CVA = cerebrovascular accident.

Tone

Assessment of tone is an often overlooked, underutilized, and misunderstood component of the neurologic examination. Tone is, however, central to the neurologic examination and should be assessed and taught. Tone is the summation of the contributions that the muscles provide within a joint to maintain baseline position. Many neurologic problems manifest with an increase or decrease in joint tone. The **technique** to most effectively assess tone is one in which the examiner places one hand proximal to the joint, the other distal to the joint to be assessed **(Fig. 7.6)**. Passively and with a gliding smoothness, fully flex and extend the patient's elbow, fully circumduct the wrist, or circumduction* of the ankle. Perform this in three to five cycles, then repeat in the opposite direction. In our opinion, the best overall site and procedure is circumduction of the wrist. To optimize the sensitivity of the examination, the joint being examined must be as passive as possible. An excellent method to optimize the passive aspect is to instruct a patient to repetitively tap contralateral hand on their thigh, in order to distract them.

Upper motor neuron (UMN) damage manifests with increased tone on the side contralateral to damage. The increased tone is **spastic**, i.e., agonists and antagonists are equally involved. The classic **clasp-knife** phenomenon, in which there is severe resistance initially that dramatically decreases with passive motion, of spastic paralysis may be present. Examples of diseases with spasticity include cerebrovascular accident (CVA) and head trauma. **Basal ganglia** damage manifests with increased tone on the side ipsilateral to damage. This increased tone is **rigid**, i.e., involves an imbalance between agonists and antagonists, and manifests with **cogwheel** rigidity. In severe cases, it is profoundly akin to resistance provided in trying to bend a lead pipe, hence the term "**lead-pipe**" rigidity. The best sites for tone assessment include flexion and extension of the elbow; circumduction of the wrist; and circumduction of the ankle. Examples of diseases with rigidity include Parkinson's disease and the effects of neuroleptic agent use. **Myotonic dystrophy** manifests with increased tone in which there is the inability to relax a muscle contraction **(Fig. 7.7)**. An excellent method to assess for this is to instruct the patient to squeeze your hand for 10 seconds, then to rapidly release and spread out the fingers. A patient with myotonia is unable to perform this rapidly. The company myotonic dystrophy keeps includes the classic male pattern baldness and an acquired atrophy of the sternocleidomastoid and facial muscles with bilateral ptosis. Also noted are profound proximal muscle weakness and abnormal flexion of the thumb on the *thenar eminence percussion test* **(Fig. 7.8)**. For this test, place the patient's hand neutral and

Figure 7.6.

Technique to perform tone assessment at elbow **(A)**, wrist **(B)**, and ankle **(C)**.

 **TIPS**

- Place one hand on proximal to joint, the other distal
- Passively fully, and with a gliding smoothness, flex and extend at elbow **(A)**
- Passive circumduction at the wrist **(B)**
- Passive circumduction at the ankle **(C)**
- Perform three to five cycles, then repeat in opposite direction
- Instruct patient to tap hand on thigh, which distracts the patient
- Normal: smooth gliding action
- Rigidity: cogwheel sensation
- Spasticity: clasp-knife phenomenon
- Contracture: no movement because of primary joint problem

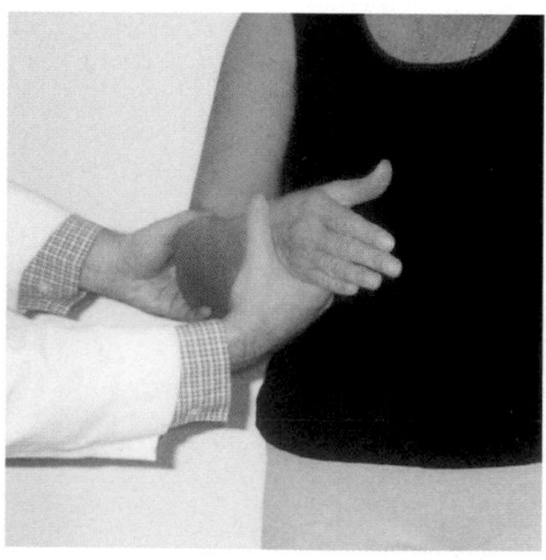

A

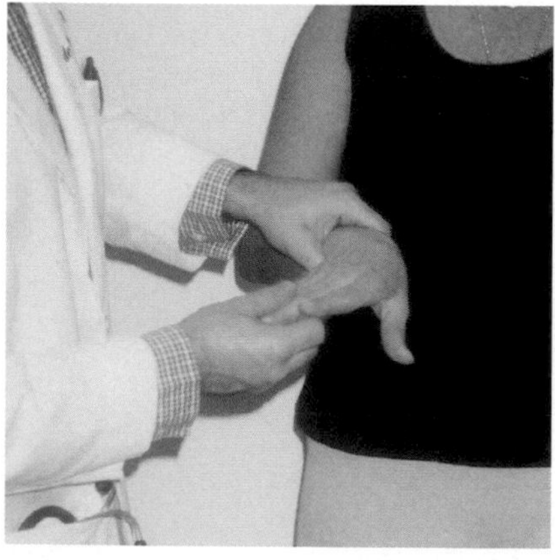

B

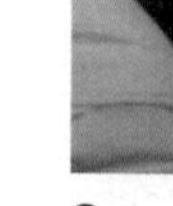

C

*Passive dorsiflexion and plantarflexion may be used at ankle instead of circumduction.

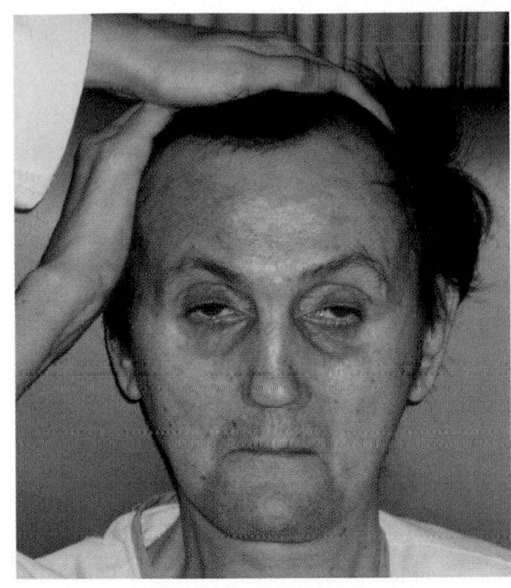

Figure 7.7.

Facies of myotonic dystrophy. Sad appearing, bilateral ptosis, and male pattern alopecia.

TIPS

- Inspect hair distribution and muscles of the face, head, and neck
- Myotonic dystrophy: muscle atrophy of the facial muscles (masseter or temporalis) and the sternocleidomastoids
- Myotonic dystrophy: male pattern balding, which is important in that if no balding, myotonic dystrophy is highly unlikely

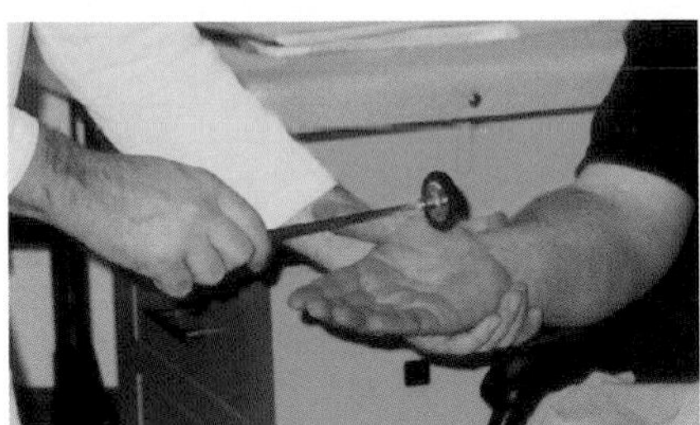

Figure 7.8.

Technique for the thenar eminence percussion test. Excellent confirmatory test for myotonia.

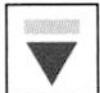

TIPS

- Hand neutral, forearm supinated
- Use a plexor to tap over thenar muscle
- Normal: thumb mildly bounces upward
- Myotonia: thumb moves upward, i.e., it flexes slightly

forearm supinated, tap on the thenar muscle **(Fig. 7.9)**. A finding that is of historical importance only is the *tongue percussion test* in which the percussion of the midline corsal tongue feels stiff, i.e., the test is positive. Finally, the patient will have systolic heart failure. **Cerebellar problems** manifest with a marked decrease in tone, ipsilateral to the damage. The tone about the joints is inappropriately loose or floppy and upon performing reflexes, there is **pendulum swinging**, i.e., the arm or leg swings to and fro several times with patellar and triceps reflexes. The baseline stance of the patient is with hand slightly flexed and bilateral pes planus is noted.

Reflexes

Although the term **deep tendon reflexes (DTR)** is best known as an integral part of the medical vernacular, they are best referred to as **muscle stretch reflexes (MSR)** because they impact on the spindle cells in the muscle, not the tendons. Because DTR is universally recognized, we will use that term and its acronym. These reflexes are a set of techniques that the lay public expects a physician to perform. These tests are especially useful with a patient who has increased or decreased tone and has concurrent paresis. Two fundamental components to the assessment and measurement of DTR include: first, a complete relaxation of the joint and, second, the use of a reflex hammer. Several different reflex hammers are demonstrated in **Fig. 7.10**. Although the finger is the most portable and convenient to use, our favorite is the Queens Square hammer (Fig. 7.10). Obtain DTRs from two to three sites in both upper and lower extremities; compares side-to-side.

Sites for *DTR measurement* include the biceps (C5), pectoralis major (C7), triceps (C7), quadriceps (L4), Achilles (S1), and the plantar (S1). The technique for **biceps reflex**: with the patient sitting, elbow in 90 degrees of flexion and the forearm neutral between supination and pronation, grasp the elbow, with the thumb on the olecranon and the index finger to press on, and stretch the biceps tendon **(Fig. 7.11)**. Tap a hammer on the finger overlying the tendon of the biceps where it inserts on the proximal forearm (mediate percussion). The technique for **triceps reflex**: with the patient standing or sitting, support the arm so that it is parallel to floor, then flex the forearm (dangled) to 90 degrees; use the hammer to tap over the proximal triceps aponeurosis **(Fig. 7.12)**. The technique for **pectoralis major reflex**: with the patient supine, arm at the side, approximately 20 degrees of humeral abduction, place your hand over the top of acromion, fingers toward the back, thumb

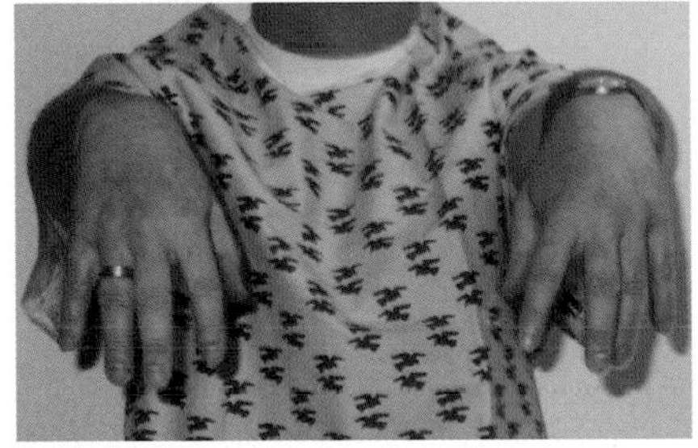

Figure 7.9.

Stance of hypotonia.

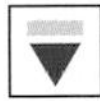

TIPS

- Instruct patient to stand with arms at 90 degrees of forward flexion, forearms pronated
- Hypotonia: able to perform, but the pronated hands are flexed almost to 90 degrees
- Concurrent bilateral pes planus and even mild out toeing

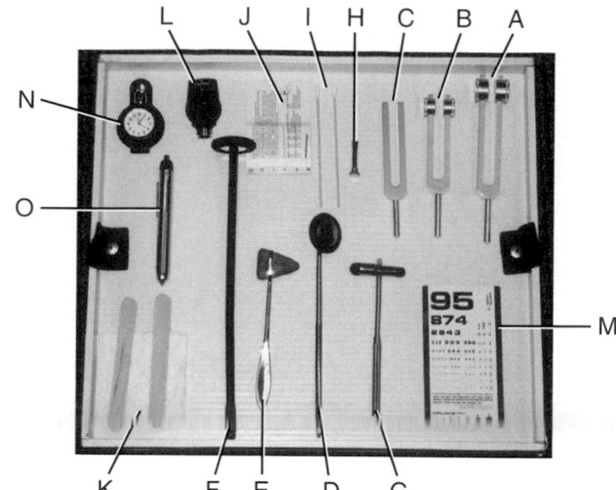

Figure 7.10.

Some tools for a neurologic examination. **A.** Tuning fork, 128 Hz. **B.** Tuning fork, 256 Hz. **C.** Tuning fork, 512 Hz. **D.** Babinski plexor. **E.** Taylor plexor. **F.** Queen's square plexor with plastic handle (recommended by us). **G.** Bucks or modified Dejerine plexor. **H.** Camel hair brush. **I.** Cotton-tipped swab. **J.** Set of monofilaments. **K.** Tongue blades. **L.** Opthalmoscope head. **M.** Pocket Snellen chart. **N.** Pocket watch. **O.** Penlight.

 **TIPS**

- Queen's square hammer: circular structure on a flexible stick; this is highly satisfactory in all endeavors
- Taylor hammer: tomahawk-shaped, may use either the flat or the pointed side, adequate
- Bucks hammer: two-headed, structures
- Fingertip: the most portable of hammers

over the tendon of the pectoralis major; then tap on the thumb that is transmitted to the tendon **(Fig. 7.13)**. The technique for the **quadriceps reflex**: with the patient sitting, legs hanging over the table at 90 degrees of flexion (Fig. 7.14A) or supine with the knees flexed to 20 degrees (Fig. 7.14B), tap over the infrapatellar ligament **(Fig. 7.14)**. The technique for the **Achilles reflex**: with the patient kneeling on a chair or supine **(Fig. 7.15)**, gently stretch the gastrocnemius tendon by passively dorsiflexing the foot and striking the distal Achilles tendon with the reflex hammer (Fig. 7.15). The technique for the **plantar reflex**: with the patient kneeling on a chair, gently stretch the gastrocnemius tendon by passively dorsiflexing the foot and striking the plantar foot

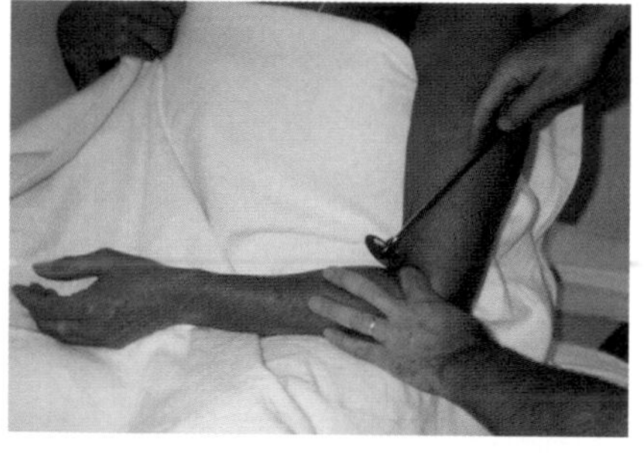

Figure 7.11.

Technique for biceps reflex. Use mediate percussion to perform. Here, a Queen's square hammer is used.

 **TIPS**

- Assessment of cervical root 5
- Patient is sitting, the elbow is in 90 degrees flexion, the forearm neutral between supination and pronation
- Grasp the elbow, thumb on the olecranon, second digit on the biceps tendon
- Tap hammer over the finger overlying the tendon of the biceps where it inserts on the proximal forearm (mediate percussion)
- Note biceps brachii contraction and flexion of the forearm

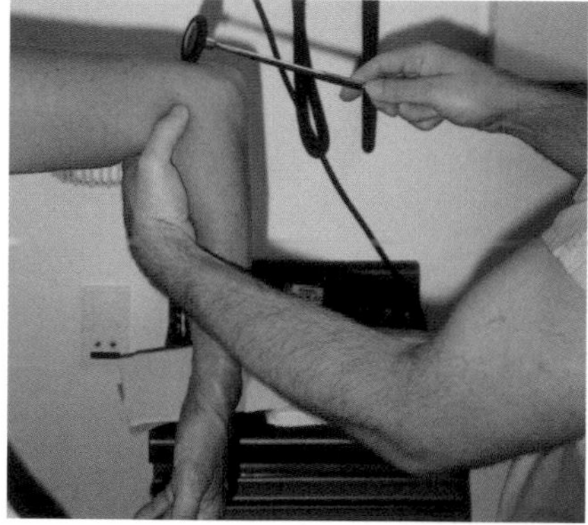

Figure 7.12.

Technique for triceps reflex. Use direct percussion to perform. Here, a Queen's square hammer is used.

 **TIPS**

- Assessment of cervical root 7
- Patient standing or sitting, the arm is supported by examiner so that it is parallel to floor
- Note that the forearm is then flexed to (dangled at) 90 degrees
- Use hammer to tap over the triceps aponeurosis
- Note triceps contraction or extension at the elbow

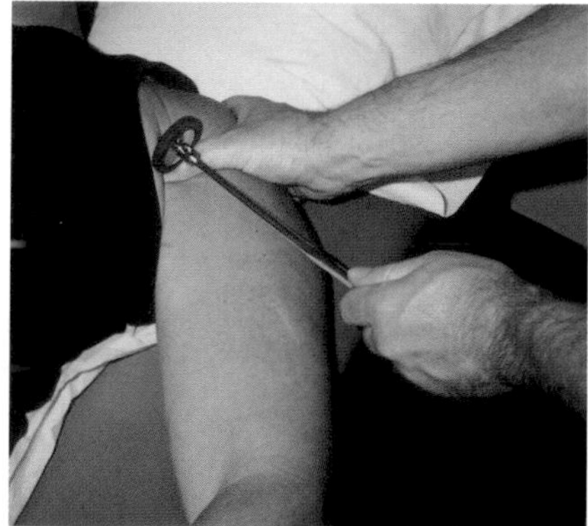

Figure 7.13.

Technique for pectoralis major reflex. Use mediate percussion to perform. Here, a Queen's square hammer is used.

 **TIPS**

- Assessment of C7
- Patient is supine, arm at side, approximately 20 degrees of abduction
- Place hand over top of acromion, fingers toward the back, thumb over the tendon of the pectoralis major
- Tap on thumb, to transmit the tap to the tendon
- Note contraction of the pectoralis major or adduction of the humerus

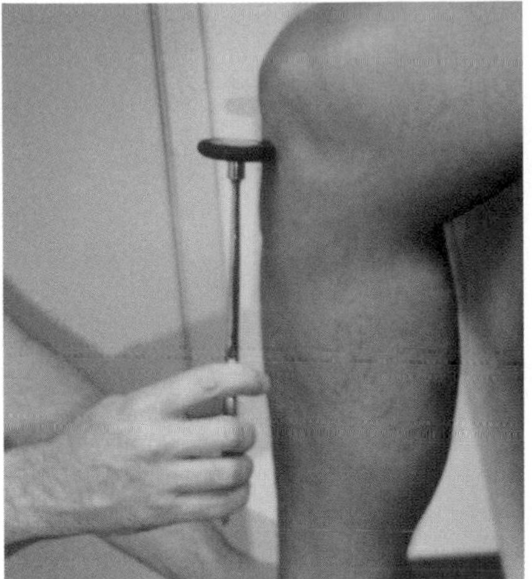

A

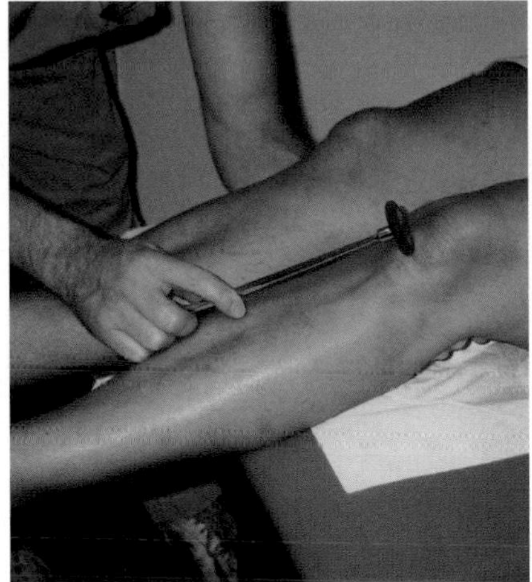

B

Figure 7.14.

Technique for quadriceps reflex. **A.** Patient sitting. **B.** Patient supine. Use direct percussion to perform. Here, a Queen's square is used.

 **TIPS**

- Assessment of L4 (lesser extent roots L2 and L3)
- Patient sitting, legs hanging over the table side: 90 degrees of flexion **(A)** or supine with knee flexed to 20 degrees **(B)**.
- Tap the hammer over the infrapatellar ligament
- Note quadriceps contraction and extension of knee

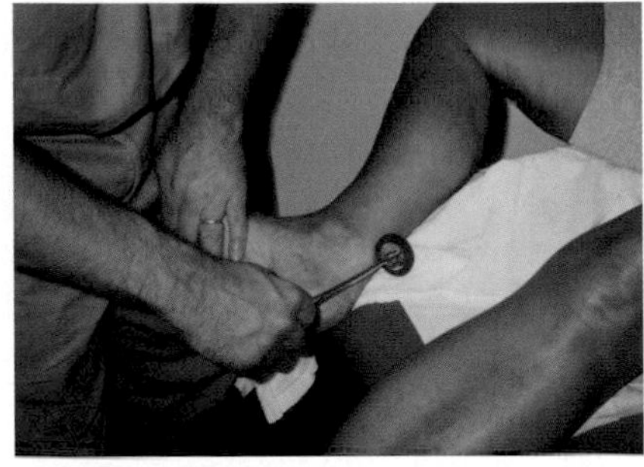

Figure 7.15.

Technique for Achilles reflex, patient kneeling. Mild passive dorsiflexion of the foot at ankle; here, a Queen's square hammer is used.

 **TIPS**

- Assessment of S1
- Patient is kneeling on a chair; may also be sitting or supine
- Gently stretch the tendon by passively dorsiflexing the foot
- Strike the distal Achilles tendon with the hammer
- Note gastrocnemius contraction and plantarflexion of foot

with the reflex hammer **(Fig. 7.16)**. We find the plantar reflex to be the superior maneuver, for S1.

Grading for DTR is on a 0 to 4 scale **(Table 7.3)**, in which 0 is absent, 1+ is barely present, 2+ normal, 3+ is brisk but without clonus, and 4+ is brisk with clonus. An excellent rule to interpret reflexes is that reflexes that are graded 0 or 4+ are abnormal until proved otherwise, whereas, reflexes that are graded 1+, 2+, or 3+ are normal until proved otherwise. To confirm that reflex is absent, the reflex procedure should be performed while the patient is performing **Jendrassik's maneuver (Fig. 7.17)**. The technique for Jendrassik's maneuver is one in which the patient holds hands before in front and mightily squeezes them together; then repeat the reflex assessment during this. **Upper motor neuron damage** manifests with hyperreflexia (3+ or 4+); **lower motor neuron damage** and primary muscle problems manifest with hyporeflexia (1+ or 0). **Clonus**, the rhythmic involuntary alternation of joint movement can also be assessed and demonstrated by passively stretching a joint. These include passive wrist dorsiflexion or passive ankle dorsiflexion. Recall, clonus means that the reflex is

Table 7.3. Deep Tendon Reflex (DTR) or Muscle Stretch (MSR) Grading

Grade	Interpretation
0*	No reflex present
1+	Minimal contraction of muscle; no joint movement
2+	Contraction of muscle with mild movement of joint
3+	Significant muscle contraction with brisk joint movement
4+	Significant muscle contraction with brisk joint and clonus or crossover to contralateral side

*If 0, repeat after doing the Jendrassik maneuver; if now present, the reflex is truly 1+.

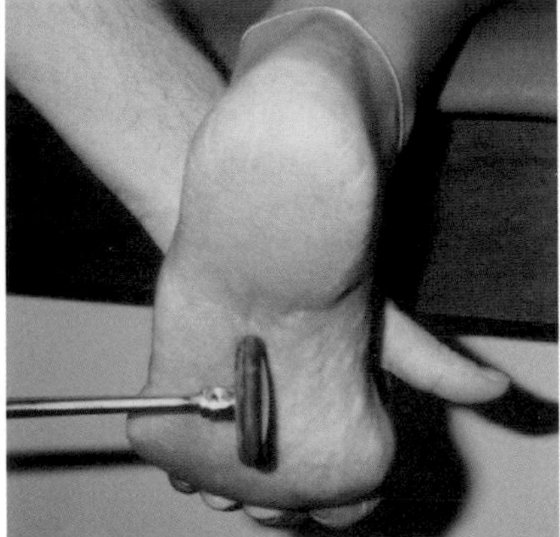

Figure 7.16.

Technique for plantar reflex. Direct percussion. Queen's square hammer is used here.

 **TIPS**

- Assessment of S1
- Patient kneeling on a chair; may also be sitting or supine
- Stretch the tendon by passively dorsiflexing the foot
- Strike the plantar foot with the hammer
- Note any contraction of the gastrocnemius and plantarflexion of foot

TEACHING POINTS

OVERALL POWER, TONE, AND REFLEXES

1. Power = strength.
2. Power is graded from 0 to 5: 0 = no movement; 5 = normal; system is satisfactory for proximal muscle grading, but not for distal muscles.
3. Use two muscle groups from the upper and two muscle groups from the lower compare upper versus lower and side-to-side.
4. Tone is the baseline summation of all muscle activity within a joint when passive.
5. Hypotonicity: usually cerebellar dysfunction.
6. Hypertonicity: usually cogwheel rigidity or spasticity.
7. Hypertonicity does not equal hyperreflexia.
8. Reflexes are graded 0 to 4: 0 and 4 are almost always abnormal; 1, 2, 3 are often normal.
9. Use two reflexes from the upper extremity and two reflexes from the lower extremity; compare upper versus lower and side-to-side.

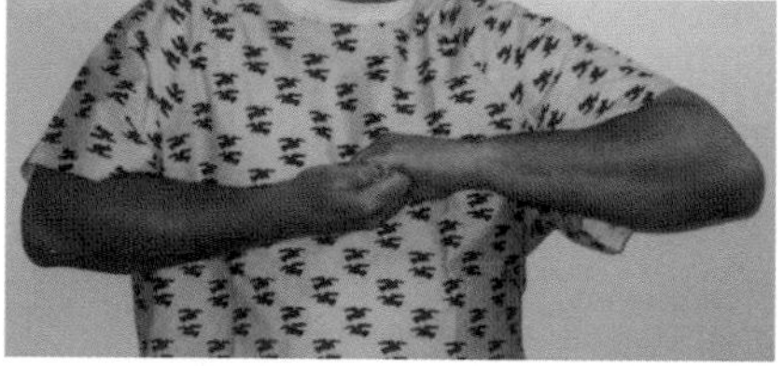

Figure 7.17.

Technique for Jendrassik's maneuver to increase sensitivity of deep tendon reflexes (DTR), also known as the muscle stretch reflexes (MSR).

TIPS

- The patient is holding hands before her and is instructed to squeeze mightily
- Repeat the lower extremity reflexes
- Perform on patient with a 0 reflex; may become present, i.e., 1+, with this maneuver

indeed 4+. In addition to the grading of reflexes, the **contraction** and the **relaxation** phases of the reflex movement need to be assessed. **Hypothyroidism** manifests with reflexes that have a delayed relaxation phase. **Hypotonia** manifests with pendulum swinging with the triceps and the patellar reflexes, i.e., the contraction and relaxation phases continue over and over. Of final note, in **lower spinal cord transection injury** (L2, L3, or L4), the quadriceps reflex paradoxically flexes the knee. This grossly unusual and pathologic reflex is called Boyle's sign.

Anal Wink and Cremasteric Reflexes

Two unique peripheral reflexes that are extremely important in the evaluation of spinal cord injuries and low back pain are the **anal wink** and the **cremasteric reflex**. After an **acute spinal cord injury**, presence of the reflexes indicates a favorable prognosis; in the **setting of low back pain**, their absence suggests cauda equina syndrome or central spinal cord compression. (See Chapter 12 for further details.)

CRANIAL NERVE EXAMINATION

Smell is the function of **cranial nerve I**, a purely sensory nerve. Smell deficits are usually nonspecific; however, **viral rhinitis** manifests with overall decrease in smell sense. The company it keeps includes cough, serous rhinitis, and sore throat. **Unilateral frontal lobe tumor** manifests with unilateral, ipsilateral loss of smell; the company it keeps includes a change in behavior and olfactory hallucinations. Determining smell requires two vials, one for each nostril, of different odiferous materials, e.g., one of ground coffee and a second of vanilla. A useful tool for assessing smell sensation is the University of Pennsylvania Smell Identification Unit (UPSIT), which is commercially available. Overall, this set of tests is rarely performed.

Vision is the function of **cranial nerve II**, another purely sensory nerve, which is extensively discussed in the chapter on eye examination. Recall, a magnificent method to detect visual function is that of the **rotating black and white drum** in which **blindness** results in no nystagmus; however, **feigned blindness** or normal vision manifests with involuntary, optokinetic horizontal nystagmus.

Cranial nerves III, IV, and VI, all purely motor nerves, are assessed together. Deficits of these purely motor nerves manifest as a strabismus, the patient complaining of "double vision." To assess these nerves, start from the baseline of a patient with a natural gaze at a point of light at least 2 meters before the patient in the horizontal plane. This is called a Hirschberg test for strabismus. Place one finger in horizontal gaze plane, 20 to 25 cm anterior to the midline of the patient's face. Also place the thumb of the other hand on the chin to prevent head movement (Fig. 15.2). The patient follows the finger in two diagonal and horizontal axes. **Cranial nerve III**, oculomotor nerve, supplies the superior rectus, inferior rectus, inferior oblique, and medial rectus muscles. **Cranial nerve III deficit** manifests with multiple extraocular motor defects and a baseline gaze of a walleye (exotropia) or exophoria (Fig. 15.3). A walleye or an exophoria is caused by the fact that the lateral rectus remains intact and, therefore, will dominate the eye. Also, a ptosis will be present on the affected side. **Cranial nerve IV**, trochlear nerve, is the smallest of all of the cranial nerves and innervates the superior oblique muscle. **Cranial nerve IV deficit** manifests with a paralysis (tropia) or weakness (phoria) to nasal and inferior (down and in) eye movements. A not uncommon reason for this is a step-off fracture of the infraorbital rim (Fig. 1.24) and basilar skull fracture with trochlear nerve damage. In addition, Brown's syndrome of superior oblique tenosynovitis results in a deficit without CN IV problem. **Cranial nerve VI**, abducens nerve, innervates the lateral rectus muscle. **Cranial nerve VI deficit** manifests with a cross-eye paralysis (Fig. 15.4) (esotropia) or weakness (phoria) of lateral movement. Furthermore, when performing active extraocular movements, use the **axes of motion** described in Fig. 15.2. **Box 7.1** contains a method to remember these. Perform the range of motion (ROM) of the eyes with eyes closed if the patient has photophobia.

Box 7.1.

Rules of Extraocular Movements

1. All recti muscles move the eyeball out, except one—the medial.
2. All obliques muscles move eyeball nasal, opposite to superior or inferior.
3. Superior oblique muscle (SO) = 4; lateral rectus (LR) = 6; all the rest are 3.

Cranial nerve V, trigeminal nerve, is a mixed motor and sensory nerve. Motor is to the temporalis, pterygoid and masseter muscles. To assess the motor function, place a sterile tongue depressor between the molar teeth of the maxilla and mandible **(Fig. 7.18)**. The patient gently bites on the blade as the examiner gently pulls blade outward. Palpate the masseter and temporalis muscles. To assess sensory function, touch the skin lightly with a cotton-tipped swab over the skin of V1, V2, and V3 **(Fig. 7.19)**. **Cranial nerve V deficits** manifest with weakness to bite and even atrophy of the temporalis and the masseter muscles and decreased sensation in V1, V2, and V3 sites. The company it keeps includes weakness to movement of the jaw from side-to-side, which indicates pterygoid muscle problem and confirms a CN V deficit. **Tic douloureux** manifests with hyperesthesia and pain on touching the affected branch, usually the V2 or V3 areas. This is due to inflammation, trauma, or infiltration of the trigeminal ganglion, e.g., multiple sclerosis or Lyme disease.

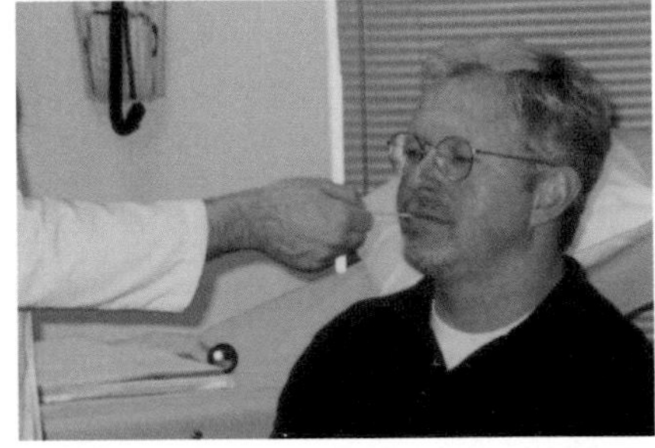

Figure 7.18.

Technique to assess masseter strength as a method to assess motor function of cranial nerve V.

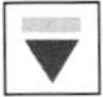 **TIPS**

- Place sterile tongue depressor between the molars of the maxilla and mandible on one side
- Patient gently bites the blade; examiner attempts to pull it outward
- Palpate masseter and temporalis muscle
- Repeat on other side
- Cranial nerve V deficit: weakness, ipsilateral, extremely rare
- Myasthenia gravis: weakness, bilateral
- Landry Guillain-Barré polyneuritis: no weakness

Cranial nerve VII, the facial nerve, is also a mixed nerve—motor to the facial muscles, including the orbicularis oris and oculus, the frontalis muscle; and sensory to the lobe of the ear and to the lateral and anterior taste buds. To assess motor function, have the patient actively **smile**; to assess the function of the orbicularis oris muscle, have the patient **growl** or **puff out cheeks (Fig. 7.20)**. The growl and the "puff out" of cheeks tests are the best two, because both false-positive and false-negative findings occur with a smile. The second component required to assess the function of cranial nerve VII is for the patient to actively and against resistance **close the eyes**. This is to assess the orbicularis oculus muscle. Testing the function of orbicularis oris and orbicularis oculus muscles is required to satisfactorily assess the function of cranial nerve VII **(Fig. 7.21)**. In addition, it is important to note the function of the frontalis

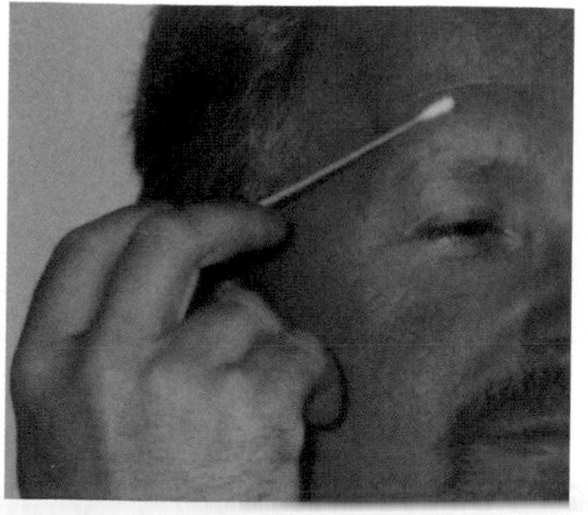

A

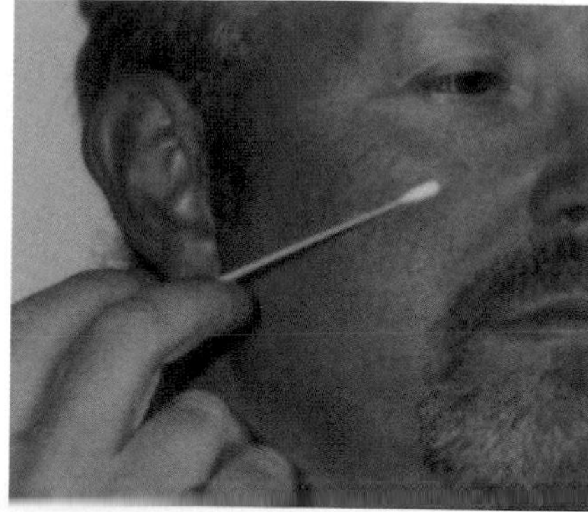

B

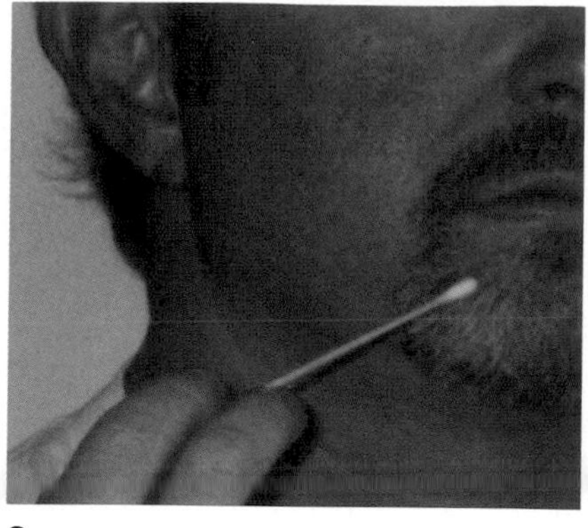

C

Figure 7.19.

Technique to assess sensory component of cranial nerve V. **A.** V1. **B.** V2. **C.** V3.

TIPS

- Touch lightly with cotton-tipped swab in middle of V1, V2, and V3 areas
- Tic douloureux: severe pain on touching in V1, V2, or V3 distribution, usually V2 or V3
- V1 or V2 or V3 problem: decreased sensation

muscle **(Fig. 7.22)**. To assess this, instruct the patient to look upward with both eyes in order to furrow the forehead (brow). The sensory examination of cranial nerve VII is far less important and will not be discussed other than to state that taste is partially served by cranial nerve VII. **Ramsay-Hunt syndrome** manifests with clusters of vesicles in dermatome of CN VII. This is due to herpes zoster of the geniculate ganglion. **Central cranial nerve VII deficit** manifests with droop when smiling and when showing teeth (growl) on the side contralateral to the UMN* lesion. **Peripheral cranial nerve VII deficit** manifests with a droop when smiling, when showing teeth (growl), and weakness to closure of the eye and a marked decrease in brow wrinkling with eyebrow elevation, all unilateral and ipsilateral to the damage. Long-standing peripheral cranial nerve VII palsy may have a Bell's phenomenon—a synkinesia in which the eye on the affected side rolls upward. Obviously, the overall examination is difficult to perform if the patient has received botulinum toxin injections in the past.

Cranial nerve VIII is the purely sensory auditory nerve. To assess this nerve, use the Weber and the Rinne tests. With the **Weber test**, apply a vibrating tuning fork (512 Hz is best, but 256 Hz is acceptable) to the base of the mastoid process **(Fig. 7.23)**. When the patient can no longer hear the sound of

Figure 7.20.

Active smile **(A)** or puff out cheeks **(B)** tests. These effectively use the orbicularis oris muscle. A deficit is either ipsilateral peripheral or contralateral central cranial nerve VII damage. **A.** Patient has right weakness

TIPS

- Actively smile **(A)** or "puff-out" **(B)** using the orbicularis oris muscle
- Peripheral cranial nerve VII deficit (LMN): ipsilateral inability to smile
- Central cranial nerve VII deficit (UMN): contralateral inability to smile
- Growl or cheek puff out is the superior maneuver

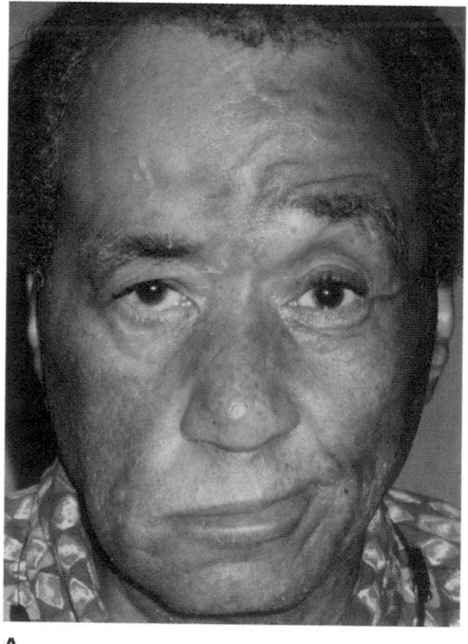

A

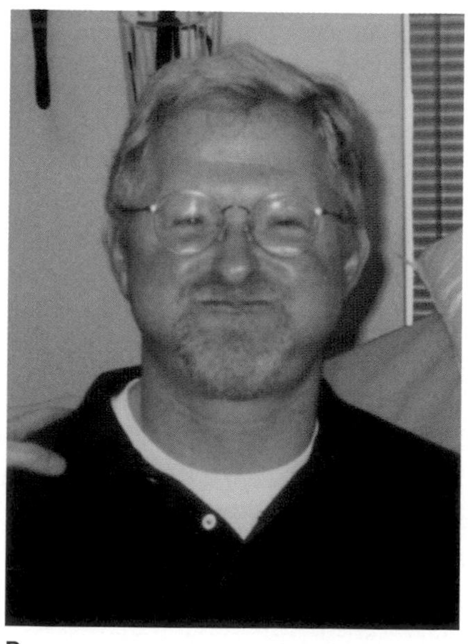

B

*UMN = upper motor neuron.

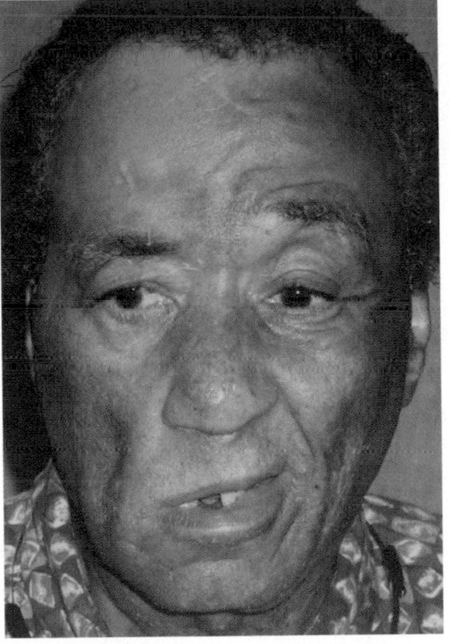

A

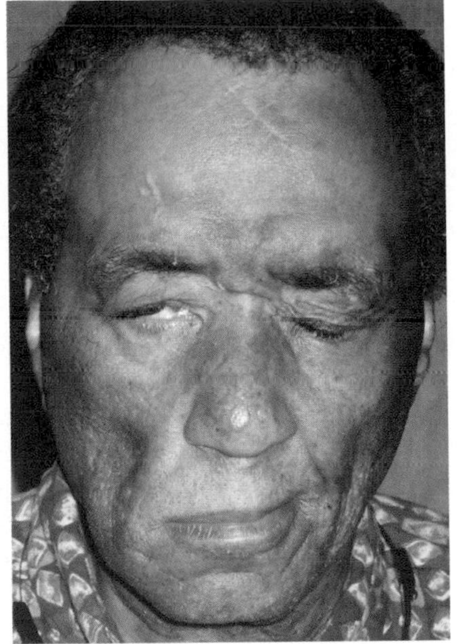

B

Figure 7.21.

Peripheral cranial nerve VII deficits. **A.** Smile, right weakness. **B.** Close eyes, right weakness. Note the Bell's phenomenon.

TIPS

- Actively close eyes tightly using the orbicularis oculus muscle
- Peripheral cranial nerve VII deficit (LMN): unilateral, ipsilateral inability to close eye
- Peripheral cranial nerve VII deficit (LMN): eye rolls upward when attempt is made to close the eye (Bell's phenomenon), a synkinesia
- Central cranial nerve VII deficit (UMN): normal ability to close eyes

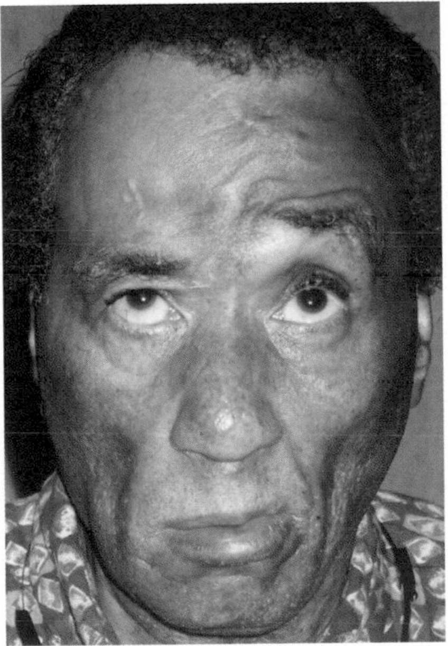

Figure 7.22.

Frontalis muscle function. A deficit is caused by an ipsilateral cranial nerve VII defect; central VII does not result in any deficit to eye closure.

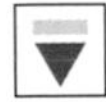

TIPS

- Patient instructed to look upward without lifting head
- Normal: furrowed brow bilaterally
- Peripheral cranial nerve VII deficit (LMN): unilateral, ipsilateral loss of forehead wrinkling
- Central cranial nerve VII deficit (UMN): normal ability to wrinkle forehead
- One of the best methods to assess peripheral cranial nerve VII function

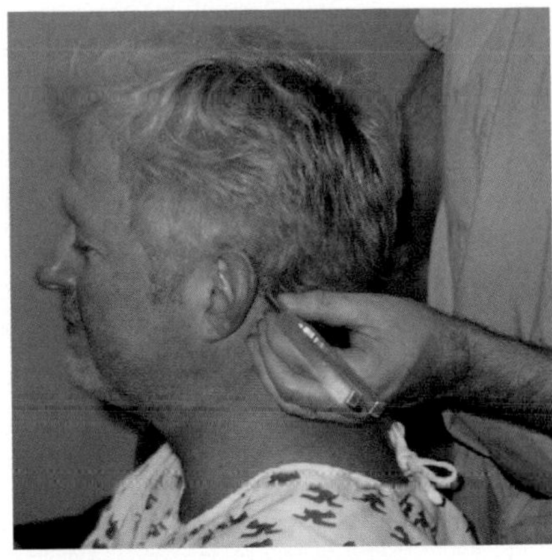

A

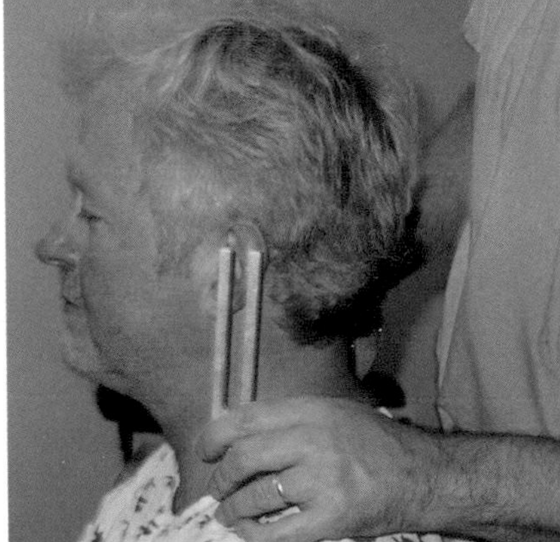

B

Figure 7.23.

Technique for Weber test, using a 512-Hz tuning fork. Satisfactory bedside method to differentiate conductive from neurosensory hearing defects. **A.** On mastoid process, **B.** Next to ear.

TIPS

- Apply vibrating tuning fork (512 Hz is best; 256 Hz is less useful) base to the middle of forehead or the vertex of head
- Ask patient when sound is extinguished in each ear
- Normal: time to extinguish, equal to both ears
- Unilateral conductive: sound present longer on side of defect (bone conduction longer than air)
- Unilateral neural: sound present longer on side opposite defect

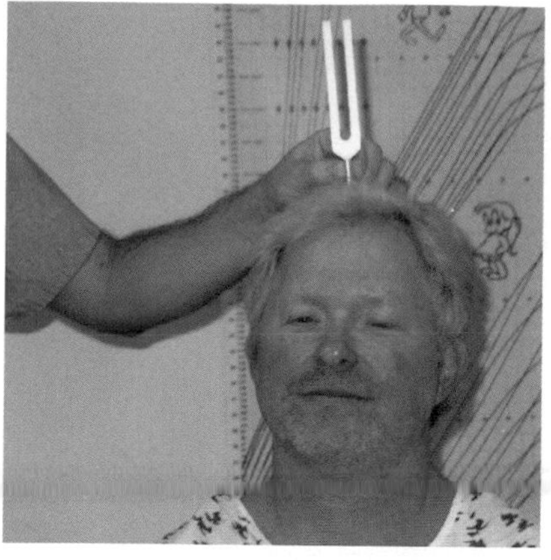

A

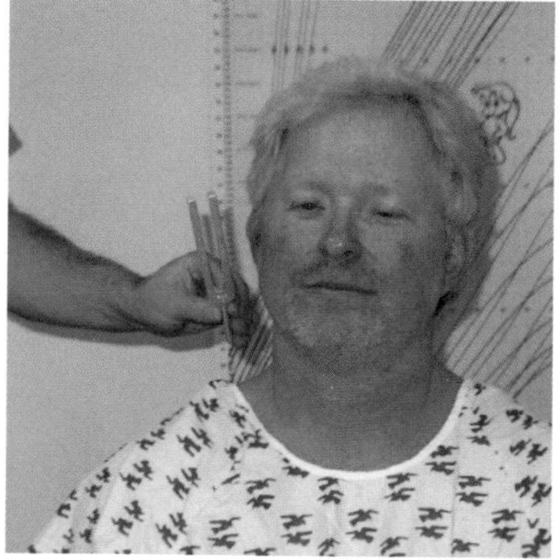

B

Figure 7.24.

Technique for Rinne test, using a 512-Hz fork. Excellent bedside method to differentiate conduction from neurosensory hearing defects. **A.** On top of head. **B.** Next to ear.

TIPS

- Apply vibrating tuning fork (512 Hz is best, a 256 Hz is less useful) base to the mastoid process
- At point when the patient can no longer hear the tuning fork, remove fork to a site adjacent to external auditory meatus
- Normal: sound heard through air longer than through the mastoid (bone)
- Conductive loss: sensation through air less than through bone (air extinguished before bone)
- Neural loss: equal loss of bone and air conduction

the fork, remove it and place it adjacent to the external auditory canal. Although in the original description the fork should remain perpendicular to the canal, we have found this to be fastidious. With the **Rinne test**, apply a vibrating tuning fork (512 is best, 256 Hz is satisfactory) to the middle of the vertex of the head or the middle of the forehead **(Fig. 7.24)**. Ask the patient to state when sound is extinguished in both ears. Normally, the time is equal. **Cranial nerve VIII deficits** manifest with decreased hearing as assessed by Weber and Rinne tests using either a 512- or 256-Hz tuning fork. Often, concurrent problems with vertigo, tinnitus, and ataxia are also present. **Conductive hearing loss** manifests with diminished auditory acuity. A Weber test reveals that the sensation through air is less than through bone, i.e., air is extinguished before the mastoid bone, the Rinne test reveals sound present longer on the side of the conductive deficit. *Conductive hearing loss* is caused by recurrent otitis media, otosclerosis, or tympanic membrane damage. The company it keeps includes significant findings on otoscopic imaging. **Neural hearing loss** manifests with diminished auditory acuity. A Weber test reveals that the sensation is equally diminished through bone and through air; the Rinne test reveals sound present longer on the side opposite the neural defect. Neural deficits are caused by presbyacusis, loud noise trauma, or medicine-related damage to hair cells, including exposure to the life-saving aminoglycoside antibiotics. Related symptoms include increasing age, exposure to agents that can cause this, and a remarkable paucity of abnormal findings on external and middle ear examination.

Cranial nerves IX, the glossopharyngeal, and **X**, the vagus, are assessed together because they have similar functions and both are mixed sensory and motor. A deficit of IX or X manifests with deviation of the uvula at baseline or with an active "Ahhhh." See **Table 7.4** to differentiate **unilateral paresis** from **unilateral plegia** from **bilateral plegia** of the posterior pharynx musculature. This is a relatively poor test in that many false-positive findings result. Thus, if it is an isolated finding, it may be a variant of normal or is caused by dryness in the posterior pharynx. Specific features of a cranial nerve X **deficit** include a loss of the *oculocardiac reflex*, i.e., loss of heart rate slowing on gentle application of mild pressure with fingertips over the patient's closed eyes. This is a rarely used test. **Vocal changes** specific to CN IX or X deficits include difficulty in stating the "K," hard "C," or the "Q" sound. This is hyponasal speech of cranial nerve IX and X mischief. One great method to assess for hyponasal speech is to have the patient state the word "Kentucky" three times. In hyponasal speech, this sounds like en/u/EEE, whereas normal is Ken/TUCK/e. In addition, the patient often reports fluid goes through the nasopharynx when swallowing. A specific type on unilateral CN X is **Ortner's syndrome**, which is left unilateral recurrent laryngeal nerve damage. This is due to compression of the nerve caused by left atrial enlargement or thoracic aortic aneurysm. The company it keeps includes dysphagia caused by extrinsic compression on the esophagus and, often, the irregularly irregular rhythm of atrial fibrillation. The vocal change is one in which it is harsh and hoarse.

Table 7.4. Uvular Movements to Assess for Cranial Nerve IX and X Deficits

Diagnosis	Baseline position	Active AHHHHH
Normal	Hangs low in midline	Elevated in midline
Paresis, unilateral	Hangs low in midline	
Plegia, unilateral	Hangs low, deviated away from lesion	Elevated but deviates further away from lesion
Plegia, bilateral	Uvula midline, low	No elevation

CN IX and X deficits are highly correlated with swallowing dysfunction. It is necessary to look for other cranial nerve deficits at brainstem, including CN XI and CN XII. If upper motor neuron cranial nerve deficits are noted, the condition is called **pseudobulbar palsy**; if lower motor neuron cranial nerve deficits are noted, the condition is called **bulbar palsy**. Pseudobulbar palsy is most common today; whereas, 50 years ago at height of polio, bulbar palsy was most common.

Cranial nerve XI, the spinal accessory nerve, is purely motor; it innervates the trapezius and the sternocleidomastoid muscles. **Cranial nerve XI deficits** manifest with decreased power to shoulder shrugging. In addition, often noted is a winged scapula as demonstrated by the technique of the *push-out* forward test **(Fig. 7.25)**. For this technique, the patient pushes a hand against the hand of the examiner in an attempt to perform a push-up against resistance. Observe the placement of the vertebral surface of the scapula. Also noted is atrophy of the trapezius. As CN XI also innervates the **sternocleidomastoid muscle** there may be ipsilateral decreased strength to head rotation, and atrophy of the sternocleidomastoid muscle. To assess this, place hands on the sides of the patient's head and instruct the patient to actively rotate the head to the right and to the left **(Fig. 7.26)**. Often, concurrent cranial nerve IX or X and XII deficits are noted, as is an ipsilateral Horner's syndrome. One of the most common reasons for the development of cranial nerve XI palsy is a gunshot wound to the neck.

Cranial nerve XII, the hypoglossal nerve, which also is purely motor, innervates the tongue musculature. To assess cranial nerve XII, instruct the patient to actively protrude tongue three times and note any deviation from midline **(Fig. 7.27)**. Normally, the patient can perform this without deviation from midline. *Lower motor neuron* (*LMN*) cranial nerve XII deficits manifest

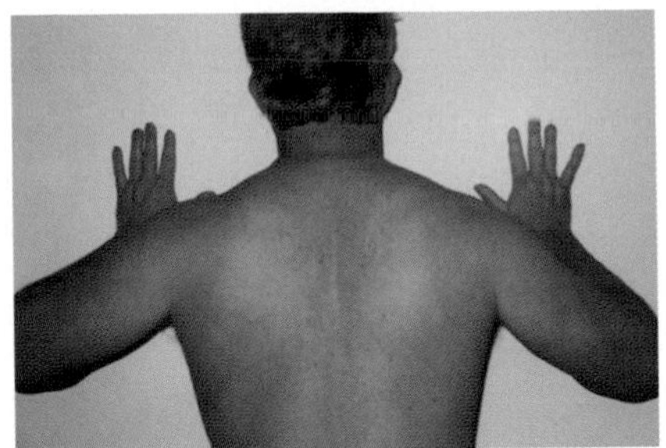

Figure 7.25.

Technique for push-out forward test for assessment of trapezius and serratus anterior.

 **TIPS**

- Patient pushes hand against the hand of examiner or the side wall
- Note the location of the vertebral border of the ipsilateral scapula, before and during the procedure
- Normal: scapula does not deviate, i.e., does not wing
- Trapezius weakness: winging, especially of the upper (superior) angle of the scapula
- Serratus anterior weakness: winging, the entire vertebral border of the scapula
- Perhaps the most sensitive method to assess cerebral nerve XI

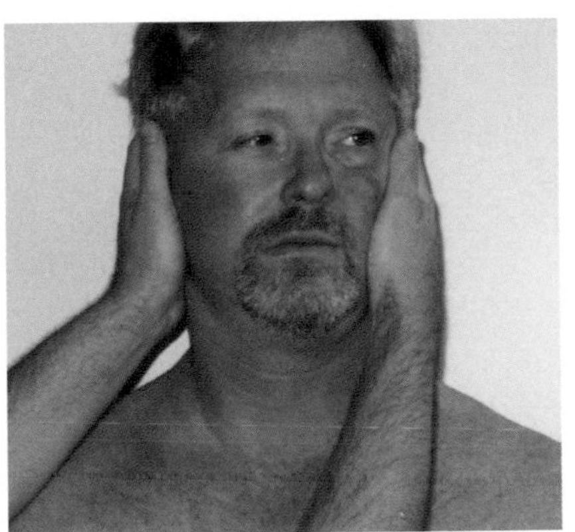

A

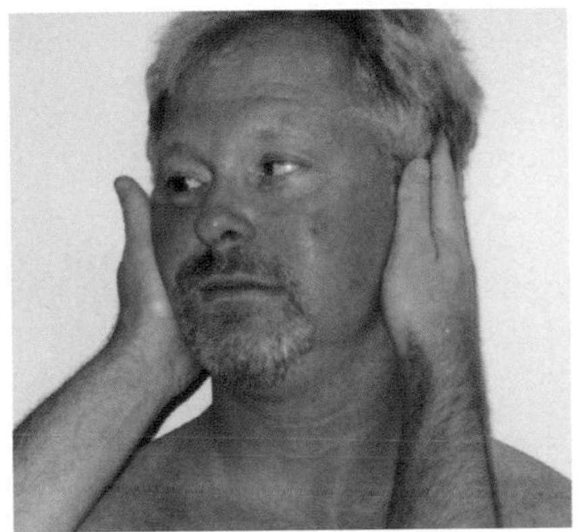

B

Figure 7.26.

Technique to assess sternocleidomastoid and cranial nerve XI: actively rotate head against resistance, left **(A)** and then right **(B)**.

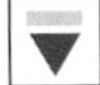 **TIPS**

- Place hands on sides of patient's head
- Instruct patient to rotate left and then right; apply resistance
- Cerebral nerve XI damage: ipsilateral weakness often with sternocleidomastoid atrophy
- Note any concurrent trapezius deficit
- Requires a severe deficit of the nerve to manifest

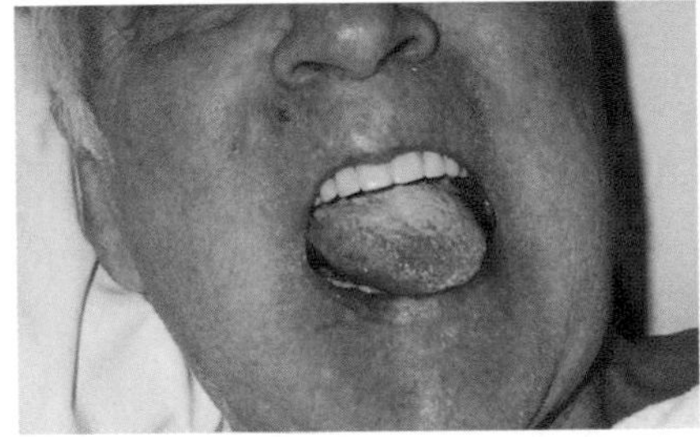

Figure 7.27.

Dinkler's sign of an old peripheral cerebral nerve XII palsy. There is also atrophy of the tongue musculature.

 **TIPS**

- Actively protrude tongue thrice
- Note any tongue deviation
- Normal: able to actively protrude tongue in midline, no change from first to third time
- Cerebral nerve XII damage (LMN): deviation of the tongue to the side of the damage; usually tongue muscle atrophy and, if acute, fasciculations in tongue are present

TEACHING POINTS

CRANIAL NERVE EXAMINATION

1. Vanilla or freshly ground coffee are excellent sources for smell when testing cranial nerve (CN) I examination. This is rarely used today.
2. Snellen chart is used to screen CN II; perform on each eye. This is complemented by visual field assessment.
3. CN III, CN IV, and CN VI are assessed together during eye active ROM. Recall the teaching aphorism of SO4, LR6, all the rest CN3.
4. Look for a concurrent ptosis because this may indicate a CN III problem or, if ptosis associated with a miosis, the presence of Horner's syndrome.
5. All recti muscles move the eye outward, except the medial rectus.
6. The obliques move the eye inward (nasally) and opposite to superior or inferior names.
7. Look for company specific to the deficits: multiple eye deficits and ptosis, more likely a CN III deficit.
8. CN V best assessed by palpating the masseter muscle and sensation to V1, V2, and V3.
9. CN VII central involves the mouth muscles only—contralateral to lesion.
10. CN VII peripheral involves mouth, eye, and forehead muscles—ipsilateral to the lesion.
11. CN VIII sensory has auditory, and vestibular components.
12. CN IX and CN X are always assessed together.
13. Swallowing in which the fluid reproducibly goes into nose: CN IX and CN X deficits.
14. The company of CN IX and CN X palsies includes problems with other brainstem nuclei, including CN XI and CN XII, i.e., problems with shoulder shrugging or dysarthria.
15. CN XI palsy that is solitary is rare, usually as the result of direct trauma to the area, e.g., gunshot wound to upper neck.
16. Relatively easy to examine CN XI: all motor involving two large muscles—the sternocleidomastoid and the trapezius.
17. Tongue always points to the side of the lesion on protrusion.

SO = superior oblique; LR = lateral rectus; CN = cranial nerve.

with weakness to tongue protrusion, i.e., the tongue deviates to side of damage with atrophy of the tongue on that side. *Upper* ***or*** *lower motor neuron* cranial nerve XII deficit has company of a dysarthria to the LU/LU or La/La/La (tongue-specific) sounds. In this tongue-specific dysarthria, they sound like ooou, oOa, aaAA, i.e., a mashed-potato, peanut-butter type diction.

GAIT **(see Table 7.12)**

The **normal gait** in a human being is a thing of elegant beauty. It integrates an incredible number of sensory and motor components into a free-flowing movement: the ability to walk. It is also a foundation on which a directed

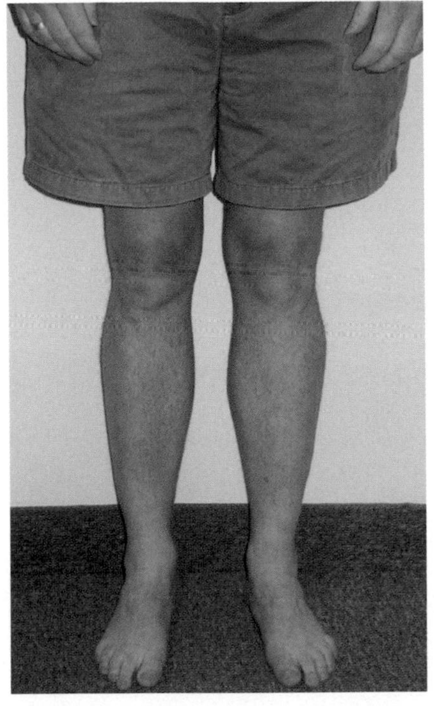
A

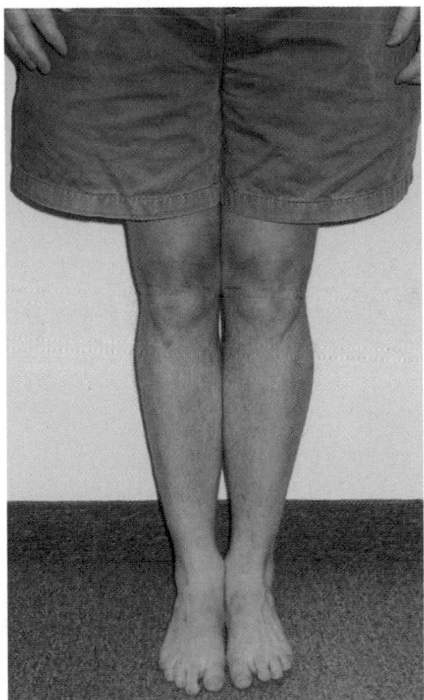
B

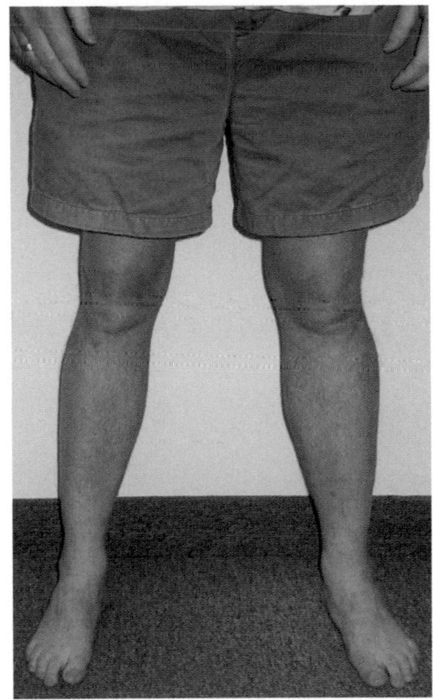
C

Figure 7.28.

Stance. A baseline position for gaits. **A.** Normal-based gait. **B.** Narrow-based gait. **C.** Wide-based gait.

TIPS

- Instruct patient to stand normally in a relaxed manner
- Note the location of feet relative to the anterior superior iliac spines (ASIS)
- This is classic anatomic position; the ASIS is an excellent point of reference
- Normal: each foot beneath the ASIS **(A)**
- Narrow-based gait: feet placed inside the ASIS, e.g., in Parkinson's disease **(B)**
- Wide-based gait: feet placed outside of the ASIS—ataxia **(C)**

neurologic examination can be best performed. **Normal gait** manifests with feet directed forward, directly below to slightly medial to the anterior superior iliac spine **(Fig. 7.28A)**; each arm swings alternating with the feet, such that left arm and right leg move together, then right arm and left leg. Abnormal gaits are either **narrow-based gaits**, in which the feet are placed **medial** to the anterior superior iliac spine **(Fig. 7.28B)**; or **wide-based gaits**, in which the feet are placed **lateral** to the anterior superior iliac spine **(Fig. 7.28C)**.

Profound proximal muscle weakness often manifests with a **waddling gait**. A **cerebrovascular accident** or other damage to the **upper motor neuron** areas manifests with a **spastic, hemiparetic gait. Parkinson's disease** manifests with a **shuffling–type gait. Cerebellar damage** or peripheral **sensory** damage manifests with an **ataxic gait. Common peroneal nerve damage** manifests with a **steppage–type** gait. **Ankylosing spondylosis** or paraspinal spasm manifests with a **poker gait**, in which the patient is straight as a poker. **Hip degenerative joint disease** manifests with an *antalgic gait*, in which there is a unilateral limp, the affected leg adducted and externally rotated to minimize pain with each step. (See Chapter 12 for further details.) For each of these gaits, the descriptors of **tone**, **reflexes**, and **power** will be described and discussed. A summary of these features is outlined in Table 7.12.

Waddling-type Gait

Profound proximal muscle weakness manifests with a **waddling gait** that is normal to narrow based. In order for the patient to maintain an erect posture, maximal use is made of gluteal muscles, which results in an accentuation of the lumbar lordosis. On overall inspection, the patient uses the rails on walls or sturdy objects to maintain an erect posture. The company it keeps includes moderate to significant proximal muscle weakness (usually grade 2, 3, 4) and a decreased ability to stand from a seated position, also

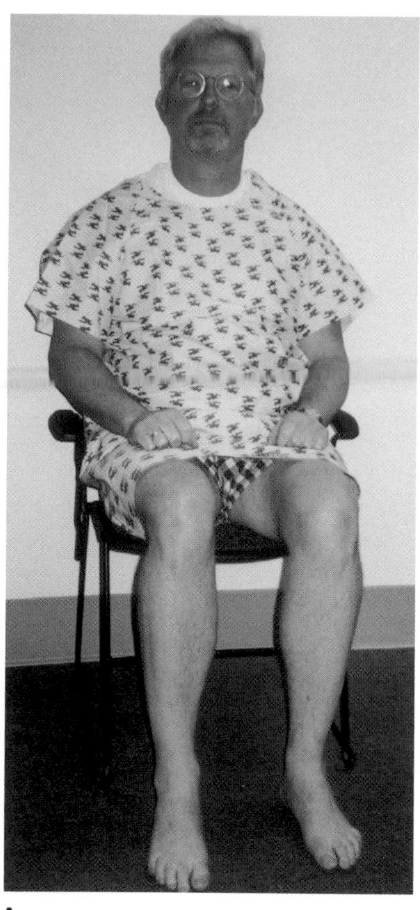
A

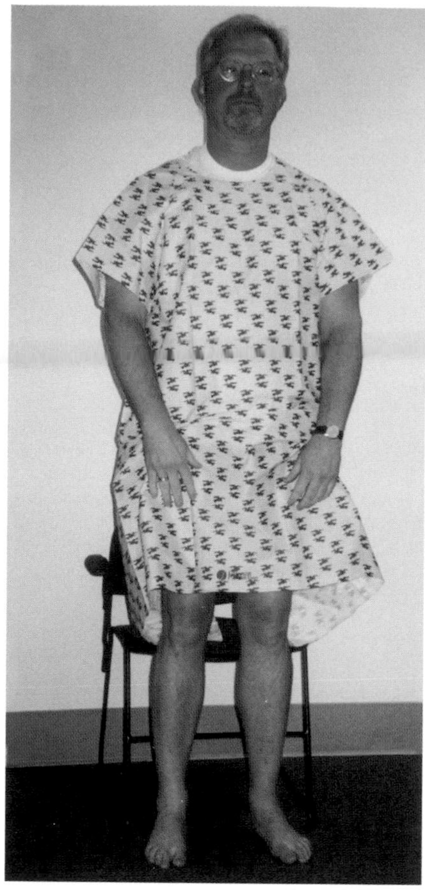
B

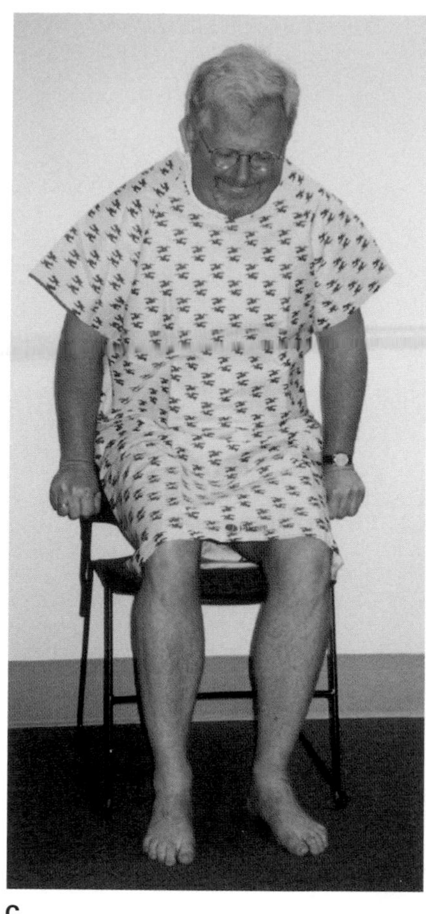
C

Figure 7.29.

Technique for sit-to-stand test to assess for proximal muscle weakness. **A**, **B**. Normal. **C**. Weakness, i.e., patient uses arms to stand.

 **TIPS**

- Instruct patient to stand from an armchair
- Note ability to perform with or without use of upper extremities
- Count number of times able to perform over a 15-second period
- Elegant in its simplicity
- Described by Csuka and McCarty, 1985
- Normal: at least three times without using the hands or arms
- Proximal muscle weakness: unable to perform without using arms or hands

known as a positive **Csuka-McCarty test**, first described in 1985 **(Fig. 7.29)**. For this test, instruct the patient to stand erect from an armchair. Note any use of the arms and the number of times over a 15-second period that this can be performed. This is an elegant test in its simplicity and grand to quantify and to follow-up proximal muscle strength. *Normal* is to be able to perform the test at least three times without using the arms. Also present is a positive tripod or Gowers' sign, in which the patient cannot stand from a prone position without the use of upper extremities (this is an archaic test that we do not recommend) and those manifestations specific to the underlying cause. Please refer to **Table 7.5** for extensive discussion.

Spastic Hemiparetic Gait

A **cerebrovascular accident** or other damage to the **upper motor neuron** areas, e.g., from head trauma or intracranial neoplasia, manifests with a **spastic**, narrow-based **hemiparetic gait**, forearm supinated with elbow flexed and held to the trunk, and knee slightly flexed **(Table 7.6)**. Circumduction and forward push or "pseudodrag" of the foot contralateral to the UMN lesion are noted. The overall spastic hemiparetic gait is narrow based, the side contralateral to the damage has foot placement medial or inside to the ASIS. The knee is slightly flexed and the hand or forearm is supinated, with the elbow flexed and adjacent to the trunk. The company it keeps includes unilateral spasticity-hypertonicity to wrist, ankle, and elbow; unilateral **hyperreflexia**

TEACHING POINTS

WADDLING GAIT

1. Waddling gait indicates significant proximal muscle weakness.
2. The standing from chair test is an excellent functional assessment of the proximal muscle.
3. Many of the entities that manifest with proximal muscle weakness can be defined by physical examination.

Table 7.5. Waddling-type Gait Features

Diagnosis	Manifestations
Duchenne muscular dystrophy	Pseudohypertrophy of muscles, especially gastrocnemius
Myotonic dystrophy	Frontal balding (Fig. 7.7) Bilateral ptosis Strap and facial muscle atrophy Myotonia
Polymyositis	Mild tenderness in muscles Cramping and ache in muscles
Dermatomyositis	Nontender muscles Heliotropic rash about the periorbital areas (Fig. 7.31) Gottron's papules on dorsum of fingers (Fig. 7.30)
Hypothyroidism	Goiter or scar on neck (Fig. 1.64) Delayed relaxation phase of reflexes Alopecia, with thickened hair Queen Anne's sign of lateral eyebrow loss (Fig. 1.63) Weight gain Macroglossia
Hyperthyroidism	Goiter with bruit (Fig. 1.68) Lid lag (Fig. 1.67) Distal onycholysis (Plummer's nails) (Fig. 1.69) Mild, diffuse hyperreflexia Tremor Tachycardia
Myasthenia gravis	Bilateral ptosis Hanging jaw sign Weakness, all manifestations worse in afternoon Weak tongue protrusion Swallowing dysfunction with fluids going into the nasopharynx Diplopia with strabismus
Polymyalgia rheumatica	Jaw claudication Monocular blindness Palpable temporal artery, sometimes even serpinginous (Fig. 7.32)

Table 7.6. **Features of a Spastic Hemiparetic Gait (Related Symptoms)**

Feature	Contralateral side	Ipsilateral side
Tone	Increased, spastic in nature	Normal
Reflexes	3+ to 4+ Clonus in ankle and wrist	1+ to 2+ No clonus
Power	2–4/5 to upper and lower	5/5 upper and lower
Hoffman maneuver	Involuntary flexion of digits 1, 2, 4, 5	No involuntary flexion
Tromner maneuver	Involuntary flexion of digits 1, 2, 4, 5	No involuntary flexion
Babinski's sign	Involuntary abduction of toes Involuntary dorsiflexion of toes	Voluntary withdrawal of toes Voluntary flexion of toes
Oppenheim maneuver	Involuntary abduction of toes Involuntary dorsiflexion of toes	Nonspecific
Chaddock maneuver	Involuntary abduction of toes Involuntary dorsiflexion of toes	Voluntary withdrawal of foot
Stransky maneuver	Involuntary abduction of toes Involuntary dorsiflexion of toes	Nonspecific
Active smile	Loss of nasolabial fold Unable to bring corner of mouth upward	Accentuated nasolabial fold Able to bring mouth corner upward
Puff out cheeks	Unable to puff out cheek	Able to puff out cheek
Active show of teeth (growl)	Unable to show teeth	Able to show teeth
Close eyes tightly	Able to perform	Able to perform
Wrinkle up forehead	Furrows in brow present	Furrows in brow present
Uvula	Midline	Midline
Uvula with AHHH	Elevated, deviated to side of lesion	Elevated, deviated to side of lesion
"Kentucky"	e/uck/EEE	e/uck/EEE
Pronator drift	Involuntary drift into pronation of forearm from a baseline of arm forward flexed and supinated	Able to maintain supinated position
Barre's sign	Involuntary drift to extension of knee from a baseline of prone with leg, at knee flexed to 90 degrees	Able to maintain knee flexion

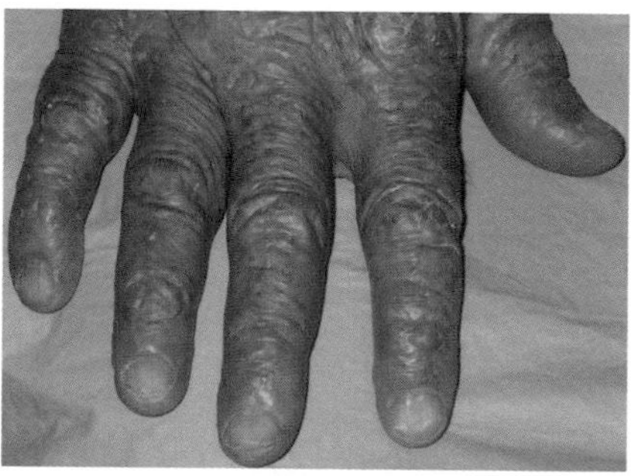

Figure 7.30.

Classic Gottron's papules on the dorsum on the fingers of this patient with dermatomyositis.

 **TIPS**

- Inspect skin on dorsal hands and fingers
- Dermatomyositis: erythematous papules and plaques on the dorsal skin of the hands (Gottron's sign)
- Part of waddling gait evaluation

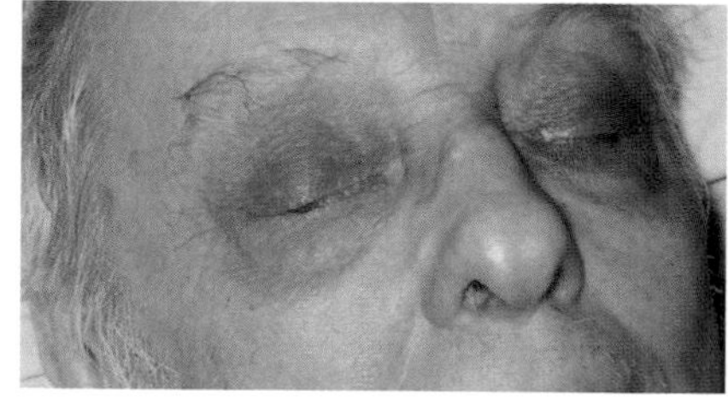

Figure 7.31.

Classic heliotropic rash about the eyes of this patient with dermatomyositis.

 **TIPS**

- Inspect the skin around the eyes
- Dermatomyositis: heliotropic colored rash in the periorbital areas
- Part of waddling gait evaluation

often with clonus; and decreased power, i.e., **paresis**, on the entire affected side. In addition, there is involuntary flexion of digits with the **Hoffman or Tromner** maneuver **(Fig. 7.33)**. For the *Hoffman's maneuver*, grasp the patient's third finger with the thumb on the palmar side of the middle phalanx, index finger on the dorsal side of the distal phalanx. Flex the digit at the distal interphalangeal (DIP) joint and acutely release. For the *Tromner's maneuver*, the examiner snaps thumb upward and hits the palmar pad of the patient's third digit. Normally, there is no other digit finger flexion. In addition, there is involuntary flaring and dorsiflexion of toes noted with the maneuvers of **Chaddock, Stransky**, and **Oppenheim**. For *Chaddock maneuver*, use the middle knuckle or a plexor to stroke the skin over the lateral foot, from the mid–fifth metatarsal to the calcaneus bone; another variant is to tap eight to ten times over the lateral malleolus. For *Stransky's maneuver*, the examiner grasps the fourth and fifth toes and passively abducts the toes; then, acutely releases this passive abduction **(Fig. 7.34)**. Normally, the other toes remain unchanged. For *Oppenheim's maneuver*, use the knuckles on fingers 2 and 3 to stroke from the infrapatellar area to the ankle on the anterior tibial surface **(Fig. 7.35C and D)**. Although we rarely perform Babinski's maneuver, because it is more than a noxious stimulus applied to the foot—it can be obnoxious—it is important to know as many clinicians often use it for diagnostic benefit. For *Babinski's maneuver*, use the thumb, a tongue blade, or the handle of a plexor to stroke the skin on the plantar aspect of the foot. The path of the stroke is on the lateral foot, commencing posterior and then extending across the plantar metatarsal heads (Fig 7.35A and B). A **pronator drift**, i.e., the inability to maintain a forward flexed, supinated upper extremity on the side contralateral to the UMN lesion, is also noted **(Fig. 7.36)**. The technique for pronator drift is one in which the patient stands with arms forward flexed to 90 degrees and the forearms fully supinated. Normally, the patient is able to maintain this position. There is a **Barre's pyramidal sign**, i.e., the inability to maintain a flexed knee in a prone position on the side contralateral to the UMN lesion **(Fig. 7.37)**. In addition, there is weakness to smile and growl on the contralateral side (central cranial nerve VII), **dysarthria** (mashed-potato or peanut-butter stuck in mouth type of

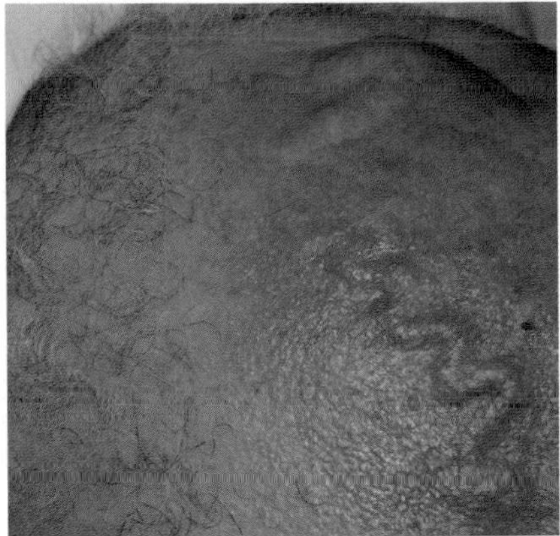

Figure 7.32.

Temporal arteritis: an enlarged, tender, and serpiginous temporalis artery.

TIPS

- Palpate the temporalis artery immediately anterior to the tragus of auricle
- Normal: pulse present; nontender; no nodules
- Temporal arteritis: tender; may have nodules; may have a diminished or even absent pulse; artery serpiginous
- Part of evaluation of waddling gait

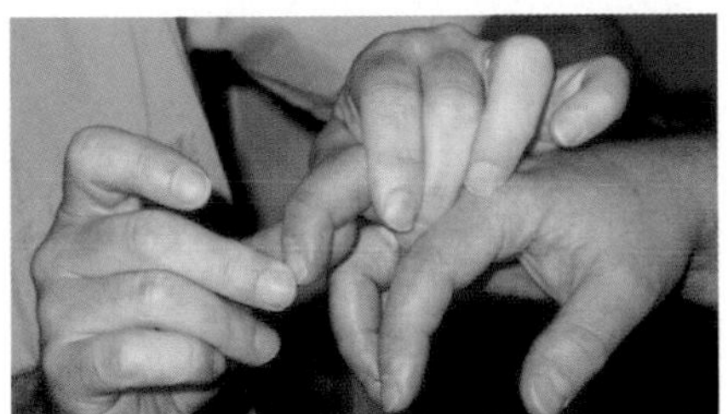

A

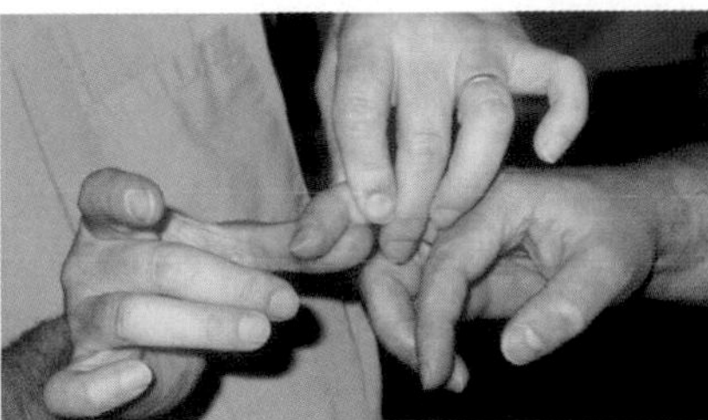

B

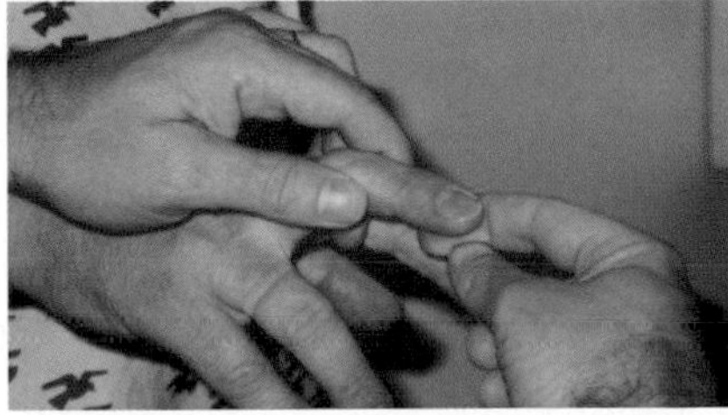

C

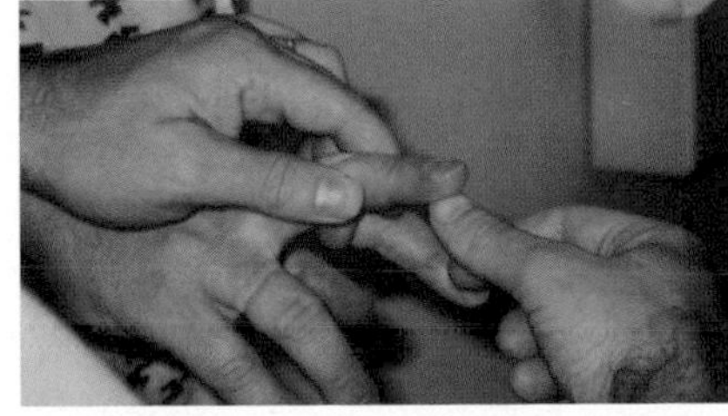

D

Figure 7.33.

A and **B**. Hoffman's maneuver. **C** and **D**. Tromner's maneuver. Both are excellent methods to assess for contralateral UMN complications.

TIPS

- Support the patient's hand, middle finger; hand neutral
- **A** and **B**. Hoffman's maneuver: grasp the patient's third finger with thumb on palmar side of middle phalanx, index finger on dorsal (plate) side of distal phalanx
- Flex **(A)** the digit at the DIP and acutely release **(B)**
- **C** and **D**. Tromner's maneuver: examiner snaps up thumb and hits the palmar pad of the patient's third digit
- Normal: no finger flexion
- Upper motor neuron problem: abnormal reflexive flexion of thumb and fifth digit

TEACHING POINTS

SPASTIC AND SCISSOR GAITS

1. Spastic gaits are associated with 3+ or 4+ reflexes and abnormal reflexes (e.g., Hoffman's and Chaddock's maneuvers).
2. Most of the Babinski signs and correlated reflexes are associated with up-going toes and are caused by contralateral upper motor neuron (UMN) damage.
3. Hoffman's maneuver is the easiest and best upper extremity abnormal UMN reflex.
4. Chaddock and Stransky maneuvers are the best and easiest to perform lower extremity abnormal UMN reflex.
5. Scissors gait is truly a bilateral spastic hemiparetic gait; it has a much higher incidence of falls and of significant swallowing dysfunction and is associated with pseudobulbar palsy.

diction), **dysphonia** of upper motor neuron cranial nerve problems, and potentially significant swallowing defects. All of these are on the side opposite to the intracranial event.

A **scissors gait** is bilateral spastic hemiparesis with severe limitation of gait, unsteady in nature, and legs cross over each other when walking forward. A major difference is often the marked brainstem involvement; often, with a scissors gait, will be bilateral cranial nerve VII damage, multiple, bilateral brainstem deficits, and thus **pseudobulbar palsy**. This gait is due to cerebral palsy or multiple cerebrovascular accidents or marked head trauma.

Ataxic Gaits

Cerebellar ataxia, peripheral sensory (proprioceptive) ataxia, and **vestibular ataxia** manifest with a wide-based, unsteady gait **(Table 7.7)**. The ataxic gait is one that is wide-based, feet placed lateral to the ASIS, arms dangling to the sides, and the patient is very, if not severely, unsteady. As such, there is a great risk for falls; thus the examiner must zealously monitor the patient during exam. **Cerebellar ataxia** manifests with minimal arm swinging

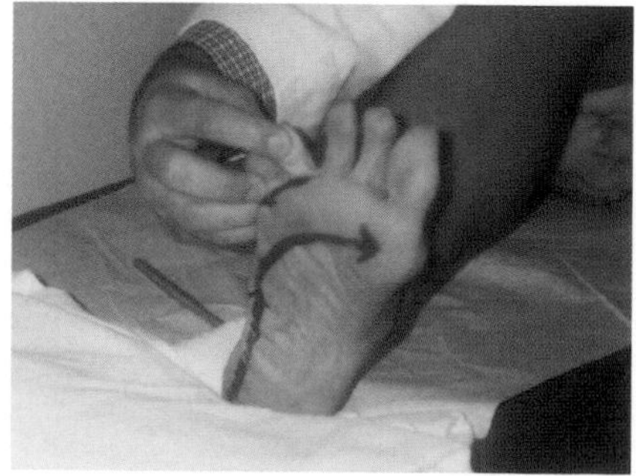

A

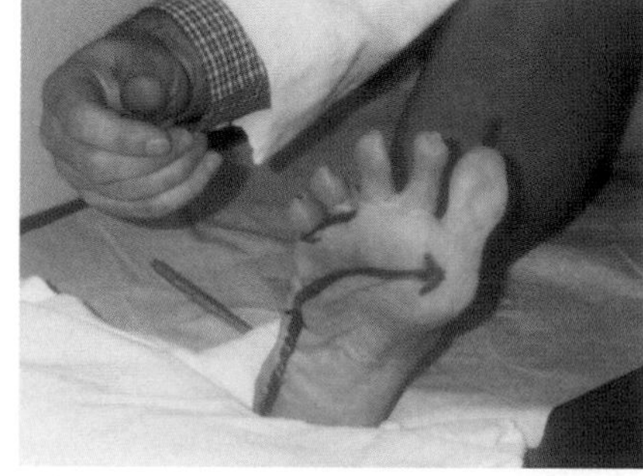

B

Figure 7.34.

Techniques for foot signs of upper motor neuron (UMN) release. **A, B.** Stransky maneuver.

TIPS

- **A, B.** Stransky maneuver: grasp the fourth and fifth toes; passively abduct the toes, then acutely release them
- Normal: toes remain unchanged, i.e., no flaring or upward movement
- Upper motor neuron damage: toes on the foot contralateral to damage flare out and dorsiflex involuntarily within 5 seconds of the procedure

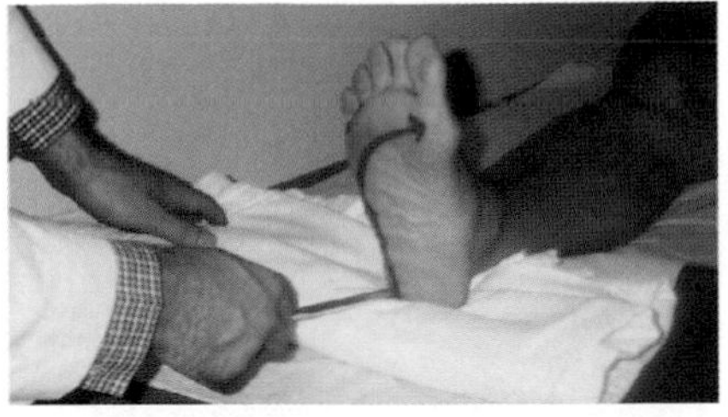
A

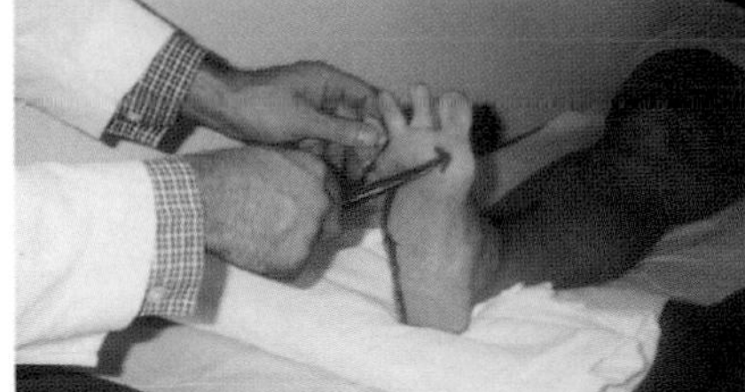
B

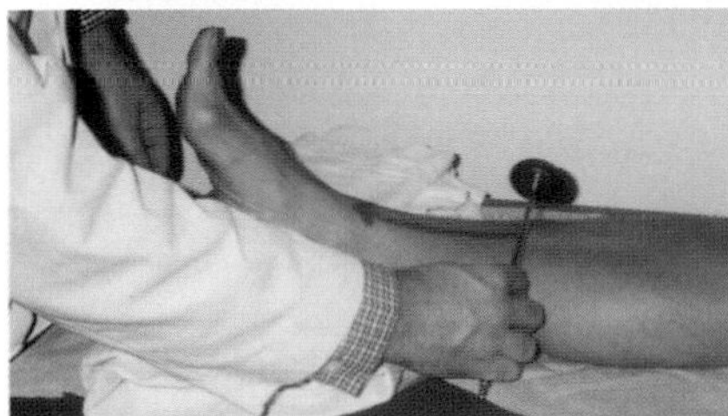
C

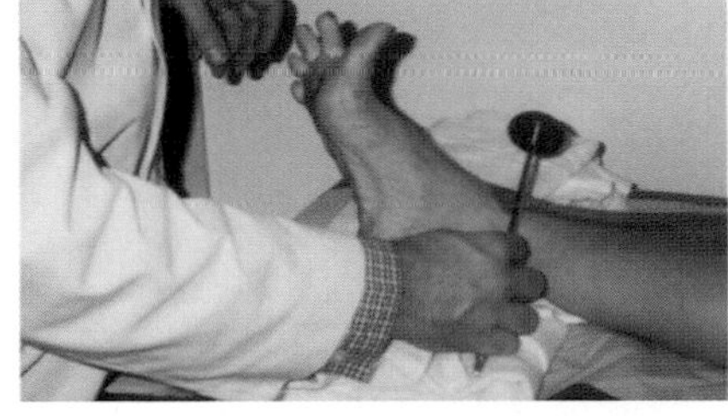
D

Figure 7.35.

Technique for foot signs of upper motor neuron (UMN) release. **A and B.** Babinski maneuver. **C and D.** Oppenheim maneuver.

TIPS

- **A, B.** Babinski maneuver: use the thumb, a tongue blade, or a pleximeter handle to stroke the skin of the plantar aspect of the foot
- The path of "stroking" is as detailed on the plantar foot-lateral plantar foot, then across the plantar metatarsal heads
- **C, D.** Oppenheim maneuver: use a tongue blade or knuckles 2 and 3 to stroke superior to inferior on the anterior tibial surface
- Normal: withdrawal, toes flex, no flaring outward of the toes
- Upper motor neuron damage: toes flare out (abduct) and dorsiflex involuntarily within 5 seconds of the procedure on the side contralateral to the lesion

(Wartenberg's sign). There is diffuse hypotonia as manifested by "floppy" joints, the hands flop and flex when arms are forward flexed and kept at 90 degrees, and bilateral pes planus **(Fig. 7.38)**. The company cerebellar ataxia keeps includes an inability to perform a **tandem walk**, in which the patient is instructed to walk across the room on an imaginary line **(Fig. 7.39)**. This test has high sensitivity, but very poor specificity. In addition, the presence of greater than two beats of horizontal and/or vertical or even rotatory **nystagmus** occurs in cerebellar ataxia. Also present is **dysdiadochokinesis**, which is an inability to perform rapidly alternating actions such as rapid alternation between supination and pronation *or* the **finger march** method of rapidly touching thumb to tip of finger 5, then 4, then 3, then 2, then 3, then 4, then 5 for a set of three times *or* rapidly crossing feet in front of each other **(Fig. 7.40)**. A final, quite excellent method is twiddling one's thumbs, forward then backward then forward. The sensitivity of the examination increases when distracting the patient. In addition, in cerebellar ataxia often present is **dysmetria**, i.e., inability to judge distances; thus, the patient is unable to touch the index finger to the examiner's finger, as it moves to various points in front

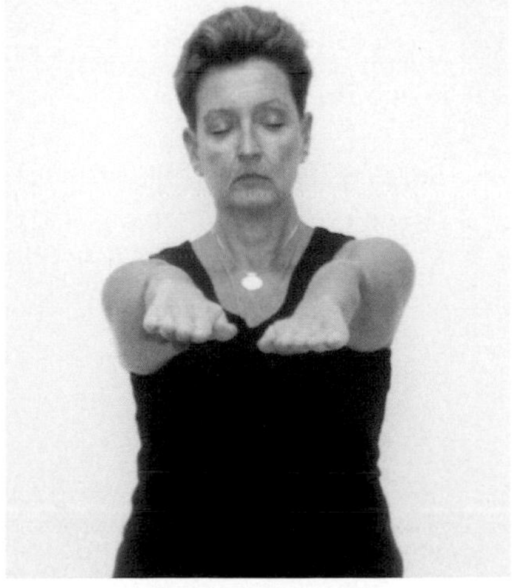
A

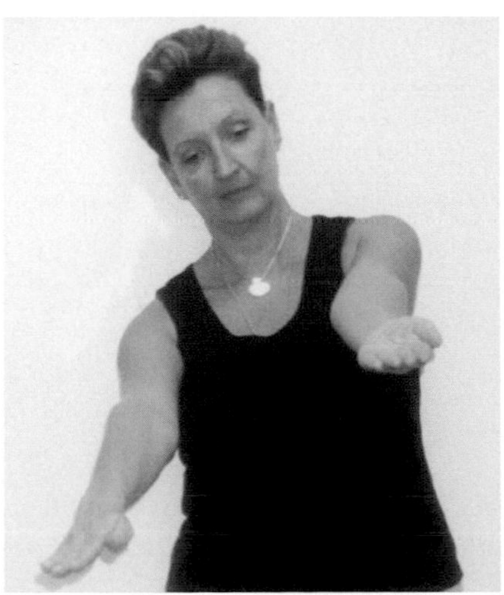
B

Figure 7.36.

Technique for pronator drift sign: the inability to maintain a forward flexed, supinated upper extremity on the side contralateral to the upper motor neuron (UMN) lesion.

TIPS

- Patient stands with arms forward flexed to 90 degrees and forearms fully supinated
- Normal: able to maintain
- Upper motor neuron deficits: involuntary pronation of the arm on the contralateral side
- Excellent example of company, especially useful in mild hemiparesis

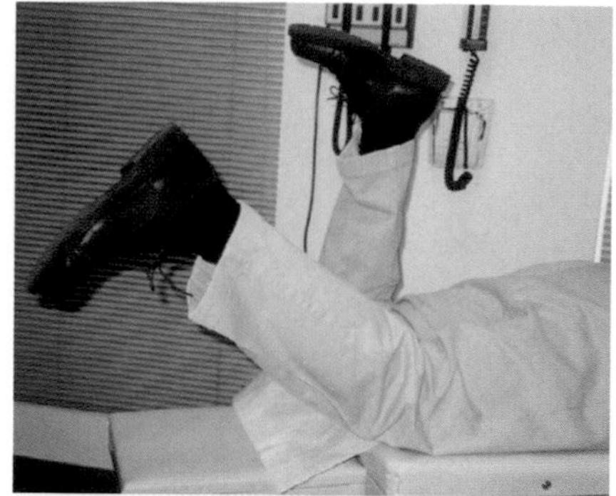

A

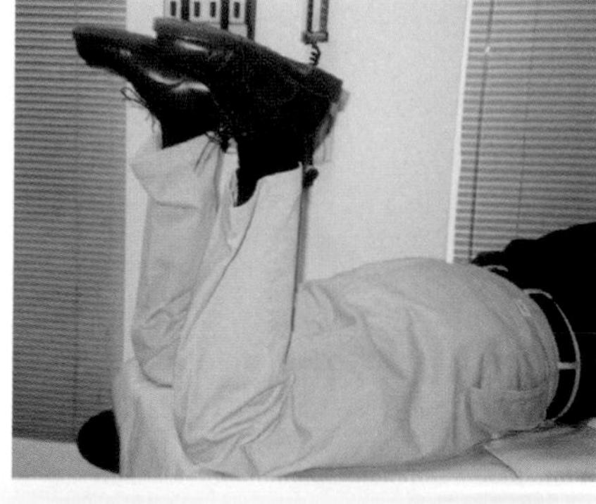

B

Figure 7.37.

Technique for the Barre's test: the inability to maintain a flexed knee in a prone position on side contralateral to the upper motor neuron (UMN) lesion. **A.** Leg flexion. **B.** Unable to maintain position.

 **TIPS**

- Patient is prone with knees flexed to 90 degrees
- Instruct patient to maintain this position
- Normal: able to maintain position
- Upper motor neuron deficit: involuntary extension of knee on side contralateral to lesion
- Excellent example of company that a finding keeps, especially useful in moderate hemiparesis when the patient cannot stand

of patient **(Fig. 7.41)**. We do not recommend the traditional finger-to-nose approach because it is far too optimistic in that a poor result can read to a finger accidentally stuck into the eye. The lower extremity can also be used to assess for toe to finger on both sides. Furthermore, the assessment for

Table 7.7. Ataxia: Features of Each Type

Physical examination	Cerebellar	Sensory	Vestibular
Tone	Hypotonia Pes planus Pendulum reflexes	Normal tone	Normal tone
Romberg	Nonspecific	Unsteady from heels	Unsteady
Tandem walk	Unsteady	Unsteady	Unsteady
Looking at feet when walking	No change	Improvement	No change
*Diadochokinesis (rapid alternating movements)**	Dysdiadochokinesis	Normal	Normal
Metria	Dysmetria	Normal	Normal
Synergia (smooth, gliding motion)	Asynergia	Normal	Normal
Tremor	Intention tremor	No tremor	No tremor
Nystagmus	>2 beats horizontal and vertical or even rotatory	<2 beats horizontal	>2 beats horizontal
Sit next to patient in bed (truncal ataxia)	Unsteady	Steady	Steady
Handwriting	Wild, messy	Baseline	Nonspecific
States "Kentucky"	"enthucha"	"Kentucky"	"Kentucky"
Sensation, monofilament	Intact	Stocking or stocking-glove deficit	Intact
Sensation, 256-Hz tuning fork	Intact	Stocking or stocking-glove deficit	Intact
Dix-Hallpike maneuver	Nonspecific	Nonspecific	Precipitates nausea, vertigo, nystagmus

*e.g., twiddle thumbs.

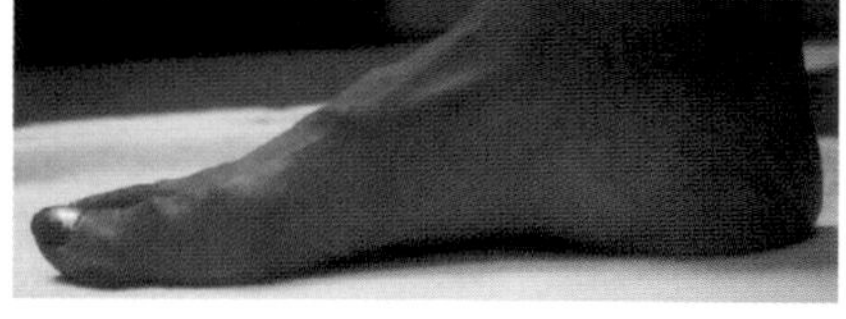

Figure 7.38.

Cerebellar ataxia: pes planus, bilateral. A clear feature of hypotonia.

 **TIPS**

- Note the presence of bilateral pes planus and moderate outtoeing in this individual with hypotonia

TEACHING POINTS

ATAXIA

1. Cerebellar ataxia does not improve with use of visual cues; sensory ataxia does so improve.
2. Ataxia is a wide-based gait.
3. An early sign of cerebellar ataxia: a loss of arm swinging (Wartenberg's sign).
4. Unilateral cerebellar lesion manifests with ipsilateral findings: ataxia, dysmetria, asynergia, dysdiadochokinesis.
5. Cerebellar ataxia manifests with wide-based stance, dysmetria, asynergia, dysdiadochokinesis, intentional "tremor," nystagmus, and hypotonia.
6. Sensory ataxia manifests with wide-based stance; with the Romberg test, a tilt from the heels, sensory deficits in the feet.
7. Hypotonia is not equal to hyporeflexia.
8. Hypotonia manifests with pendulum-type reflexes and type "floppy" joints.
9. There are three types of ataxia: cerebellar, sensory (proprioceptive), and vestibular.

asynergia, i.e., inability to perform complex actions in a smooth, gliding manner, is of tremendous importance in cerebellar ataxia **(Fig. 7.42)**. To assess this, the patient glides heel up and down the anterior tibial surface, which is repeated three times, or the patient slides the index finger up and down the anterior humeral surface, also repeated three times. Normally, this can be done and, thus, the patient has the ability to integrate multiple motor activities, which is called synergy. In our view, the one best method for synergy is swinging a baseball bat, or rapid twiddling of thumbs. Other company includes a **tremor of intention**, which is often a mixture of the staccato, abrupt, nonsmooth movements indicative of asynergia and concurrent significant dysmetria. The patient often has severe difficulty in stating the sounds of K, Q, or hard C (Celtic). When such a patient states the word "Kentucky" it sounds like "enthucha." There is also a **scanning speech**, in which the pattern is a soft, slow monotone, with multiple mistakes, with a sudden burst of rapid increased volume speech. Finally, the patient has very wild handwriting. A rule of thumb for handwriting is if it is very tight and neat there is less likelihood of cerebellar disease; if wild and messy, it is of little diagnostic importance (especially for a patient who is a physician). In severe cerebellar disease, there may even be **truncal ataxia**, i.e., the patient cannot maintain a sitting posture when the examiner sits next to the patient on the side of bed. The sensory examination in pure cerebellar ataxia is usually without deficit. **Cerebellar damage** can be from a stroke, in which case the manifestations are on the ipsilateral side to the injury, from acute or chronic ethanol use, or be caused by multiple sclerosis, in which there is bilateral involvement.

Sensory (also known as proprioceptive) **ataxia** manifests with a marked decrease in sensation to feet as assessed using a cotton-tipped swab, a 256-Hz tuning fork, or the monofilament tests. In addition, a *Romberg test** is often markedly positive, in which the patient is unsteady and sways from the heels to either direction **(Fig. 7.43)**. Recall, there are specific levels or steps in performing a Romberg. The first is baseline, with the patient standing with feet apart; the next level is when the patient places feet together, but

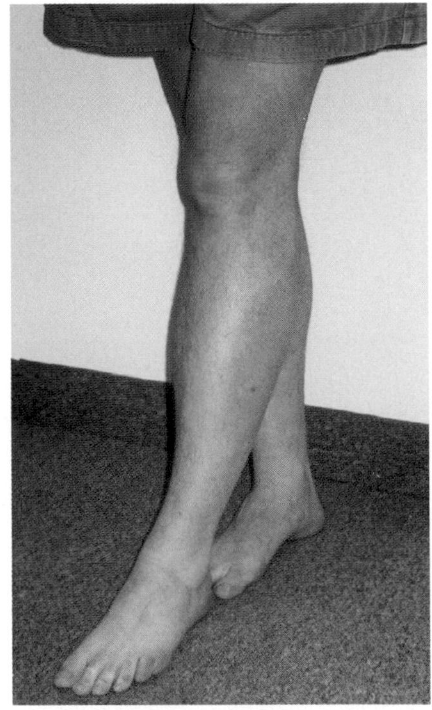

Figure 7.39.

Cerebellar ataxia: tandem walk. A highly sensitive, but nonspecific, method to assess for mild ataxia.

 **TIPS**

- Instruct patient to attempt to walk toe to heel across the room as if on an imaginary tightrope
- Mild ataxia: able to ambulate, but unable to perform this activity

*Romberg first described this to assess for tabes dorsalis.

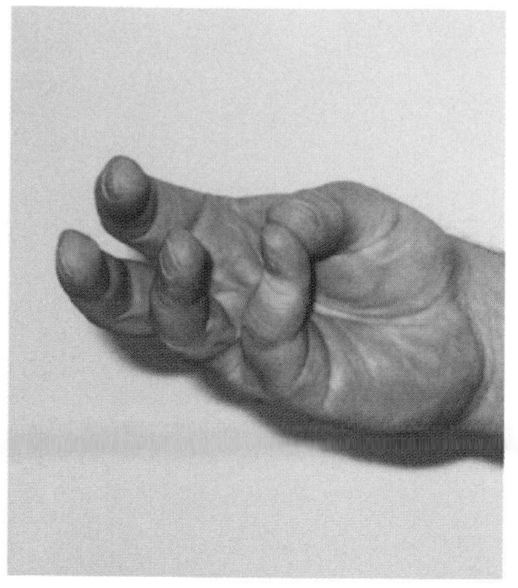
A

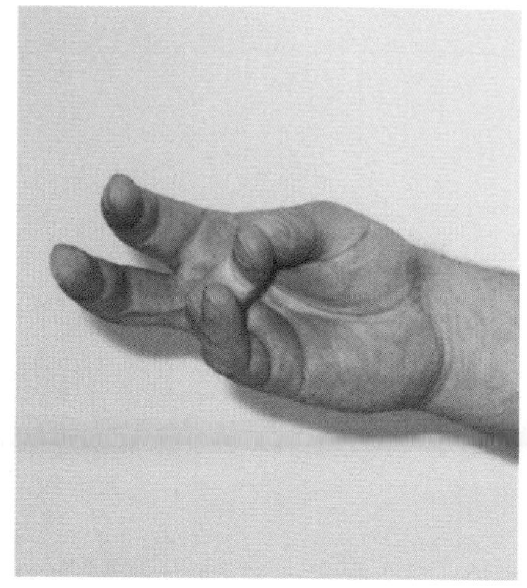
B

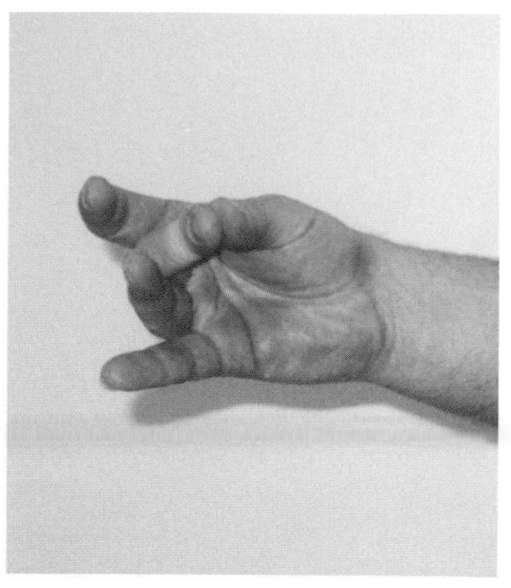
C

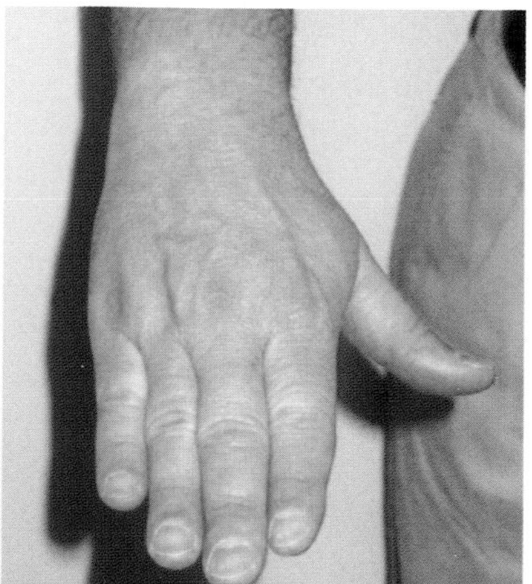
D

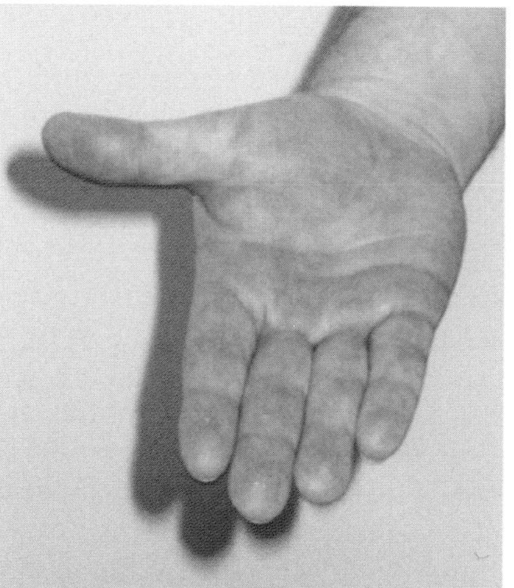
E

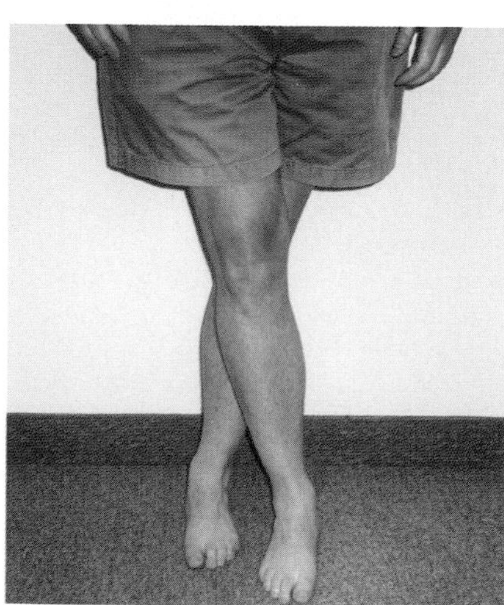
F

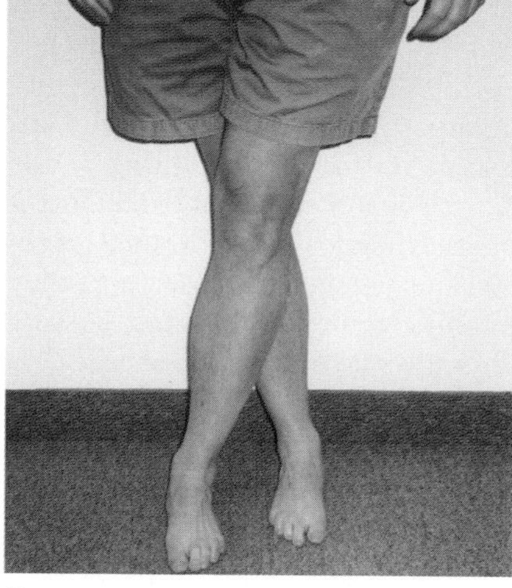
G

Figure 7.40.

Techniques to assess diadochokinesis. **A, B, C.** Finger march method. **D** and **E.** Forearm supination or pronation. **F** and **G** Crossing over of feet method. Note any decreased ability to perform these rapidly alternating movements, i.e., dysdiadochokinesis. Excellent measure of cerebellar function.

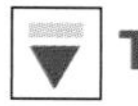

TIPS

- **A, B, C.** Finger march. Instruct patient to tap thumb to fingertips 5, 4, 3, 2, then thumb to fingertips 2, 3, 4, 5; repeat cycle three times *or*
- **D, E.** Hand or wrist in neutral position, alternate between full pronation and full supination three times *or*
- **F, G.** Actively cross feet in front of each other
- Normal: diadochokinesis, the ability to perform these rapidly alternating activities
- Cerebellar disease: inability to perform this activity—unilateral, ipsilateral or bilateral dysdiadochokinesis

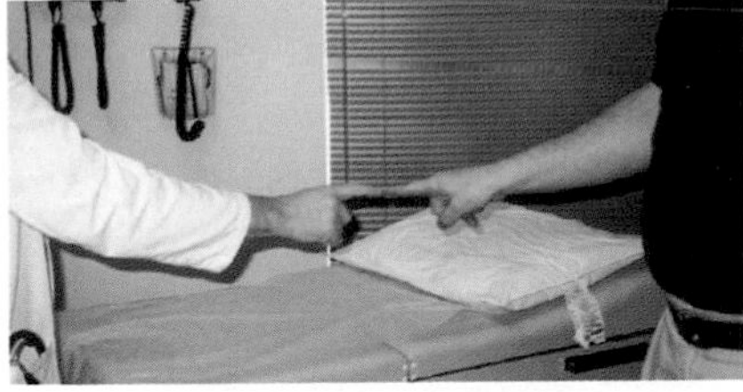

A

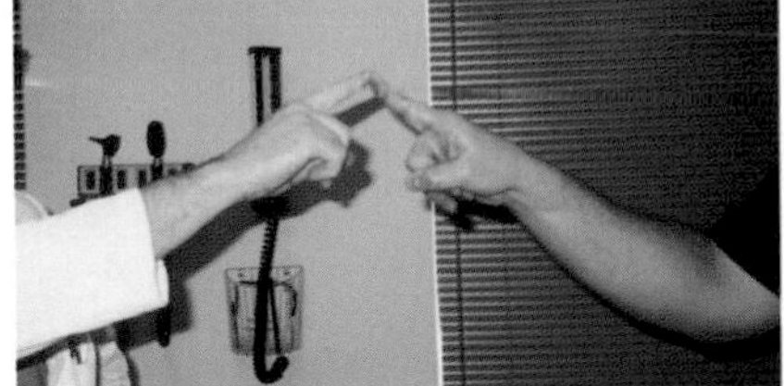

B

eyes remain open; the third level is when the patient forward flexes the arms to 90 degrees with the forearms pronated; the fourth level is with the eyes closed; and the final level is with stress applied to the outstretched arms. *Normal* is no drifting to one side or the other. To perform the Romberg test, always stand near the patient to save the patient from any potential falls. In sensory ataxia, there is marked improvement of the gait disturbance when the patient looks at the floor and feet. In a sensory–type ataxia, the patient has normal metria, diadochokinesis, synergy of movement, normal tone, and no nystagmus or tremor of intention. Every physician who cares for patients at risk for sensory ataxia, e.g., patient with diabetes mellitus, should be adept at using monofilaments. These are used bilaterally on the plantar foot and the palmar hand. Use monofilaments to gently dimple the skin over several sites on the plantar foot and palmar hand. **(Fig. 7.44)**. This technique for monofilaments is from the National Leprosy Foundation United States

Figure 7.41.

Technique to measure metria: the ability to judge and voluntarily move hand to specific locations. Here, the finger-to-finger test is an excellent measure of cerebellar function.

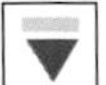

TIPS

- Instruct patient to touch finger to your finger
- Move finger to a new spot, patient moves finger to it
- Perform on each side, from each visual field
- Repeat process with patient's other hand
- Normal: able to judge distances—metria
- Cerebellar dysfunction: difficult to judge distances and, thus, point past objects—dysmetria
- Dysmetria is a contributor to the "tremor" of intention

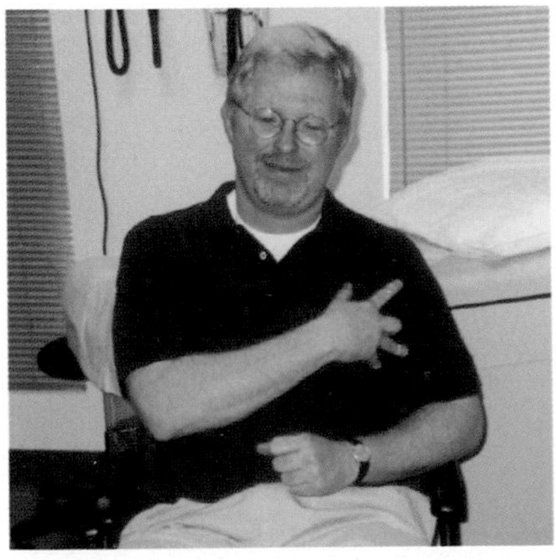

A_1

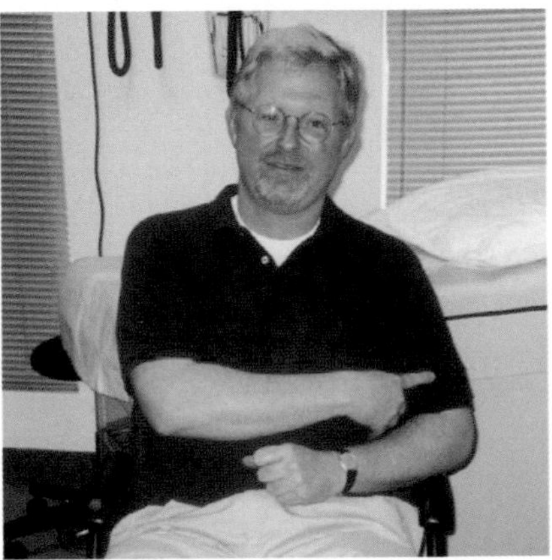

A_2

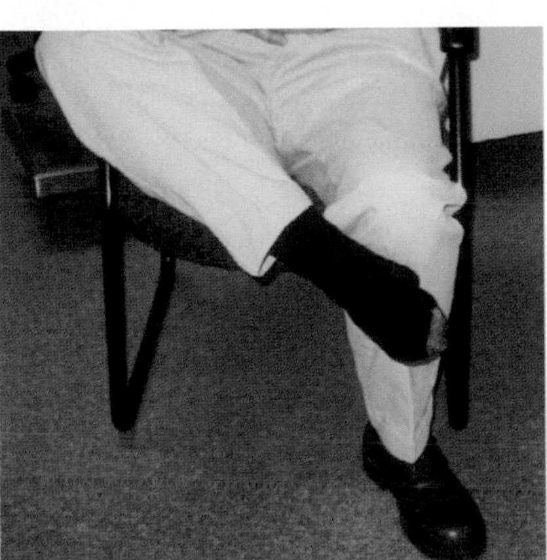

B_1

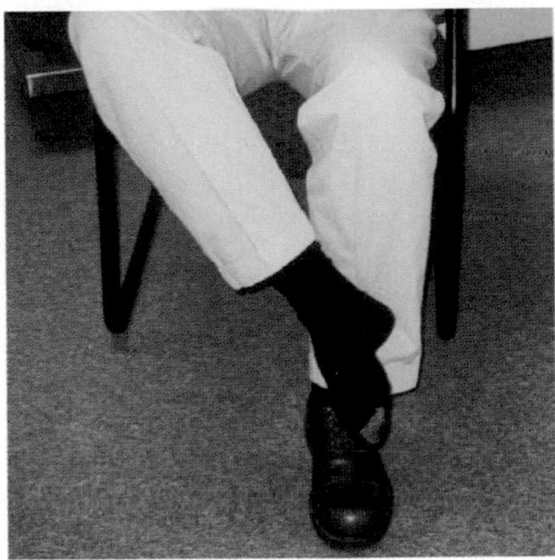

B_2

Figure 7.42.

Technique to assess synergia. **A.** The index finger glides up and down the ulnar forearm. **B.** The heel glides up and down the anterior tibia. These are excellent measures of cerebellar function.

TIPS

- Patient sitting
- **A_1 and A_2.** Patient slides finger up and down the anterior humeral surface; repeat cycle three times
- **B_1 and B_2.** Patient slides (glides) heel up and down the anterior tibial surface; repeat cycle three times
- Cerebellar dysfunction: unable to perform a glide—asynergia. Contributes to the large amplitude tremor of intention
- Normal: able to perform as a glide—synergia

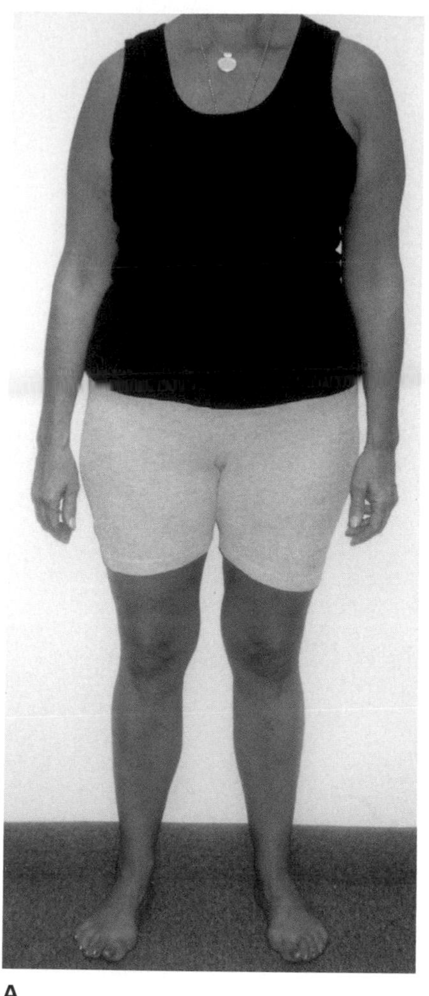
A

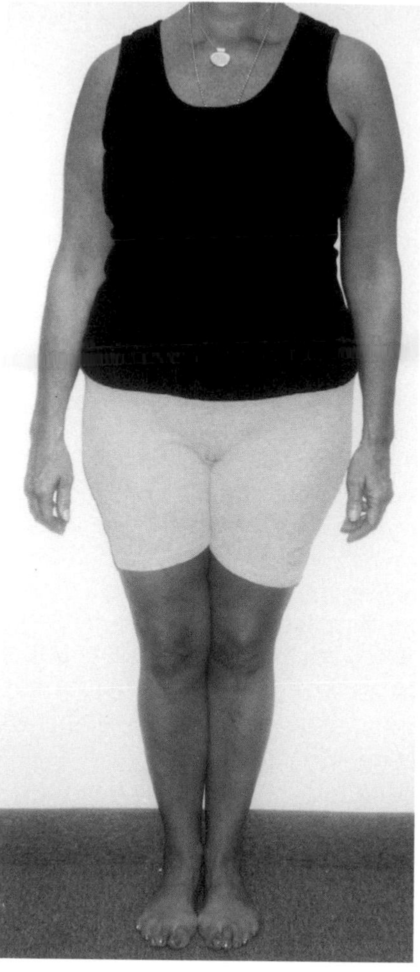
B

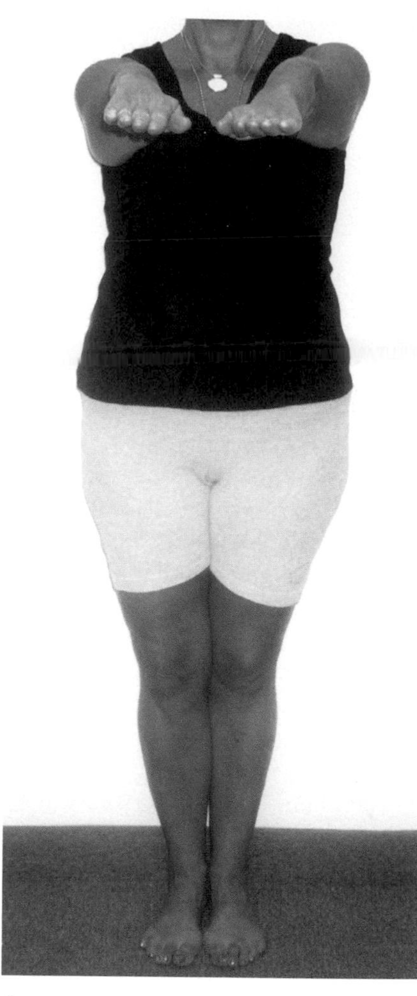
C

Figure 7.43.

The four levels of stress for the Romberg maneuver. **A.** Baseline anatomic position. **B.** Level one: stance: put feet together. **C.** Level two: actively forward flex arms, forearms pronated. Level three: close eyes. Level four: examiner places stress on the forward flexed arms (not shown). Must monitor patient closely to prevent falls; once patient lists or drifts to one or either side, record and state which level and terminate the test.

TIPS

- Baseline: Patient standing with feet apart **(A)**
- Patient places feet together, keeps eyes open **(B)**
- Actively puts arms in forward flexion of 90 degrees, forearms pronated **(C)**
- Closes eyes
- Place downward stress on patient's forward flexed arms
- Patient attempts to maintain the arms in position
- Note any drift to either or both sides at the heels
- Ataxia, especially sensory: loss of ability to maintain position from the heels; the drift is from the feet
- Once patient lists or drifts to one or either side, record and state which level and terminate the test
- *Caution:* Stand near patient to save the patient from any potential fall

Public Health service (USPH). Use of monofilaments is an excellent way to test various reproducible sites; monofilaments of various sized diameters should be used. *Vibratory sensation* should also be measured in all cases **(Fig. 7.45)**. The technique that we recommend is to use a 256-Hz tuning fork, although a 128-Hz tuning fork is adequate. The 256 Hz is best to assess Pacinian and Meissner's corpuscles. Assessment of vibratory sensation is termed "pallanesthesia." The fork is placed, in the following order, over the (1) tips on the first and second toes, (2) head of the second metatarsal, (3) dorsum of foot at Lisfranc's joint, (4) medial malleolus, (5) patella, and, finally, (6) greater tuberosity of the femur. The examination is complete when the patient can sense the vibration of the tuning fork.

Ataxia of vestibular origin manifests with a wide based, unsteady gait with significant nystagmus, vertigo, nausea, vomiting, and tinnitus. This can be remarkably severe. In performing the Romberg test, the patient often is unsteady; often unable even to attempt a tandem walk, with no improvement when looking at the feet. If caused by benign positional vertigo, the *Barany-Dix-Hallpike-Nylen maneuver* will reproduce the vertigo, nausea, and the

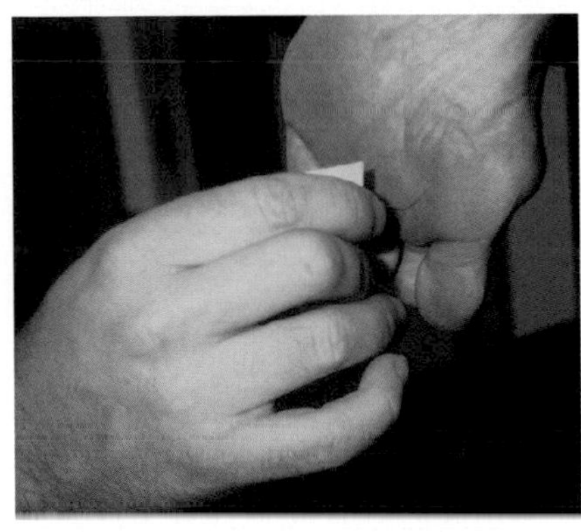

Figure 7.44.

Technique for use of monofilament to gently dimple skin to test fine touch sensation. Excellent method to assess and grade sensory deficits, if present.

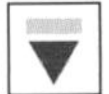 **TIPS**

- Use monofilaments to gently dimple the skin over several sites on the plantar foot
- Monofilaments are excellent to test various reproducible sites; use various diameter (intensity) monofilaments
- Sensory ataxia, e.g., from diabetes mellitus: stocking or stocking-glove deficit
- Peripheral neuropathy: deficit in a specific nerve distribution

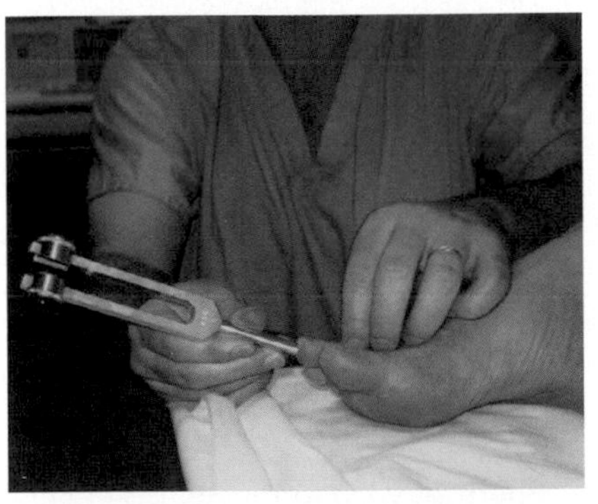

A

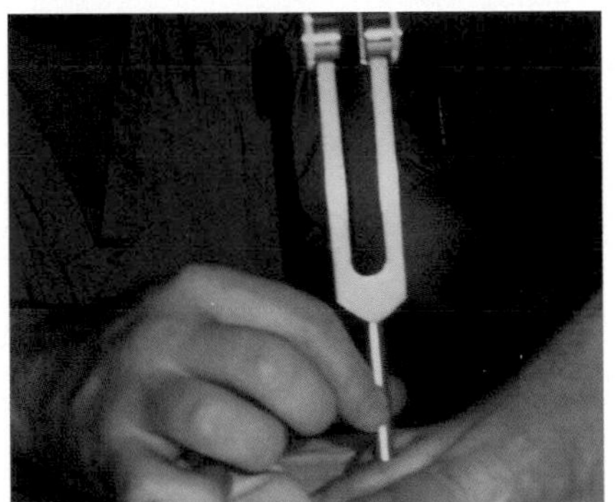

B

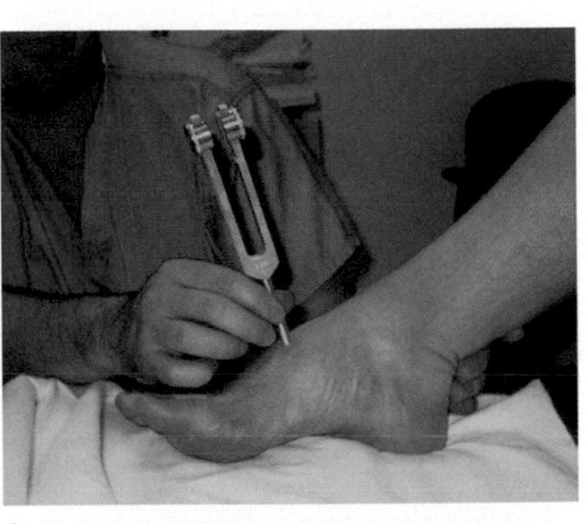

C

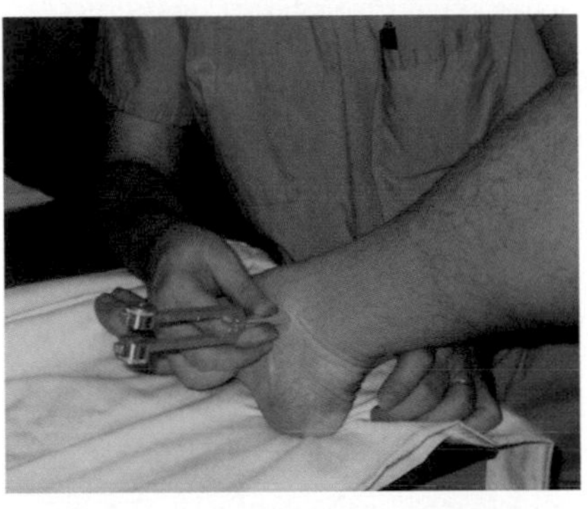

D

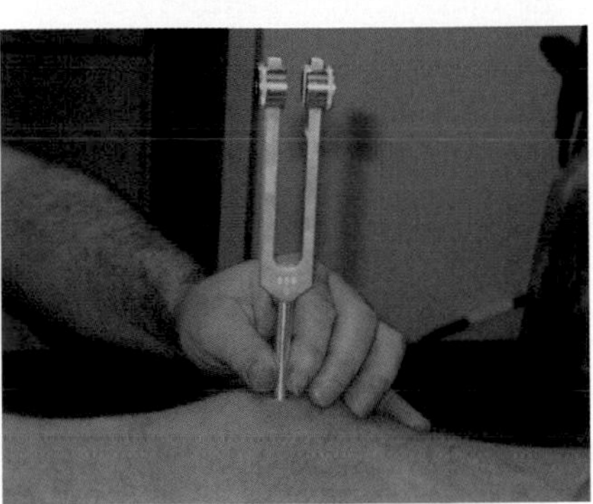

E

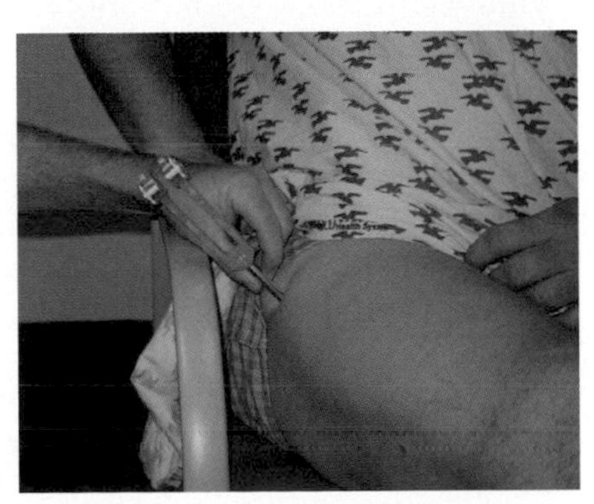

F

Figure 7.45.

Technique for vibratory sensation assessment. An excellent complementary test to monofilaments or cotton-tipped swab testing.

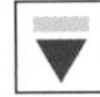 **TIPS**

- Vibratory sensation is an excellent surrogate for proprioception
- Use a 256-Hz tuning fork
- Note sites and order of tuning fork placement: **A.** First or second digit tip. **B.** Head of second metatarsal. **C.** Over Lisfranc's joint. **D.** Medial malleolus. **E.** Patella. **F.** Greater trochanter of femur.
- Sensory ataxia, e.g., from diabetes mellitus: stocking or stocking-glove deficit

Figure 7.46.

Technique for Barany-Dix-Hallpike-Nylen maneuver for benign positional vertigo. Excellent screening test for this type of vestibular ataxia.

TIPS

- Patient supine, head over side of table **(A)**
- Extend patient's head at neck 25 to 30 degrees and rotate head to right or left for 30 seconds **(B)**
- Assist patient to rapidly assume a sitting position, maintain for 1 minute **(C)**
- Repeat the procedure with the head rotated to other side **(D)**
- Normal: no nausea, vomiting, vertigo, nystagmus
- Benign positional vertigo: marked nausea, vomiting, vertigo, and nystagmus acutely develop
- Must have a *stable neck*

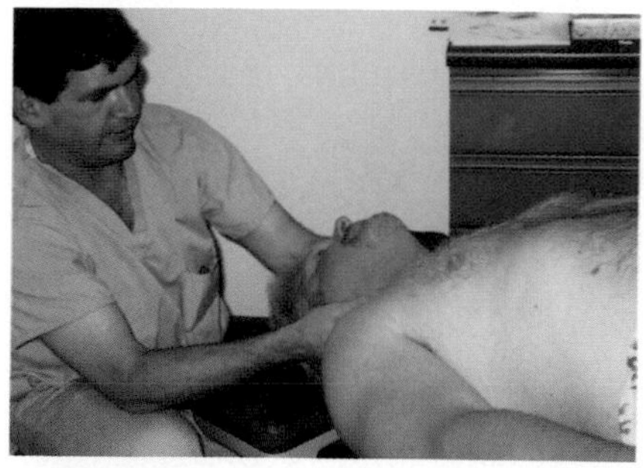

A

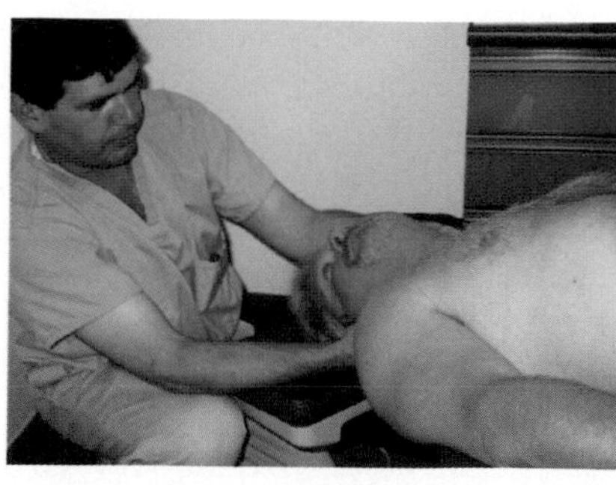

B

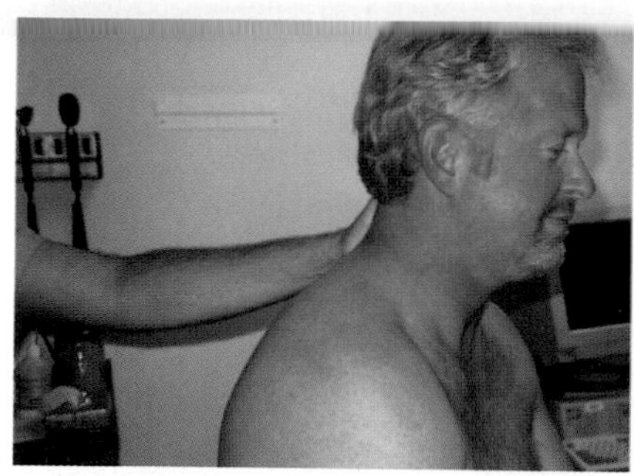

C

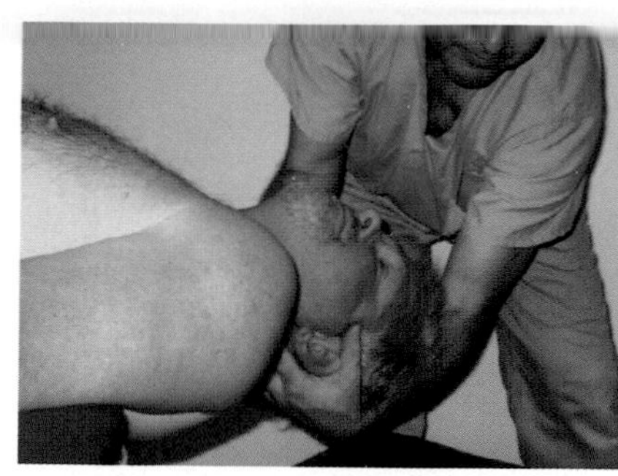

D

nystagmus **(Fig. 7.46)**. For this technique, with the patient supine, head over the end of the table, extend the head at the neck 25 to 30 degrees and rotate the head left or right 15 degrees for 30 seconds. Then, help the patient assume a sitting position and maintain it for 1 minute. Repeat the procedure with the head rotated to the other side. The development of vertigo makes BPV likely. In vestibular ataxia there are no sensory deficits seen to hands or feet and no signs of cerebellar dysfunction.

Shuffling Gait

Parkinson's disease manifests with a **shuffling–type gait** that is narrow based, shuffling, hunched over, with the elbows slightly flexed. Overall, the gait itself is steady. The company it keeps includes marked **bradykinesia**, i.e., inability rapidly to start and to stop an activity. In addition is seen a **marche a petit pes** or **festination**, a slow steady speeding up of all movements once the ambulation has commenced. An example of this is the late Pope John Paul II who suffered from the disease Parkinson described. Other company includes an increase in tone throughout the body, which is either *cogwheel rigidity* or, in severe cases, *lead-pipe rigidity.* Although the elbow is the traditional site used and the site taught to assess cogwheel rigidity, we find circumduction of the wrist (Fig. 7.6) is the one best site to assess cogwheel rigidity. One further site is circumduction of the ankle. Further features include a flat expressionless facies and a fine oscillating, "pill-rolling" type tremor at rest in both hands and feet. *Myerson's sign,* in which the patient blinks each time that the examiner taps the forehead with finger, is a finding of advanced disease, often associated with dementia **(Fig. 7.47)**. To elicit Myerson's sign, gently tap over the midpoint between the supraorbital areas and observe the eyes for blinking. Normally, the blink is extinguished after four to five taps. In Parkinson's disease, the blink is not extinguished until after the tenth tap. In addition, the patient has a small, tight handwriting and the soft,

TEACHING POINTS

SHUFFLING OR PARKINSON'S TYPE GAIT

1. Narrow-based stance and gait.
2. Rigidity is cardinal feature of this problem.
3. Cogwheel rigidity is less intense than lead-pipe rigidity.
4. Unilateral basal ganglia lesion manifests with ipsilateral findings of pill-rolling tremor, cogwheel rigidity, bradykinesis, and shuffle on side.
5. Parkinson's manifests with a gait that is narrow based; tremor at rest, cogwheel rigidity, bradykinesis, hypophonia, and flat facies.
6. The patient with Parkinson's has a flat facies, a soft, slow low voice, and a lag time to start speech.
7. Dementia overlaps with Parkinson's disease; thus, necessary to perform mental status examination and frontal release tests on any patient with a shuffling gait.
8. Shy-Drager syndrome is Parkinson's with decreased autonomic function.
9. Decreased autonomic function: urinary or stool incontinence, orthostatic hypotension without any reflex tachycardia, an absence of sweating, and no skin pruning in water; if seen in a patient with gait disturbance, think Shy-Drager.
10. Classic example of Parkinson's gait is that of the late Pope John Paul II.
11. Essential tremor can be mistaken for Parkinson's tremor.
12. Essential tremor affects head and neck (yes-yes); Parkinson's affects hands and feet.
13. Essential tremor affects the voice: gravelly, oscillating type; think of the late Katharine Hepburn.

slow speech pattern of hypophonia. In this pattern, there is a lag period at outset and the speech becomes progressively faster in a grouping; it is festinating. As with the assessment of handwriting in cerebellar disease, its utility is that if the writing is large and robust the clinician should seriously question the diagnosis of Parkinson's disease. **Shy-Drager syndrome** is a variant of that described by Parkinson in that it manifests with Parkinson's disease and orthostatic hypotension without any appropriate reflex tachycardia. The company it keeps includes the diffuse loss of sweating, the loss of erectile

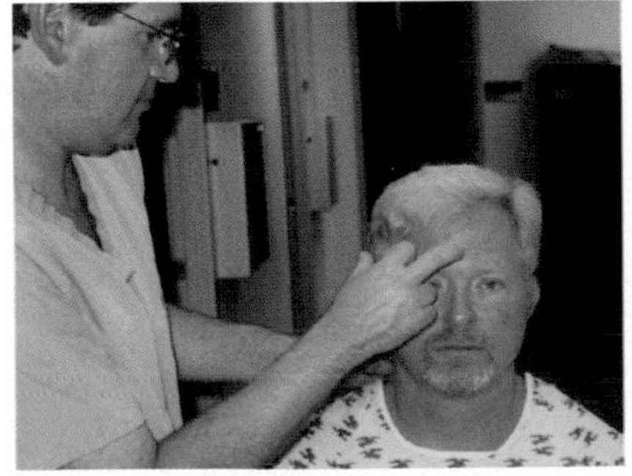

A

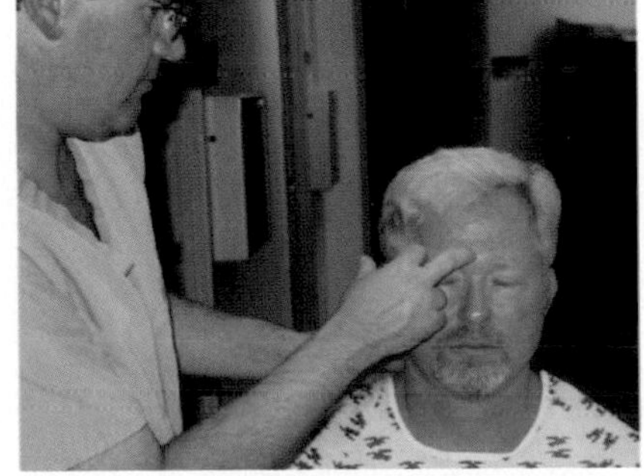

B

Figure 7.47.

Technique for Myerson's sign of Parkinson's disease with dementia.

TIPS

- Tap gently with middle finger over the midpoint between both supraorbital areas
- Normal: blink extinguished after the third or fourth tap
- Parkinson's with dementia—blink with repetitive taps, even after the fourth, fifth, or even tenth tap

Table 7.8. Tremor: Company they Keep

Physical examination	Parkinson's	Essential
Gait	Shuffling, with festination	Normal
Location of tremor	Hands and feet	Head and neck
Descriptors of tremor	"Pill rolling"	"Yes-yes"
Speech	Soft, lag time at outset of response	Oscillates gravelly
	Festination-slow, quickens with use	No festination Can be robust
	Carries minimal emotion	Can carry emotion
Tone	Cogwheel rigidity	Normal
Face	Flat emotionless	Carries emotion and expression
Myerson's sign	Blink with >4 taps	Blink extinguished <4 taps
Handwriting	Tight, small, slow	Baseline
Orthostatic parameters	If Shy-Drager: decreased BP, no increase in HR	No decrease in BP or increase in HR
Pruning of skin when immersed in water	If Shy-Drager: no wrinkling/pruning	Normal pruning
Sweating	If Shy-Drager: minimal to none	Normal sweating

BP = blood pressure; HR = heart rate.

function, and no "skin pruning" when the hands are placed in warm water for several minutes. All of these are caused by concurrent systemic autonomic degeneration. **Dementia** with frontal release signs (Table 7.13) and cognitive impairment may also be present.

Parkinson's syndrome can be idiopathic or caused by medications (chronic neuroleptic use) in which the manifestations are bilateral; if caused by a CVA involving the basal ganglia, the manifestations are unilateral and ipsilateral to the damage.

Although in essential tremor the patient does not have a shuffling gait, **essential tremor** can often be confused with early Parkinson's disease **(Table 7.8)**. Essential tremor is different in that, although it occurs at rest, unlike Parkinson's, it affects the head and neck to a much greater extent. Often, a nodding yes-yes or no-no is present. In addition, essential tremor has an impact on the voice itself, with an oscillation of speech. Essential tremor has no other complications. Think of the late Katharine Hepburn as an example of a person with essential tremor.

Steppage Gait

Common peroneal nerve damage manifests with a **steppage–type** gait. This is normal-based, and quite steady but the patient needs to lift the foot by flexing at the knee, i.e., "step up," because of profound weakness to dorsiflexion of the foot at the ankle involved. The company it keeps includes weakness to ankle **dorsiflexion** at the tibiotalar joint, weakness to **great toe extension**, and weakness to foot **eversion**. It is important to know all three motor tests for the common peroneal nerve to uncover an early and, perhaps yet reversible, lesion **(Table 7.9)**. In severe, advanced cases, the baseline position of

TEACHING POINTS

STEPPAGE GAIT

1. Common peroneal nerve damage results in steppage gait.
2. Sciatica, especially if piriformis syndrome, can cause common peroneal nerve problem.
3. Anterior and lateral leg compartments are involved in the common peroneal nerve; therefore, weak ankle dorsiflexors (deep peroneal) and ankle evertors (superficial peroneal).
4. Often a baseline position of out-toeing and plantarflexion in severe, advanced common peroneal nerve damage.
5. Achilles and plantar reflexes intact in isolated common peroneal nerve damage, but are diminished if sciatic nerve related.
6. Always palpate the fibular head or radiograph the fibula/knee if any suspicion of fibular head or neck fracture.
7. Look for company in the ear, nose, and throat examination. Tongue: atrophic glossitis for vitamin B_{12} deficiency, Teeth-Burton's lines for lead intoxication.
8. Look for company in nail plates for the transverse white lines of lead or arsenic ingestion.
9. Sensory exam is pivotal: dorsal foot deficit, common peroneal; plantar foot deficit, tibial nerve; both, sciatic nerve problem.

the foot is plantar flexed and laterally rotated because of the **anterior** and **lateral** leg compartment muscle **atrophy** (see Chapter 13). Also, there is **decreased sensation** of the **dorsum** of foot. A normal Achilles reflex is elicited because it is supplied by a different nerve, the tibialis (S1). **Common peroneal nerve** damage that is bilateral can be caused by Charcot-Marie-Tooth syndrome, peripheral neuropathies from diabetes mellitus, vitamin B_{12} deficiency, excessive ethanol ingestion, heavy metal intoxication, lead intoxication, or thyroid disease. If unilateral, trauma or compression to the nerve at the neck of the fibula, fracture of the fibular neck, piriformis syndrome, or sciatica are potential causes. See **Table 7.10** for physical examination features.

Poker Gait

Ankylosing spondylosis or paraspinous spasm manifests with a classic straight as a **poker gait**, and a stiff, straight-back stance **(Table 7.11)**. **Ankylosing spondylitis** manifests with limited ROM of thoracic and lumbar spine, sacroiliac joint tenderness, a straight lumbar spine, FABER (F = forward flexion of the

Table 7.9. Motor Examination of the Common Peroneal Nerve

Examination	Compartment	Nerve
Dorsiflexion	Anterior	Deep peroneal
Great toe extension	Anterior	Deep peroneal
Eversion	Lateral	Superficial peroneal

Table 7.10. Causes of Common Peroneal Damage

Diagnosis	Unilateral/Bilateral	ENT examination	Sensory examination	Company it Keeps
Charcot-Marie-Tooth	Bilateral	Nonspecific	No deficits	Autosomal dominant syndrome Hands may also be involved
Lead intoxication	Bilateral	Burton's stippled lines on the tartar of teeth	Stocking-glove deficit	Mees' lines in nail plates Anemia with pale nail beds
Arsenic ingestion	Bilateral	Nonspecific	Stocking-glove deficit	Aldrich–Mees' lines in nail plates
Vitamin B_{12} deficiency	Bilateral	Atrophic glossitis	Stocking-glove deficit	Anemia with pale nail beds
Fibular fracture	Unilateral	Nonspecific	Dorsum of foot, deficit	Concurrent lateral ankle sprain
Piriformis (Sciatic nerve)	Unilateral	Nonspecific	Dorsum and/or plantar foot deficit	Sciatica May have multiple L5, S1 deficits All distal to knee
Hypothyroid	Bilateral	Goiter Alopecia Thickened skin Macroglossia	Stocking-glove deficit	Delayed relaxation phase in deep tendon reflexes

ENT = ear, nose, and throat.

Table 7.11. Poker Gait Manifestations

Physical examination	Ankylosing spondylitis	Paraspinous strain
Schober maneuver	<5 cm change with forward bend	Unable to forward bend
Site of tenderness	Sacroiliac joints	Paraspinal muscles, spasm
Lumbar spine with forward flexion	Straight at outset, straight with maximal forward bend	Lumbar lordosis at outset, minimal forward bend tolerated, no change in lordosis
Knee-to-chest	Sacroiliac tenderness	Paraspinal tenderness
FABER	Sacroiliac tenderness	Paraspinal tenderness
Nerve deficits	None	None, may have in rare cases, radicular-type pain
Chest expansion	Limited	Normal
Dermatologic	Erythema nodosum	Nonspecific
Cardiovascular	Diastolic murmur at base (AI)	Nonspecific
History	Age at onset: <40 years Insidious progression Present for >3 months Morning stiffness Activity improves Calin: >4/5 yes, AS	Acute onset after lifting Poor posture

AI = aortic insufficiency; AS = ankylosing spondylitis; FABER = F = forward flexion of the hip, AB = abduction of the hip, ER = external rotation of the hip.

TEACHING POINTS

POKER GAIT

1. A non–neurologic.based gait disturbance.
2. Spasm of paraspinal muscles or ankylosing spondylitis is the most common reason for poker gait.
3. Evaluate as with low back pain.
4. FABERE maneuver is an excellent first step in evaluation.

hip, AB = abduction of the hip, ER = external rotation of the hip) with tenderness at the sacroiliac joints, and a positive Schober's test (Fig. 12.13). Each of these examination sets are described in detail in Chapter 12. **Paraspinous strain** manifests with tenderness and spasm in the paraspinal muscles.

MENTAL STATUS EXAMINATION

The ability to perform a reproducible, brief, yet complete mental status examination (MSE) is fundamental to the physical examination. **Delirium** is an acute confusional state and mandates aggressive acute evaluation. **Dementia** is insidious in onset, progressive in nature, and has more chronic manifestations of confusion. Delirium and dementia, irrespective of their underlying cause, manifest with a decrease in the score on the mini-mental status examination and a loss of a sense of **location** (place), **being** (person), and **time**. Dementia can also manifest with Myerson's sign (Fig. 7.47), and the sucking, snout, and

Table 7.12. Tone, Reflexes, and Power for the Most Common Gaits

Type	Tone	Reflexes	Power	Etiology
Waddling	Decreased	Decreased	Decreased	Proximal muscle weakness
Spastic	Increased	Increased	Decreased	UMN CVA
Ataxic	Decreased Normal	Variable	Normal	MS Cerebellar dysfunction Sensory deficit
Steppage	Normal	Decreased,* locally	Decreased, locally	Common peroneal nerve damage
Shuffling	Increased, rigid	Normal	Normal	Parkinsonism
Poker	Normal	Normal	Normal	Ankylosing spondylosis

CVA = cerebral vascular accident; MS = multiple sclerosis; UMN = upper motor neuron.
*There is no specific reflex for common peroneal nerve.

TEACHING POINTS

MENTAL STATUS EXAMINATION

1. Delirium is an acute change in the mental status examination (MSE) that mandates acute evaluation and management.
2. Dementia is chronic changes in MSE.
3. Physical examination for both delirium and dementia must include orientation to person, place, time (alert and oriented times 3), and, most importantly, a standardized MSE.
4. Dementia examination also includes gait assessment.
5. Assessment for Parkinson's or vitamin B_{12} deficiency (atrophic glossitis) and examination for the frontal release signs of snout, sucking, grasp, and retention of glabellar (Myerson's reflex).

grasp reflexes **(Table 7.13)**. All of these abnormal reflexes are markers for significant diffuse frontal lobe damage, but each finding is present only in a few patients with dementia and, thus, is of limited value. Because Parkinson's disease and vitamin B_{12} deficiency are two of the treatable causes of dementia, the examination must also include assessment for these, e.g., gait assessment, tongue inspection for atrophic glossitis.

SENSORY EXAMINATION

Sensory examination is an interesting component to the neurologic examination in that it is inherently **subjective**, i.e., the patient reports the outcome. In most cases, this is either to confirm a **peripheral neuropathy**, e.g., carpal tunnel syndrome or stocking-glove neuropathy, or to serve to define the patient's primary problem **(Table 7.14)**. For deficits of **fine touch**, we recommend the use of a camel-hair brush or a monofilament as tools. These measure the peripheral nerves and the anterior spinothalamic tracts. The monofilaments are of tremendous benefit diagnostically and, thus, this is the method of choice.

Table 7.13. Frontal Release Signs

Sign	Procedure	Finding	Sensitivity (%)
Sucking	With finger, stroke upper lip from philtrum to side	Sucking movement of lips	5
Snout	Tap philtrum with fingertip several times	Puckering or pursing of lips	25
Grasp	Patient's hand is extended palmar side up Place digits 2 and 3 transversely on the palm of the patient's hand	Slow involuntary flexion of the fingers	

TEACHING POINTS

SENSORY EXAMINATION

1. Vibratory examination: highly myelinated dorsal columns of spinal cord; 256-Hz tuning fork.
2. Superficial pain: lateral spinothalamic tracts; broken tip of swab.
3. Fine touch: anterior spinothalamic tracts; cotton-tipped swab or monofilament.

Please refer to extensive description on page 187 and in Fig. 7.44 for monofilament use. For deficits of **superficial pain**, we recommend the use of the broken end of a cotton-tipped swab as a tool in performing this technique. This measures the function of the peripheral nerves and the lateral spinothalamic tracts. For deficits in **vibration**, we recommend the use of a 256–Hz tuning fork (Fig. 7.45). This measures the function of the peripheral nerves and the **dorsal columns** of **the spinal cord. Parietal lobe damage** to be damage manifests with diminished stereognosis and diminished graphesthesia. *Stereognosis* is assessed by placing a common object in palm of hand, e.g., a key; the patient should be able to state what it is without looking at it. Likewise, *graphesthesia* is assessed by "drawing," with a cotton–tip applicator, a number on palm, e.g., "8."

INVOLUNTARY MOVEMENTS (Table 7.15)

Tics manifest with brief, repetitive, irregular stereotyped movements, i.e., normal muscle actions occurring at inappropriate times. Examples include

Table 7.14. Sites for the Sensory Examination

Nerve root	Skin surface over
C2	Upper half auricle
C4	AC joint
C5	Deltoid
C6	Thenar eminence
C7	Palmar third digit
C8	Palmar fifth digit—hypothenar side
T1	Medial epicondyle
T4	Nipples
T7	Xiphoid process
T10	Umbilicus
T12	Inguinal ligament
L1	Inguinal ligament
L2	Proximal anterior thigh
L3	Medial patella
L4	Medial malleolus
L5	Dorsal foot
S1	Plantar foot
S2	Popliteal fossa
S3, 4, 5	Perineum

AC = acromioclavicular joint.

Table 7.15. Tremor and Other Involuntary Movements

Movement	Rhythm	Amplitude	Company it Keeps	Diagnoses
Physiologic tremor	Regular fast	Very low	Accentuated with anxiety Distal, e.g., hands	Normal anxiety
Intention tremor	Irregular	High	Cerebellar dysfunction	Cerebellar
Essential tremor	Regular fast	Moderate	Gravelly voice Head and neck	Basal ganglia
Pill-rolling tremor	Regular fast	Moderate	Parkinson's hands and feet	Parkinsonism Neuroleptic use
Asterixis	Irregular	High	Inability to maintain a specific position Encephalopathy	ESLD CO poisoning
Tic	Irregular repetitive	Nonspecific	Purposeful action, abnormal spontaneous time, e.g., wink, shrug	Normal-variant
Myoclonus	Nonrepetitive Rapid Not predictable	Nonspecific	Involves the limbs, e.g., a kick	
Chorea	Brief, nonrepetitive	Nonspecific	Purposeless action, e.g., flinging of arm Upper extremity	Huntington's chorea St. Vitus' dance (rheumatic fever)
Athetosis	Slow, writhing	Nonspecific	Alternates between two poles: e.g., flexion/extension; supination/pronation	Cerebral palsy
Hemiballism	Nonrepetitive Irregular	High violent flailing	Purposeless unilateral; always involves shoulder	CVA of basal ganglia
Dyskinesis	Repetitive Bizarre	Nonspecific	Bizarre Tongue, jaw Mouth	Neuroleptic side effect

ESLD = end–stage liver disease; CVA = cerebral vascular accident; CO = carbon monoxide.

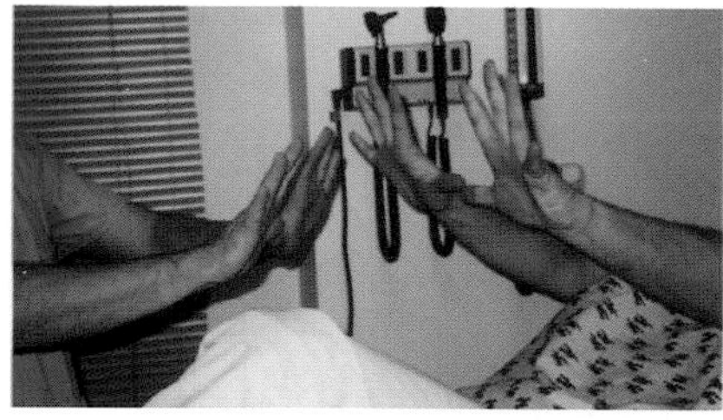

Figure 7.48.

Method to detect asterixis. Note that the patient is instructed to maximally dorsiflex hands with fingers spread apart and maintain that position for 60 seconds.

TIPS

- Patient holds hands dorsiflexed with fingers spread out for 60 seconds or foot dorsiflexion
- Maintains the position of dorsiflexion
- Asterixis: irregular flapping of both hands because of inability to maintain the position

winking or shoulder shrugging. **Chorea** manifests with brief, nonrepetitive, purposeless movements, most prominent in the upper extremities; chorea is associated with rheumatic fever (St. Vitus' dance), cerebral palsy, or the progressive hereditary syndrome of Huntington's chorea. **Hemiballism** manifests with flailing, almost violent, purposeless movements, most often involving the shoulder. Because hemiballism is unilateral, it is usually caused by a stroke involving the ipsilateral basal ganglia. **Athetosis** manifests with slow, writhing-type, purposeless movements. These movements alternate between two extremes: flexion or extension, adduction or abduction; most often in the face and upper extremities. These movements are most commonly caused by cerebral palsy. **Dyskinesis** manifests with repetitive bizarre movements of the tongue, jaw, and mouth, e.g., lip-smacking. This is most commonly caused by the medication side effects of neuroleptics. **Myoclonus** manifests with nonrepetitive, rapid, nonpredictable movements, usually of the limbs, e.g., a kick. **Asterixis** manifests with flapping, irregular movements when the patient attempts to maintain a specific position of wrist dorsiflexion or ankle dorsiflexion **(Fig. 7.48)**. The technique we recommend to assess for asterixis is to hold the hand dorsiflexed with fingers spread apart for 60 seconds. Normally, the position can be maintained. **Encephalopathy** manifests with irregular flapping of the hands; this occurs because the patient cannot maintain the position. Of interest, is that the technique can also be performed with the patient's feet dorsiflexed at ankles. Asterixis is caused by encephalopathy, most often end-stage liver disease. **Tremor** manifests with a rhythmic repetitive movement. Different tremor types have different manifestations. **Physiologic** tremor is low amplitude, usually in the distal extremities and brought on by maintaining a position, e.g., holding out hands. Often is caused by anxiety or excess catecholamines. **Parkinsonian tremor** is low to moderate amplitude, usually present at rest, and has an oscillatory component. The company it keeps are those of Parkinson's disease. **Essential tremor** is moderate amplitude, often involving the neck, with a characteristic mild yes-yes or no-no action, but no concurrent parkinsonian features. Finally, **cerebellar tremor** is high amplitude and is accentuated by voluntary goal-oriented actions, e.g., turning off the light switch; hence the term, "intentional tremor."

Annotated Bibliography

Overall

AIDS to the Examination of the peripheral nervous system, 4th ed. WB Saunders, Edinburgh, 2000.
The masterful work on peripheral nerve examination.

Cohen SN. The neurologic examination. Part 1: Practical points. *Hosp Med* 1987;(Sept): 21–40.
Basic review of the examination of the 12 cranial nerves; satisfactory discussion and illustrations. We do not test the gag reflex as a basic part of the cranial nerve examination.

Cohen SN. The neurologic examination. Part 2: Practical points. *Hosp Med* 1987;(Oct): 27–42.
Very basic review of the motor, sensory, and cerebellar examination. A potpourri of tests and findings; we do not use a safety pin or any pin or needle to assess for pain. The illustrations for the snout and glabellar tests are adequate.

Dawson DM. Entrapment neuropathies clinical overview. *Hosp Pract* 1995:37–44.
Summary of evaluation, including some aspects of physical examination and some features of management of several peripheral neuropathies: carpal tunnel syndrome, ulnar neuropathy, thoracic outlet syndrome, and anterior and posterior interosseous syndromes.

Dodelson R. Checkup and Chovostek. *N Engl J Med* 1963;268:199.
Brief, but useful, paper that restates the procedure and outcomes of this test for tetany and its underlying hypocalcemia.

Hall GW. Neurologic signs and their discovers. *JAMA* 1930;95(10):703–707.
Delightful set of vignettes about the individuals who described some of the neurologic signs, including Argyll Robertson, Romberg, Brudzinski, Babinski, Kernig, Oppenheim, and Horner.

Horner JF. Ueber eine form von ptosis, Klin Monatsbl. F. Augenh. 1869;7:193–198.
The original description of Horner's syndrome and sign.

Medical Research Council (Great Britain). Aids to the examination of the peripheral nervous system. *Memorandum no. 45,* 1st ed. London: Her Majesty's Stationery Office, 1976.
The one best reference for peripheral nervous system examination; required reading for any primary care physician; any teacher should obtain a copy for reference. A document of great importance to the teacher.

Nolan MF, Brownlee HJ. Neurologic examination: a strategy to enhance the diagnostic yield. *Consultant* 1996;(Feb):323–329.
Fundamental aspects to the neurologic physical examination are described in this paper; descriptively good; the specifics on the examination techniques are relatively sparse in the paper.

Robertson DA. Pupillary reflex. *Edinburgh Medical Journal* 1868;14:696.
The original description of this finding in tertiary syphilis.

Trousseau A. *Clinique medicale de l'hotel dieu de Paris,* Vol. 2. Paris: JB Balliere, 1861.
The classic article that describes this procedure; used thumb compression of the brachial artery, as the sphygmotonometer would not be invented for another 30 years.

Mental Status Examination

Attia J, Hatala R, Cook DJ, Wong JG. Does this adult patient have acute meningitis? *JAMA* 1999;282:175–181.
A metaanalysis of studies in the French and English literature; 10 studies involving 824 patients were included in the "study." The three findings of fever, neck stiffness, and altered mental status had sensitivities of 85%, 70%, and 67%, respectively. The presence of all three had a sensitivity of almost 100%. The studies included were relatively heterogeneous and of modest quality at best.

Brudzinski J. Berlin klin Wehnschr. 1916;53:686.
The original description of this sign to diagnose meningitis; sensitivity of 97%; found a sensitivity of 57% for Kernig's sign.

Folstein MF. "Mini-mental status." A practical method for grading the cognitive state of patients for the clinician. *J Psych Res* 1975;12:189–198.
A grand paper in which an instrument to quantitatively assess the mental status of a patient is described. This tool is used by primary care physicians at least once daily, if not hourly.

Kernig W. St. Petersb med. Wchnschr. 1882;7:398.
The original description of this sign to diagnose meningitis; sensitivity of 84%.

Molloy AK. Primitive reflexes in Alzheimer's disease. *J Am Geriatr Soc* 1991;39:1160.
Performed specific physical examination tests on 136 patients with Alzheimer's disease. Sensitivities include 28% palmomental reflex; 25% snout reflex; 17% grasp reflex; and 5% sucking reflex.

Thomas RJ. Blinking and release signs: are they clinically useful? *J Am Geriatr Soc* 1994;42: 609–613.
Describes the procedures for Myerson's sign and the reflexes for snout, grasp, sucking, and palmomental—all of some use in the assessment of severe dementia.

Walker MC, O'Brien MD. Neurological examination of the unconscious patient. *JR Soc Med* 1999;92:353–355.
Succinct, well-written review of some of the physical examination markers useful in the evaluation of a patient who is comatose. Included in this bibliography as a reference for further reading on this topic.

Power

Csuka M, McCarty DJ. Simple method for measurement of lower extremity muscle strength. *Am J Med* 1985;78:77–81.
Wonderful report of a test that is elegant in its simplicity; it is an excellent, functional method to assess proximal muscle strength, but instructs the patient to stand without using arms of a chair. Useful for diagnosis and for follow-up; a method to assess power objectively.

Wallace GB, Newton RW. Gowers' sign revisited. *Arch Dis Child* 1989;64:1317–1319.
Nice description of Gowers' sign. From a recumbent position, first procedure is for patient to roll over prone, then pull legs under the trunk, and, finally, walk the hands up the legs, in order to stand up.

Reflexes

Boyle RS: Inverted knee jerk: A neglected localising sign in spinal cord disease. *J Neurol Neurosurg Psychiatry* 42:1005–1007, 1979.
Describes what is Boyle's sign: paradoxic flexion of knee with patellar tap.

Jendrassik E. Beitrage zur Lehre von den Shnen-reflexen. *Deutsch Arch Klin Med* 1883;33: 177–199.
The original description of this procedure to accentuate normal reflexes.

Lanska DJ, Lanska MJ. John Madison Taylor (1855–1931) and the first reflex hammer. *J Child Neurol* 1990;5:38–39.
Although the Taylor hammer is not our favorite reflex hammer, this is an excellent history paper regarding a truly innovative and inventive physician who clearly deserves the accolades received in this paper.

Wartenberg R. *The Examination of Reflexes.* Chicago: Yearbook Medical Publishers, 1945.
Excellent discussion of the DTR.

Cranial nerves

Adour KK, Byl FM, Hilsinger RL, et al. The true nature of Bell's palsy: analysis of 1000 consecutive patients. *Laryngoscope* 1978;88:787–801.
Excellent review of the manifestations of Bell's palsy: facial palsy, multiple lower cranial nerve problems, facial pain (60%), dysguesia (57%), and hyperacusis (30%).

Bell C. On nerves, giving an account of some experiments on their structure and functions, which led to a new arrangement of the system. *Philos Trans R Soc London B Biol Sci* 1821;111: 398–424.
The original description of this peripheral cranial neuropathy.

Brazis PW. Palsies of the trochlear nerve: diagnosis and localization—recent concepts. *Mayo Clin Proc* 1993;68:501–509.
Extremely complete, erudite, and dense discussion of the pathoanatomy, history, and physical diagnosis of the trochlear nerve.

Hanson MR. Clinical evaluation of cranial nerves VIII through XII. *Hosp Med* 1996;(Jan): 32–35.
Overview of the physical examination of the lower cranial nerves, VIII–XII; descriptions of the techniques are well illustrated but simplistically described. Includes cranial nerve VIII: watch ticking, the use of a 256-Hz tuning fork for assessment; cranial nerves IX and X: assessment of uvula with "phonation," and the gag reflex; cranial nerve XI: sternocleidomastoid and the trapezius, as manifested by winging of scapula; and cranial nerve XII: tongue protrusion.

Hayden GF. Olfactory diagnosis in medicine. *Postgrad Med* 1980 67(4):110–118.
The clinical utility of smell in the diagnosis of disease, including odors on the breath, in the urine, specific to the skin, and in the sputa, vomitus, vaginal discharge, and stool.

James DG. All that palsies is not Bell's. *JR Soc Med* 1996;89:184–187.
An erudite discussion of rare or unusual causes of peripheral cranial nerve palsies. Of tremendous importance in that it provides a set of entities that can be diagnosed and even treated, thus, there are specific causes for a peripheral cranial nerve VII.

Ohye RG, Altenberger EA. Bell's palsy. *Am Fam Phys* 1989:40(2):159–165.
Nice review of this not uncommon peripheral cranial neuropathy; based on a specific case, reviews the symptoms and signs of this disorder. A terse description of management techniques is also included.

Pope C. The diagnostic art of smelling. *Am J Med* 1928;34:651–653.
Great overall paper using the sense of smell in diagnosis.

Gait Overall

Kurent JE, Sudarsky L. Gait disorder in the elderly. *Consultant* 1995;(June):783–788.
Highly satisfactory discussion of gaits and disturbances of gait in the geriatric population; nonspecific, but interesting information.

Gait-steppage

Charcot JM, Marie P. Peroneal muscle atrophy. *Rev Med* 1886;6:97.
The first description of this specific peripheral neuropathy that impacts on the common peroneal nerve.

Pickett JB. Localizing peroneal nerve lesions. *Am Fam Phys* 1985;31(2):189–196.
Excellent review of the clinical anatomy of the sciatic and the common peroneal nerve; reviews that superficial peroneal nerve is sensory to the dorsum of foot; the deep peroneal nerve is the web space between the digits 1 and 2 on the dorsum of the foot. Excellent anatomic basis for statements.

Tooth HH. The peroneal type of progressive muscular atrophy. Thesis for doctorate of medicine in the University of Cambridge, 1886.
The first description of this specific peripheral neuropathy that impacts on the common peroneal nerve.

Gait-ataxic

Dix MR, Hallpike CS. The pathology, symptomatology, and diagnosis of certain common disorders of the vestibular system. *Proc R Soc Med* 1952;45:341–354.
A paper describing this stress test for vertigo.

Holmes G. Clinical symptoms of cerebellar disease. Lecture III. *Lancet* 1922;(Jul 28):59–65.
Original lecture series on cerebellar physical diagnosis; describes diadochokinesis and adiadochokinesis as, "frequently unable to perform rapidly alternating movements;" hypotonia; dysmetria; asynergia as, "dissociation in time and force of muscle contraction;" also describes the gait and stance of a patient with cerebellar disease as, "reels in all directs like a drunken man;" the speech, "slow, drawling, and monotonous character of the voice, the unnatural separation of the syllables and the slurred, jerk and often explosive manner in which they are uttered;" and nystagmus. The best of the four lecture series.

Gait-spastic

Babinski J. Sur le reflexe cutane plantaire danse certaines affections organiques du systeme nerveaux central. *Comptes Rendus des Seances de la Societe de Bioloie* 1896;3:207.
First description of extension on the metatarsus in a patient with paralysis; very preliminary.

Babinski J. Du phenomene des orteils et de sa valeur semiologique. *La Semaine Med* 1898; 18:321–322.
A lecture in which Babinski refined and further delineated the manifestations of the test itself, including specifics on techniques and the abnormal extension of the great toe.

Babinski J. De l'abduction des orteils (signe de l'eventail). *Rev Neurol* 1903;11:1205–1206.
Babinski added the outcome of toe flaring to the abnormal extension.

Grant R. The neurological assault on the great toe (1893–1911). *Scott Med J* 1987;32:57–59.
Fascinating read describing the history behind the methods of Babinski, Oppenheim, Chaddock, Stransky, and others to place a noxious stimulus on the foot to observe the response of the great toe.

Oppenheim H. Monatschr. F. Psychiat. U. Neurol. 1902;12:421.
The original description of this derivative of Babinski's sign.

Wartenberg R. The Babinski reflex after fifty years. *JAMA* 1946;135(12):763–767.
Overall description of the Babinski reflex and its utility over the course of five decades.

Gait Parkinsonian

Ahlskog JE. Diagnostic steps for suspected Parkinson's disease.
A review of the physical examination to diagnose Parkinson's disease; specifics on therapy also included.

Calne DB. Diagnosis and treatment of Parkinson's disease. *Hosp Pract* 1995;(Jan):83–87.
A review of the features to diagnose Parkinson's disease; some aspects on therapy are also described. Includes description of supranuclear palsy and Shy-Drager syndrome.

Hallett M. Classification and treatment of tremor. *JAMA* 1991;266(8):1115–1117.
An approach to the evaluation of tremor, including tremor at rest, postural tremor, kinetic tremor, and other tremors.

Sandroni P, Young RR. Tremor: classification, diagnosis and management. *Am Fam Phys* 1994;50(7):1505–1512.
Nice, clinically based classification of tremors, with emphasis on tremors at rest, postural tremor, and intention tremor. Excellent differential diagnosis of each type and discussion of entities that can be tremor-like, e.g., the nonrhythmic tremor-like entity, asterixis.

Thomas RJ: Blinking and release reflexes: Are they clinically useful? *J Am Ger Soc* 1994;42: 609–613.
Study looking at the sensitivity of many of the classic findings of dementia.

Gait Waddling

Buzzard EF. The clinical history and post-mortem examination of five cases of myasthenia gravis. *Brain* 1905;28:438–483.
A classic and extensive discussion of the manifestations and descriptive features of this disorder.

Drachman DB. Myasthenia gravis. *N Engl J Med* 330(25):1797–1800.
Excellent paper that reviews the pathophysiology and the clinical features of myasthenia gravis, the features of which include diplopia and swallowing dysfunction.

Kinnier-Wilson SA, Bruce AN, eds. *Neurology,* 2nd ed. London: Butterworth and Co., 1955: 726–1731.
Nice review, including such manifestations as hanging jaw; repetitive tests of EOM (extraocular movements) looking for ptosis by repetitive movement.

Schneiderman H. Trident tongue of myasthenia gravis. *Consultant* 1994;34:367–368.
Case-based report with images describing this rare finding in myasthenia gravis. Fascinating discussion—clearly a related symptom. Reviews the findings and emphasizes the import of repetitive testing to unmask a nascent paresis. Counting to 40 to unmask a nasal phonation (akin to nasal regurgitation), ROM of eyes to axis, and ptosis testing.

Sensory

Lehman LB. An approach to the evaluation and management of lesions of the peripheral nervous system. *Resident and Staff Physician* 5–14.
Good overall review of these common problems, including carpal tunnel, cubital tunnel, tarsal tunnel, Guyon's tunnel, meralgia paresthetica; discusses Tinel's sign and other physical examination maneuvers to define disease.

8

Knee Examination

PRACTICE AND TEACHING

SURFACE ANATOMY

Anterior

The **quadriceps muscle** and the patella are the major structures of the anterior knee **(Fig. 8.1)**. The quadriceps inserts on the anterior tibial tuberosity and acts in knee extension; its nerve is the femoral. The **patella** is located in the tendon of the quadriceps. The *quadriceps tendon* extends from the muscle to the inferior pole of the patella, whereas the *patellar ligament* extends from the inferior pole of the patella to the anterior tibial tuberosity. The patella serves as a pulley in the groove between the two femoral condyles. It is stabilized medially by the vastus obliquus medialis and laterally by the lateral patellar facet or lateral femoral condyle. Although the inferior pole of the patella crosses over the joint, the patella is mainly over the femur. The posterior patella sustains high compression loads and bears significant stress, especially when the patient walks down stairs. The largest of the four heads of the quadriceps is the **vastus obliquus medialis** (VOM). Problems can occur when there is quadriceps atrophy, which results in a relatively greater loss of both VOM function and thus a loss of the

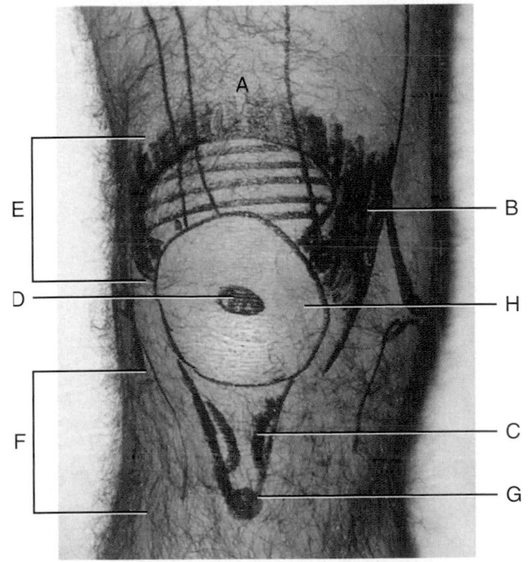

Figure 8.1.

Anterior knee surface anatomy. **A.** Quadriceps muscle components: vastus obliquus medialis (VOM) very large component. **B.** Suprapatellar bursa: deep to quadriceps tendon. **C.** Infrapatellar bursa: adjacent to patellar ligament. **D.** Prepatellar bursa: on point of patella. **E.** Quadriceps tendon: proximal to, and including, patella. **F.** Patellar ligament: distal to patella. **G.** Anterior tibial tuberosity. **H.** Patella.

TIPS

- Quadriceps muscle: VOM is a large component
- Suprapatellar bursa: deep to quadriceps tendon, above the patella
- Infrapatellar bursa: adjacent to patellar ligament, below the patella
- Prepatellar bursa: on point of the patella
- Quadriceps tendon: proximal to, and including, the patella
- Patellar ligament: distal to the patella
- Anterior tibial tuberosity
- Patella overlies the femur

TEACHING POINTS

SURFACE ANATOMY

1. The patella is proximal to the joint itself.
2. The patella normally moves medial with knee extension and lateral with knee flexion relative to the underlying femur. Note how your own patella moves with knee extension and flexion (it migrates medially with full extension); thus, no need to memorize.
3. The medial cruciate ligament (MCL) and medial meniscal (MM) are intimately related and intercalated; therefore, a significant tear of one often will result in a concurrent tear of the other.
4. The lateral collateral ligament (LCL) and the lower meniscal (LM) are distinct entities; therefore, each can tear individually.
5. The anterior cruciate ligament (ACL) is a foundation of the internal knee.
6. The ACL runs in close proximity to MM and MCL; if a severe sprain in one, the other two are often involved.
7. Several bursae in anterior knee: suprapatellar, prepatellar, and infrapatellar, any one of which can become irritated and cause mischief.
8. Quadriceps tendon is, by definition, from the muscle edge to inferior pole of patella; patellar ligament is, by definition, from inferior pole of patella to anterior tibial tuberosity.
9. Popliteal fossa is defined by hamstrings on the medial superior side, biceps femoris on the lateral superior side, and heads of gastrocnemius on inferior side.
10. Popliteal fossa contains several unnamed bursae, the tibialis nerve, and the popliteal artery.
11. Severe ACL tears and definitely any ACL and posterior cruciate ligament (PCL) tear (knee dislocation) can damage structures of the popliteal fossa, i.e., the popliteal artery and tibialis nerve.
12. Damage to the fibular head or neck can result in damage to the common peroneal nerve; this nerve runs adjacent to the fibular neck.
13. The MCL attaches the femoral condyle to the tibial condyle; it prevents inappropriate valgus (abduction) at knee.
14. The semimembranosus muscle (the medial knee flexor) is the larger of the two hamstrings and crosses two joints; the hip and the knee.
15. The most effective method to find the pes anserine bursa is to palpate the semitendinosus muscles and trace the muscle and its tendon distally to the site where it inserts on the medial tibia.
16. The LCL attaches the femoral condyle with the head of the fibula; it prevents inappropriate varus (adduction) at the knee.
17. The menisci move posteriorly with flexion of the knee and anteriorly with extension of the knee.

normal medial movement of the patella with extension. Thus, quadriceps atrophy is a root cause of patellofemoral syndrome. Finally, three bursae are located in the anterior knee: the suprapatellar bursa deep to the quadriceps tendon, the prepatellar bursa at tip of patella, and the infrapatellar bursa adjacent to the patellar ligament.

Posterior

The knee flexors comprise the major component of the posterior knee. These include, on the medial side, the two hamstrings, the semimembranosus and semitendinosus muscles; and, on the lateral side, the two heads of the **biceps femoris muscle**. The **semimembranosus muscle**, which acts in knee flexion and hip backward flexion, originates at the ilium and inserts on the medial tibia; the nerve is the sciatic. The muscle is remembered by being "M"(membranosus, medial, muscular); it crosses two joints, the hip and the knee. The **semitendinosus muscle**, which originates on the proximal femur, acts in knee flexion. It inserts on pes anserine; the nerve is sciatic. The semimembranosus is shorter, tendinosus, and immediately lateral to the semimembranosus muscle. The **pes anserine** (German = goose foot) is the confluence of the sartorius, gracilis, and semitendinosus tendons as they merge to insert on the medial proximal tibia. Recall, the sartorius muscle is the lateral border of the femoral triangle. The **pes anserine bursa** is located immediately deep to this confluence.

The two heads of **biceps femoris**, which originate on the proximal femur and insert on the lateral proximal tibia, act in knee flexion; the nerve is sciatic. They are located in the lateral knee and posterior thigh. These muscles are often overlooked as sites of mischief and are infrequently discussed in physical diagnosis curricula. The **popliteal fossa** is formed by the semimembranosus muscle and biceps femoris superiorly and the gastrocnemius muscle on the medial and lateral posterior tibia. Components of the popliteal fossa include the tibial nerve, the popliteal artery and its branches, and the posterior tibial and dorsalis pedis arteries.

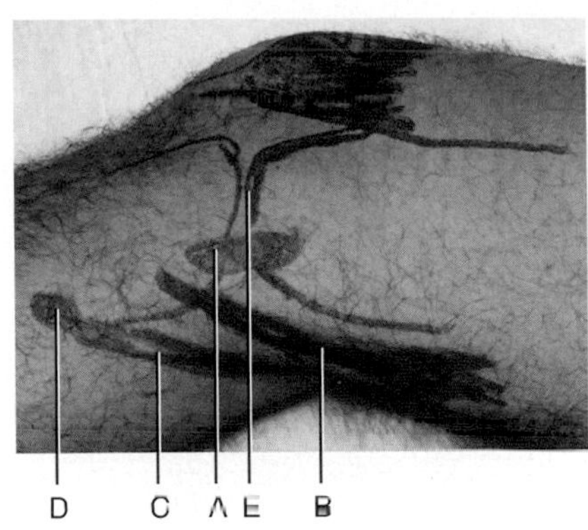

Figure 8.2.

Medial surface anatomy, knee extended. **A.** Medial collateral ligament. **B.** Semimembranosus muscle. **C.** Semitendinosus muscle. **D.** Pes anserine. **E.** Medial meniscus muscle.

TIPS

- Medial collateral ligament: midposterior joint line between the tibia and the femur
- Semimembranosus muscle: inserts on tibia barely across the joint line
- Semitendinosus muscle: inserts with gracilis and sartorius at pes anserine, 5 to 6 cm distal to the joint line on tibia
- Medial meniscus is anterior to the MCL when knee extended

Medial and Lateral

The **menisci** are smooth discs of cartilage found between the femur and the tibia; **medial** in the medial knee compartment; **lateral** in the lateral knee compartment. The menisci are posterior with the knee flexed and anterior in the joint line with the knee extended. They provide support for the smooth glide of the tibiofemoral joint itself. The **collateral ligaments** provide some internal stability to the knee. The **medial collateral ligament** (MCL) is a broad band that extends from the femoral condyle to the tibial condyle on the medial knee; it prevents inappropriate valgus displacement at the knee **(Fig. 8.2)**. The MCL has a superficial layer and a deep layer that merges with the posterior knee joint capsule; its fibers are intimately intercalated with the underlying medial meniscus. The MCL is in the midposterior joint line.

The **lateral collateral ligament** (LCL) is a narrow band of tissue that extends from the lateral condyle of femur to fibular head; it functions to prevent inappropriate varus at the knee **(Fig. 8.3)**. The LCL is in the midposterior joint line. It is independent of the lateral meniscus. The *iliotibial band (ITB)* is a direct

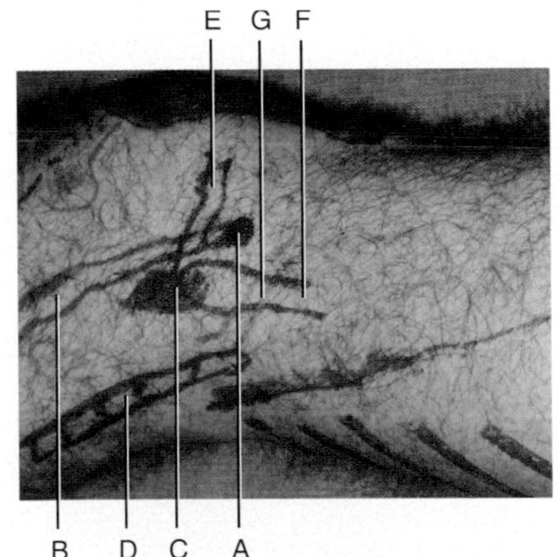

Figure 8.3.

Lateral surface anatomy, knee extended. **A.** Gerdy's tubercle. **B.** Iliotibial band. **C.** Lateral collateral ligament. **D.** Biceps femoris muscle. **E.** Lateral meniscus muscle. **F.** Fibula. **G.** Common peroneal nerve.

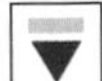

TIPS

- Iliotibial band: direct extension of gluteus maximus from lateral thigh. Its insertion site is Gerdy's tubercle on the lateral tibia. It is anterior to both the LCL and fibula.
- Lateral collateral ligament: fibula to femur
- Biceps femoris muscle: inserts on the proximal lateral posterior fibula
- Lateral meniscus muscle is in joint line, anterior to LCL when knee is extended
- Common peroneal nerve wraps around the neck of the fibula; innervates anterior and lateral compartments of the leg

extension of the gluteus maximus muscle onto the lateral thigh. The insertion site of the ITB is Gerdy's tubercle on the lateral tibia. This tubercle is anterior to both the LCL and the fibula. The LCL, which extends from the fibula to the femur, prevents excessive or inappropriate knee varus. The biceps femoris muscle, discussed above, inserts on the fibula. The lateral meniscus muscle, found in the joint line, is anterior to the LCL when the knee is extended. The common peroneal nerve wraps around the neck of the fibula and innervates the anterior and lateral compartments of the leg and foot.

The **cruciate ligaments,** a foundation of the knee, cross over, i.e., cruciate. The **anterior cruciate ligament** (ACL) inserts on the anterior aspect of tibia and is closely applied to the medial meniscus and MCL to prevent inappropriate rotation and to prevent inappropriate anterior subluxation of the tibia on the femur. The **posterior cruciate ligament** (PCL) prevents inappropriate posterior subluxation of the tibia on femur and, thus, prevents knee hyperextension.

KNEE RANGE OF MOTION

Passive

Passive range of motion (ROM) of the knee includes **flexion** to 140 degrees and **extension** to –5 degrees, **varus** (adduction) of 0, and **valgus** (abduction) of 3 to 5 degrees **(Table 8.1)**. To effectively assess varus and valgus, the lower

TEACHING POINTS

RANGE OF MOTION (ROM)

1. Perform ROM, passive and then active, on both knees.
2. Internal and external rotation, although rarely performed, is best assessed when the knee is in 90 degrees of flexion.
3. Varus and valgus motion: best assessed when the knee is in full extension.
4. Minimal internal and external rotation is normal; if greater than minimal, consistent with intrinsic knee complications.
5. Slight (2–5 degrees) valgus at the knee is normal.
6. Flexion and extension, valgus and varus, internal and external rotation all measure function of the tibiofemoral joint.
7. Significant valgus or varus motion of one knee at baseline indicates damage to one of the collateral ligaments: acute MCL sprain or tear: valgus deformity; acute LCL sprain or tear: varus deformity.
8. Genu recurvatum at baseline increases the risk for a cruciate ligament sprain.
9. Genu valgus = abduction = knock-kneed.
10. Genu varus = adduction = bow-legged.

Table 8.1. Passive Range of Motion (ROM) of Knee

Motion	Patient position	Normal
Knee flexion	Patient supine	140 degrees
Knee extension	Patient supine or sitting	0–5 degrees
Valgus	Knee extended	<5 degrees
Varus	Knee extended	None
Internal rotation	Knee flexed to 90 degrees	<5 degrees
External rotation	Knee flexed to 90 degrees	<5 degrees

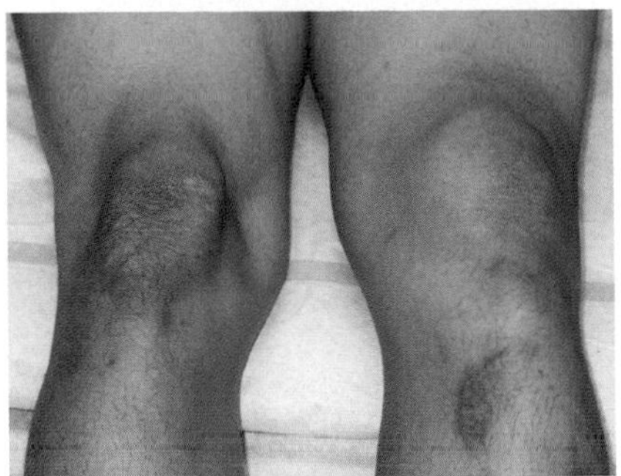

Figure 8.4.

Knee effusion. Note the bulge of fluid present. Effusion is modest to large in size.

 **TIPS**

- Knee fully extended, leg parallel to the floor
- Note the sites to the inferior sides of the patella
- Normal: concave (dimples) on inferior side of patella
- Effusion: flat or convex (bulging) on inferior sides of the patella

extremity should be in full extension. Furthermore, although not routinely performed, passive **internal** and **external rotation** of the knee is normally <2 degrees. To assess rotation effectively, the knee should be in 90 degrees of flexion.

Active

The two components of active ROM are flexion and extension. Active **flexion**, which is to 140 degrees, is performed by the **four flexors**: semimembranosus and semitendinosus muscles, and the biceps femoris. All knee flexors are innervated by the sciatic nerve. Active **extension** is to –5 degrees by the four extensors (i.e., the four heads of the **quadriceps** muscle) **(Table 8.2)**. All extensors are innervated by the femoral nerve.

KNEE SWELLING

An effusion, that is, an intraarticular fluid collection, manifests with an increase or decrease in the **passive ROM** at the joint **(Figs. 8.4** and **8.5)**. On inspection, the normal concavity or dimpling of the inferior sides of the patella is replaced with a **bulging** of fluid or flattening of the dimple on the distal, deep medial or lateral aspect of the patella. The patella is **ballotable** or a **bulge sign** is seen medial, lateral, or on both sides. To perform ballottement have the patient's knee extended, place the web of the hand over the distal quadriceps and place a gentle force on the patella. Feel for fluid and look for a bulge **(Fig. 8.6)**. In addition, a bulge or flattening of the concave area behind and adjacent to the patella develops on the other side of the area deep to the patella on **fluid displacement**. In this procedure, fluid is "milked" by applying pressure with the thumbs or index fingers to make the skin over the joint line

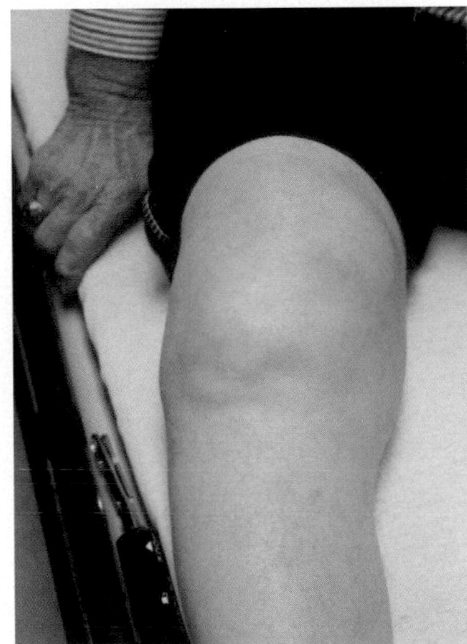

Figure 8.5.

Massive knee effusion. This patient has severe neuropathy and very advanced degenerative joint disease.

 **TIPS**

- Inspect knee for effusion
- Effusion: large bulge deep to the patella bilaterally

Table 8.2. Active Range of Motion (ROM) of Knee

Action	Muscles	Nerves
Active flexion	Biceps femoris Semimembranosus Semitendinosus	Sciatic (S1, L5)
Active extension	Quadriceps	Femoral (L4)

Figure 8.6.

Technique for ballottement of the patella. **A.** View from top. **B.** View from side.

TIPS

- Note the knee is extended, leg parallel to floor
- Place web of hand between thumb and index finger on the suprapatellar area
- Perform ballottement on the patella: place discrete mild downward push on the patella with index finger or thumb
- Inspect sides for bulge
- Effusion: ballottement can be performed and a bulge is seen on both sides of the inferior aspect of patella

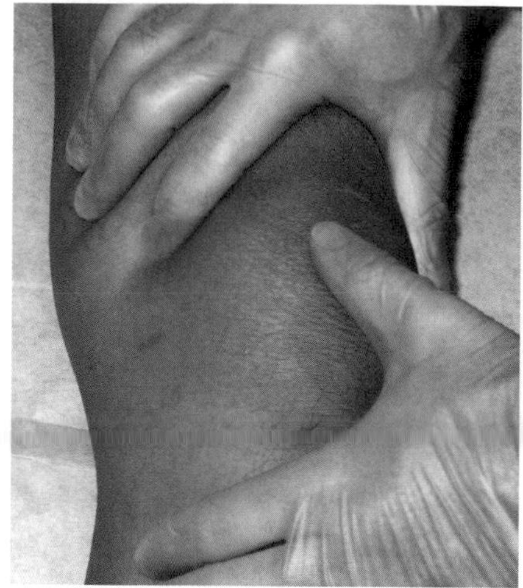

A

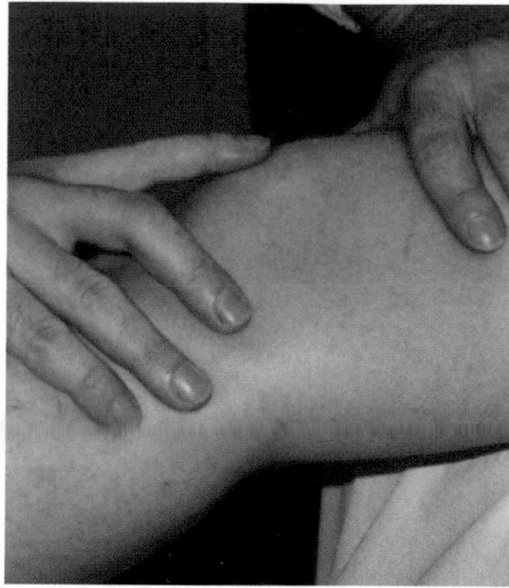

B

Box 8.1.

Causes of Knee Swelling

Effusion
Infrapatellar bursitis
Prepatellar bursitis
Suprapatellar bursitis
Patella fracture
Quadriceps strain
Patellar ligament

taut **(Fig. 8.7)**. Observe for fluid collection displacement to the other side. These techniques have no reported specificities or sensitivities; however, in our view, they should be **performed in the order described above**. For all of these techniques, the knee should be fully extended with the leg parallel to the floor.

Anterior

Swelling specific to the anterior knee has a discrete set of potential diagnoses **(Box 8.1** and **Table 8.3)**. **Suprapatellar bursitis** manifests with a diffuse and doughy swelling in the area immediately superior to the patella, but has minimal impact on motion. Usually unilateral, it can be bilateral; if bilateral, consider a systemic cause. **Prepatellar bursitis** manifests with discrete swelling at the point of the patella, often with pain at the site with active extension **(Fig. 8.8)**. Usually bilateral, this occurs in certain occupations, e.g., roofers; if unilateral, consider a septic cause. **Infrapatellar bursitis** manifests with swelling and tenderness adjacent and deep to the patellar ligament, with a modest degree of pain over the site with active extension **(Fig. 8.9)**. Usually bilateral, this is seen especially in occupations that require repeated kneeling, e.g., the clergy.* Unilateral infrapatellar bursitis may be septic. **Quadriceps tear** manifests with swelling and tenderness in the distal quadriceps and patella baja, i.e., an inferiorly displaced patella; **patellar ligament tear** manifests with swelling and tenderness distal to the patella and a patella alta, i.e., a superiorly displaced patella; **patellar fracture** manifests with widening of the patella,

*Hence the term, "clergy person's knee."

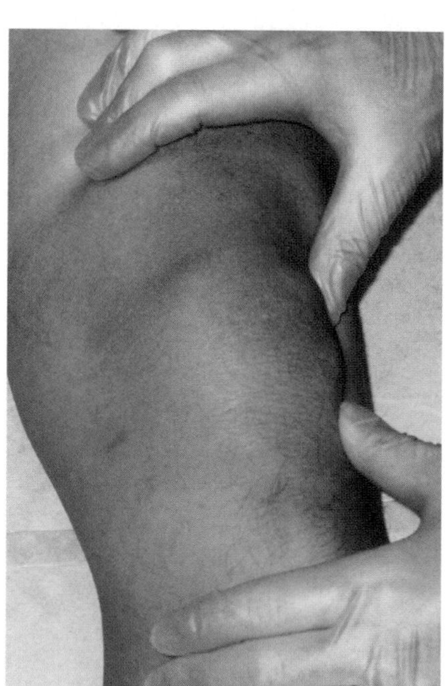

Figure 8.7.

Technique for fluid displacement to assess for a small effusion.

TIPS

- Knee extended, leg parallel to floor
- Apply thumbs to the medial or lateral knee to make the skin taunt
- Observe for flattening or bulging on the opposite side, deep to the patella
- Mild effusion: fluid displacement to the other side

Table 8.3. Anterior Knee Swelling Syndromes

Diagnosis	Location	Synonyms	Patellar Location	Acuity
Suprapatellar bursitis	Superior to the patella Diffuse, doughy Unilateral, nondominant knee	Houseperson's knee	Normal	Subacute
Prepatellar bursitis	At point of patella Bilateral, if occupation related Unilateral, septic	Roofer's knee	Normal	Acute
Infrapatellar bursitis	Inferior to the patella, deep to the patellar ligament Bilateral	Clergyperson's knee	Normal	Subacute
Patellar fracture	Diffusely over the patella		Normal Patella is widened	Acute
Quadriceps muscle tear	Superior to the patella	Clinton syndrome	Patella baja	Acute
Patellar ligament tear	Inferior to the patella		Patella alta	Acute
Osgood-Schlatter	Anterior tibial tuberosity		Normal	Acute, adolescents
	Heterotopic bone formation		Normal	Chronic
Patellar dislocation, medial	Patella medial to medial condyle of femur		Medial	Trauma Acute
Patellar dislocation, lateral	Patella lateral to lateral condyle of femur		Lateral	PFS or trauma acute

PFS = patellofemoral syndrome.

tenderness, swelling, and a marked decrease in active knee extension; **patellar dislocation**, lateral or medial, manifests with gross dislocation of the patella.

A **quadriceps muscle or tendon tear** manifests with unilateral, acute painful swelling of the distal quadriceps **(Fig. 8.10)**. The company it keeps includes ecchymosis, a patella baja, and a marked decrease in the ability to actively extend the knee. Furthermore, a flaccid mass is noted in the quadriceps muscle, the flaccid mass increases in size with active knee extension. This is due to trauma. **Patellar ligament tear** manifests with unilateral painful swelling, with patella alta and a marked decrease in active extension at the knee. Due to jumping with knee hyperflexed.

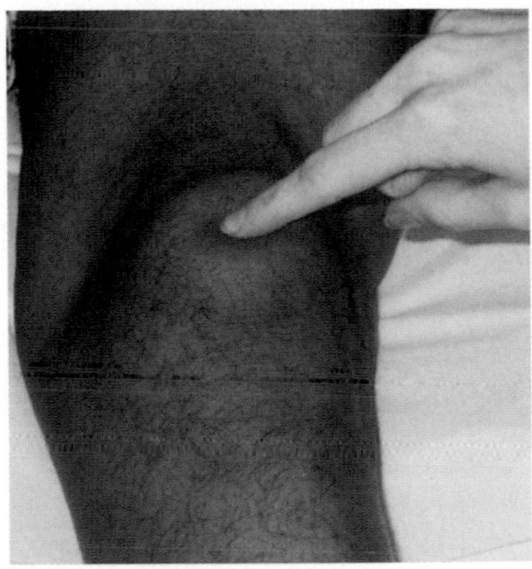

Figure 8.8.

Prepatellar bursitis. Discrete swelling and tenderness on the point of the patella; the swelling is fluctuant.

TIPS

- Palpate the anterior knee
- Prepatellar bursitis: discrete swelling and tenderness over the point of the patella
- Roofer's knees: bilateral
- Septic prepatellar bursitis: unilateral

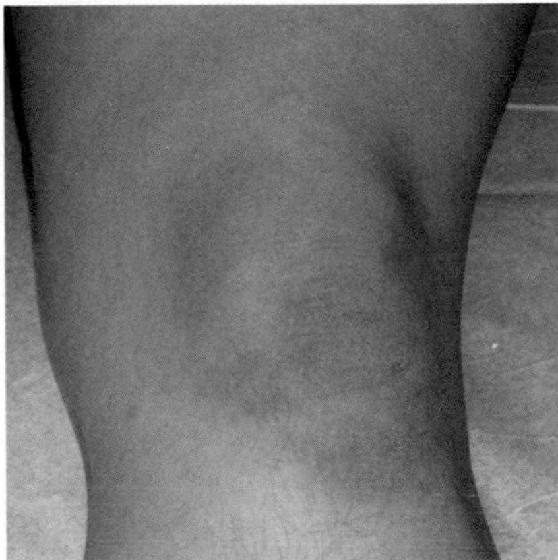

Figure 8.9.

Infrapatellar bursitis. Swelling and tenderness deep to the infrapatellar ligament. Note the callus over the site.

TIPS

- Palpate the anterior knee
- Infrapatellar bursitis: swelling and tenderness deep to the infrapatellar ligament
- Clergyperson's knees: bilateral complications
- Septic infrapatellar bursitis: unilateral

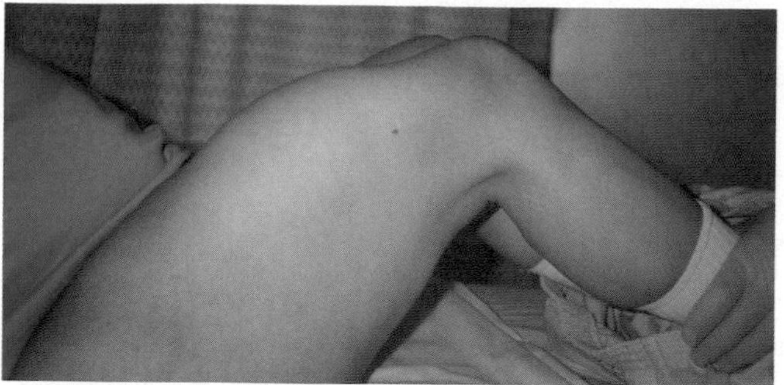

Figure 8.10.

Old quadriceps tear. Patella baja with a mass of noncontracting quadriceps muscle after a tear of the quadriceps.

 **TIPS**

- Note location of patella relative to the joint line
- Normal: inferior pole crosses the joint line
- Old patellar ligament tear: patella alta
- Old quadriceps tear: patella baja

Osgood-Schlatter disease, in the adolescent, manifests with marked tenderness and pain in the patellar ligament at its insertion—the anterior tibial tuberosity. **Osgood-Schlatter** disease in an adult manifests with a nontender, bony prominence at the anterior tibial tuberosity **(Fig. 8.11)**. This is due to inflammation at the site of tendon insertion.

Patellofemoral syndrome is very common, perhaps the most common reason for knee problems today. The patient has pain in anterior knee, especially when knee flexed for a long time (e.g., a long movie; hence the term by Newell of "moviegoers" knee) or pain with walking down stairs. In the normal setting, the patella usually migrates laterally with flexion and medially with extension. If the patella is inappropriately lateral in extension, the underlying femoral condyle femur jams into the overlying patella. This is especially evident while walking down stairs or walking or running downhill. The most common reason for this inappropriate laterality of the patella with extension is quadriceps atrophy, especially of the large medial head the VOM. This commonly occurs after knee injuries if no quadriceps rehabilitation or maintenance program has been initiated. Patellofemoral syndrome, therefore, is a constellation of findings related to the inappropriate laterality of the patella with extension. The company patellofemoral syndrome keeps includes an **increase in Q (quadriceps) angle**. Measurement of the Q angle is performed to objectively assess the magnitude of patellar lateralization **(Fig. 8.12)**. Normal Q angles are <10 degrees in boys, men, and prepubescent girls; <15 degrees in women. If the angle is indeed >15 degrees, it is consistent with, but not diagnostic of, patellofemoral syndrome. **Inspection of the quadriceps** may reveal general atrophy of the quadriceps and specific atrophy of the VOM. Severe patellofemoral syndrome manifests with a positive **apprehension sign** in which the patient grimaces or contracts the quadriceps when a medial to lateral stress is placed on the patella. In addition to pain, a complication of patellofemoral

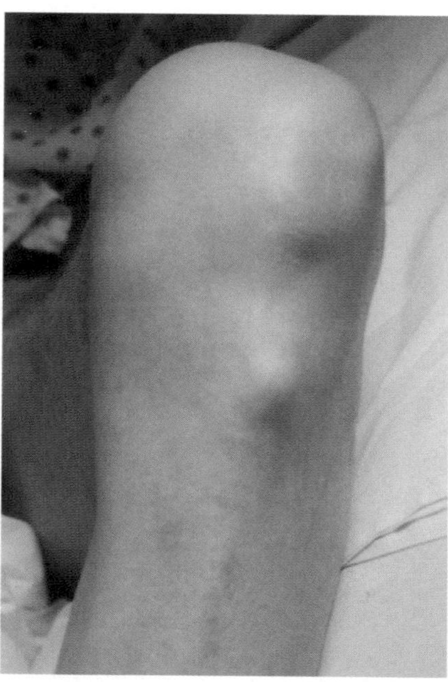

Figure 8.11.

Osgood-Schlatter disease, old: a nontender, exostosis over the anterior tibial tuberosity.

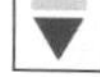 **TIPS**

- Osgood-Schlatter disease, healed: prominent boney nodule on the anterior tibial tuberosity

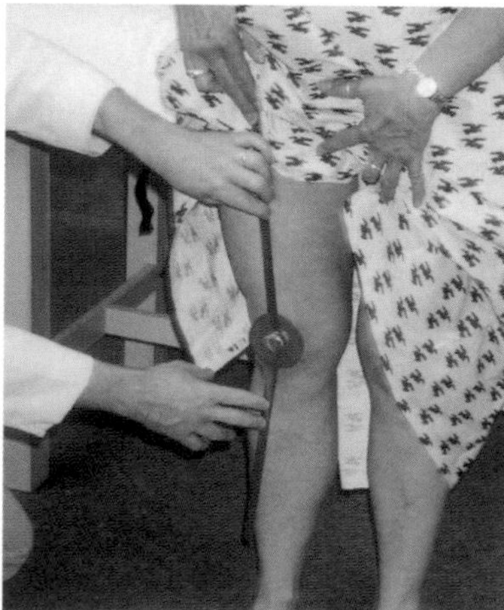

Figure 8.12.

Technique for Q-angle measurement. The knee is in extension; here, the Q angle is normal. Here, using a goniometer.

 **TIPS**

- Leg at knee in full extension
- One line (in figure, the top arm of the goniometer): from the anterior superior iliac spine (ASIS) to the center of the patella
- One line (in figure, the bottom arm of the goniometer): from the center of the patella to the anterior tibial tuberosity
- Measure angle between the two lines
- Normal: Q angle <10 degrees
- Patellofemoral syndrome: Q angle >10 degrees; atrophy of the quadriceps and VOM

TEACHING POINTS

KNEE SWELLING

Anterior Swelling

1. Quadriceps muscle tear: patella baja, pain, and swelling; audible rip.
2. Patellar ligament tear: patella alta, pain, and swelling.
3. Suprapatellar bursitis: diffuse swelling of area superior to patella, mild pain, normal patellar height.
4. Prepatellar bursitis: discrete swelling over the point of the patella, normal patellar height.
5. Patellar fracture: diffusely swollen and exquisitely tender widened patella, normal patellar height.
6. Infrapatellar bursitis: discrete tender swelling deep to the patellar ligament, normal patellar height.
7. Osgood-Schlatter disease (in adolescent patient): discrete swelling and tenderness at anterior tibial tuberosity, site of patellar ligament insertion.
8. Trauma-related patellar dislocation = patella dislocated medially, i.e., medial to the medial femoral condyle.
9. Severe patellofemoral syndrome = patella dislocated laterally, i.e., lateral to the lateral femoral condyle.
10. Acute inability to walk: patellar dislocation, quadriceps muscle or tendon tear, patellar fracture, or patellar ligament tear.

Posterior Swelling

11. Baker's cyst: fluctuant, nontender mass, transilluminable.
12. Popliteal artery aneurysm: pulsatile mass, nontransilluminable; has a bruit.

syndrome is acute patellar dislocation in the lateral direction. Patellofemoral syndrome without significant quadriceps atrophy or with a fixed laterally displaced patella should lead to a **lateral facet disorder** as the underlying cause.

Posterior causes of knee swelling are less common than those of anterior knee swelling. **Baker's cyst** manifests with a mass that, on transillumination, diffusely lights up. This is due to chronic effusion that evaginates posteriorly; it was first described by Adams, not Baker, in 1840. **Popliteal artery aneurysm** manifests with a pulsatile mass that is not transilluminble; on auscultation, it reveals a bruit. **Deep venous thrombosis** manifests with swelling and edema of the affected lower extremity that is documented by inspection and measurement of the circumference 15 cm above and below the center of the patella. The classic feature of pain on squeezing the posterior compartment of the leg (Homan's sign) is so nonspecific and nonsensitive as to make it clinically useless. The physical examination in the diagnosis of deep venous thrombosis is suboptimal.

Medial Knee (Tables 8.4 and 8.5)

Semimembranosus strain manifests with pain (sometimes severe), swelling, and ecchymosis in the medial knee and thigh. The pain increases with the *hamstring squeeze test* in which the bellies of the hamstring muscles are palpated and gently squeezed at a site 10 to 12 cm proximal to the knee joint

Table 8.4. Overall Knee Examination: Medial Knee

Procedure	Contusion	Pes anserine bursitis	Hamstring pull	MCL sprain	Medial meniscus tear
Inspection	Ecchymosis on bone	Swelling at site	Ecchymosis medial-posterior thigh	Swelling at medial joint line	Swelling at medial joint line
Palpation	Tender	Tender	Tender	Tender	Tender
Valgus stress	-	-	-	Medial pain and laxity	-
Varus stress	-	-	-	-	Medial pain
Cross-legged test	-	-	Pain medial thigh	-	Unable to perform
Tenderness displacement	-	-	-	Medial joint line pain; no change in location Flexion or extension	Pain anterior with extension, posterior with flexion of knee
McMurray external rotation	-	-	-	-	Medial click posterior horn of MM
McMurray internal rotation	-	-	-	-	Medial click anterior horn of MM
Apley distraction	-	-	-	+, Medial pain	-
Apley grind	-	-	-	-	+, Medial pain

MCL = medial collateral ligament; MM = medial meniscus.

(**Fig. 8.13**). In addition, the patient is acutely unable to walk on that extremity. This is often an acute injury related to running. **Pes anserine bursitis** manifests with pain and tenderness over the medial tibia, 5 to 7 cm distal to the joint line. The pain increases at pes anserine with the hamstring squeeze test. This strain is often caused by running with flat shoes, hyperpronating while running, or pes planus, which recurrently overstretches the hamstrings and irritates the pes anserine and its bursa.

Sprain of the MCL manifests with tenderness over the posterior medial joint line and a positive **valgus stress test**. For the test, place stress on the medial knee by applying valgus force on the tibia. Multiple variants of this test include supine, with the examiner's flexed knee under the patient's knee (**Fig. 8.14**). Other variants include with the patient sitting, leg stabilized under the examiner's arm; sitting, foot on examiner's thigh; supine or sitting, examiner's thigh as a pivot point; and the patient in the prone position (**Fig. 8.15**). It is important for the clinician to be comfortable with performing and teaching each of these variants and remember that each maintains the fundamental concepts of the valgus stress test: with the patient's knee flexed at 20 to 25 degrees, palpate the site of

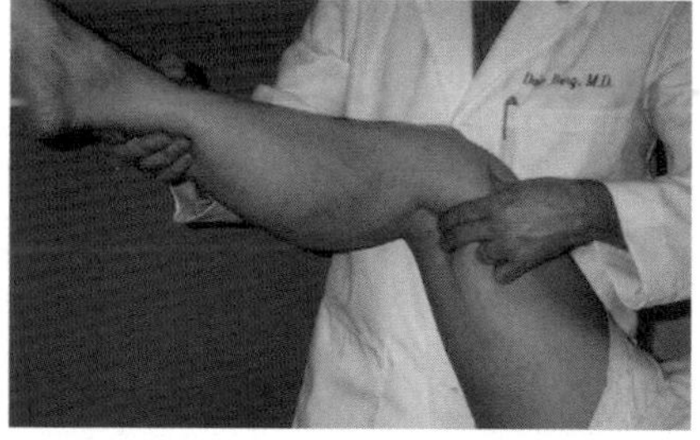

Figure 8.13.

Technique for the hamstring squeeze test. Excellent method to assess the hamstrings (semimembranosus) and pes anserine (semitendinosus).

TIPS

- Patient supine, knee flexed to 20 degrees
- Gently palpate the bellies of the hamstrings 10 to 12 cm proximal to the joint line
- Pes anserine bursitis: pain on the proximal medial tibia
- Semimembranosus strain: pain in the medial thigh up to the groin

Table 8.5. Medial and Lateral Knee Problems

Medial diagnoses	Lateral diagnoses
Hamstring pull or strain	Biceps femoris strain
Pes anserine bursitis	Iliotibial band syndrome
Medial collateral ligament sprain	Lateral collateral ligament sprain
Medial meniscus	Lateral meniscus
Blunt trauma or contusion	Fibular head fracture

Table 8.6. Evidence to Support the Physical Examination: Meniscal Tears

Test	Study	Sensitivity (%)	Specificity (%)
Joint line tenderness	Fowler, et al	85	-
	Noble, et al	79	-
	Barry, et al	76	43
McMurray	Fowler, et al	29	-
	Noble, et al	63	-
	Barry, et al	56	100
	Evans, et al	16	98
Apley grind	Fowler, et al	16	
Multiple tests:			
McMurray, Apley grind, Payr, and Steinmann	Muellner, et al	96.5	87

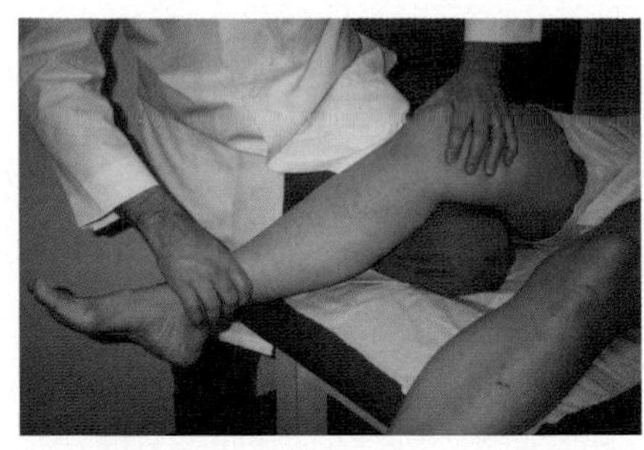

Figure 8.14.

Technique for valgus or varus stress test. Position of knee at 20 degrees flexion, examiner's knee under patient's knee.

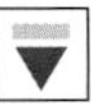

TIPS

- Knee flexed to 20 degrees
- Palpate the medial joint line, especially the posterior aspect
- Apply valgus stress to the tibia
- Excellent style for the bedridden patient
- MCL sprain: tenderness of the posterior joint line, laxity of the line
- Lateral meniscal sprain: tenderness at the lateral compartment

the joint line and apply valgus stress to the tibia. MCL sprain is due to valgus trauma to knee; also described in use of whipkick in the breast stroke.*

A **medial meniscal tear** manifests with pain in the medial compartment (Bohler's sign) when performing the **varus stress test**, a positive **tenderness displacement** test in which the patient reports maximal pain at posterior aspect of joint line when the knee is flexed, more anterior when the knee is extended **(Table 8.6)**. For the **cross-legged maneuver**, instruct the patient to sit cross-legged, i.e., in the typical yoga meditation position. The inability to do so is nonspecific; the ability to perform makes a medial meniscal tear highly unlikely (Payr's sign) **(Fig. 8.16)**. **McMurray's maneuver** will elicit a click or thud in the medial knee compartment **(Fig. 8.17)**. As this maneuver is moder-

*Hence the term by Kennedy of "breast stroke" knee.

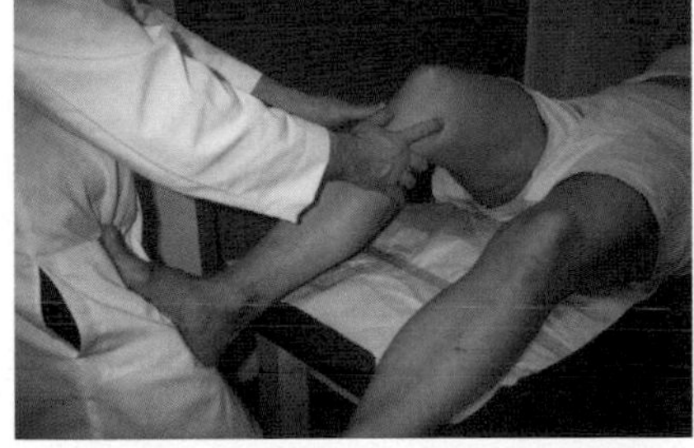

A

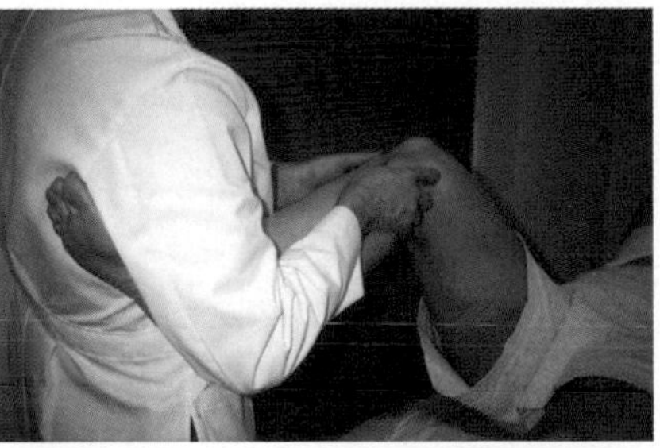

B

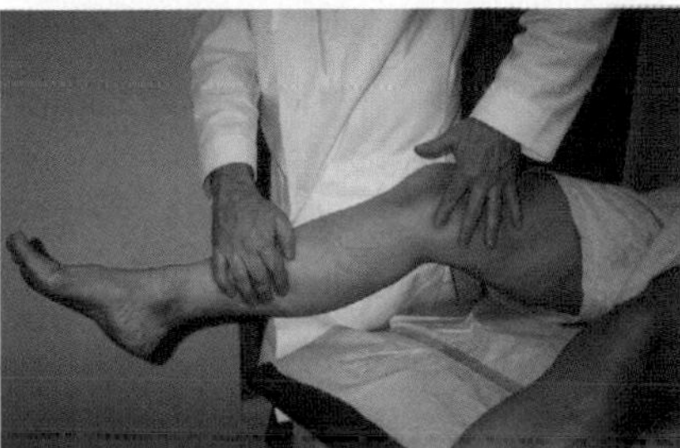

C

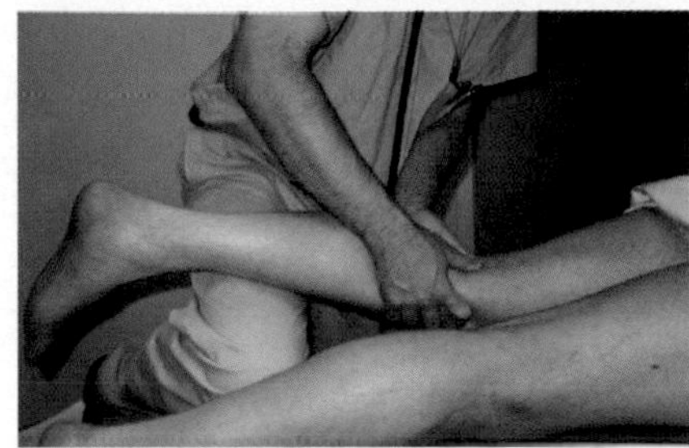

D

Figure 8.15.

Other positions for valgus or varus stress test and Lachman maneuver. **A.** Placing foot on thigh. **B.** Placing foot under arm: stabilizes the knee at 20 degrees; easy to use "W" configuration. **C.** From side, using the examiner's thigh as a pivot point: excellent for a bedridden patient. **D.** Prone position: easy to use "W" configuration.

TIPS

- Use various styles and positions for different patients
- All have the same fundamentals: 20 degrees of flexion; know the landmarks
- The prone position is excellent for obese patients
- The "W" configuration of the index fingers on the MCL and LCL sites, with the thumbs on the anterior tibial tuberosity

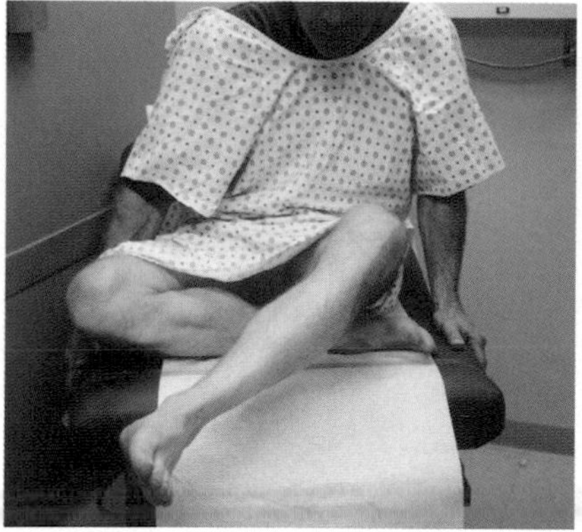

Figure 8.16.

Technique for the crossed-leg test. When instructed to sit cross-legged, the patient is unable to do so using the left knee.

TIPS

- Instruct patient to sit cross-legged
- Medial meniscal tear: unable to perform; if able to perform this procedure, highly unlikely to be a medial meniscal tear

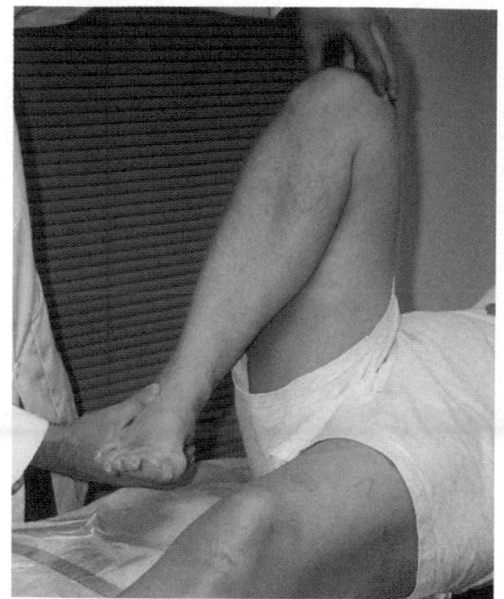

A

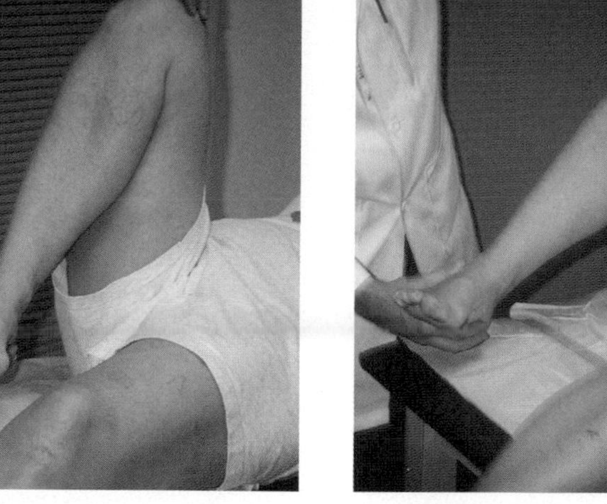

B

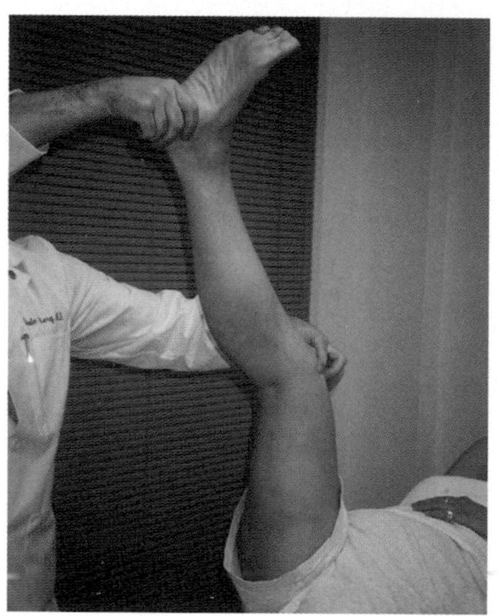

C

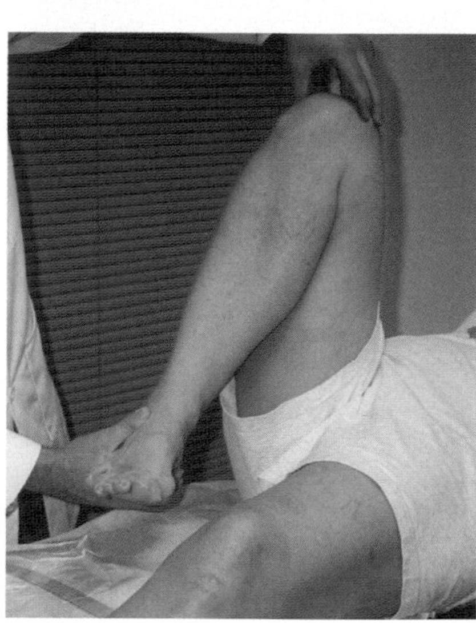

D

Figure 8.17.

Technique for McMurray maneuver. **A.** Grasp foot at ankle and maximally internally rotate ankle, place other hand over knee to feel the medial and lateral joint lines and flex the knee maximally. **B** and **C.** Continue in internal rotation of the ankle; extend the knee maximally. **D.** Then, passively flex the knee. This set is repeated with ankle maximally externally rotated.

TIPS

- Grasp foot at ankle and maximally internally rotate ankle
- Place other hand over knee to feel the medial and lateral joint lines
- Flex and extend the knee maximally
- The click, thud, or pop of a meniscal tear will occur at the extremes of flexion and extension—the last 5 to 10 degrees of flexion and extension
- Repeat cycle three times
- Medial meniscal tear: medial click audible or thud palpable
- Lateral meniscal tear: lateral click audible or thud palpable

TEACHING POINTS

MEDIAL KNEE EXAMINATION

1. Best position to examine the knee is at 20 degrees of flexion—the position in which the knee is most at jeopardy for injury, thus increases or optimizes the sensitivity of the examination.
2. Pes anserine bursa is immediately deep to the confluence of the three tendons of the gracilis, sartorius, and semitendinosus muscles, as they insert on the proximal medial tibia, approximately 5–10 cm distal to the joint line.
3. The pes anserine and its bursa are best found by palpating the semitendinosus muscle and tracing it to its insertion.
4. Risk factors for pes anserine bursitis include running with flat shoes, pes planus, and hyperpronation with running. A common weekend runner type injury, especially if in a runner who is wearing ill-fitting, flat running shoes.
5. The semimembranosus muscle crosses two joints: the hip (backward flexor) and the knee (flexor). In a tear, there is an acute inability to ambulate.
6. Because the medial collateral ligament (MCL) and the medial meniscal (MM) are intimately related, a significant sprain of one will result in a sprain of the other; therefore, it is difficult to differentiate a significant MCL from an MM—they are concurrent.
7. Any second- or third-degree tear of the MCL has a concurrent MM damage.
8. Acute medial pain that radiates into the medial thigh while running: think hamstring pull (semimembranosus strain).
9. If subacute or recurrent medial pain in the area below the knee after running and able to walk on it but with discomfort: think pes anserine bursitis.
10. The symptom of clicking or locking: think medial meniscal damage.
11. Recurrent bilateral medial pain after swimming the breast stroke: incorrect whip kick use, with resulting mild damage to the MCL.

ately difficult to perform, it should be the last maneuver in this set used to evaluate a patient with medial knee discomfort. The maneuver requires the examiner to apply a rotational force to the knee by first externally rotating the foot at the tibiotalar joint and then passively, maximally extending and flexing the leg at the knee three times; this set is repeated with the ankle passively internally rotated. It is important to know two different styles in performing the McMurray test; the technique and results are the same, but the styles are so different that it may look like two different examinations. The first of these styles is with the examiner at the foot of the bed or table looking at the patient while performing the technique; the second is with the examiner at the patient's side. A final point regarding McMurray's maneuver is that it should go to the extremes of flexion and extension when performing; any injury more serious will manifest with **knee locking**, i.e., the acute inablity to flex or extend from 10 degrees of flexion and, thus, makes performing the McMurray test irrelevant. The **Apley distraction** test **(Fig. 8.18)** is used to assess collateral ligament sprains, whereas the **Apley grind (Fig. 8.19)** is used to assess meniscal tears (see Figs. 8.18 and 8.19 for specifics on technique). Meniscal tears are trauma-related.

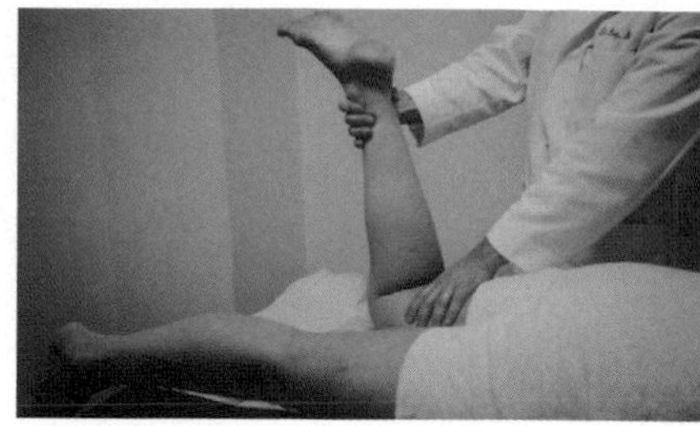
A

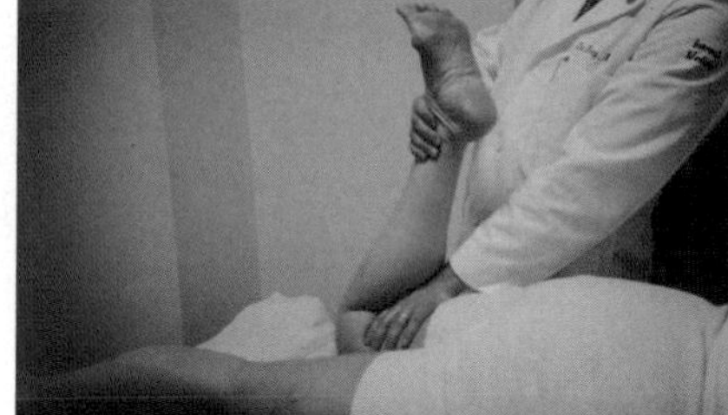
B

Figure 8.18.

Technique for Apley distraction test **A.** Baseline. **B.** Flexion to 120°. Useful in assessing for collateral ligament sprains.

 **TIPS**

- Patient prone, knee flexed to 90 degrees
- Grasp the ankle and hold the distal posterior thigh
- Pull upward on the leg, then passively flex the leg at the knee
- Normal: passive flexion to 140 degrees
- MCL sprain: medial joint pain
- LCL sprain: lateral joint pain
- Least useful of the maneuvers

Lateral Knee (Table 8.7)

Biceps femoris strain manifests with pain, swelling, and ecchymosis in the posterior lateral knee and lateral thigh **(Fig. 8.20)**. The pain increases to the lateral thigh with muscle palpation. An excellent site to examine the muscle is 10 cm proximal to the knee.

Fibular neck fracture manifests with point tenderness over the lateral fibula, a positive squeezing together of the fibula and tibia 15 cm distal to the knee. There is often a concurrent lateral ankle sprain. It is important to assess the common peroneal nerve by evaluating the active extension of the hallux and dorsal foot sensation, specifically between toes 1 and 2. Such common peroneal nerve damage manifests with weakness to great toe extension, decreased sensation to the dorsum of the foot, and weakness to foot dorsiflexion (see Chapter 13).

Iliotibial band syndrome and bursitis manifest with pain in the anterior lateral knee, from Gerdy's tubercle (lateral tibia) into the lateral thigh and gluteal muscle of buttock **(Fig. 8.21)**. Pain is noted in the area with ambulation. Furthermore, the discomfort is reproduced with the **hyperabduction test** (Fig. 8.21). In this, the patient is in a decubital position and maintains the hip in backward flexion and abduction. Finally, there is pain with *Ober's maneuver.* This is best performed with the patient in a lateral decubital position with the asymptomatic leg down. Forward flex the hip on the side down and backward flex the hip on the side up; then, attempt to adduct the leg so that the knee touches the table. Normally, this can be performed (see Chapter 12). Noble reports that 52% of long distance runners have ITBFs.

Sprain of the LCL manifests with tenderness over the posterior lateral joint line (Figs. 8.14 and 8.15) and a positive **varus stress test.** For this test, place stress on the lateral knee by applying varus force on the tibia. The multi-

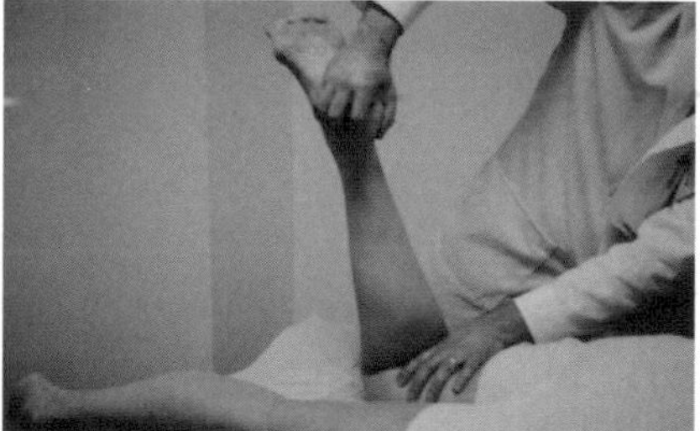

Figure 8.19.

Apley grind test. Useful in assessing for meniscal tears.

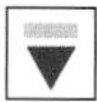 **TIPS**

- Patient prone, knee flexed to 90 degrees
- Grasp foot at calcaneus and place downward force on knee, first to medial compartment then to lateral compartment
- Lateral meniscus tear: lateral compartment pain
- Medial meniscus tear: medial compartment pain
- Least important of the maneuvers

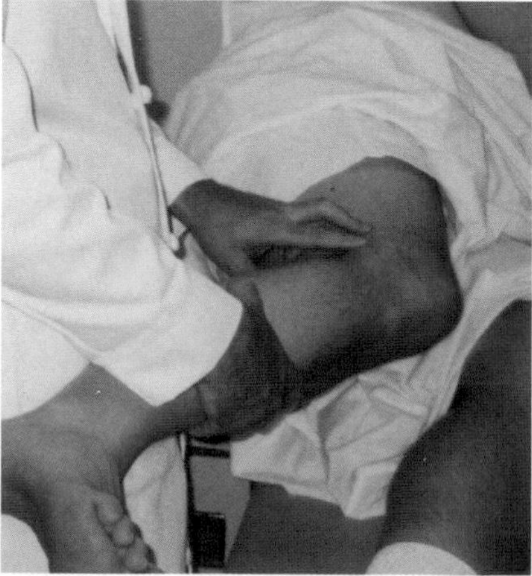

Figure 8.20.

Biceps femoris strain. Tenderness in the posterior lateral thigh.

 **TIPS**

- Knee flexed to 20 degrees, lower extremity parallel to floor
- Palpate the posterior lateral superior popliteal fossa
- Biceps femoris strain: tenderness in posterior lateral knee to the lateral thigh

Table 8.7. Overall Knee Examination: Lateral Knee

Procedure	Biceps femoris strain	Fibular fracture neck	LCL sprain	Lateral meniscus tear	Iliotibial band syndrome
Inspection	Swelling posterior thigh	Swelling fibular head	Swelling lateral joint line	Swelling lateral joint line	-
Palpation	Tender posterior thigh	Tender fibular head	Tender lateral joint line	Tender lateral joint line	Tender lateral thigh
Squeeze	-	+ Lateral knee	-	-	-
Varus stress	-	-	Pain in lateral joint line, laxity	-	-
Valgus stress	-	-	-	Pain in lateral compartment	-
Tenderness displacement	-	-	-	Lateral joint line pain, no change in location Flexion or extension	-
McMurray external rotation	-	-	-	Lateral click—anterior horn of LM	
McMurray internal rotation	-	-	-	Lateral click—posterior horn of LM	
Thigh abduction hyperextension test	-	-	-	-	+ Pain
Apley distraction	-	-	Lateral pain	-	-
Apley grind	-	-	-	Lateral pain	-

LCL = lateral collateral ligament; LM = lateral meniscus.

ple variants discussed above in the valgus stress test (Figs. 8.14 and 8.15) are easily used here also. Be comfortable with each one of these variants and always remember that each maintains the fundamental concepts of the varus stress test: knee flexed at 20 to 25 degrees, palpate the site of the condyles, and apply varus stress to the tibia. A **lateral meniscal tear** manifests with pain in the lateral compartment (Bohler's sign) when performing the **valgus stress test**, a positive **tenderness displacement** test in which the pain in flexion is maximal posteriorly; the pain becomes maximal anteriorly on extension because of a meniscal tear; **McMurray's maneuver** will elicit a click or thud in lateral knee compartment.

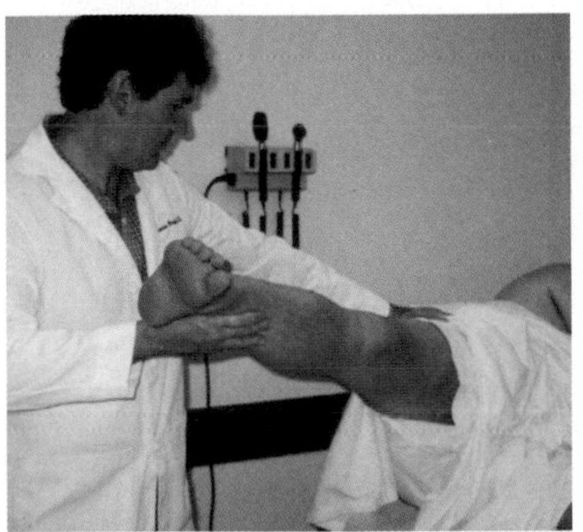

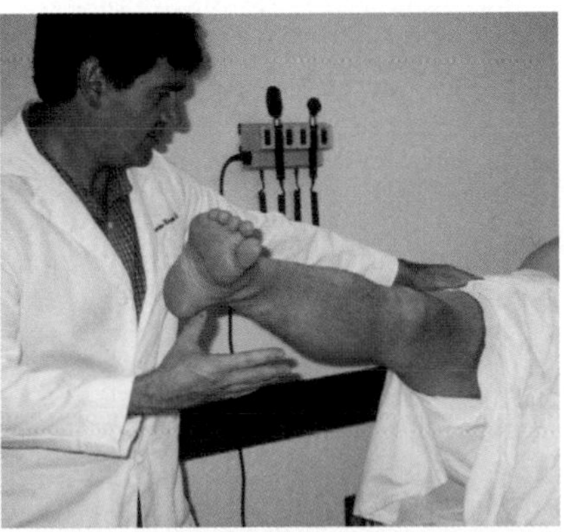

Figure 8.21.

Technique for the hyperabduction test. Useful to assess for iliotibial band syndrome.

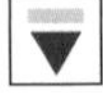

TIPS

- Patient in lateral decubitus position, asymptomatic side down
- Passively backward flex and abduct the side up
- Instruct patient to maintain position; acutely let go
- Normal: a small amount of discomfort in lateral thigh
- LCL sprain: tenderness over the lateral joint line
- ITB syndrome: significant tenderness in lateral thigh from Gerdy's tubercle to the gluteal muscle

TEACHING POINTS

LATERAL KNEE EXAMINATION

1. Best position to examine the knee is at 20 degrees of flexion—the position in which the knee is most at jeopardy for injury, thus increases or optimizes the sensitivity of the examination.
2. Iliotibial band is the direct extension of the gluteal muscles. This covers the lateral thigh and inserts on Gerdy's tubercle on the tibial condyle. As such, it will snap over the condyle of the femur with repeated flexion of the knee, especially if the thigh is moderately externally rotated. This snapping over the lateral femoral condyle results in irritation to the connective tissue in the band and to its adjacent bursa or will cause biceps femoris strain.
3. Methods to confirm the diagnosis of iliotibial band (ITB) is to perform the thigh hyperextension or abduction test and the Ober maneuver.
4. The lateral cruciate ligament (LCL) and the lateral meniscal (LM) are discrete, distinct entities; therefore, it is possible to have a severe tear of one without damaging the other.
5. Direct trauma to the lateral knee, e.g., a football helmet to the knee, can result in contusion or fibular fracture. Either can cause common peroneal nerve damage.
6. Common peroneal nerve damage: pain or tingling on the dorsum of the foot and weakened dorsiflexion of the toes and foot.
7. The best tests for mild common peroneal damage are assessing sensation at the dorsum of the web between the first and second toes and the strength to great toe dorsiflexion.
8. Lateral pain after acute trauma to the lateral knee: think of fibular fracture or common peroneal nerve damage.
9. Lateral knee pain after ankle sprain: think of fibular neck fracture.

CRUCIATE LIGAMENTS EXAMINATION

Acute or Unstable Cruciate Ligament Sprains

Acute cruciate ligament sprains or tears often manifest with an unstable knee, i.e., an injury that without proper treatment can progressively worsen and result in severe, perhaps even limb-threatening sequelae. Although the sprains may be partial, damage to the cruciate ligaments is associated with a greater risk of the knee being unstable. The cruciate ligaments cross over each other and provide a significant degree of internal support and strength to the knee joint. This is particularly true of the ACL. The **anterior cruciate ligament** is large; it has a significant vascular supply, attaches to the anterior tibia, and prevents both rotatory movement at the tibiofemoral joint and abnormal anterior movement of the tibia on the femur. The **posterior cruciate ligament**, although not as large, provides a function that is complementary to the ACL. It also prevents rotation at the tibiofemoral joint and abnormal posterior movement of the tibia on the femur. If one cruciate is damaged, there is often damage to other internal structures of the knee, including its sibling cruciate. A general rule is that the more structures damaged within the knee, the more likely the injury is unstable.

Acute cruciate ligament sprains (either ACL or PCL) manifest with five cardinal historical features: first, **acute swelling** caused by significant effusion within 1 hour of the injury, often within minutes. Second, **severe pain** in the knee. Third, an **audible** (often to both the patient and to teammates) **pop** at the time of the injury. Fourth, the acute **inability to walk** or bear weight on the joint, "feels like it is going to go out, doc." Finally, the development of a **clinched fist** when an attempt is made to perform any of the classic stress maneuvers to diagnose this entity. On **inspection** of the knee, a **severe ACL** tear will manifest with an **anterior sag of the tibia** on the femur **(Fig. 8.22)**. A **severe PCL** tear will manifest with **anterior sag of the femur** on the tibia. Concurrent, acute collateral ligament damage manifests with a valgus or varus deformity. Any significant cruciate ligament tear or suspected knee dislocation (Kennedy) requires assessment of **neurovascular status** of the leg distal to the knee. It is extremely important to assess this because severe damage can manifest with damage to the popliteal artery and to the tibialis nerve. The **popliteal artery** damage manifests with diminished or even absent **dorsalis pedis** and **posterior tibialis** pulses and a delayed **capillary refill** in the great toe, measured by the time required to return the blanched area to pink (>6 seconds). **Tibialis nerve** damage manifests with diminished sensation on the **plantar aspect of the foot** and weakness to **great toe flexion**.

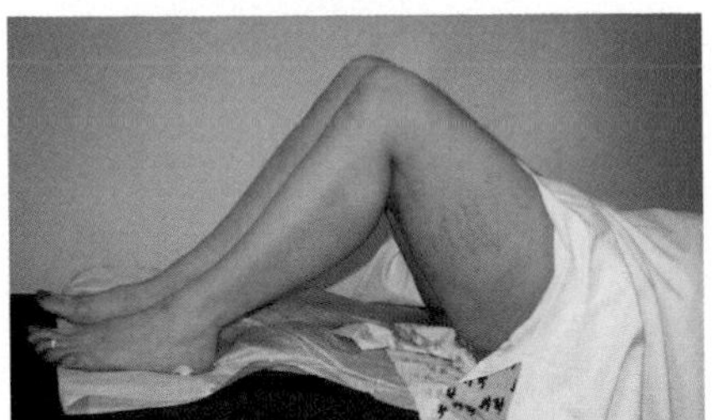

Figure 8.22.

Technique for anterior sag; if sag present, consistent with severe anterior cruciate ligament tear.

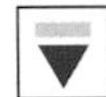

TIPS

- Knee flexed at 90 degrees
- Inspect the knee from the side, specifically where the tibia is located
- Mild ACL sprain: no sag
- Severe ACL sprain: sag present in which tibia is sagging anterior on the femur, concurrent effusion
- Mild PCL sprain: no sag
- Severe PCL sprain: sag present in which tibia is sagging posterior on the femur, concurrent effusion
- Most specific, but least sensitive, test

Stable or Chronic Anterior or Posterior Cruciate Ligament Sprains

Anterior cruciate ligament sprains, when severe, manifest with an **anterior sag** (sensitivity, <10%; specificity, 99%); if moderately severe, a positive **anterior drawer (Fig. 8.23)**, in which the tibia subluxates >5 mm anteriorly on the femur (sensitivity, 30%; specificity, 95%) **(Table 8.8)**; and a positive **Lachman maneuver**, performed at 25 degrees of flexion, in which the tibia is subluxed >5 mm anteriorly on the femur (sensitivity, 75%; specificity, 95%) (see Table 8.8). Several positions are used to perform a Lachman maneuver, including the examiner's knee under the patient's knee, the patient's foot on the examiner's thigh, the patient's foot under the examiner's arm, and the prone position **(Fig. 8.24)**. In addition, the **pivot shift test** is positive in ACL sprains (sensitivity, 82%; specificity, 98%) **(Fig. 8.25)**. ACL tears are trauma-related, often rotational trauma to knee.

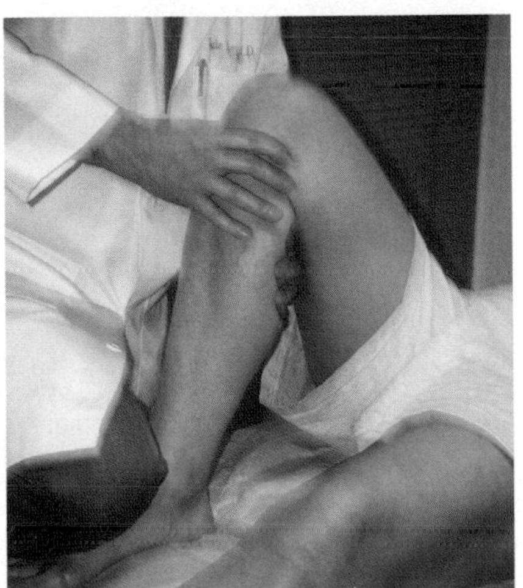

A

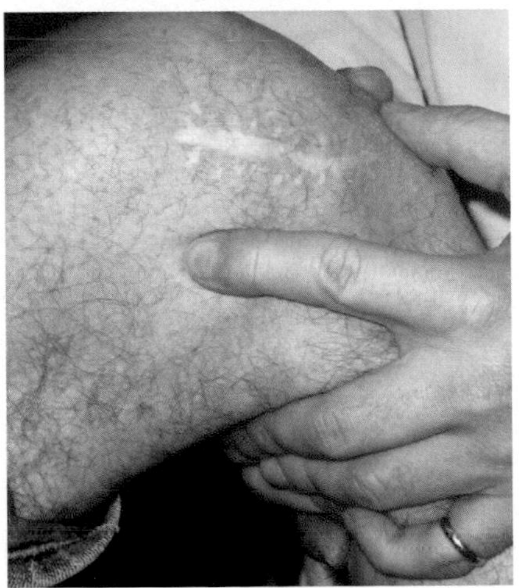

B

Figure 8.23.

Technique for assessing the anterior drawer sign. **A.** Knee flexed at 90 degrees. **B.** Here, the sign is present because of a severe ACL tear.

TIPS

- Knee flexed at 90 degrees, stabilized by holding foot
- Normal: no subluxation or <5 mm of movement
- Mild ACL sprain: no subluxation or <5 mm of movement
- Moderately severe ACL sprain: >5 mm of anterior subluxation and a soft endpoint (positive)
- Sensitivity: 30%
- Specificity: 95% (see Table 8.8)

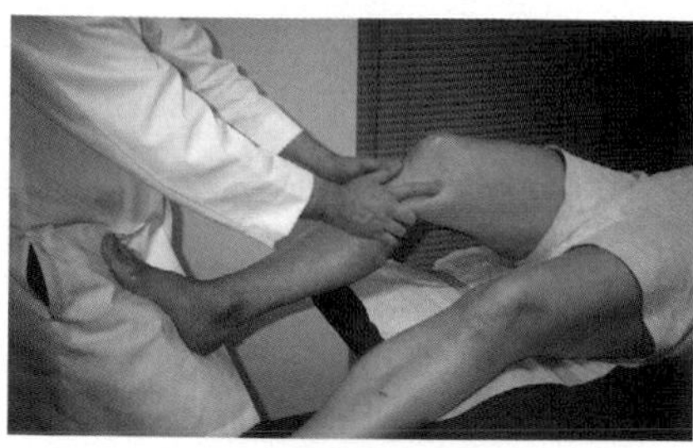

Figure 8.24.

Technique for Lachman maneuver. Knee flexed at 20 degrees; note the foot on examiner's thigh position used here. See Figs. 8.14 and 8.15 for other styles.

 **TIPS**

- Knee flexed to 20 degrees
- Use the "W" configuration
- Use hands to place posterior to anterior stress on the knee
- Normal: no subluxation or <5 mm of movement
- Mild or any ACL sprain: >5 mm anterior subluxation and a soft endpoint (positive)
- Sensitivity: 75%
- Specificity: 95% (see Table 8.8)

Table 8.8. Evidence to Support the Physical Examination: ACL Tears

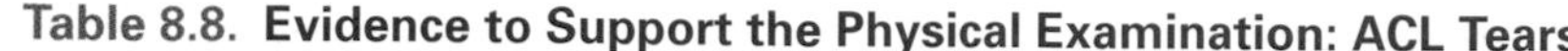

Test	Study	Sensitivity (%)	Specificity (%)
Anterior drawer	Solomon, et al	-	-
	Noble, et al	79	-
Lachman	Fowler, et al	29	-
	Noble, et al	63	-
	Barry, et al	56	100
	Evans, et al	16	98
Apley grind	Fowler, et al	16	-
Pivot shift	Katz, et al	82	[illegible]

Most of the examinations involve placing stress on the tibia to subluxate it anteriorly; the difference in sensitivity is based on the anatomic consideration that the menisci move posteriorly with knee flexion and anteriorly with knee extension. Thus, a patient with a completely torn ACL, but with a completely intact set of menisci may have a negative anterior sag and drawer, but a positive Lachman maneuver. The anterior sag and anterior drawer are better tests for an unstable knee (they require an ACL and a meniscus) and are not as sensitive for an ACL. DeHawen reports that meniscal tears accompany 60–70% of ACL tears.

Posterior cruciate ligament sprain, if severe, manifests with a **posterior sag**; if moderately severe, with a positive **posterior drawer sign** in which the tibia subluxates >5 mm posteriorly on the tibia **(Fig. 8.26)**. In addition, a positive Lachman maneuver is noted with the patient in the prone posterior position **(Fig. 8.27)** and a positive recurvatum (Godfrey's) test **(Fig. 8.28)**, in which there is posterior displacement of the tibia on the femur. It is **uncommon** to diagnose an isolated PCL tear. A final test for PCL is the *quadriceps active test* of Daniel. In this the patient actively extends knee from a baseline of 90-degree flexion. In PCL tear, there is posterior subluxation of the tibia.

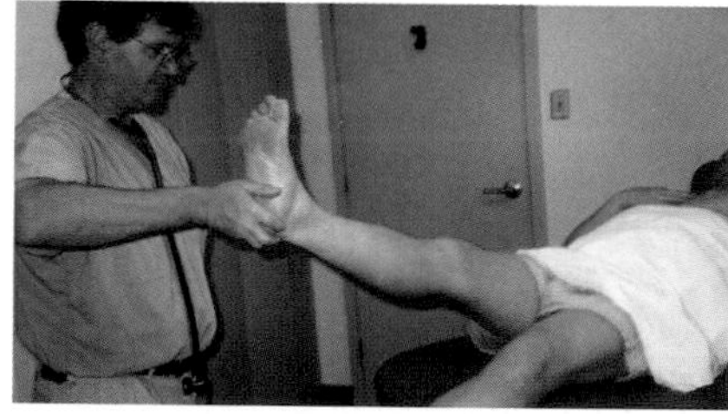

A

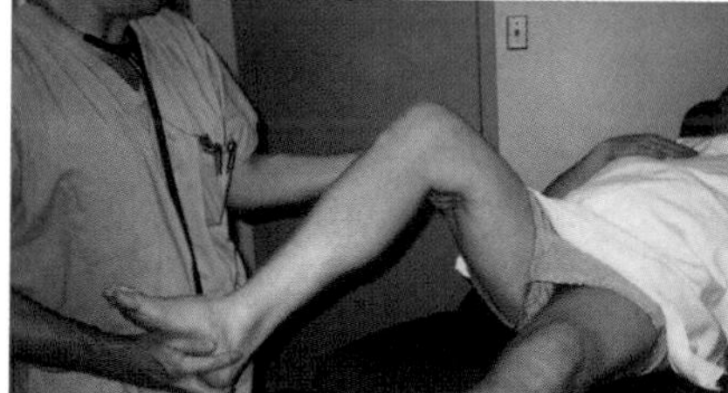

B

Figure 8.25.

Technique for pivot-shift test. **A.** Passively hyperextend the leg at the knee. **B.** Apply valgus force and concurrently passively flex the knee. Highly satisfactory for an anterior cruciate ligament (ACL) tear.

 **TIPS**

- Patient supine
- **Step one (A)**: passively hyperextend knee
- Passively abduct leg at hip
- Inspect for any anterior subluxation of tibia on femur (Galway-MacIntosh step)
- **Step two (B)**: passively apply valgus force to the knee while flexing the knee
- Palpate for movement of the tibia on the femur (i.e., a reduction of step one).
- Normal: no subluxation
- ACL tear: anterior subluxation as in step 1, but may be subtle; step 2: a palpable shift (reduction) with pivot

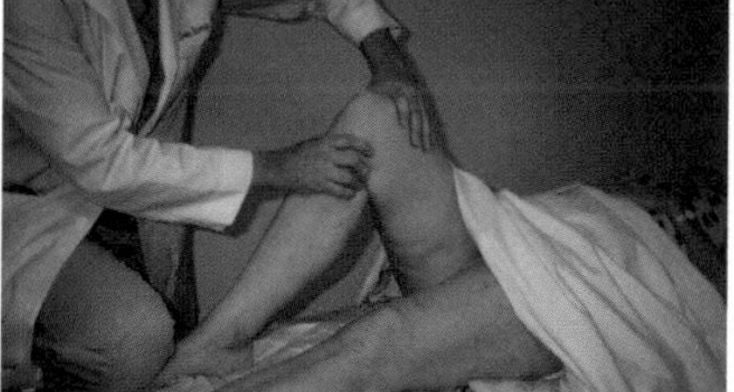

Figure 8.26.

Technique for posterior drawer sign. Satisfactory test for posterior cruciate ligament (PCL) tear.

 **TIPS**

- Knee flexed to 90 degrees
- Condyles in line at outset
- Place moderate pressure over the anterior tibial tuberosity with thumbs
- Normal: no or <5 mm of posterior movement of tibia on femur
- Moderately severe PCL sprain: >5 mm of posterior subluxation of tibia on femur, with a shelf present

TEACHING POINTS

UNSTABLE KNEE: CRUCIATE LIGAMENT TEARS

1. The anterior cruciate is the major ligament of the internal knee.
2. The anterior drawer sign has a sensitivity that is lower than the Lachman sign.
3. An anterior drawer sign or anterior sag indicates anterior cruciate ligament damage with concurrent meniscal damage; recall, the menisci move posteriorly with flexion and, thus, if intact, often prevent a Lachman's sign even with an anterior cruciate ligament (ACL) tear.
4. Anterior cruciate ligament normally prevents rotation and inappropriate anterior movement of the tibia on the femur.
5. Posterior cruciate ligament normally prevents rotation and inappropriate posterior movement of the tibia on the femur.
6. Concurrent lesions to ACL tears are common: medial meniscus tear, medial collateral ligament tear, known as the unhappy triad of O'Donaghue.
7. Cardinal features of an acute, significant ACL sprain include acute swelling, marked pain, and marked instability, including the inability to bear weight on the joint.
8. Always assess the neurovascular status of the lower extremity distal to the knee in cases of a significant cruciate injury: palpate the pulses of the dorsalis pedis and posterior tibialis to assess the patency of the popliteal artery and assess the sensory function of the plantar foot and toe plantar flexion for function of the tibialis nerve.

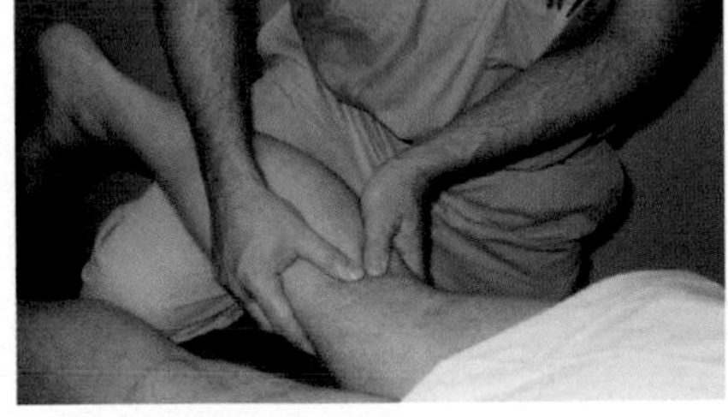

Figure 8.27.

Technique for prone Lachman maneuver. Excellent test for an anterior or posterior cruciate ligament (PCL) tear.

 **TIPS**

- Patient prone, standard procedure for prone test at 30 degrees, except attempt to subluxate tibia posterior on the femur
- Normal: no subluxation
- PCL sprain: >5 mm posterior tibial subluxation and pain

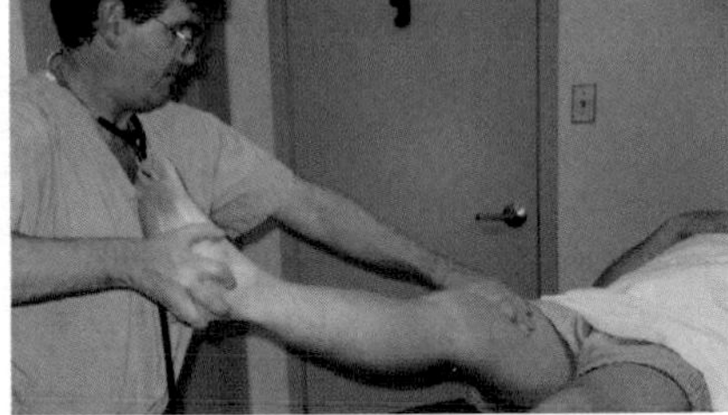

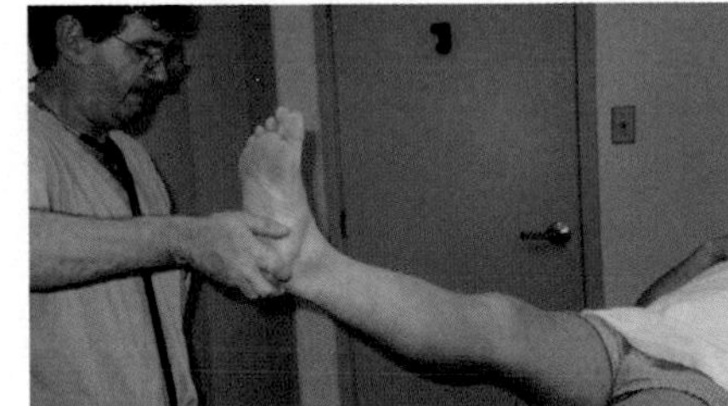

Figure 8.28.

Technique for recurvatum test (Godfrey's) for posterior cruciate ligament sprains.

 **TIPS**

- Patient supine
- Grasp the lower extremity at the heel
- Passively forward flex leg with the knee in full extension; add varus stress and external rotation at the knee
- Normal: no subluxation
- PCL sprain: posterior displacement of tibia on the femur

Annotated Bibliography

Apley AG. The diagnosis of meniscus injuries: some new clinical methods. *J Bone Joint Surg* 1947;29(1).

Clearly a classic with an excellent review of the knowledge and theory of meniscal damage at that time—state of the art. Describes the various Apley tests and variations, with excellent diagrams. A joy to read. Interesting bibliography.

Bullek DD, Scuderi CR. Getting your patient back in action after a meniscal tear. *J Musculoskel Med* 1994;11(5):68–76.

Describes some of the history and physical examination for meniscal tears; McMurray, Apley grind, and Steinmann tests; as well as treatment and rehabilitation in moderate detail.

Evans PJ, Bell D, Frank C. Prospective evaluation of the McMurray test. *Am J Sports Med* 1993;21: 604–608.

Prospective study of 104 patients about to have arthroscopy and 60 students without pathology. McMurray test was poor for lateral meniscal tears (PPV 29%), but was good in the diagnosis of medial meniscal tears (specificity, 98%; sensitivity, 16% for the thud medially). It has fair interobserver reproducibility and is best for the diagnosis of tears involving the posterior aspect of the meniscus.

McMurray TP. The semilunar cartilages. *Br J Surg* 1942;29: 407–414.

A classic. A delight to read the original description in this 1940 Robert Jones Memorial lecture of the Royal College of Physicians. Fascinating discussion of pathoanatomy and pertinent historical and examination techniques, including the one bearing his name.

Muellner T, Weinstable R, Schabus R, et al. The diagnosis of meniscal tears in athletes. *Am J Sports Med* 1997;25:7–12.

Interesting prospective study of 93 athletes in Vienna. Used surgery as a gold standard; magnetic resonance imaging (MRI) was performed after the examination and before surgery on 36/93 athletes, the balance having a clinical examination only. Examination included joint line tenderness, Bohler sign, McMurray's test, Steinmann test, Apley grind test, and the Payr sign. Using these techniques, overall results for lateral and medial tears include positive predictive value (PPV), 91.5; negative PPV 99; sensitivity, 96.5%; and specificity, 87%. Values for MRI: PPV 96, NPV 91.5; sensitivity, 98%; and specificity, 85.5%, respectively. Elegantly demonstrates the need for reproducible tests, recognizable outcomes, and clustering of tests that are important to diagnose the lesions. Tremendous bibliography included.

Solomon DH, Simel DL, Bates DW, et al. Does this patient have a torn meniscus or ligament of the knee? *JAMA* 2001:286(13):1610–1620.

A metaanalysis type review of the value of specific procedures to diagnose ACL, PCL, and meniscal tears. Used 23 articles to determine that, for ACL tears, the likelihood ratio (LR) for a positive anterior drawer: 3.8 (CI 0.7–22); a negative: 0.3 (0.05–1.5); a positive Lachman maneuver 25 (CI –2.7–651), and negative test 0.1 (0.0–0.4) and the composite: 25 (2.1–306), negative test: 0.04 (0.01–0.48). Demonstrated the pivot shift but gave vanishingly little evidence to support its use. For meniscal tears, McMurray sign for a positive examination had a LR of 1.3 (0.9–1.7) and, for a negative examination, a LR of 0.8 (0.6–1.1). Satisfactory, albeit terse, description of some of the procedures and a nice bibliography. Concluded that several different examination techniques used together are better than one technique. Problem is the lack of assurance that all papers performed examination the way that it was described in the paper.

Strobel M, Stedtfeldt HW. Meniskusdiagnostik. In: Strobel M, Stedtfeldt HW, eds. *Diagnostik des Kneigellenks.* Berlin: Springer Verlag, 1990:166–180.

Describes the Bohler, Payr, and Steinmann tests.

Posterior Cruciate Ligament Tears

Allen AA, Harne CD. When your patient injures the posterior cruciate ligament. *J Musculoskel Med* 1996;13(2):44–55.

Excellent overview of the history and physical examination, including pathoanatomic considerations. Tests included are the posterior drawer and Godfrey's test; a nice overview and excellent bibliography. Perhaps the best paper on PCL tears to date.

Baker CL, Norwood LA, Hughston JC. Acute combined posterior cruciate and posterolateral instability of the knee. *Am J Sports Med* 1984;12:204–208.

Forty patients in the study, gold standard arthroscopy, posterior drawer: sensitivity, 86%; specificity, not done.

Barry OCD, Smith H, McManus F, et al. Clinical assessment of suspected meniscal tears. *Ir J Med Sci* 1983;152:149–151.

Forty-four patients in the study, gold standard arthroscopy or arthrotomy, Joint line tenderness: sensitivity, 76%; specificity, 43%; McMurray, 56%; specificity, 100%; effusion: sensitivity, 35%; specificity 100%.

Cooper DE, et al. The PCL and posterolateral structures of the knee: anatomy, function and patterns of injury. *AAOS Instructional Course Lectures* 1991;40:249–270.

Emphasizes that, in patients with PCL deficit, the tibia may be posterior at outset of examination, i.e., sag to begin with, and, therefore, movement is not a drawer.

PPV=positive predictive value; NPV=negative predictive value.

Daniel DM, et al. Use of the quadriceps active test to diagnose PCL and measure posterior laxity of the knee. *J Bone Joint Surg* 1988;70(3):386–391.

Using 92 subjects (67 with PCL damage and 25 with no damage), the knee was placed in 90 degrees of passive flexion, and the patient was instructed to actively extend the knee against resistance. A posterior translation of the tibia indicated a PCL tear. Sensitivity, 97%; specificity, 100%.

Fowler and Lubliner

In a study of 80 patients with chronic knee pain, gold standard arthroscopy: sensitivity joint line tender, 85%; McMurray, 29%; Apley, 16%; specificity, not done.

Loos WC, Fox JM, Blazina ME, et al. Acute posterior cruciate ligament injuries. *Am J Sports Med* 1981;9:86–92.

Fifty-nine patients, gold standard was arthroscopy: physical examination sensitivity, 51%; specificity, not done.

Noble J, Erat K. In defense of the meniscus: a prospective study of 200 patients. *J Bone Joint Surg Br* 1980;62:7–11.

A study of 200 patients, acute and chronic, gold standard arthroscopy: sensitivity for joint line tenderness, 79%; McMurray, 63%; specificity for joint line tenderness, 11%; McMurray, 57%.

Anterior Cruciate Ligament Tears

Donaldson WF III, et al. A comparison of acute ACL examinations. Initial examination under anesthesia. *Am J Sports Med* 1985;13:5.

Lachman maneuver has a sensitivity of 99% for ACL tears; also there is marked swelling; Lachman maneuver is superior.

Donaldson WF, Warren RF, Wickiewicz T. A comparison of acute anterior cruciate ligament examinations: initial versus examination under anesthesia. *Am J Sports Med* 1985;13:5–10.

Using 101 patients, gold standard of arthroscopy or arthrotomy. Anterior drawer sign sensitivity: 70%; pivot shift sensitivity, 35%; Lachman maneuver sensitivity, 99%; no specificities were performed.

Feagin JA, Cooke TT. Prone examination for ACL insufficiency. *J Bone Joint Surg Br* 1989; 71(5):863.

Prone test for ACL assessment, may be easier in patients with thick thighs or examiners with small hands.

Galway HR, MacIntosh DL. The lateral pivot shift: A symptom and sign of ACL insufficiency. *Clin Orthop* 1980;147:45–50.

A description of this test for ACL integrity.

Gurtler RA, Stine R, Torg JS. Lachman test evaluated: quantification of a clinical observation. *Clin Orthop* 1987;216:141–150.

Using 75 patients, gold standard arthroscopy, Lachman maneuver sensitivity for ACL, 100%.

Hardaker WT, Garrett WE, Bassett FH. Evaluation of acute traumatic hemarthrosis of the knee joint. *South Med J* 1990;83:640–644.

Using 101 patients with acute injury to knee and an acute effusion hemarthrosis (i.e., clinical suspicion of ACL tear relatively high); gold standard arthroscopy: anterior drawer sensitivity, 18%; pivot shift sensitivity, 29%; Lachman maneuver sensitivity, 74%.

Houghton JC.: Classification of knee ligament instabilities I. The medial compartment and the cruciate ligament. *J Bone Joint Surg* 1976;58:159.

Nice description of valgus stress and the fact that the anterior drawer has a sensitivity of 77% in an ACL tear.

Katz JW. The diagnostic accuracy of ruptures of the ACL comparing the Lachman test, anterior drawer and pivot shift test in acute and chronic knee injuries. *Am J Sports Med* 1986; 14:88–91.

Retrospective study that compared the accuracy of Lachman sign and anterior drawer sign in the diagnosis of ACL tears. Gold standard was arthroscopy. In acute injuries (n = 9) (<2 weeks): Lachman sensitivity, 77.7%; anterior drawer, 22.2%; all specificity of >95%. In subacute injuries (n = 13) (>2 weeks): Lachman sensitivity, 84.6%; anterior drawer, 53.8%.

Lee JK, Yao L, Phelps CT, et al. Anterior cruciate ligament tears: MR imaging compared with arthroscopy and clinical tests. *Radiology* 1988;166:861–864.

Using 41 patients, gold standard was arthroscopy: anterior drawer, 78%; Lachman sensitivity, 89%; specificities for both, 100%.

Liu SH, Osti L, Henry M, Bocchi L. The diagnosis of acute complete tears of the anterior cruciate ligament. *J Bone Joint Surg Br* 1995;77:586–588.

Using 38 patients and gold standard arthroscopy: sensitivities; anterior drawer, 63%; pivot shift, 95%; Lachman sign sensitivity, 72%; specificities not done.

Solomon DH, Simel DL, Bates DW, et al. Does this patient have a torn meniscus or ligament of the knee? *JAMA* 2001;286(13):1610–1620.

A metaanalysis type review of the value of specific procedures to diagnose ACL, PCL, and meniscal tears. Used 23 articles to determine that for ACL tears, the LR for a positive anterior drawer, 3.8 (CI 0.7–22); a negative anterior drawer, 0.3 (0.05–1.5); a positive Lachman sign, 25 (CI 2.7–651); negative test, 0.1 (0.0–0.4); and the composite, 25 (2.1–306); negative Lachman sign, 0.04 (0.01–0.48).

Demonstrated that the pivot shift gave little evidence to support its use. For meniscal tears, McMurray sign for a positive examination had a LR of 1.3 (0.9–1.7) and for a negative examination a LR of 0.8 (0.6–1.1). Satisfactory, albeit terse, description of some of the procedures; nice bibliography; concluded that several different examination techniques used together are better than one technique. Problem is the lack of assurance that examinations reported in all papers were performed as described in the paper.

Torg JS, Conrad W, Kalen V. Clinical diagnosis of anterior cruciate ligament instability in the athlete. *Am J Sports Med* 1976;4:84–93.

Dr. Torg names Lachman test for his mentor John W. Lachman, professor of orthopedics at Temple University P. from 1956 to 1989. Specifically describes the outcome of a palpable or visible anterior subluxation of the tibia in relation to the femur with a soft or mushy endpoint for an ACL tear. Dr. Lachman taught this test to his students but never claimed to have been the originator of the test named for him. Documents the need to stabilize the knee at 20 to 30 degrees of flexion to perform the Lachman maneuver.

Wroble RR, Lindenfeld TN. The stabilized Lachman test. *Clin Orthop* 1988;237:209–212.

Describes the modifications of the Lachman maneuver when a flexed knee is placed beneath the patient's knee to stabilize. Makes a plea for reproducibility and quantification of outcomes.

Anterior Knee

Dandy DJ. Arthroscopy in the treatment of young patients with anterior knee pain. *Orthop Clin North Am* 1986;17:221–229.

An exhaustive list of common and rare causes of anterior knee pain. Excellent.

Dunn JF. Osgood-Schlatter disease. *Am Fam Phys* 1990;41(1):173–176.

Overview of pathogenesis, diagnosis, and treatment of this common disease.

Hughston JC, Deese M. Medial subluxation of the patella as a complication of lateral retinacular release. *Am J Sports Med* 1988;16:383–388.

Description of the dimple sign of vastus obliquus medialis atrophy.

Larson WG, et al. Patellofemoral disorders: physical and radiologic evaluation. Part I. and Part II. *Clin Orthop* 1984;185:165–186.

Excellent review of the mechanisms to develop patellofemoral syndrome (PFS)—patellofemoral joint disturbances.

Newell SG, Bramwell ST. Overuse injuries to the knee in runners. *Phys Sport Med* 1984; 12(3):81–92.

One of first times the term "theatre knee" was used for patellofemoral syndrome.

Osgood RB. Lesions of the tibial tubercle occurring during adolescence. *Boston Medical Surgical Journal* 1903;148:114.

A classic.

Ruffin MT, Kiningham RB. Anterior knee pain: the challenge of patellofemoral syndrome. *Am Fam Phys* 1993;47(1):185–194.

Examination overview is more general than that for anterior pain, but the descriptions and diagrams are well detailed. Includes apprehension test, Q angle, Ober's maneuver, Lachman maneuver, and the anterior drawer sign. In addition, describes thigh measurement for atrophy, which is excellent for anterior knee pain. Nice differential diagnosis for anterior knee pain, including for adolescents and adults. Excellent bibliography.

Schlatter C. Verletzungen des schnabelformigen fortsatzes der oberen tibia epiphyse. *Beitr Klin Chir* 1903;38:874.

A classic.

Posterior Knee

Adams M. Chronic rheumatic arthritis of the knee joint. *Dublin Journal of Medical Science* 1840;27:520.

Perhaps the first description of a popliteal cyst; therefore, one might argue that the eponym should be Adams.

Baker WM. Formation of synovial cysts in the leg in connection with disease of the knee joint. *St. Bartholomew's Hospital Report* 1887;13:245.

Classic description.

MacGuire AM, Cassidy JT. Popliteal cysts. *Am Fam Phys* 1985;32(6):139–144.

Deftly written review of the pathogenesis and manifestations of popliteal cysts.

Medial Collateral Ligament

Houghton JC.: Classification of knee ligament instabilities. I. The medial compartment and the cruciate ligaments. *J Bone Joint Surg* 1976;58:159.

Nice description of the valgus stress test.

Kennedy JC, Hawkins RJ. Breaststroker's knee. *Phys Sports Med* 1974;2: 33–38.

First description of this not uncommon syndrome.

Pecina. The knee. In *Overuse Injuries of the Musculoskeletal System.* 161–220.

In-depth, magnificent review of common and uncommon overuse syndromes of the knee. Pathophysiology, mechanisms, and manifestations are all described in great detail. Exceptional discussions of patellofemoral joint syndrome, breaststroker's knee, and iliotibial band syndrome. A must for those who have a keen interest in this topic. Bibliography is splendid.

Lateral Collateral Ligament

Houghton JC.: Classification of knee ligament instability. II: The lateral compartment. *J Bone Joint Surg* 1976;58(2):179.

Describes the varus stress test.

Nicholas JA. Injuries in sports—recent developments. *Orthop Clin North Am* 1977;8(3):523.

Nice overview of varus and valgus stress tests.

Noble CA. The treatment of ITBFS. *Br J Sports Med* 1979;13:51–54.

The prevalence of iliotibial band friction syndrome (ITBFS) in long distance runners is 52% Also describes the Noble test.

Renne RJ. The iliotibial band friction syndrome. *J Bone Joint Surg* 1975;57A:1110–1111.

One of the first times the term ITBFS was used. Also described the Renne test.

Acute Knee Injuries

DeHaven KE. Diagnosis of acute injuries with hemarthrosis. *Am J Sports Med* 1980;8:9–14.

Meniscal tears accompany ACL tears in 60% to 70% of cases; is evidenced by locking or clicking.

Flanagan JP, et al. Primary care of the acutely injured knee. *Journal of Musculoskeletal Medicine* 1992; 9(11):29–41.

Overview of basic and some advanced techniques in history and physical examination. Solid standard overview.

Kennedy JC. Complete dislocation of the knee joint. *J Bone Joint Surg* 1963;45(5):889.

Classic review of a serious injury; details vascular and nerve damage risk.

Schenk RC, Rodriguez F. Office evaluation of the acutely injured knee. *Journal of Musculoskeletal Medicine* 1992;9(2):17–34.

Brief review of specific history and physical diagnostic tests useful in the diagnosis of common outpatient ligamentous and meniscal injuries. Very good images of McMurray maneuver and several other useful techniques in physical examination. Very well-written paper for diagnostic information.

Warme WJ, et al. Teton Village Clinic, Jackson Hole Wyoming: ski injury statistics, 1982 to 1993. *Am J Sports Med* 1995;23:597–600.

Incidence of injuries were MCL, 60%; ACL, 16.5%; combined MCL and ACL, 20%.

Zarin B, Fish DN. Knee ligament injury. In Nicholas JA, Hershman EB, eds. *The Lower Extremity and Spine in Sports Medicine,* Vol 1. St Louis: CV Mosby, 1995:825–864.

A grading system for MCL sprains: I. Stretch (tenderness); II. Partial tear (tender with <5 mm laxity); III. Complete tear (tender with >5 mm laxity).

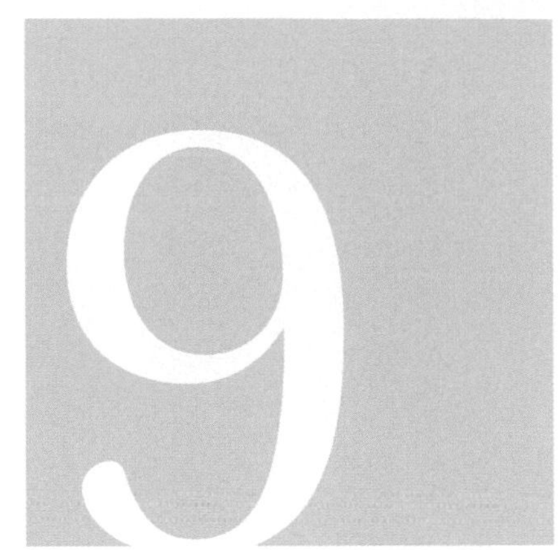

Shoulder Examination

PRACTICE AND TEACHING

ANTERIOR SURFACE ANATOMY

(Figs. 9.1 and 9.2)

The **lesser tuberosity** of the humerus, is on surface anatomy, immediately lateral to the coracoid process of the scapula; this is the insertion site of the subscapularis muscle. The **bicipital groove** is between the more medial lesser tuberosity and the more lateral greater tuberosity. This groove is the site of the long head of the biceps tendon as it runs from its origin on the supraglenoid tubercle above the glenohumeral joint. Refer to Fig. 9.2 for mechanism to find landmarks. The **subscapularis** muscle is a component of the rotator cuff. It originates on the anterior scapular surface, inserts on the lesser tuberosity of the humerus, has the infrascapular (C5) nerve, and acts in internal rotation of the humerus. The **biceps brachii** muscle has a long and a short head. The **long head** originates on the supraglenoid tubercle, inserts on the proximal volar ulna, and has the musculocutaneous (C5/6) as its nerve. It acts in forward flexion of the humerus, as a flexor of the arm at the elbow, and it is a

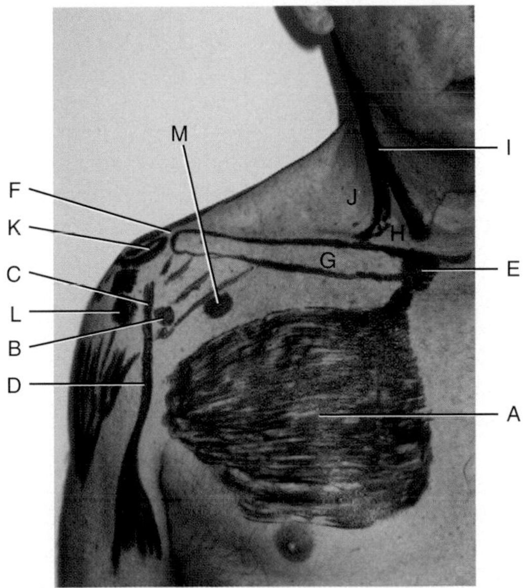

Figure 9.1.

Surface anatomy of the anterior shoulder and arm—to the elbow. **A.** Pectoralis major. **B.** Lesser tuberosity of humerus. **C.** Bicipital groove. **D.** Long head biceps brachii. **E.** Sternoclavicular joint. **F.** Acromioclavicular joint. **G.** Clavicle. **H.** Supraclavicular fossa. **I.** Sternocleidomastoid muscle. **J.** Anterior scalene muscles. **K.** Deltoid muscle. **L.** Greater tuberosity of humerus. **M.** Covacoid process.

TIPS

- Pectoralis major muscle: the major adductor of the humerus
- Lesser tuberosity of humerus: insertion site of subscapularis
- The bicipital groove: bounded by the lesser tuberosity and greater tuberosity
- Long and short heads of the biceps brachii: both flex elbow and supinate forearm; long head forward flexes the humerus
- Sternoclavicular joint and acromioclavicular joint both contribute to the ROM above the horizontal plane
- Supraclavicular fossa is a site to assess lymph nodes
- Sternocleidomastoid muscle acts to rotate the head

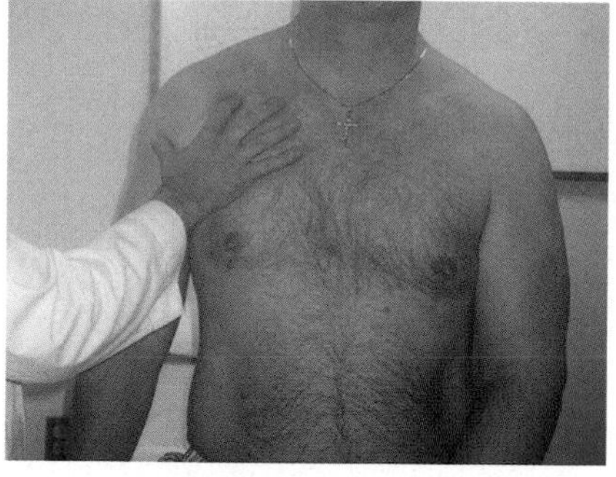

A

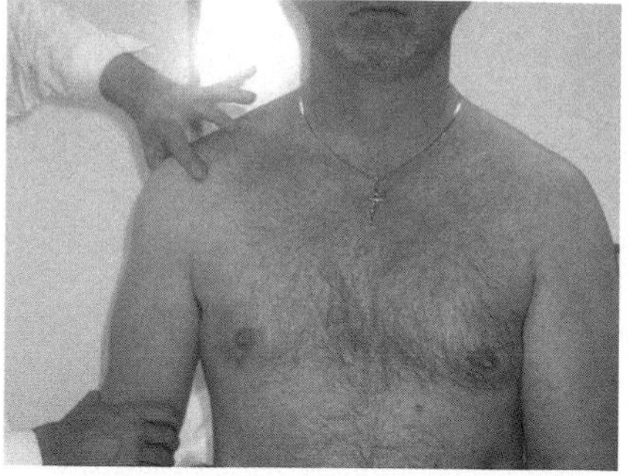

B

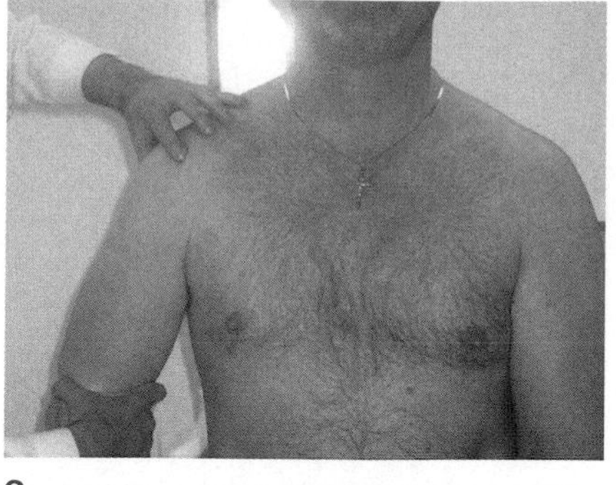

C

Figure 9.2.

Technique and mechanism to find landmarks on the anterior humerus. Step 1: Remember to have patient in a neutral position; palpate the coracoid, lesser tuberosity, and bicipital groove. Step 2: Passively internally rotate the arm to feel the greater tuberosity.

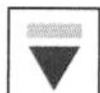 **TIPS**

- **Step 1: (A) and (B)**
- Note the position of the patient: arm at side, forearm at side, neutral between supination and pronation
- Passively backward flex the arm to about 20°, palpate the coracoid
- Note that the lesser tuberosity is immediately lateral to coracoid **(B)**
- **Step 2: (C)**
- Passively internally rotate the arm; the greater tuberosity will move under the fingers
- Then, externally rotate the arm, the lesser tuberosity will move under the fingers

supinator of the forearm. The **short head** is similar, except that it originates on the coracoid process and acts only to flex arm at the elbow and supinate the forearm. The **pectoralis major** muscle originates on the lateral sternum and inserts on the proximal medial humerus; its nerve is derived from the roots of C7 and it acts in adduction of humerus. The **sternoclavicular joint**, the **clavicle**, the **acromioclavicular joint**, and the coracoid process are bony landmarks in the area of the anterior shoulder. The **coracoid process** is a useful as a guide to locate the lesser tuberosity, and for the anterior approach in glenohumeral joint injection and, in a glenohumeral joint injury, whether the humerus is dislocated or subluxed. It is also the insertion site of the pectoralis minor muscle and the origin of the short head of the biceps brachii. Enlarged **supraclavicular lymph nodes** are in the fossa formed in the medial aspect immediately superior to the clavicle. This has been called Virchow's or Troisier's node. Specifically, when the node is enlarged and filled with metastasis it is the node of Troisier. Although the eponym is unimportant, knowledge that this is a site of potential metastatic disease is important. The **sternocleidomastoid** muscle originates on the mastoid of the cranium and inserts on the sternum and medial clavicle; its nerve is cranial nerve XI (CNXI) and it acts in head rotation. The **anterior scalene** muscles are readily demonstrable in the anterior neck. Deep to these, although not palpable, the positions of the **brachial plexus**, the **subclavian artery**, and the **subclavian vein**; each of which are often of great importance to the examining physician.

POSTERIOR SURFACE ANATOMY

(Fig. 9.3)

The **supraspinatus** muscle originates on the posterior scapula, above the scapular spine; it inserts on the greater tuberosity; its nerve is the suprascapular (C5); and it acts to abduct the humerus. The **infraspinatus** muscle originates on the posterior scapula below the scapular spine; it inserts on the greater tuberosity; its nerve is infrascapular (C5); and it acts in external rotation of the humerus. The **teres minor** muscle is similar to the infraspinatus except its nerve is axillary. **(Table 9.1)**.

The **trapezius** and **levator scapulae** are more superficial muscles. The trapezius has three discrete components. The upper one third originates on the cervical spinous processes, inserts on superior angle of scapula; its nerve is CNXI, and it acts to **elevate or shrug the scapula** and shoulder and to abduct the humerus at the scapulothoracic joint. The lower two thirds originate on the lower cervical and upper thoracic spinous processes and insert on the mid to lower scapula; its nerve is CNXI, and it acts in backward flexion of the scapula

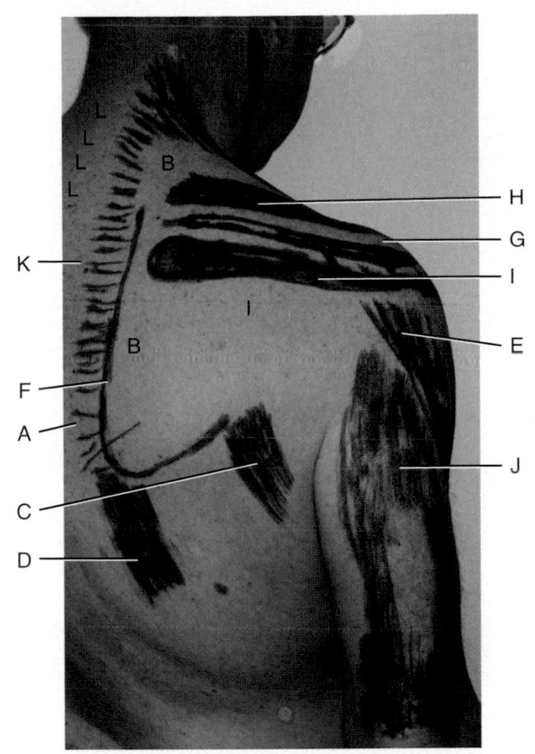

Figure 9.3.

Posterior shoulder surface anatomy landmarks. **A.** Rhomboid muscle. **B.** Trapezius muscle. **C.** Teres major. **D.** Latissimus dorsi. **E.** Posterior deltoid muscle. **F.** Vertebral border of scapula. **G.** Spine of the scapula. **H.** Supraspinatus muscle. **I.** Infraspinatus muscle. **J.** Triceps muscles. **K.** Paraspinous muscle. **L.** Spines of vertebrae.

TIPS

- Rhomboid muscle works with the middle trapezius to retract (backward flex) the scapula
- Trapezius muscle contributes to the stability of the cervical spine and the shoulder; scapular elevation with the levator scapula; and scapular retraction (backward flexion) with the rhomboid
- Teres major and latissimus dorsi, with the subscapularis, result in internal rotation; teres major and latissimus dorsi with the long head of the triceps and the posterior deltoid, result in backward flexion
- Posterior deltoid muscle works in external rotation and backward flexion
- Spine of the scapula is used to differentiate the supraspinatus from infraspinatus muscles
- Triceps muscle extends the arm at the elbow and, with latissimus dorsi, teres major, and posterior deltoid, backward flexes arm

(retraction). The **levator scapula** originates on the cervical spinous processes; it inserts on the superior angle of scapula; its nerve is composed of the roots of C2, C3, and C4; and it acts in scapular elevation and, thus, extreme shoulder abduction. The **rhomboid muscles** originate on thoracic spinous processes and insert on the mid medial scapula; the nerve is dorsal scapular, roots of C4, and C5. These muscles act in **backward flexion** (retraction) of scapula. The **teres major** originates on the dorsal inferior angle of scapula; inserts on the lateral scapula; its nerve is subscapular (C6/7); and it acts to backward flex the humerus. The **latissimus dorsi** muscle originates on the spinous processes of the thoracic vertebrae 7-12; inserts on proximal humerus; its nerve is thoracodorsal (C6, C7, and C8); and it acts, with the subscapularis muscle, to provide **internal rotation** of the humerus and, with the long head of the triceps and the posterior deltoid muscles, to provide **backward flexion** and adduction of the humerus. The posterior **deltoid** muscle originates on the clavicle and acromion; it inserts on the lateral mid humerus; its nerve is axillary; and it acts in abduction and backward flexion of the humerus and, with the infraspinatus

Table 9.1. Rotator Cuff Muscles

Muscle	Location	Insertion	Action*	Innervation	Pain site
Supraspinatus	Posterior scapula above the spine	Greater tuberosity	Abduction 0–30 degrees	C5 Suprascapular	Posterior lateral
Infraspinatus	Posterior scapula above the spine	Greater tuberosity	External rotation Weak abductor	C5 Infrascapular	Posterior lateral
Teres minor	Posterior scapula above the spine	Greater tuberosity	External rotation	C5 Axillary	Posterior lateral
Subscapularis	Anterior scapula	Lesser tuberosity	Internal rotation Weak adductor	C5	Anterior

*On humerus.

Box 9.1

Thoracic Spine Levels of the Medial Scapula

Level	Landmark
T2	Superior angle of the vertebral spine of the scapula = insertion of levator scapula
T3	Spine of the scapula
T4/T5	Site of insertion of rhomboid
T7	Inferior angle of the vertebral spine of the scapula = insertion of latissimus dorsi

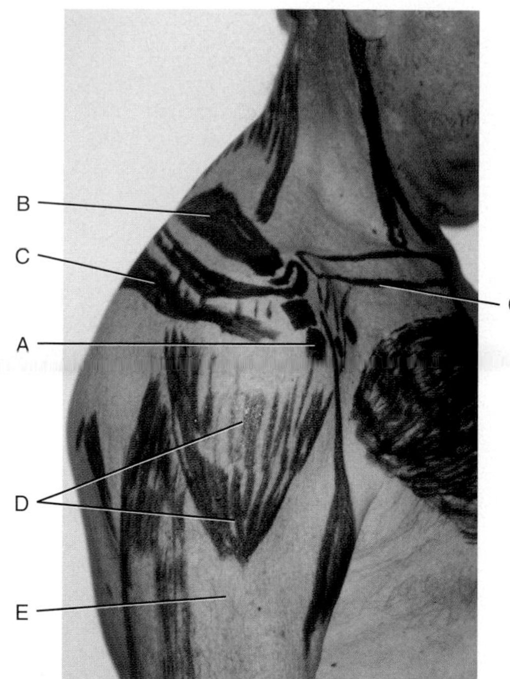

Figure 9.4.

Lateral shoulder surface anatomy and landmarks. **A.** Greater tuberosity of the humerus. **B.** Supraspinatus muscle and tendon. **C.** Infraspinatus muscle and tendon. **D.** Deltoid muscle. **E.** Humerus.

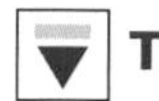 **TIPS**

- Greater tuberosity: insertion of supraspinatus, infraspinatus, and teres minor muscles
- Deltoid muscle: large, meaty triangle-shaped muscle draped around the acromion and overlying all of the structures

and teres minor muscles, to provide **external rotation** of the humerus. The **triceps muscle** long head originates on the proximal humerus; it inserts on the proximal ulnar aspect via the triceps aponeurosis; its nerve is radial (C7); and it acts to extend arm at elbow and, with the posterior deltoid, the latissimus dorsi, and the teres major, to provide **backward flexion**. The **vertebral border of the scapula** normally is found equidistant from the spinous processes top-to-bottom and side-to-side. With any difference between the two sides, consider an extrinsic muscle problem. The spine of scapula is at level T3, the inferior angle of scapula at T7. See Box 9.1.

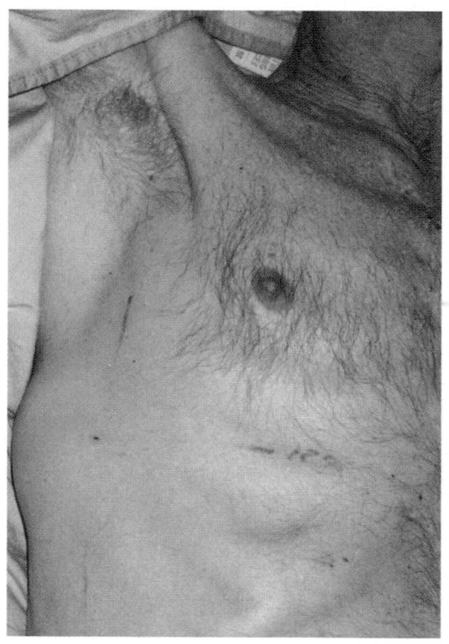

Figure 9.5.

Visible axillary lymph node enlarged because of lung carcinoma metastatic to the node. Note also the visible nodule present, a metastatic deposit from the primary lung tumor.

 **TIPS**

- Note any enlarged axillary nodes
- Look for visible nodes when examining the patient with lung cancer, breast cancer, and arm cellulitis

LATERAL SURFACE ANATOMY (Fig. 9.4)

The **greater tuberosity** of the humerus is the insertion site of the supraspinatus, infraspinatus, and teres minor muscles. The **supraspinatus** muscle originates on the posterior scapula, above spine; it inserts on greater tuberosity; its nerve is suprascapular (C5); and it acts to abduct the humerus. The **infraspinatus** muscle originates on the posterior scapula below the spine; it inserts on the greater tuberosity; its nerve is the infrascapular (C5); and it acts in external rotation: **Teres minor** muscle is similar, except it has the axillary nerve (Table 9.1). The **deltoid** muscle overlies the rotator cuff. The deltoid originates on clavicle and acromion, inserts on the lateral mid humerus, has the axillary nerve, acts to abduct and backward flex the humerus, and works with the infraspinatus to externally rotate the humerus. The **subacromial bursa** is a potential space lined with synovium that lies between the rotator cuff muscles and the deltoid.

The **axilla** is a pyramidal-shaped structure with the following boundaries: Anterior is the pectoralis major; posterior are the latissimus dorsi and teres major; medial is the serratus anterior; and lateral is the humerus. The apex is the intersection of the scapula, clavicle, and first rib. This is a structure that contains lymph nodes and may have palpable sebaceous cysts, lipomas, or nodes **(Fig. 9.5)**. To palpate the axilla and its contents, **(Fig. 9.6)**, the examiner passively abducts arm to 40°, places the tips of the fingers on the medial side, that is on the chest wall to the apex of the pyramid. Passively adduct the arm, and slip the fingers upward on the medial wall searching for any lumps and bumps. Palpation repeated in the anterior, lateral and posterior walls.

TEACHING POINTS

SHOULDER SURFACE ANATOMY

Anterior

1. The biceps brachii muscles are the hamstrings of the upper extremity; the long head is like the semimembranous as it crosses two joints; the short head is like the semitendinous as it crosses only the elbow.
2. The long head biceps brachii contribute to elbow flexion, forearm supination, and forward flexion of humerus; the short head, only to elbow flexion and forearm supination.
3. The pectoralis major is major adductor of the arm.
4. The subscapularis muscle inserts on the lesser tuberosity and, thus, is included in the differential diagnosis of anterior shoulder problems.
5. The brachial plexus is located deep to the anterior scalene muscles above the clavicle; thus, this is a site of potential entrapment.
6. Bicipital tendonitis usually results from a secondary cause; always look for another reason for the syndrome.

Posterior

1. The trapezius muscle, upper portion, contributes to shoulder shrug or elevation; lower portions, to scapular retraction and shoulder stabilization.
2. The triceps muscle extends the arm at the elbow and backward flexes the humerus.
3. The latissimus dorsi and the teres major are extrinsic muscles that act to internally rotate (with the subscapularis) and backward flex (with posterior deltoid and long head of the triceps), the humerus.
4. The posterior deltoid muscle contributes to external rotation (with the infraspinatus and the teres minor), and backward flexion (with the latissimus dorsi, the teres major, and the long head of the triceps) of the humerus.

Lateral

1. Greater tuberosity is the insertion site of the supraspinatus, infraspinatus, and teres minor muscles.
2. The deltoid muscle is large, meaty, triangle-shaped muscle draped over the acromion; it acts in forward flexion, abduction, and backward flexion of the humerus.
3. Between the rotator cuff and the deltoid muscle is the large subacromial bursa.

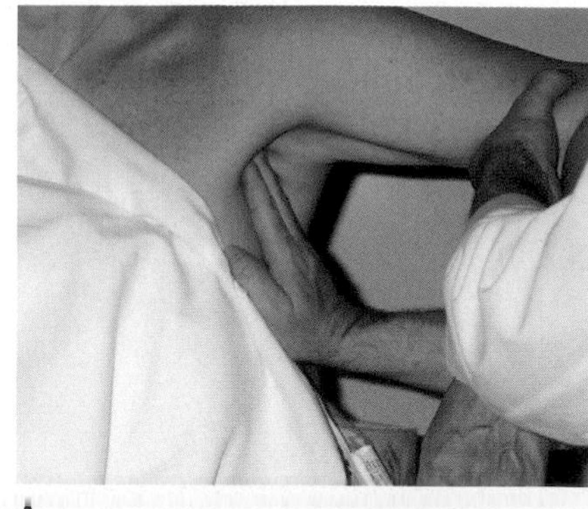
A

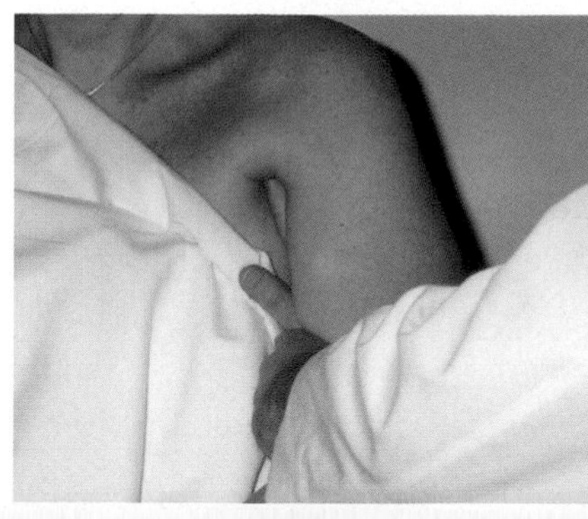
B

Figure 9.6.

Technique to perform axillary examination. **A.** Arm abducted, examiner places hand with fingers slightly flexed into axilla and **B.** passively adducts the arm in the scapular plane.

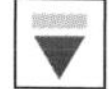
TIPS

- **Step 1:**
- Baseline the patient's arm is abducted 40 degrees and slightly forward flexed
- Gently place the tips of digits on the medial side (on the chest wall) at the apex of the pyramid **(A)**
- **Step 2:**
- Gently passively adduct the arm, allowing the fingers to painlessly migrate superiorly into the apex
- Palpate the medial wall for lump and bumps **(B)**
- Palpate all 4 walls of axilla

NEUROLOGIC EXAMINATION

It is always useful to assess the patient for any neurologic deficits. It is very important to assess the motor activity of the five spinal roots **(C5 to T1)** and the five major distal nerves (**axillary, musculocutaneous, radial, median,** and **ulnar**) of the upper extremity **(Table 9.2)**. This should be performed in any patient with a shoulder or neck problem.

Table 9.2. Assessment of the Peripheral Nerves Involving the Upper Extremity

Root	Nerves	Muscles	Sensory	Reflex	Movements
C5	*Axillary*	Deltoid Teres minor	Lateral antecubital fossa	Biceps	Abduction, humerus
	Musculocutaneous	Biceps Brachii			Flexion, elbow
	Suprascapular *Infrascapular*	Supraspinatus Infraspinatus			Abduction, humerus External Rotation, humerus
C6	*Musculocutaneous*	Biceps	Dorsal Forearm radial side	Brachio radialis	Supination, forearm
	Radial	Brachioradialis			Supination, forearm
	Radial	Extensor carpi radialis longus			Extension, wrist
	Median	Pronator teres			Pronation, forearm
C7	*Median*	Wrist flexors	Olecranon process	Triceps	Flexion, wrist
	Radial	Triceps			Extension, elbow
	C7 roots	Pectoralis sternal head major		Pectoralis	Adduction, humerus
C8	*Median*	Superficial flexors Digits 2 - 5	Dorsal forearm, ulnar side	Finger flexion reflex	Flexion, PIP digits 2 - 5
	Anterior Interosseous	Flexor pollicis longus			"OK" tip-to-tip
	Ulnar	Long flexors Digits 4 and 5			Flexion, DIP digits 4 and 5
T1	*Ulnar*	Interossei	Ulnar side of Antecubital fossa	None	Abduction digits 2–5 Adduction digits 2–5

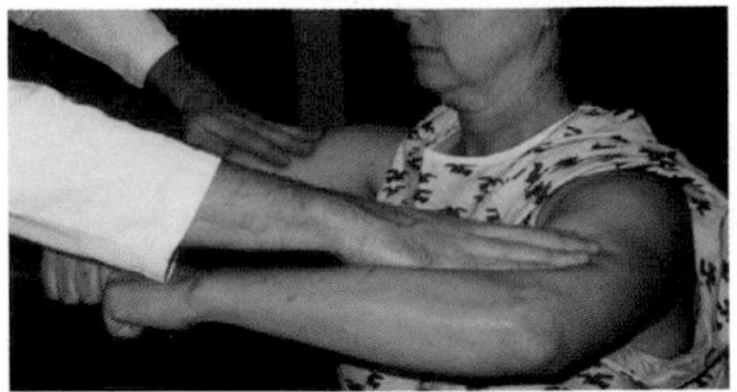

Figure 9.7.

Technique for active abduction against resistance. Assessment for C5, deltoid muscle.

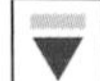 **TIPS**

- Patient actively abducts, usually with elbows in flexion
- Apply resistance to distal humerus
- C5 problem: weakness to this; may have atrophy of rotator cuff, deltoid, or biceps
- Shoulder problems decrease sensitivity and specificity

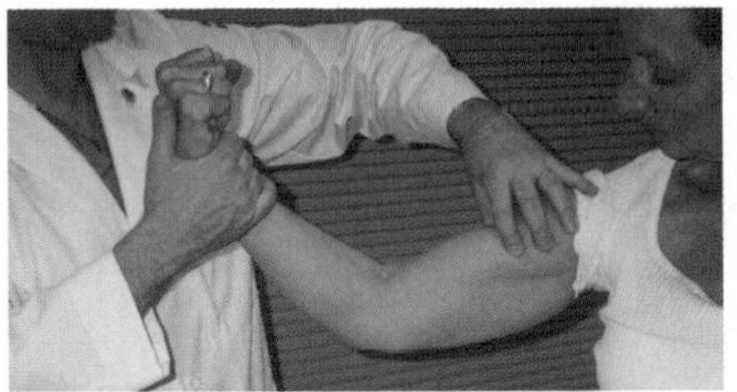

Figure 9.8.

Technique for active flexion against resistance. Assessment of C5, biceps brachii.

 **TIPS**

- Patient actively flexes arm at elbow
- Apply resistance to distal forearm
- C5 problem: weak applies pressure may have atrophy of biceps
- Complements the shoulder abduction; good if patient has a limitation to shoulder ROM

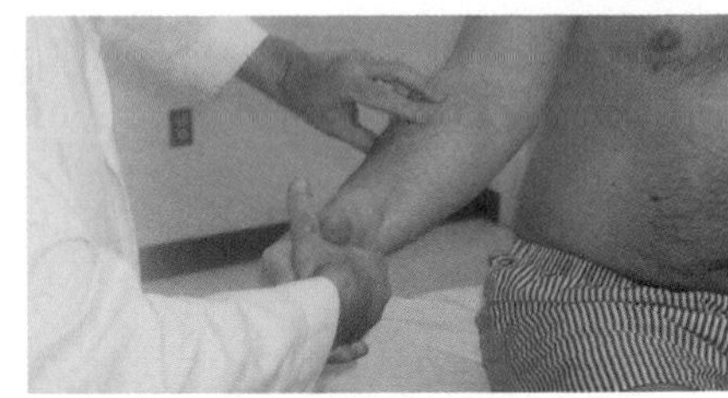

Figure 9.9.

Technique for active forearm supination against resistance, the handshaking maneuver. Assessment of C6.

 **TIPS**

- Patient actively supinates forearm
- Apply resistance by shaking hand, patient applies pressure thumb to examiners thumb
- C6 problem: weak supination; may have brachioradialis atrophy, fasciculations
- Brachioradialis is radial nerve

C5 to T1 Assessment

Cervical root 5 is assessed by examining the function of **deltoid** (axillary nerve), **supraspinatus** (suprascapular nerve), and the **biceps brachii** (musculocutaneous nerve); therefore, the best screening techniques for function are **humeral abduction** and/or arm flexion at **elbow (Figs. 9.7 and 9.8)**. C5 also innervates the infraspinatus and the subscapularis muscles; thus, active external and internal rotation of the humerus can be used to further define and assess C5 integrity. **C6 root** is most diffuse; it contributes to the **brachioradialis** muscle (radial nerve) and the **biceps brachii** (musculocutaneous), both of which act in forearm supination; to the **pronator teres** muscle (median nerve), which acts in forearm pronation; and to the **wrist extensor** muscles on radial side (radial nerve). Therefore, the best screening techniques for C6 function are **wrist extension, forearm supination**, or both **(Figs. 9.9 and 9.10)**. **C7 root** is assessed by examining the **pectoralis major** muscle, the **triceps** (radial nerve), or the **flexor carpi radialis** muscle (median nerve). Therefore, the best screening techniques for C7 are to assess the strength of extension of arm at **elbow** or **forearm pronation (Fig. 9.11)**.

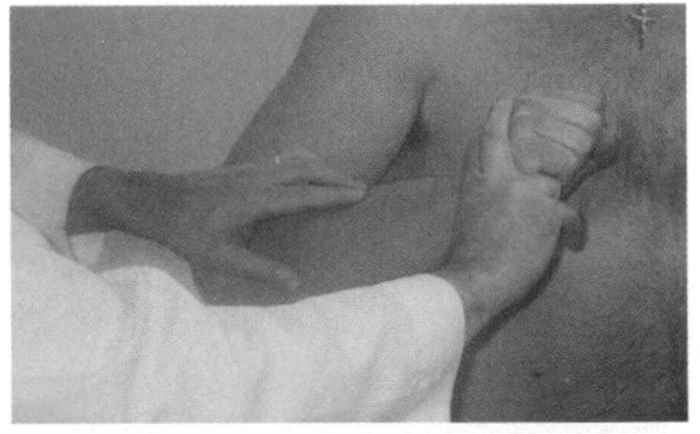

Figure 9.10.

Technique for active wrist extension against resistance. Assessment of C6 and C7.

 **TIPS**

- Patient actively extends wrist
- Apply resistance on dorsal mid metacarpal
- C6 problem: weak wrist, especially radial side, may have wrist extensor muscle atrophy, fasciculations

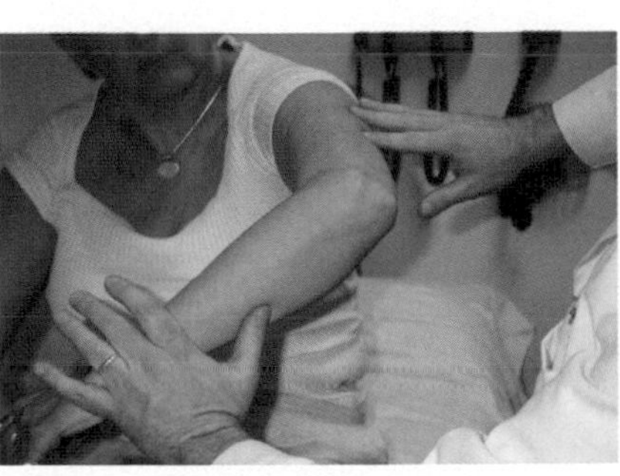

Figure 9.11.

Technique for active extension of arm at elbow. Assessment of C7 root; triceps muscle.

 **TIPS**

- Patient actively extends arm at elbow
- Apply resistance against distal forearm
- C7 problem: weakness; may have atrophy of triceps

TEACHING POINTS

BASELINE NEUROLOGIC EXAMINATION

1. Each root from C5 to T1 has discrete motor actions.
2. C4: sensory to acromioclavicular (AC) joint area; T2: to anterior axillary fold; T3: to posterior axillary fold
3. Use monofilaments or cotton-tipped swabs for sensory examination.
4. It is very important to perform to establish a baseline.

C8 root is assessed by examining the **deep finger flexors** (digits 2 and 3 anterior interosseous nerve, digits 4 and 5 ulnar nerve) and the **flexor pollicis longus** (anterior interosseous nerve). Therefore, the best screening technique for C8 is to assess **finger flexion** i.e., making a fist **(Fig. 9.12)** or **tip-to-tip "OK"** maneuver against resistance **(Fig. 9.13)**. **T1 root is** assessed by examining the **intrinsic muscles** of the hand and digits (ulnar nerve). Therefore, the best screening techniques for T1 are to assess the strength of **finger abduction** or **adduction** of digits 2 through 5 **(Figs. 9.14 and 9.15)**. (Please see also Table 10.4)

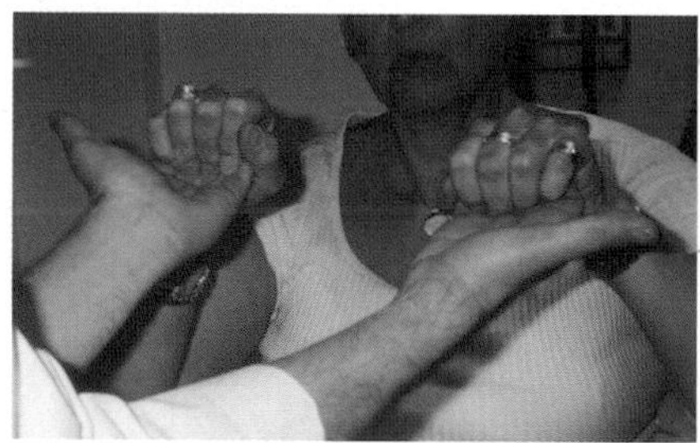

Figure 9.12.

Technique for active making a fist, finger flexion, against resistance. Assessment of C8 root.

 **TIPS**

- Patient forms a fist
- Apply resistance at fingertips
- C8 complication: weakness to making a fist; may have atrophy of long and intrinsic flexors
- C8 median nerve problem: weakness to PIP in all digits
- C8 ulnar nerve problem: weakness to DIP in digits 4 and 5

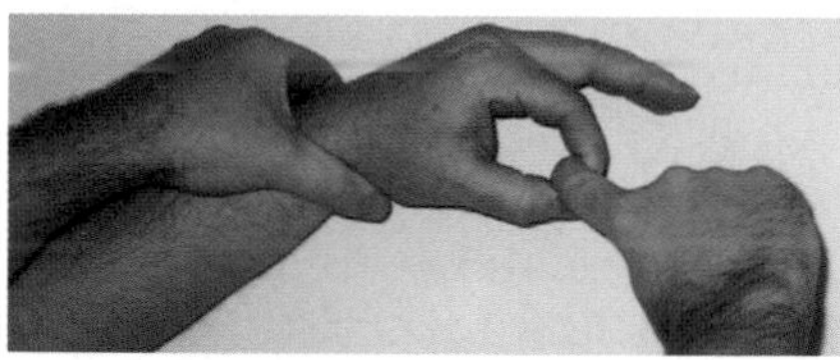

Figure 9.13.

Technique for active OK sign against resistance. Apply resistance to the tip-to-tip site to measure the median nerve, overall an assessment of C8.

 **TIPS**

- Actively perform tip-to-tip "OK" sign: flexion of both the thumb and index finger
- Apply resistance by pulling backward on the "OK" loop, at the point of the tips i.e., distal phalanges
- Normal: able to maintain the tip-to-tip "OK"
- C8 problem: weakness to tip-to-tip "OK"

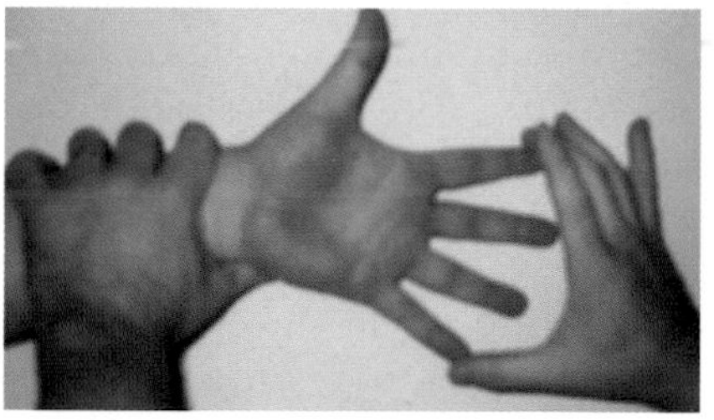

Figure 9.14.

Technique for active finger abduction against resistance. Assessment of T1.

 **TIPS**

- Patient actively abducts fingers against resistance
- Normal: able to perform
- T1 problem: weakness; may have interosseous wasting

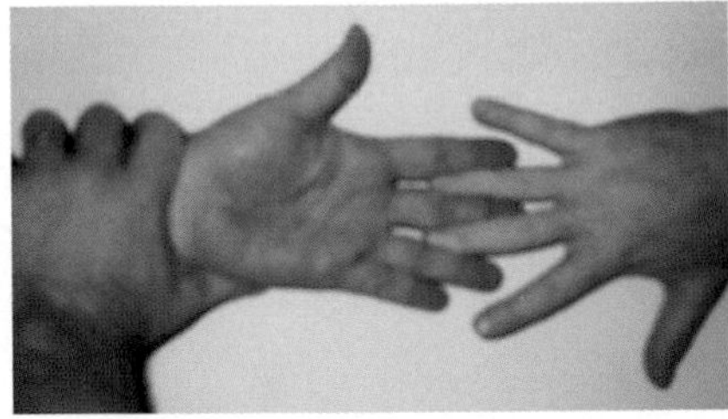

Figure 9.15.

Technique for active adduction of fingers, T1 assessment.

 **TIPS**

- Patient actively adducting fingers, with examiner's finger squeezed between them
- Normal: able to perform
- T1 problem: weakness; may have interosseous wasting
- Best overall test for T1

Box 9.2

Specific Sites for Sensory Examination of Various Roots

Root	Site; skin over the:
C4	Acromioclavicular joint
C5	Lateral antecubital fossa
C6	Dorsal forearm, radial side
C7	Olecranon process
C8	Dorsal forearm, ulnar side
T1	Medial antecubital fossa
T2	Chest wall or anterior axillary fold
T3	Posterior axillary fold

Sensory

As a companion to the motor neurologic examinations one must, also perform a screening sensory examination using a **cotton-tipped swab** or **monofilaments** to dermatomes of C4 to T2 (see **Box 9.2** for specific sites).

CARRYING POSITION

The **carrying position**, by definition, is the position of the arm at the time of patients' presentation.

Of carrying positions, the two most specific are the dead arm position and the Napoleon Bonaparte position. The **dead arm position** manifests with the forearm extended; the arm is closely held to the body and stabilized by the patient with the contralateral hand **(Fig. 9.16)**. This position is caused by either a proximal **humeral fracture** or anterior **humeral dislocation** or a burner (i.e., **stinger**). The **Bonaparte position** manifests with elbow flexed, hand in jacket, and arm adjacent to the body. Most commonly, this is caused by a posterior humeral dislocation.

Figure 9.16.

Dead-arm position.

 **TIPS**

- Patient holds arm close to body to minimize pain, supported by other hand or arm
- Consistent with an anterior glenohumeral dislocation, proximal humeral fracture, or stinger or burner

RANGE OF MOTION

Crank Tests

Crank tests are a limited set of **passive**, then **active**, range of motion (ROM) isolated to the glenohumeral joint. It is of tremendous importance to emphasize that this should be the beginning of every examination, in order to specifically assess, ROM isolated to the glenohumeral joint, and to "clear" the joint of gross problems.

Passive

This first-line examination involves the assessment of passive, then active, ROM with the shoulder and humerus in neutral position **(Fig. 9.17A)**, but

TEACHING POINTS

RANGE OF MOTION

1. Assess full range of motion (ROM) only after performing the passive and active crank test.
2. A deficit in limited active more than passive ROM indicates a muscle and tendon problem; whereas, a marked decrease in both active and passive ROM indicates a joint problem e.g., arthritis or adhesive capsulitis.
3. Full abduction of the humerus involves the glenohumeral joint with the supraspinatus and deltoid muscles to 110 degrees; the scapulothoracic joint, the upper third of the trapezius, and the levator scapulae to 170 degrees.
4. The infraspinatus muscle acts to externally rotate the humerus and to mildly abduct the humerus (Apley scratch test from above).
5. The subscapularis muscle acts to internally rotate and mildly adduct the humerus (Apley scratch test from below).

Figure 9.17.

Technique for passive crank test. **A.** Baseline. **B.** Abduction. **C.** External rotation. **D.** Internal rotation.

 **TIPS**

- Arm on patient's side with the elbow flexed to 90 degrees and forearm and wrist in a neutral position **(A)**
- Grasp the distal humerus with one hand and the distal forearm with the other hand
- Passively abduct to 30 degrees **(B)**
- Glenohumeral problem: decreased ROM
- Adhesive capsulitis: painful decreased ROM in all three directions
- First-line ROM, especially in an injured patient
- Passively externally rotate to 30 degrees **(C)**
- Passively internally rotate to 30 degrees **(D)**

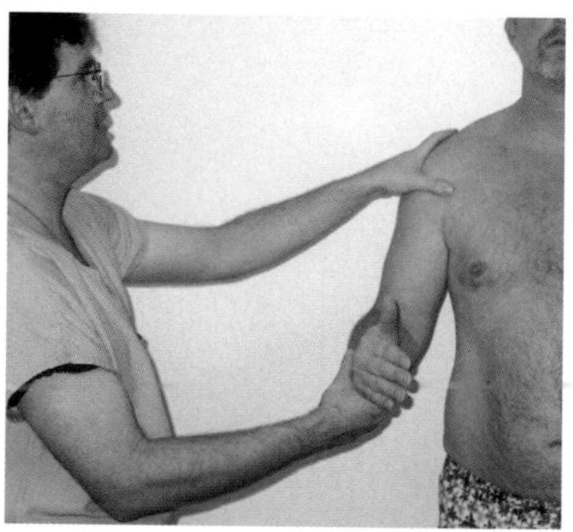

A

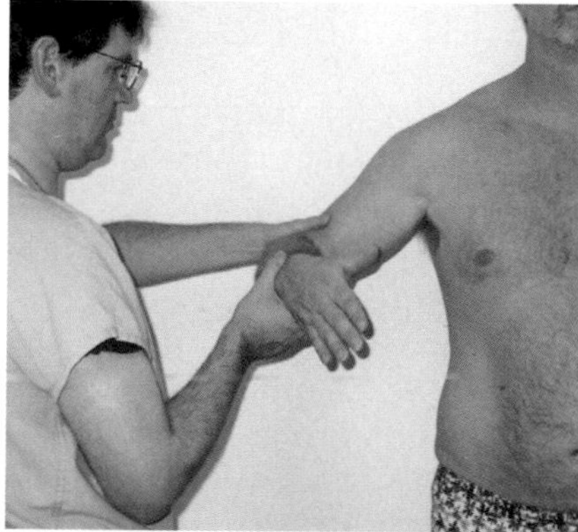

B

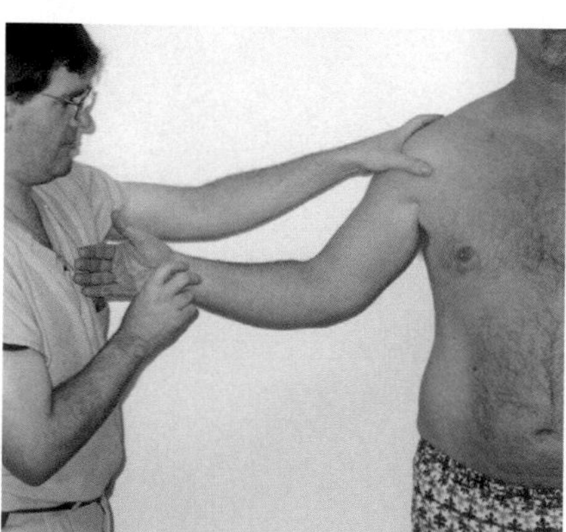

C

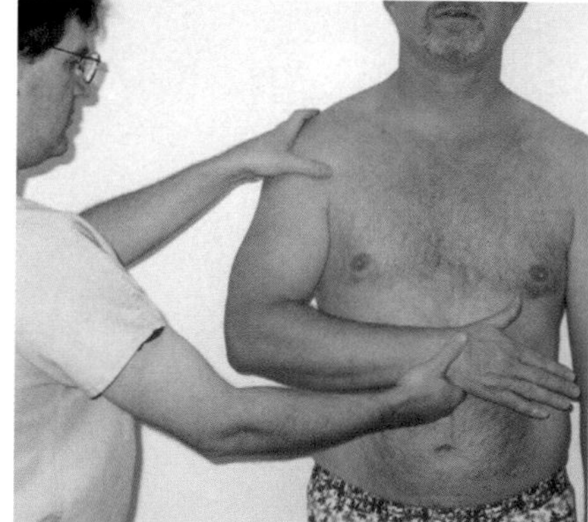

D

with the elbow flexed. **Passive abduction,** (crank-up, Fig. 9.17B) **passive external rotation** (crank out) (Fig. 9.17C) and **passive internal rotation** (crank in) (Fig. 9.17D) are performed first. **Glenohumeral joint** problems manifest with decreased ROM; **adhesive capsulitis** manifests with painful, markedly decreased ROM to all 3 components.

Active

To assess active ROM, have the individual "crank-up" **abduct against resistance** (Fig. 9.18A) to assess for **supraspinatus** or the **deltoid problems** manifest with pain or significant weakness. "Crank-out" i.e., **externally rotate against resistance** to assess the **infraspinatus** and teres minor problems which would manifest with lateral pain or significant weakness **(Fig. 9.18B)**. Finally, "crank-in" i.e., **internally rotate against resistance** (Fig. 9.18C) to assess for **subscapularis muscle** problems which would manifest with anterior pain.

Planes to Perform Range of Motion

Planes in which to perform ROM include the **coronal, scapular**, or **sagittal** plane. The **horizontal** plane i.e., a cross-section at the level of the acromioclavicular joint is useful for stress testing on the shoulder. Above this plane, the scapula thoracic joint contributes significantly to the ROM. Although the coronal and sagittal planes may seem the best planes in which to perform an examination, the truly functional plane is the scapular plane—one in which the scapulae are 30 degrees anterior to the coronal plane.

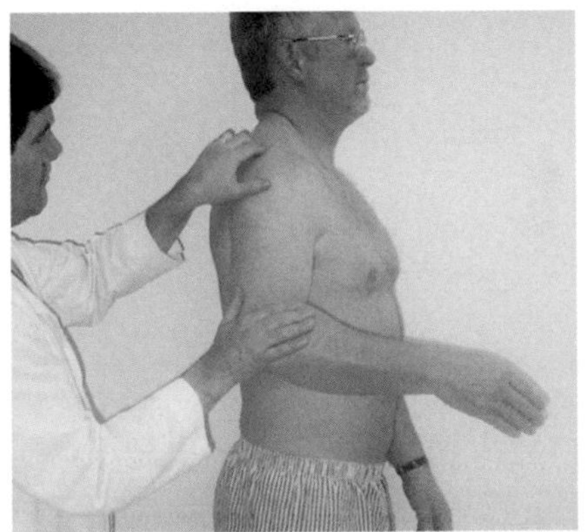

A

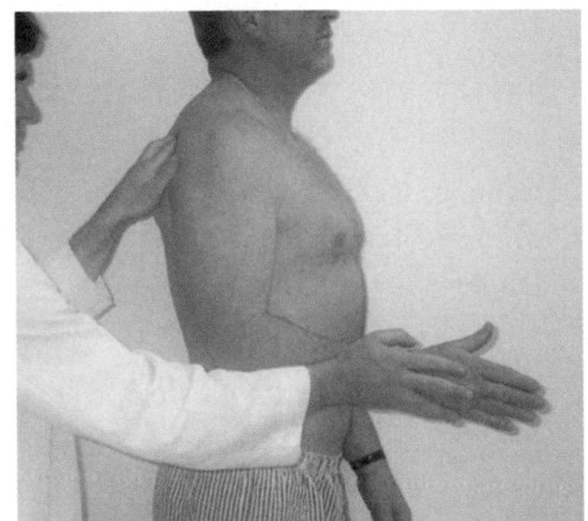

B

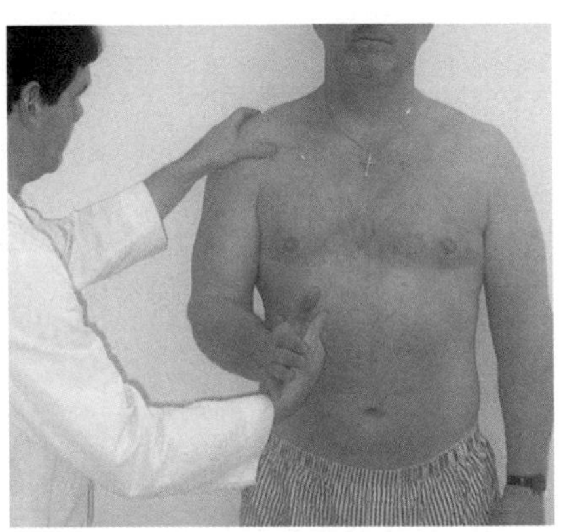

C

Figure 9.18.

Technique for active crank test. **A.** Abduction-supraspinatus. **B.** External rotation-infraspinatus. **C.** Subscapularis: internal rotation.

TIPS

- From a neutral position
- "Crank-up": Actively abduct arm, apply resistance given at the distal humerus **(A)**
- Supraspinatus problem: pain in lateral posterior shoulder, above scapular spine
- "Crank-out": Actively externally rotate against the hand on the forearm **(B)**
- Infraspinatus or teres minor problem: pain or weakness in the lateral or posterior shoulder, below the scapular spine
- "Crank-in": Actively internally rotate against the hand on the forearm **(C)**
- Subscapularis problem: pain in the anterior shoulder, weakness

Table 9.3. **Shoulder: Passive Range of Motion***

Action	Baseline position	Degrees
Forward flexion	Neutral	170
Backward flexion	Neutral	45
Internal rotation	Neutral	75
External rotation	Neutral	80
Adduction	Neutral	45
Abduction	Neutral	170

*Total, including glenohumeral and scapulothoracic joints.

Passive

Passive ROM of the entire shoulder i.e., the glenohumeral and the scapulothoracic joints includes **adduction** to 45 degrees, **abduction** to 170 degrees, **external rotation** to 80 degrees, **internal rotation** to 75 degrees, **forward flexion** to 170 degrees, and **backward flexion** to 50 degrees **(Table 9.3)**.

Active (Table 9.4)

Active **adduction** is best assessed in the scapular plane, which involves the pectoralis major muscles. Active **abduction** is best assessed in the coronal or scapular plane. The muscles involved include the supraspinatus, deltoid, levator scapula, and trapezius. Abduction in the **first 30 degrees** is exclusively the supraspinatus muscle; from **30** to **100 degrees** is the deltoid muscle; from **100** to **170 degrees** are the trapezius and levator scapula muscles (Table 9.4). (This elegant differentiation was described by Popper and Walker in 1972.) Active **external rotation** is performed as an Apley scratch test from above. Muscles involved include the infraspinatus, teres minor, and posterior deltoid. Active

Table 9.4. **Shoulder: Active Range of Motion**

Action	Extrinsic Muscles	Nerve	Intrinsic Muscles	Nerve
Forward flexion	Deltoid: anterior Biceps: long head	Axillary Musculocutaneous		
Backward flexion	Latissimus dorsi Teres major Triceps: long head Deltoid: posterior	Thoracodorsal (C7) Subscapular Radial Axillary		
Abduction 0–30 degrees			Supraspinatus	Suprascapular
Abduction 30–100 degrees	Deltoid	Axillary		
Abduction 100–170 degrees	Trapezius Levator scapulae	CNXI C2 and C3		
Adduction	Pectoralis major Deltoid-anterior	Pectoral nerve C7 Axillary		
Internal Rotation	Latissimus dorsi Teres major	Thoracodorsal Subscapular	Subscapularis	Infrascapular
External rotation	Deltoid: posterior	Axillary	Infraspinatus Teres minor	Suprascapular Axillary
Scapular elevation	Upper trapezius Levator scapula	CNXI Roots C2, C3		
Scapular retraction/extension	Rhomboid major Middle trapezius	Dorsal scapular (C4 and C5) CNXI		
Scapular protraction/flexion	Serratus anterior	Long thoracic (C5, 6, 7)		

internal rotation is performed as an Apley scratch test from below. Muscles involved include subscapularis, latissimus dorsi, and teres major. Active **forward flexion** is best performed in the sagittal plane. Muscles involved include the long head of the biceps and the anterior deltoid. Active **backward flexion** is best performed in the sagittal plane. Muscles involved include the latissimus dorsi, teres major, long head of the triceps and the posterior deltoid.

Scapular Movements

Scapular movement is at the scapulothoracic, the acromioclavicular, and the sternoclavicular joints. This set of joints provides stability when arm lower than horizontal plane; provides mobility above the horizontal plane. **Scapular elevation** involves the levator scapulae and upper one third of the trapezius muscles; **scapular forward flexion** (protraction) involves the serratus anterior muscle. **Scapular backward flexion** (retraction) involves the rhomboid muscle and middle one third of the trapezius muscle.

SHOULDER EXAMINATION: ANTERIOR

Separation of the acromioclavicular (AC) joint manifests with acute pain, tenderness, and ecchymosis over the lateral aspect of the anterior shoulder,

TEACHING POINTS

ANTERIOR SHOULDER EXAMINATION

1. Dead arm sign is present in humeral dislocation, proximal humeral fracture, or an acute burner or stinger.
2. Inspection and clavicular percussion test are quite satisfactory first maneuvers in the assessment of the anterior shoulder.
3. Acromioclavicular (AC) separation can result in damage to the suprascapular nerve (atrophy of supraspinatus muscle) or, less commonly, axillary nerve (atrophy of deltoid muscle).
4. AC separation is a relatively common entity that is assessed by inspection, palpation, crossover sign, percussion, and the AC stress test of Hutson.
5. Pectoralis major rupture is rare; knowledge of and appropriate clinical suspicion i.e., acute pain and swelling in the chest after bench pressing or water skiing is needed.
6. Apley scratch test from below is an excellent maneuver to assess the subscapularis and other muscles involved in internal rotation i.e., latissimus dorsi and teres major.
7. Yergason maneuver is effective in the evaluation for bicipital tendinitis.
8. Brachial plexopathy, from either stretching or entrapment, may be unmasked and defined by applying pressure (compression) over the anterior scalene muscles.
9. A stinger (burner) is an acute stretch of the brachial plexus.

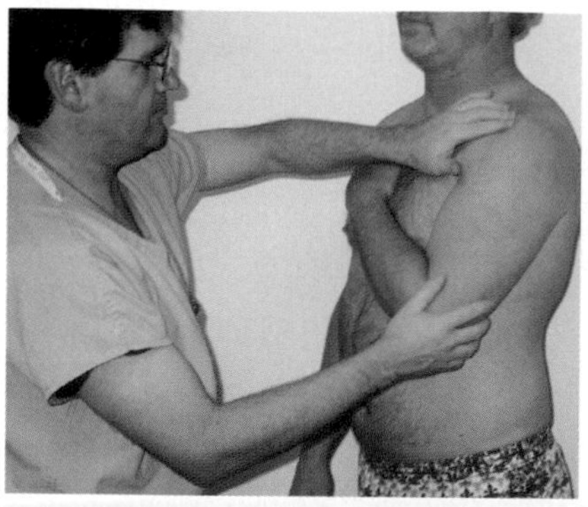

Figure 9.19.

Technique for crossover maneuver in acromioclavicular (AC) joint assessment.

 **TIPS**

- Patient actively uses arm and forearm to cross over and touch the contralateral acromioclavicular (AC) joint
- Acromioclavicular joint problem: tenderness over the AC joint

specifically and reproducibly over the AC joint itself. There is reproducible discrete tenderness over the AC joint with the **clavicle percussion sign** in which examiner percusses over midclavicle, the **cross-over test** in which the patient actively uses arm and forearm to cross over and touch the contralateral AC joint **(Fig. 9.19)** and the **acromioclavicular stress test** of Hutson in which the patient actively forward flexes the arm to 90 degrees i.e., to the horizontal plane and then the examiner passively adducts the arm in this plane to reproduce pain at the site **(Fig. 9.20)**. An **abduction arc** in which patient actively abducts humerus (Table 9.4) is normal in range, but painful over the AC joint from 140 to 170 degrees of abduction. **Complications** of AC joint separation include clavicular fracture, axillary or suprascapular nerve damage; therefore, it is important to assess the function of the deltoid and supraspinatus muscles. The usual mechanism of injury is direct blunt trauma, usually by playing a contact sports e.g., football without wearing shoulder pads or being "checked into the boards" while playing ice hockey **(Figs. 9.21 and 9.22)**. **Clavicular fracture** manifests with swelling and often a visible and palpable deformity in the clavicle, often caused by either blunt direct trauma to the area or a fall on an outstretched hand.

Sternoclavicular (SC) subluxation manifests with pain, tenderness, and ecchymosis specific and reproducible to this site. The SC joint tenderness is reproduced or increased with the **clavicular percussion test**. The company SC subluxation keeps includes rib fractures, a medial clavicle fracture, fracture of the sternum, and a pneumothorax. Therefore, the examination must include **chest wall palpation** and **chest and lungs auscultation**. The underlying mechanism is one of a direct blow to the medial clavicle e.g., hitting the upper chest wall with a steering wheel in a motor vehicle accident or being "speared" by the helmeted head of a football player **(Fig. 9.23)**.

Virchow's or Troisier's node manifests with an enlarged, nontender hard nodule or mass in the left supraclavicular fossa **(Fig. 9.24)**. This is often fixed to the underlying tissue or overlying bone. The presence of such a lymph node indicates metastatic carcinoma from the breast or from an intraabdominal source. The sensitivity of the examination is increased with cough or the Valsalva's maneuver. **Hodgkin's disease** manifests with large, matted bilateral nodes. These nodes are rubbery and, when advanced, the patient has a bullneck appearance **(Fig. 9.25)**.

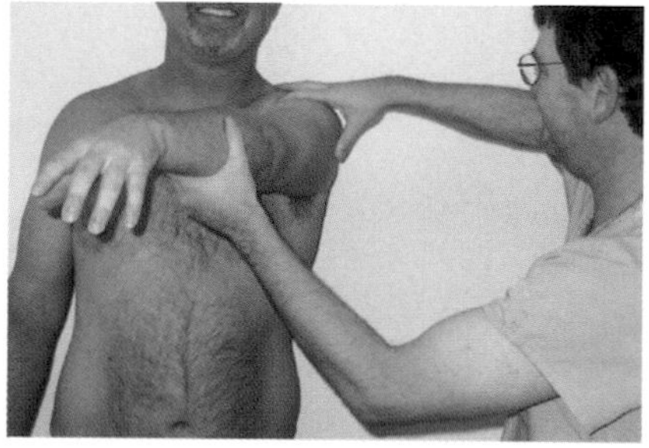

Figure 9.20.

Technique for acromioclavicular (AC) stress test of Hutson.

 **TIPS**

- Patient actively forward flexes arm to 90 degrees, that is, to the horizontal plane
- Passively adduct the arm in this plane
- Acromioclavicular joint problem: tenderness over AC joint
- Complements palpation

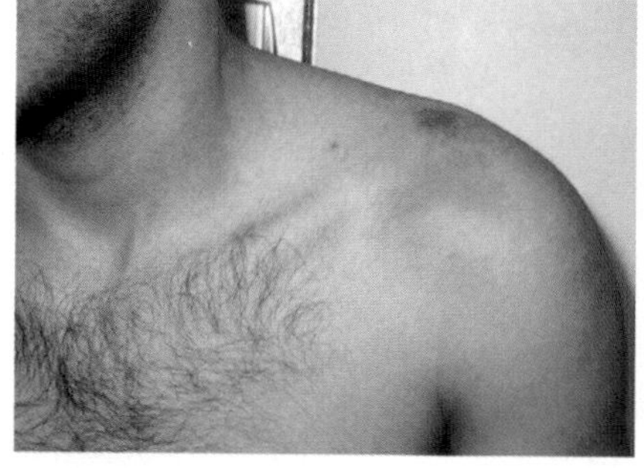

A

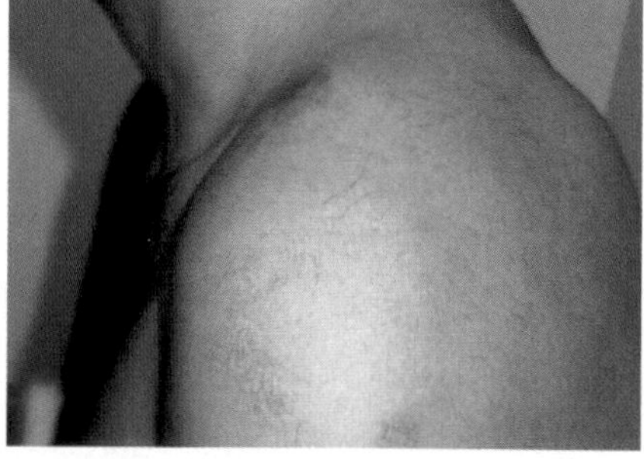

B

Figure 9.21.

Mild acromioclavicular (AC) separation in a hockey player. **A.** Front view. **B.** Side view.

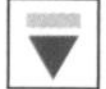 **TIPS**

- Visually inspect the anterior shoulder
- Mild AC separation: ecchymosis and swelling over the AC joint

Thoracic outlet syndrome manifests with tingling, pain and purple discoloration in the arm. The manifestations of this syndrome are especially evident in those who perform overhead activities. The company it keeps may include weakness due to brachial plexus entrapment. See brachial plexus (page 242). There is reproduction of the manifestations with **Adson's** maneuver: the patient's head and neck are extended, the head is rotated toward the side being tested, and the patient inhales maximally during the examination **(Fig. 9.26)**. In addition, the manifestations are reproduced with the **hyperabduction maneuver** in which the patient's head and neck are extended and the arm on the symptomatic side is placed in full elevation **(Fig. 9.27)**. To maximize sensitivity, the patient may be instructed to squeeze a tennis ball ten times. The company it keeps includes diminished radial pulse and venous congestion of affected hand. Thoracic outlet syndrome is most commonly the result of swelling or hypertrophy of the anterior scalene muscles or the presence of an extra cervical rib.

Bicipital tendonitis manifests with tenderness over the bicipital groove, a positive **Yergason** maneuver, in which symptoms are reproduced on active elbow flexion and forearm supination against resistance **(Fig. 9.28)**. According to Diner and coworkers, the sensitivity for this procedure is 86%. In addition, the tenderness is reproduced with active **forward flexion** of the humerus against resistance and with **active scapular forward flexion** (sometimes referred to as Speed's test) **(Fig. 9.29)**. Bicipital tendonitis is often secondary to another problem, most commonly a rotator cuff tear or tendonitis. **Long head of the biceps tendon tear** manifests with mild weakness to elbow flexion and forearm supination at the elbow and moderate weakness to **forward flexion** at the humerus **(Fig. 9.30)**. The company it keeps includes a palpable, flaccid mass of noncontracting muscle present in the belly of the biceps. **Acute** bicipital tendon tears manifest with marked swelling that is tender and ecchymosis

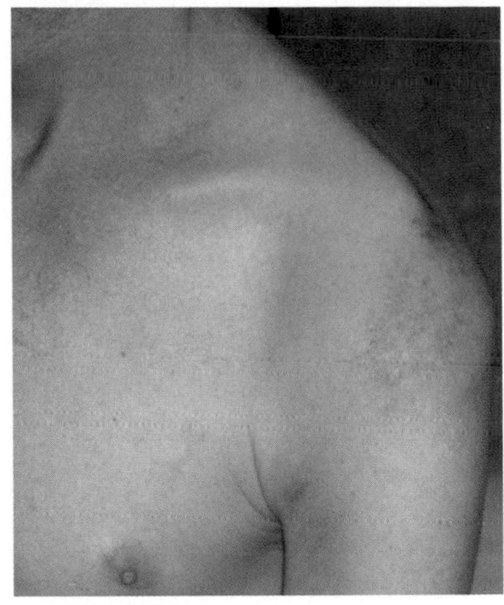

Figure 9.22.

Severe acromioclavicular (AC) separation with complication of axillary nerve damage.

 **TIPS**

- Visually inspect the anterior shoulder
- Severe AC separation: visible and palpable separation of the clavicle from the acromion

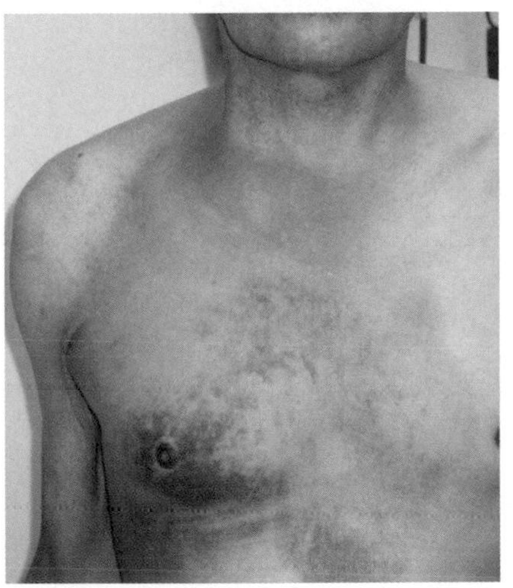

A

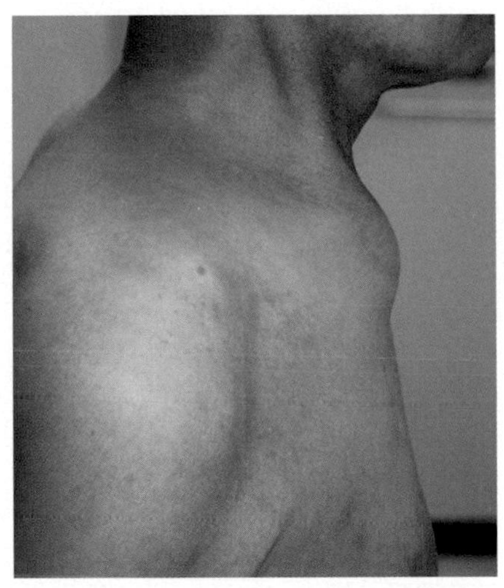

B

Figure 9.23.

Sternoclavicular separation as the result of a motor vehicle accident (MVA). May have severe sequelae. **A.** Front view. **B.** Side view.

 **TIPS**

- Sternoclavicular (SC) separation: swelling and ecchymosis over SC joint site
- Evaluate for a concurrent clavicular or rib fracture or even pneumothorax

Figure 9.24.

Troisier's node in a patient with metastatic pancreatic carcinoma.

 **TIPS**

- Virchow's or Troisier's node: left supraclavicular node hard and fixed; extremely suggestive of metastatic carcinoma

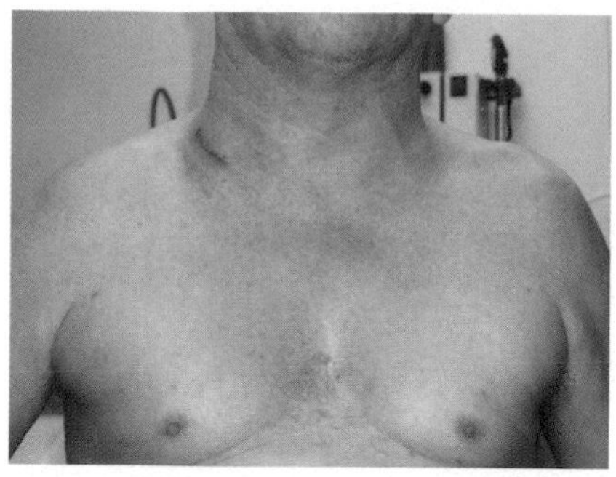

Figure 9.25.

The bullneck of Hodgkin's disease. Massive, bilateral cervical lymphadenopathy. This patient had Stage 3B Hodgkin's disease.

 **TIPS**

- Bullneck appearance to the neck due to massive cervical lymphadenopathy
- Ask patient regarding any "B" symptoms

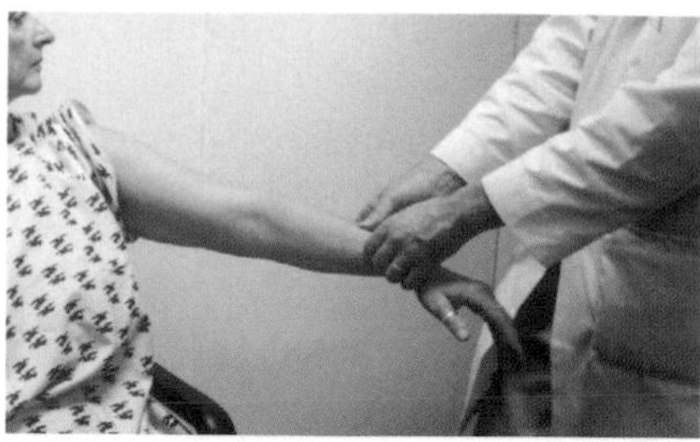

Figure 9.26.

Technique for Adson's maneuver in thoracic outlet syndrome assessment.

 **TIPS**

- Head or neck is extended; head is rotated toward the side being tested
- Patient maximally inhales and holds it
- Palpate the radial pulse; ask patient if tingling, paresthesia in affected hand. Note any purple discoloration in the hand
- Normal: no diminution of pulse; note any purple discoloration or tingling
- Thoracic outlet: diminished radial pulse, tingling in hand and, often, purple discoloration

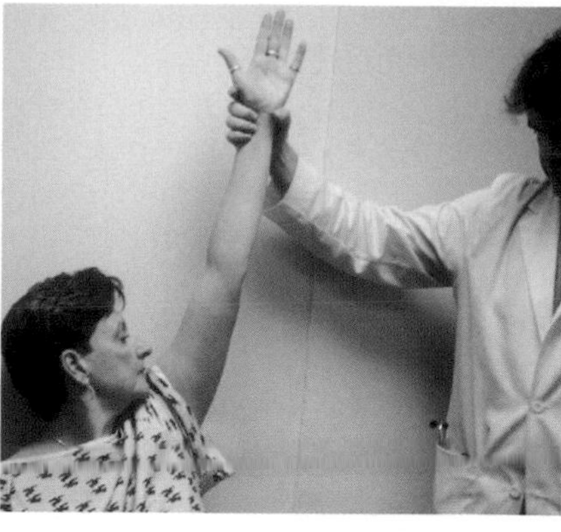

Figure 9.27.

Technique for hyperabduction maneuver in the assessment of thoracic outlet syndrome.

 **TIPS**

- Head or neck is extended; ipsilateral arm is in full elevation
- Palpate the radial pulse; ask patient if tingling, paresthesia in affected hand
- Notes any purple discoloration in the affected hand
- Thoracic outlet: diminished radial pulse, tingling in hand, and, often, purple discoloration

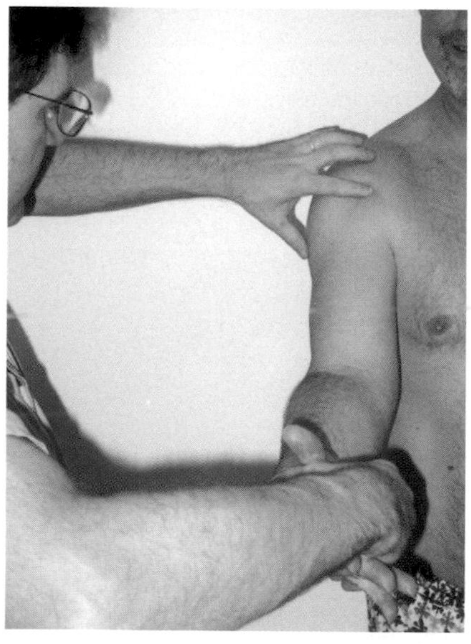

Figure 9.28.

Technique for the Yergason maneuver for assessing bicipital tendinitis.

 **TIPS**

- Patient flexes elbow and supinates the forearm or wrist against resistance
- Bicipital tendonitis: maximal pain in the bicipital groove
- Tear of the long head of the biceps muscle: increase in prominence of flaccid mass in the arm

Figure 9.29.

Technique for active forward flexion of the humerus; used to assess for bicipital tendinitis.

 **TIPS**

- Active forward flexion of arm against resistance
- Bicipital tendonitis: maximal pain in the bicipital groove
- Tear of the long head of the biceps muscle: increase in prominence of flaccid mass in the arm

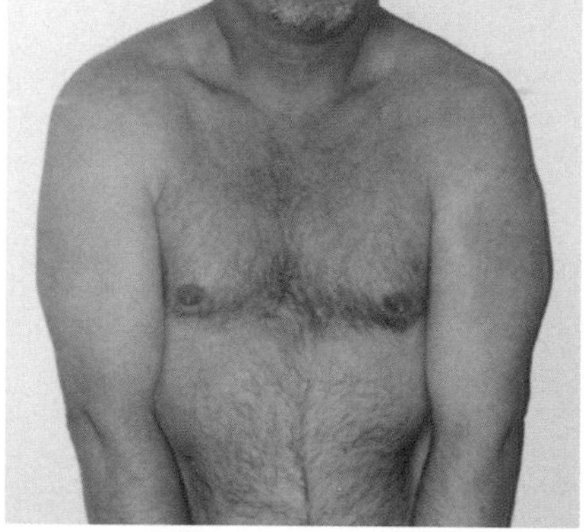

Figure 9.30.

Technique for active adduction of the humeri to assess for bicipital tendonitis.

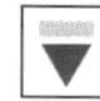 **TIPS**

- Patient actively adducts the arms, in the horizontal plane
- Press palms of hands together in midline
- Bicipital tendonitis: pain in the bicipital groove
- Pectoralis major problem: anterior chest wall pain, even a flaccid mass

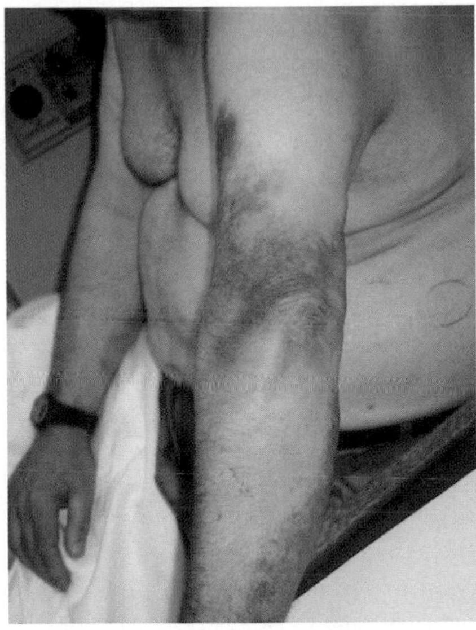

Figure 9.31.

Acute long head biceps tendon rupture. Note the large ecchymosis present in arm.

 **TIPS**

- Acute biceps tendon or muscle tear: painful with significant swelling and ecchymosis

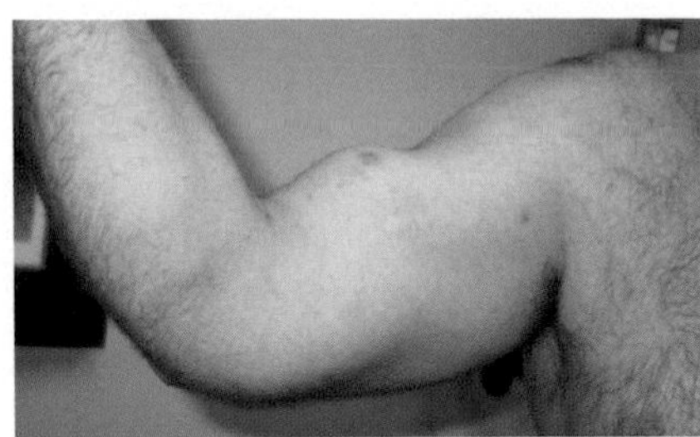

Figure 9.32.

Old tear of the long head of the biceps tendon.

 **TIPS**

- Old long head of biceps tendon tear: painless flaccid mass in the belly of biceps

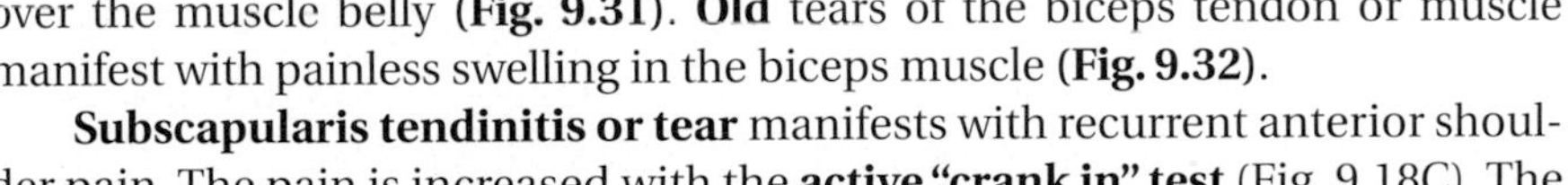

over the muscle belly **(Fig. 9.31)**. **Old** tears of the biceps tendon or muscle manifest with painless swelling in the biceps muscle **(Fig. 9.32)**.

Subscapularis tendinitis or tear manifests with recurrent anterior shoulder pain. The pain is increased with the **active "crank in" test** (Fig. 9.18C). The company it keeps includes pain is increased and limitation to motion is noted with the **scratch test from below** in which the patient is instructed to place hands and thumbs as far up on the back from below as possible **(Fig. 9.33)**. **Tenderness to palpation** is noted specific to the lesser tuberosity. Finally, in a tear there is weakness on the affected side to the **posterior lift test** (Test of Gerber and Krushell)* in which the patient performs a scratch test from below, palm placed posteriorly and presses posteriorly against the examiner's hand **(Fig. 9.34)**. A mechanism of injury for a subscapularis tear is falling with

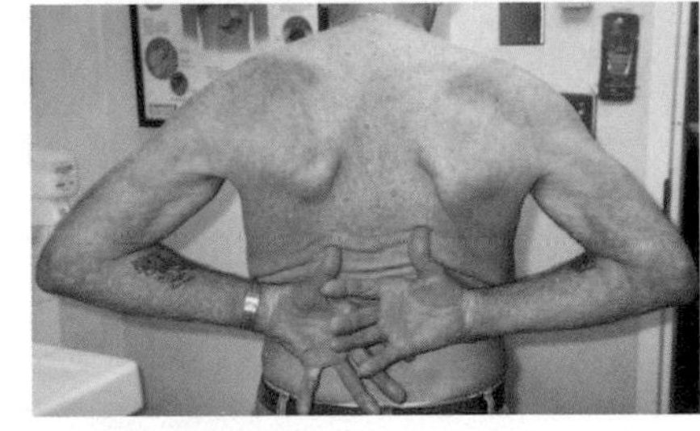

Figure 9.33.

Technique for scratch test from below. Assessment of subscapularis muscle and tendon.

 **TIPS**

- Patient actively places hands behind back with thumbs as far up on scapulae as possible
- This is a functional test of internal rotation
- Normal: T7 level bilaterally, muscles include subscapularis, latissimus dorsi, and teres major
- Subscapularis problems: anterior pain and lower thumb placement

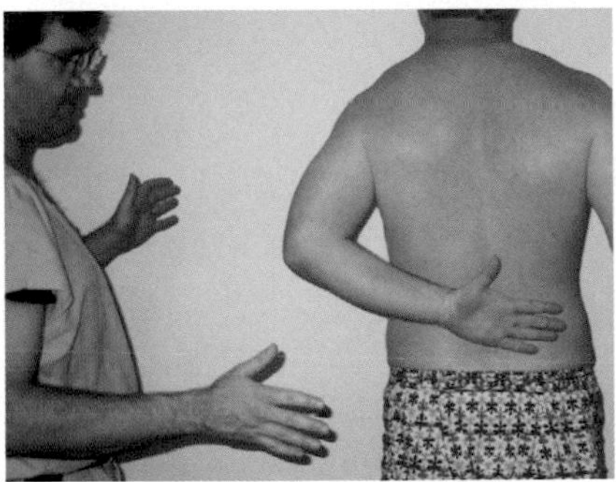

A

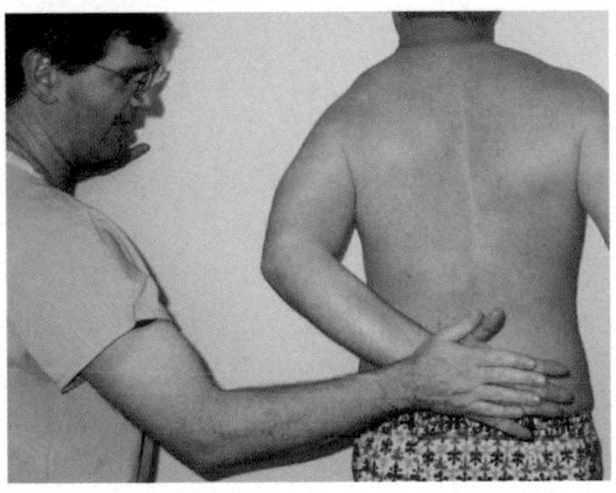

B

Figure 9.34.

Technique for posterior lift test to assess for subscapularis tear versus tendinitis.

 **TIPS**

- Apley scratch test from below, palm of patient's hand is facing posteriorly
- Place hand on patient's palm
- Patient actively attempts to press posteriorly on the examiner's hand
- Subscapularis tendinitis: anterior shoulder pain increased
- Subscapularis tear: weakness for this procedure

*Also known as, "Lift-off test of Gerber."

the elbow extended, hand outstretched, and arm in backward flexion. **Brachial plexus injury** (stinger or burner) manifests with anterior shoulder pain and an increase of the pain with palpation or application of mild pressure to the **anterior scalene area**. In addition, the patient has a **dead arm position** (Fig. 9.16) and acute weakness and numbness of the entire arm. A stinger results from the acute stretching of the brachial plexus, usually by blunt trauma involving someone pulling down on a shoulder and concurrently pushing the patient's neck to the other side e.g., a cornerback interfering with a wide receiver. Finally, thoracic outlet (see page 239) may cause this. A more common factor is the patient wearing a backpack that is either ill-fitting or too heavy "backpacker's arms," in this the symptoms are bilateral but usually milder. The cervical spine must be assessed in all cases to rule out cervical spine trauma. **Pectoralis muscle tear or strain** manifests with acute painful swelling of the anterior chest, often with ecchymosis. A flaccid mass is also noted in the belly of the muscles that becomes more prominent with **active scapular forward flexion**. A common mechanism for this uncommon entity includes, the patient was bench-pressing and felt a tear or pop or was water skiing and in the process of falling or in the process of being pulled upward felt a pop or tear.

SHOULDER EXAMINATION: LATERAL

Supraspinatus tendon tears manifest with pain in the location of the muscle, superior to the spine of the scapula in the posterior shoulder. There is reproduc-

TEACHING POINTS

LATERAL SHOULDER EXAMINATION

1. The supraspinatus and infraspinatus muscles are posterior and lateral in location; they insert on the greater tuberosity of the humerus.
2. One of the best examples of a motion that is seated in the lateral shoulder is that of overhand throwing or pitching: abduction (supraspinatus) and external rotation (infraspinatus).
3. Weakness of the rotator cuff can lead to either impingement i.e., the abnormal migration of the head of the humerus into the subacromial space or laxity i.e., abnormal displacement of the head of the humerus from the glenohumeral space.
4. The anterior apprehension, the posterior drawer, the multidirectional laxity, and Liu's crank test are all excellent examinations to perform on a patient with a significant history of rotator cuff damage who is at risk for laxity.
5. Laxity begets laxity.
6. Anterior or posterior laxity indicates a local tendon problem; multidirectional laxity indicates a systemic problem or laxity of multiple tendons.
7. The Neer and Walsh impingement and Hawkins impingement signs are excellent tests to perform for a patient with significant history of rotator cuff damage who is at risk for impingement.
8. Glenoid labrum tears are most often of superior and posterior aspect (SLAP).

Table 9.5. Features of Supraspinatus Syndromes

Diagnosis	Location	Codman's	Atrophy	Company It Keeps
Old Tear	Posterior/lateral	Passive abduction, normal Active abduction, limited	Atrophy	Drop sign at 30 Supraspinous test Weakness Jobe's sign: weakness
Acute Tear	Posterior/lateral	Passive abduction, limited Active abduction, limited	Swelling	Drop sign at 30 Supraspinous test Weakness and pain Jobe's sign: pain and weakness
Tendinitis	Lateral, slight Posterior	Passive abduction, limited Active abduction, limited	Mild atrophy	No drop sign Supraspinous test Weakness Jobe's sign: weakness Hawkins impingement: pain

tion of pain with the crank-up test (Fig. 9.18A). Of interest is that Lyons and coworkers, in 1992, looked at the evidence behind the physical examination in the diagnosis of rotator cuff tears. They determined that with examination alone performed on 42 patients had a sensitivity of 91% and specificity of 75% for rotator cuff tears. The company it keeps is specific to the underlying supraspinatus problem **(Table 9.5)**. A **complete old tear of the supraspinous muscle** manifests with a Codman's maneuver in which there is normal passive abduction but severely limited active abduction **(Fig. 9.35)**. In addition, on inspection atrophy of the supraspinatus muscle is noted **(Fig. 9.36)**. **Acute tear of the supraspinatus** tendon manifests with marked pain, tenderness, swelling, and ecchymosis to the lateral and posterior shoulder. With Codman's maneuver there is severe limitation to both active and passive abduction. **Supraspinatus tendonitis** manifests with moderate to significant lateral shoulder pain, focused especially at the greater tuberosity. With Codman's maneuver there is moderate to severe limitation to both passive and active abduction. Supraspinatus tendonitis is often associated with, and very difficult to differentiate from, a complete supraspinatus tear, but can be done by the **Hawkins impingement** maneuver

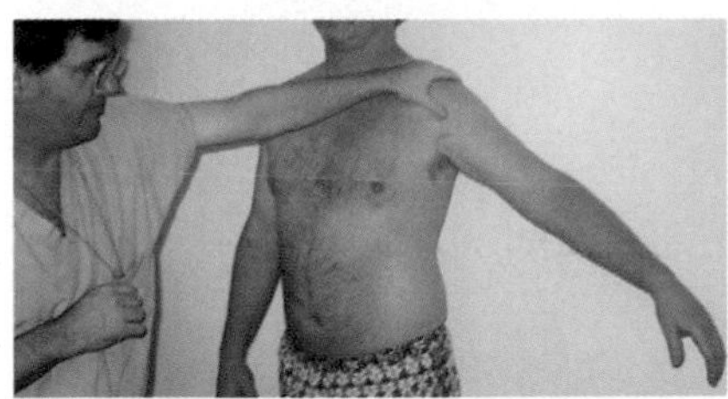

A

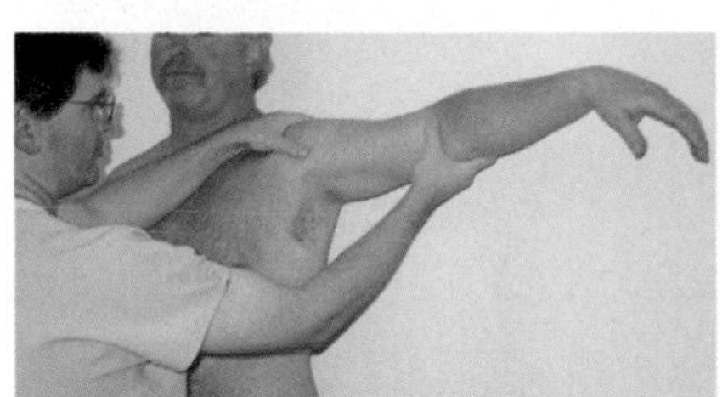

B

Figure 9.35.

Technique for Codman's maneuver in chronic supraspinatus tear. Note the limitation to active **(A)**, but not passive **(B)**, abduction.

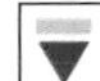

TIPS

- Places one hand on acromion of the scapula
- Instruct patient to actively abduct humerus at the glenohumeral joint
- Normal: 100 degrees of abduction
- Abnormal: <100 degrees of abduction
- Old supraspinatus tear: limitation of active **(A)** but not passive **(B)** abduction

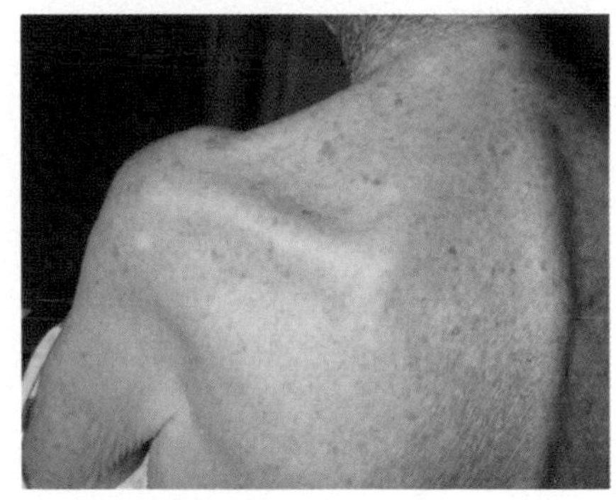

Figure 9.36.

Old rotator cuff tear, significant atrophy of the cuff muscles.

TIPS

- Inspect the shoulder from the back and side, compare with the other side
- Old supraspinatus or infraspinatus tear: atrophy with prominence of scapular spine

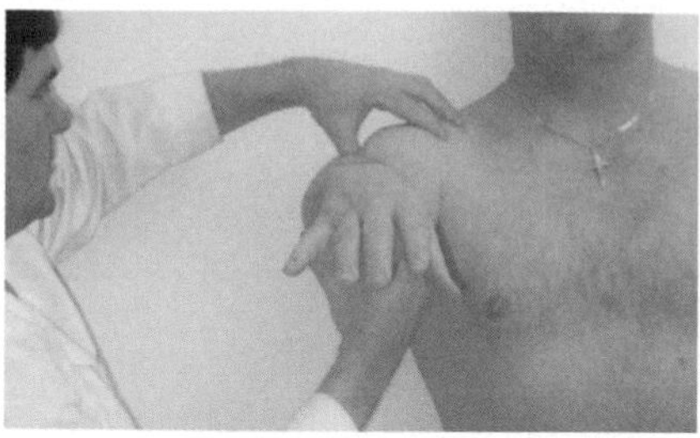

A

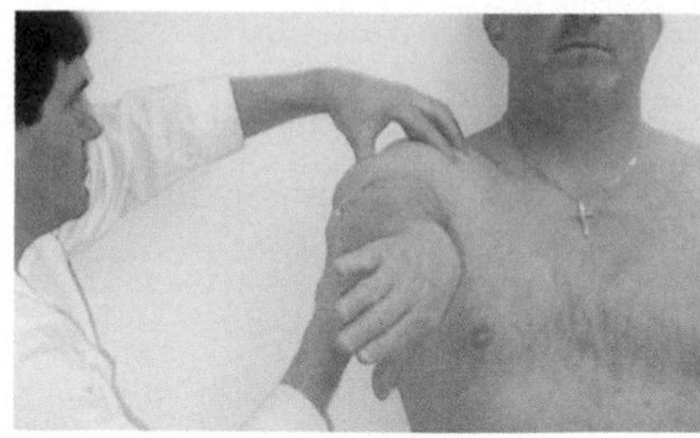

B

Figure 9.37.

Technique for Hawkins supraspinous impingement test. Excellent maneuver for the impingement of a supraspinatus tendinitis.

TIPS

- Patient standing
- Passively or actively forward flex to 90 degrees with hand in neutral position
- Grasp the distal humerus and passively internally rotate the humerus, thus jamming the greater tuberosity into the coracoacromial ligament
- Supraspinatus tendonitis pain at the lateral shoulder with this maneuver

(Fig. 9.37). With the patients arm actively forward flexed to 90 degrees and hand in neutral position, the examiner grasps the distal humerus and passively internally rotates the humerus. This technique jams the greater tuberosity into the coracoacromial ligament and any **tendinitis** reproduces the pain. The **adductor glide test** (drop sign) is one in which the patient fully abducts the arm and then slowly, gracefully adducts the arm in a steady glide. This is repeated three times **(Fig. 9.38)**. A supraspinatus **tear** causes a drop at 30 degrees. The **supraspinatus test**, in which the patient stand with an arm at 90 degrees of abduction in the scapular plane; the examiner then passively internally rotates the arm so that

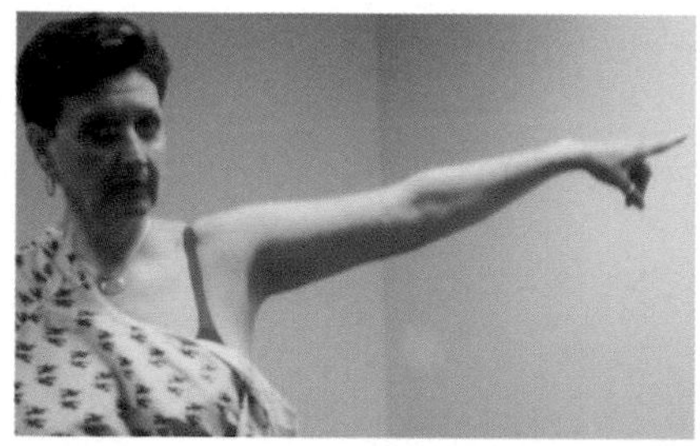

A

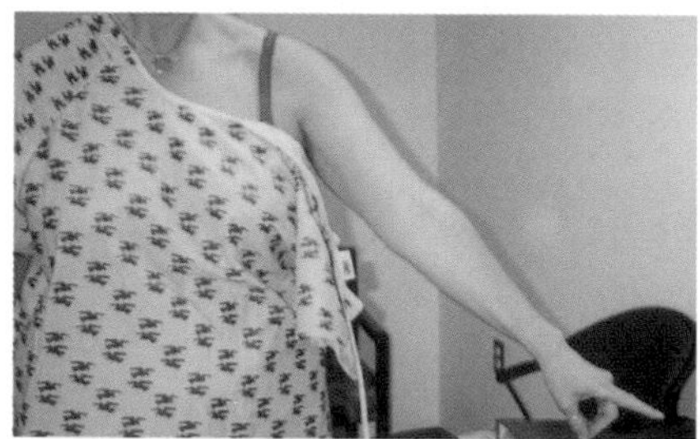

B

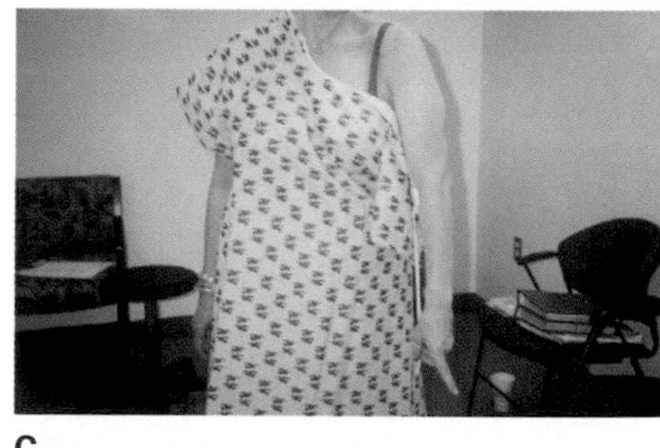

C

Figure 9.38.

Technique for adductor glide or "drop" sign for a supraspinatus tear. **A.** Full abduction. **B.** Glide to 30 degrees. **C.** Drop at 30 degrees.

TIPS

- Patient in neutral position, use the scapular plane
- Patient actively fully abducts arm
- Then patient actively adducts the arm in a slow, steady, glide
- This is repeated three times
- Normal: glide is intact
- Supraspinatus tear: drop of adduction at 30 degrees to 0
- Supraspinatus tendonitis: pain from 30 to 0 degrees, but no drop

the thumb is pointed downward and place downward pressure on the distal humerus **(Fig. 9.39)**. A **supraspinatus tear** or a tear of the **glenoid labrum** will manifest with a slip. **Jobe's test**, have the patient stand with arms and hands in neutral position; then, the examiner places the palms of hands on the patients distal humeri bilaterally and instructs the patient to actively abduct the arms against resistance **(Fig. 9.40)**. A supraspinatus tear manifests with weakness, whereas, **tendinitis** with pain (Table 9.5).

Often, there is concurrent **bicipital tendonitis** associated with the supraspinatus tear. Furthermore, concurrent tears of the infraspinatus and teres minor tendons may be present. The most common **acute mechanisms** of developing a supraspinatus tear include lifting a heavy object with the arm extended in the horizontal and then having the arm pulled anteriorly e.g., lifting a child into or out of a car seat and slipping while lifting. The most common **overuse mechanism** is repetitive overhand throwing of an object e.g., pitching a baseball without proper warm-up.

Deltoid atrophy manifests with gross atrophy of the deltoid muscle and weakness to active abduction from 30 to 100 degrees. This most commonly results from axillary nerve damage.

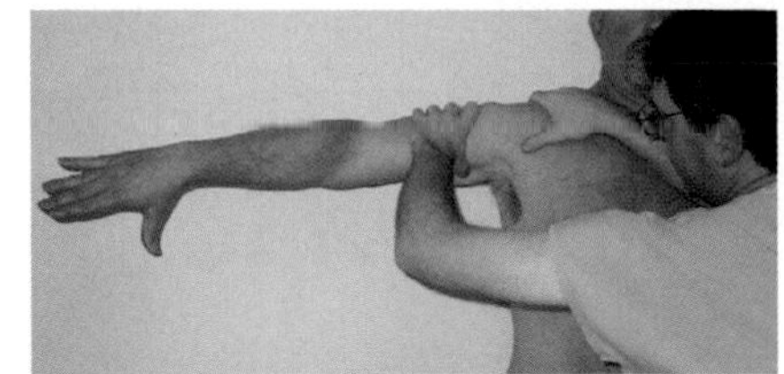

Figure 9.39.

Technique to test for a supraspinatus tear.

TIPS

- Patient stands with arm at 90 degrees of abduction in the scapular plane
- Arm is internally rotated so that the thumb is pointed downward
- Place downward pressure on the patient's distal humerus
- Supraspinatus or glenoid labrum tear: weakness and a drop
- Supraspinatus tendonitis: pain in lateral shoulder

Infraspinatus

Infraspinatus problems manifest with pain in the posterior or lateral shoulder. The **external crank test** "crank-out" (Fig. 9.18B) will reproduce the pain and localize it to an area inferior to the spine of the scapula. Also marked pain and decreased external rotation are noted with the **active scratch test from the top**. For this test, the patient actively externally rotates the arms so that the thumbs are as low on back as possible. Normal is approximately the superior angle of the scapula. Weakness is often noted to the external crank as well. As the teres minor is invariably intimately applied to the infraspinatus, it is invariably injured also. In addition, concurrent **supraspinatus** problems are very common. This is due to repetitive external rotation above the head, e.g., throwing or in volley ball.

Although it is difficult to differentiate tears of the infraspinous muscle from tendonitis, some tests do assist the clinician in this endeavor. **Infraspinatus tears** that are **old** manifest with **atrophy** of the muscle belly inferior to the spine of the scapula. Weakness to active external rotation is noted with the **scratch test from above (Fig. 9.41)**. **Infraspinatus tendonitis** manifests with no atrophy, but severe limitation to active external rotation with the **scratch test from above**.

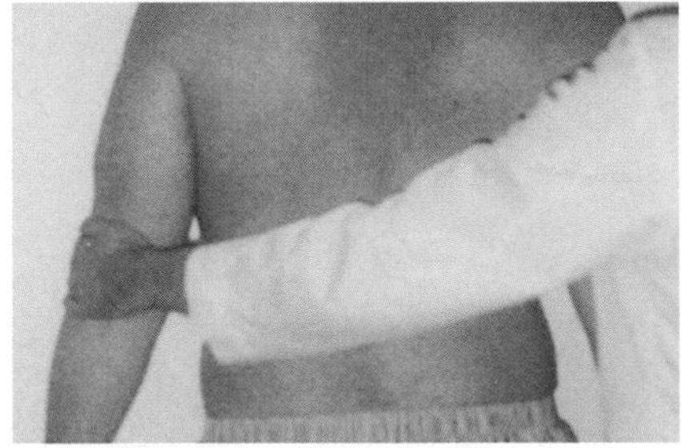

Figure 9.40.

Technique for Jobe's sign to assess a supraspinatus tear versus tendinitis.

TIPS

- Patient stands with arms and hands in neutral position
- Place palms of hand on the patient's distal arms, bilaterally
- In scapular plane, patient actively abducts arms
- Supraspinatus tear: weakness to abduction from 0 to 30 degrees
- Supraspinatus tendonitis: pain over lateral shoulder
- A derivative of the "crank-out" test

Laxity and Impingement

Weakness of the rotator cuff can lead to **laxity** i.e., abnormal displacement of the head of the humerus from the glenohumeral space or **impingement** i.e., the abnormal migration of the head of the humerus into the subacromial space. Either of these plays a role in further pathology. **Anterior laxity** of the humerus in the glenohumeral joint manifests with pain in shoulder after use and the development of patient anxiety and anterior laxity with the **anterior apprehension test**. For this test, with the patient supine, the examiner places one hand on the patient's forearm, the other hand beneath the shoulder, the examiner then gently passively abduct and externally rotates the arm to above the shoulder, horizontal plane, and then pulls upward on the humeral head **(Fig. 9.42)**. **Posterior laxity** of the humerus in the glenohumeral joint manifests with a pain in shoulder after use and posterior laxity with the **pos-**

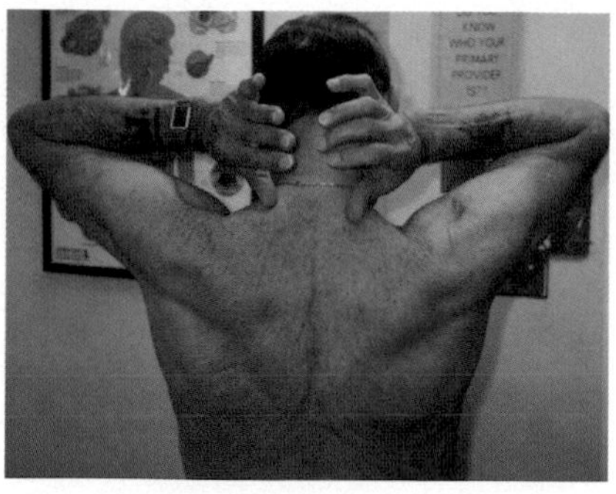

Figure 9.41.

Technique for scratch test from top to assess the infraspinatus muscle.

TIPS

- Actively externally rotate arms, scratch back from above, so thumbs are low on back as possible
- Note any atrophy of infraspinatus muscle
- Infraspinous problem: pain in posterior lateral shoulder; thumb on affected side is higher (T2 level or higher)
- Rhomboid or trapezius strain: pain over the middle one third of the vertebral side of the scapula

terior drawer test. For this test, with the patient supine, grasp the proximal forearm with one hand, flex the elbow passively to 120 degrees and forward flex the arm to 30 degrees with 100 degrees of abduction; with the other hand, surround the acromion with the second digit on the scapular spine and thumb on the coracoid. Then, forward flex the arm to 80 degrees and internally rotate the arm while concurrently applying posterior pressure to the proximal humerus. **Multidirectional laxity** manifests with recurrent pain in shoulder and a history of dislocation in past. There is a palpable clunk with the **Liu's crank test.** For this test, with the patient's arm fully forward flexed to 170 degrees, place a hand around the distal humerus, pull axially, and passively rotate the arm internally and externally. In addition, a positive **sulcus test** as described by Neer and Foster in which a sulcus develops when axial traction is placed on the humerus **(Fig. 9.43)**. Multidirectional laxity has a high incidence of recurrent humeral dislocation.

Impingement manifests with pain and limitation to both active and passive ROM. This is particularly evident and first symptomatic when the arm is above the horizontal plane. Pain is also noted at the humeral head with the **Neer and Walsh impingement sign.** This is elicited by having the patient stand, arm at 170 degrees or in maximal abduction, then grasp the distal humerus and externally rotate the arm **(Fig. 9.44)**. The company impingement keeps includes pain in the humeral head with **Hawkins impingement sign** (Fig. 9.37). Finally, a tear of the **glenoid labrum*** manifests with glenohumeral laxity, laxity either anterior or posterior, but most commonly posterior as demonstrated in the **posterior drawer** test, pain with the **supraspinatus** test (Fig. 9.39), and a clunk with **Liu's crank test (Fig. 9.45)**. In Liu's original paper the sensitivity for glenoid labrum tears was 93% (29/31), specificity was 91% (28/31), with a positive predictive value of 94% and negative predictive value of 90%. Tears are often due to over hand throwing or pitching in which the tear is in superior and often posterior labrum (SLAP)*.

*SLAP: Superior labrum anterior and posterior

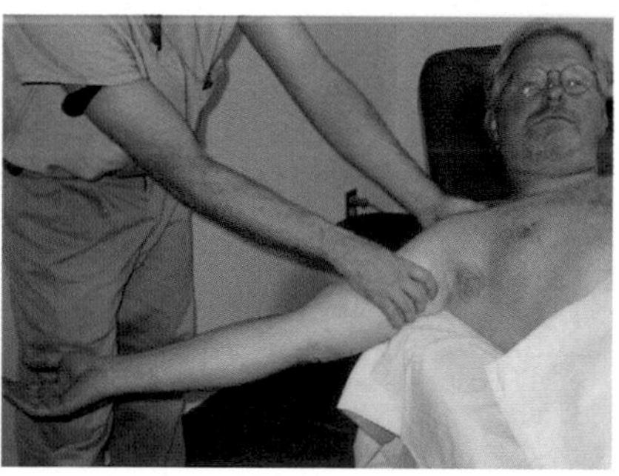

A

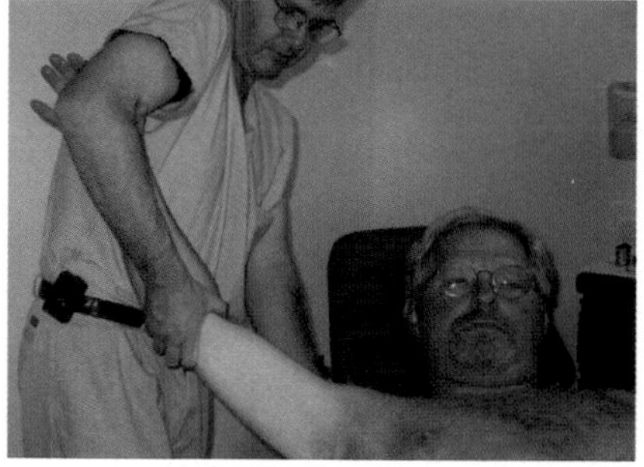

B

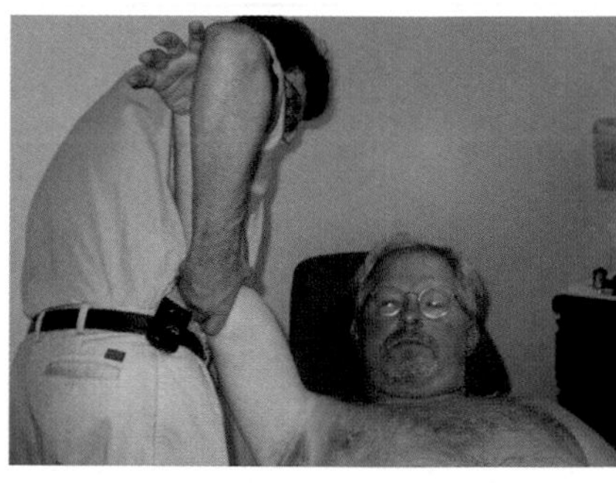

C

Figure 9.42.

Technique for anterior apprehension maneuver to assess for anterior glenohumeral laxity.

TIPS

- Patient supine
- Place one hand on patient's distal arm; the other hand beneath the shoulder
- Gently passively abduct and externally rotate the arm to above the shoulder **(A)**, horizontal plane
- Pull upward **(B** and **C)**
- Anterior shoulder laxity: patient apprehensive that the humerus is going to pop out or objective humeral subluxation or anterior pain

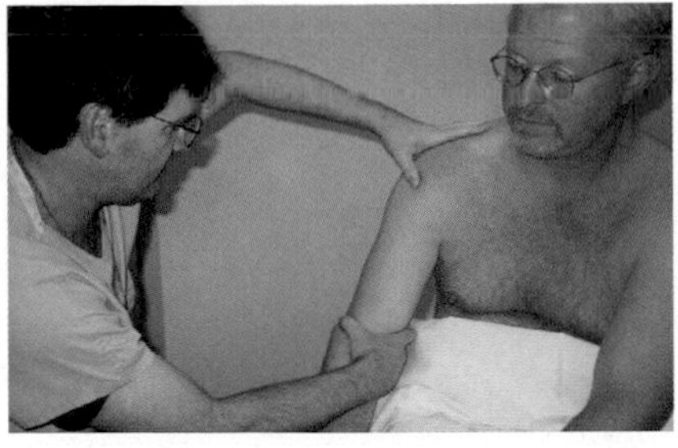
A

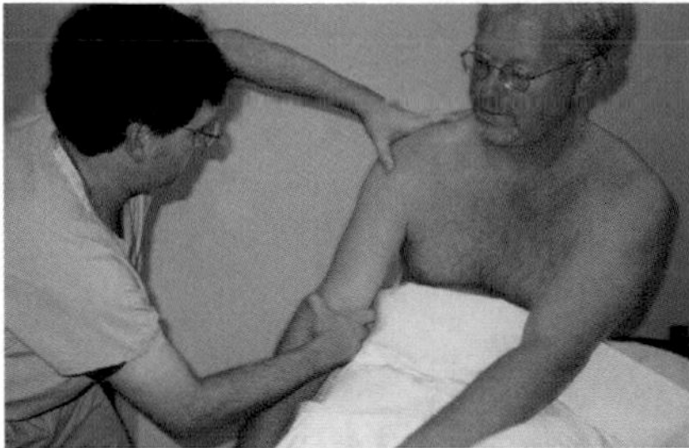
B

Figure 9.43.

Technique for multidirectional laxity stress test for severe glenohumeral laxity.

TIPS

- Grasp the distal humerus and apply significant axial traction to arm
- Normal: no sulcus formed or movement noted
- Isolated anterior or posterior laxity: no movement
- Multidirectional laxity: visible and palpable sulcus

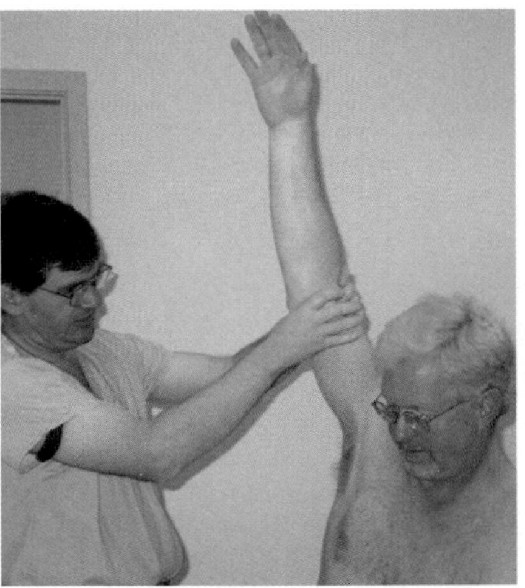
A

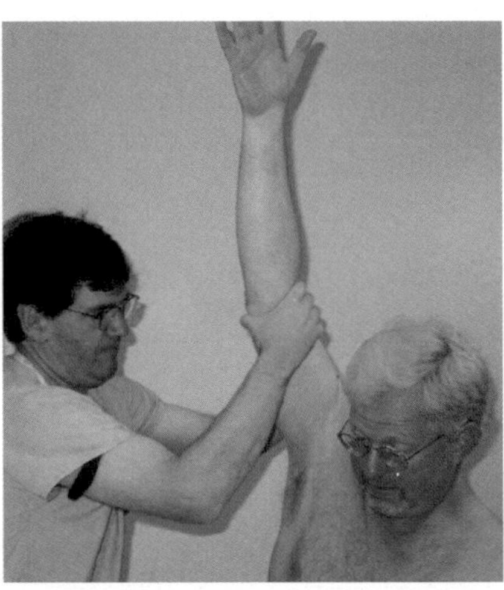
B

Figure 9.44.

Technique for subacromial impingement assessment test of Neer and Walsh.

TIPS

- Patient standing, arm at 170 degrees of, or in, maximal abduction
- Grasp the distal humerus and externally rotate the arm
- Impingement of subacromial space: significant pain and discomfort develops

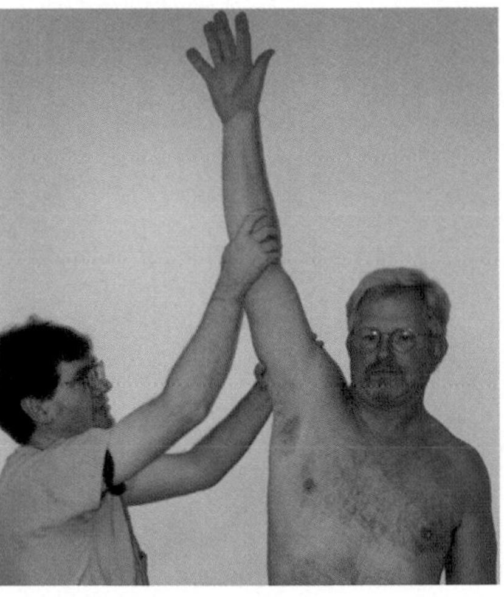
A

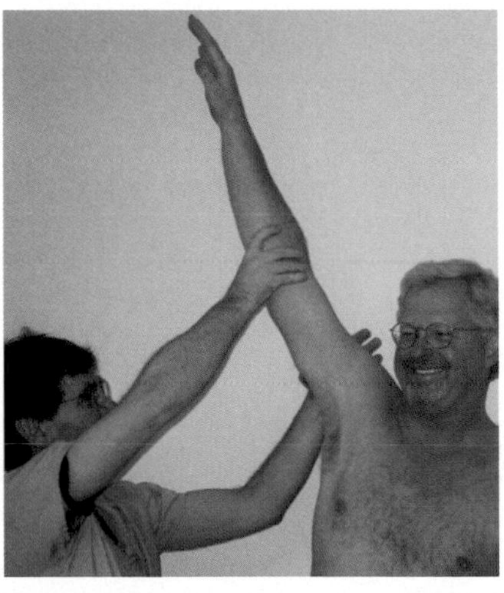
B

Figure 9.45.

Technique for Liu's crank test for laxity at the glenohumeral joint.

TIPS

- Patient's arm is fully extended to 170 degrees, forward flexed
- Place hand around the patient's distal humerus
- Pull axially, and passively rotate the arm internally and externally
- Glenoid labrum tears: a clunk over humeral head
- Most common site of labrum tear is superior and posterior

POSTERIOR SHOULDER AND NECK

The surface anatomy (Fig. 9.3) of the posterior neck and shoulder includes the **paraspinous muscles**, which are thick muscles with a high fiber to nerve ratio. These provide the muscular foundation for the neck. The **cervical spine** of seven cervical vertebrae is the boney foundation and has a lordotic curve, that partially reverses with neck forward flexion. The **thoracic spine** of 12 vertebrae is mildly kyphotic. The vertebral borders of the **scapula** should be equidistant from the vertebral bodies. Also, the muscles of the trapezius, rhomboid, serratus anterior, latissimus dorsi, and teres major contribute not only to the posterior movement of the scapula, neck, and shoulder but more importantly provide stability for the shoulder and neck (see **Table 9.6**). The **winging stress test** is an excellent screen for weakness or muscle problems involving these spe-

Table 9.6. Neck: Range of Motion

Motion	Instruction	Normal*	Muscle/nerve	Nerve
Forward flexion	"Put chin to chest"	70	Sternocleidomastoid	CNXI
Backward flexion	"Put head back"	30	Upper trapezius Paraspinous	CNXI C2–C8
Lateral bend, left and right	"Place ear to shoulder"	40	Trapezius	CNXI
Rotation, left and right	"Twist head to side"	40	Trapezius	CNXI

*Degrees.

TEACHING POINTS

POSTERIOR SHOULDER AND NECK

1. Any suspicion of cervical or thoracic spine injury must be evaluated by radiographic images of the spine. Until "cleared," the patient must be on a backboard and immobilized with a hard cervical (Philadelphia) collar.
2. Rhomboid strain is not uncommon and results in mid scapula pain with mild winging.
3. The paraspinous muscles are thick muscles with a high fiber to nerve ratio; these provide the base, i.e., the muscular foundation, for the neck and head.
4. The vertebral borders of the scapula should be equidistant from the vertebral bodies.
5. Winging of the scapula means weakness either to proximal muscle or trapezius or to serratus anterior or rhomboid.
6. The cervical spine is lordotic; the thoracic spine is kyphotic.
7. The latissimus dorsi strain manifests with lumbar back pain that is worsened with active scapular retraction or active arm backward flexion.
8. Teres major muscle strain manifests with pain in the posterior axillary fold that is worsened with active arm backward flexion.

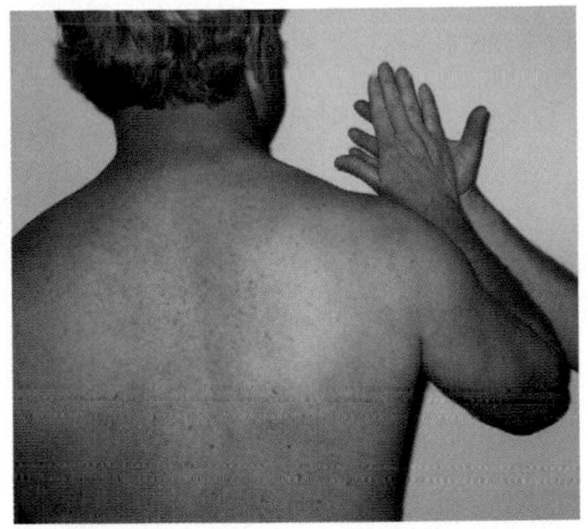
A

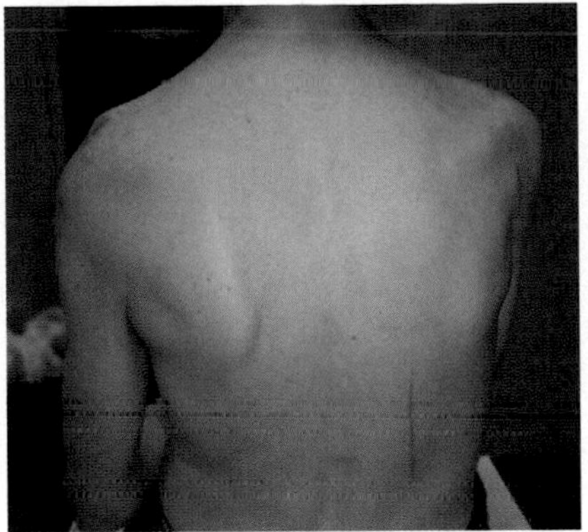
B

Figure 9.46.

Technique to stress the scapula, to assess for winging. **B.** Winging.

TIPS

- Patient standing, neutral position
- Hands in front, elbows slightly flexed
- Place hand on patient's hand as if to perform a push-up
- Normal: vertebral border, equidistant
- Posterior or medial displacement is "winging"

cific muscles **(Fig. 9.46)**. In this test, the patient is instructed to push forward against resistance. The scapula should remain stable; if movement medially the scapula is "winged." See **Table 9.7** for specific types of winging.

Trapezius strain manifests with bilateral posterior neck pain and tenderness. **Percussion** of the cervical spine elicits no tenderness, no nerve root deficits are noted in **C4 to T2**, but significant **decreased ROM** is noted to the neck with stiffness and muscle spasm. There is often concurrent **straightening** of the normal cervical lordosis. **Rhomboid strain** manifests with tenderness over the medial aspect of the inferior half of the vertebral surface of the scapula. The tenderness is exacerbated by active backward flexion of arm or backward flexion (retraction) of the scapula. There is often concurrent winging of the scapula. **Latissimus dorsi strain** manifests with tenderness over the lateral or mid to lower back. The pain and tenderness is exacerbated with active backward flexion of the arm. This is due to overuse of the muscle, e.g., excessive bowling. **Teres major strain** manifests with pain and tenderness in the posterior fold of the axilla. As with latissimus dorsi strain, this is exacerbated by active backward flexion of the shoulder.

Fractures of the cervical spine manifest with posterior neck and shoulder pain. From the outset, **before any physical examination**, if **a fracture or subluxation of the cervical spine** is suspected, **place the patient in a hard cervical immobilizer and, if indicated, a backboard, and have a radiograph taken to assess for such an injury**. The mechanism of injury may indicate that the risk for cervical spine fracture is higher. These include injury from a diving or direct trauma to the neck in a fall.

Table 9.7. Winging of the Scapula

Diagnosis	Winging	Company it Keeps
Trapezius weak	Upper angle	Cranial nerve XI deficit
Serratus anterior weak	Lower angle	Knife wound to chest or axilla
Rhomboid weak	Lower angle	Antecedent fall on outstretched hand
Proximal muscle weak	Entire vertebral surface	Waddling gait

*ROM: Range of Motion.

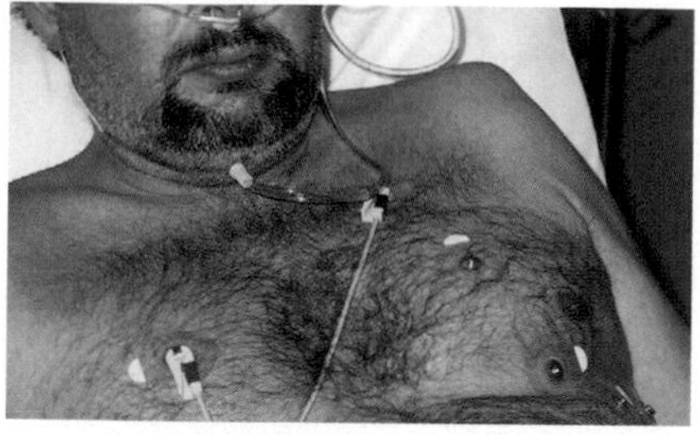

Figure 9.47.

The "square off" sign of a dislocated shoulder. This was a posterior glenohumeral dislocation that happened after a tonic-clonic seizure.

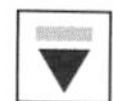 **TIPS**

- Normal: curved shoulder
- Posterior humeral dislocation: "square-off" sign, a discrete right angle is formed on the affected side

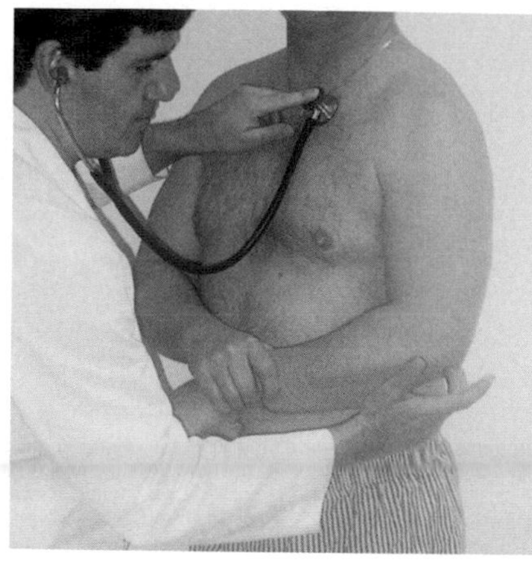

Figure 9.48.

Technique for Auenbrugger's percussion sign. This is an interesting, but rarely used, method to assess for fractures.

 **TIPS**

- Auscult over the olecranon of elbow
- Tap over the sternoclavicular joint; repeat on other, asymptomatic side
- Fracture or dislocation of humerus: decrease in sound transmission on the affected side
- Complete reduction: transmission normalizes
- Nice diagnostic test in the wild; less important since the advent of radiographs
- Recall, Leopold Auenbrugger is the "Father of percussion"

ACUTE TRAUMA

Anterior humeral dislocation manifests with acute onset of pain, tenderness, and severe limitation of passive and active ROM. The position of the arm is one of a **dead arm** (Fig. 9.16). In addition, the humerus is not palpable in the glenohumeral joint space. Furthermore, no ausculted sound is detected over the sternoclavicular joint on percussion over olecranon process of the elbow i.e., a positive **Auenbrugger's percussion sign**. Anterior glenohumeral dislocation most often results from a fall with the arm elevated in forward flexion e.g., sliding, arm first into second base or as the result of severe rotator cuff laxity. **Posterior humeral dislocation** manifests with marked pain and severe limitation of passive and active ROM. The position of the arm is one of **"Bonaparte"** On inspection of shoulder, a **square-off** sign also known as a **right angle** sign is noted in the affected shoulder **(Fig. 9.47)**. On palpation, the humerus is not palpable in the glenohumeral joint space. In addition, no ausculted sound is detected over the sternoclavicular joint upon percussion over olecranon process of the elbow i.e., a positive **Auenbrugger's sign (Fig. 9.48)**. A posterior glenohumeral

TEACHING POINTS

TRAUMA

1. "Dead arm" position sign is present in humeral dislocation, proximal humeral fracture, and acute burner or stinger.
2. Posterior glenohumeral dislocation is rare. Specific manifestations include a square-off sign and acute inability to use the arm.
3. When the humerus cannot be felt in the glenohumeral fossa, diagnosis is either glenohumeral dislocation or a fracture of the humeral head.

dislocation is usually caused by a fall or after a tonic clonic seizure. In **either type of dislocation**, damage to the neurovascular bundle is a common complication. Thus, it is of great importance to conduct a thorough and fastidious examination of **cervical roots** C5 to T1 (Table 9.2) and peripheral nerves, radial, ulnar, median, axillary, and musculocutaneous. On **reduction** of the dislocation, reassess the neurovascular status and document any changes. Auenbrugger's percussion sign will normalize after reduction. The incidence of axillary nerve damage with a dislocation is 7.8% as reported by Neviaser. **Humeral head fracture** manifests with severe limitation of ROM, pain, swelling, a dead arm position, and a positive Auenbrugger's sign.

Annotated Bibliography

Overall

Glockner SM. Shoulder pain: a diagnostic dilemma. *Am Fam Pract* 1995;51(7):1677–1687.
Excellent review of the anatomy, with emphasis on the history given by the patient to assist in evaluation. References and uses the term "Apley scratch test." Also nicely reviews the techniques of ROM, cross-over test, Speed's test, Yergason maneuver, anterior apprehension sign, posterior drawer sign, sulcus sign and the supraspinous test. The discussion of ROM is excellent with inclusion of scapular movements.

Kocher, et al. Shoulder injuries during Alpine skiing. *Am J Sports Med* 996;25:665–669.
Three-year retrospective study of skiing-related injuries at Jackson Hole, Wyoming; 39% of total injuries involved the shoulder, the most common being, in order of frequency, rotator cuff tears, anterior glenohumeral GH dislocation, acromioclavicular (AC) separation, and, clavicle fracture.

Smith DC, Campbell SM. Painful shoulder syndrome: diagnosis and management. *J Genl Intern Med* 1992;7(3):328–339.
Of all diagnoses, 60% are subacromial bursitis or supraspinatus tendonitis. Other common causes include bicipital tendonitis, rotator cuff tears, and degenerative joint disease DJD of the AC joint. Only 5% have isolated tendonitis of the long head of the biceps. Strong overview of the epidemiology of problems that present to primary care physicians.

Overall: Brachial Plexus

Campbell SM. Referred shoulder pain. *Post Grad Med* 1983;73:193–203.
Discusses cervical root 5 radicular pain that involve the superior shoulder and lateral arm.

Garth WP. Evaluation and treatment of brachial plexus injuries. *Journal of Musculoskeletal Medicine* 1994;Oct 11 (10):55–67.
Excellent, detailed discussion of the evaluation, management, and treatment of Burner or stinger. Excellent review of the manifestations of the following: isolated brachial plexus injuries, axillary nerve injuries, long thoracic and suprascapularis nerve injuries, and the dead arm syndrome (dead = numb). Occult cervical spine fractures, cervical herniation, and acute transient quadraparesis are discussed. An excellent paper.

Hershman EB. Injuries to the brachial plexus. In: Torg JS, ed. *Athletic Injuries to the Hand, Neck and Face*, 2nd ed. St. Louis: Mosby-Yearbook, 1991:338–367.
Excellent discussion of the manifestations and evaluation of injuries to the branchial plexus. Excellent reference.

Jobe, Bradley. Rotator cuff injuries in baseball. *Sports Med* 1988;6:378–387.
Describes the use of the arm in overhead positions as a risk factor for rotator cuff tears. Expands on the concept of impingement development and that instability is an integral component in development. The cycle of instability-subluxation-impingement results in further destruction of the cuff and thus more instability.

Spurling RG, Scoville WB. Lateral rupture of the cervical intervertebral discs: a common cause of shoulder and arm pain. *Surg Obs Gyn* 1944;78:350–358.
An important paper that emphasizes the importance of performing an examination of the cervical spine and neck in any patient with a shoulder complaint.

Overall: Range of Motion

Codman EA. *The Shoulder.* Boston: Thomas Todd, 1934.
A book, paid for by the author, which is a fascinating read. From his preface, "This book aims to try to teach practicing physicians, who see cases soon after the injury, how to recognize this lesion immediately and to rush the patient to a competent surgeon as promptly as if the patient had a broken arm-a much less disabiling accident." Excellent new work for the time describing rotator cuff tears, in general, and supraspinatus tears, specifically. Describes the symptoms of a supraspinatus

tear in detail, which is-common in laborers and in those at the, "time of the loosening of the teeth." Also coined the term, "frozen shoulder" for adhesive capsulitis.

DePalma AF. Loss of scapulohumeral motion (frozen shoulder) ***Ann Surg*** **1952;135:193–205.**
Good discussion of frozen shoulder syndrome.

Society of the American Shoulder and Elbow Surgeons. ***Basic Shoulder Examination—Passive and Active.***
Exhaustive list of basic active and passive ROM procedures at the glenohumeral joint.

Overall: Rotator Cuff

Jobe FW. An EMG analysis of the shoulder in throwing and pitching. ***Am J Sports Med*** **1983;11(1):3–5.**
A tantalizing study in which electromyograms (EMG) were performed during the throwing of a baseball. Five phases of activity in the rotator cuff: (1) wind-up, (2) early cocking (supraspinatus, infraspinatus, teres minor), (3) late cocking (subscapularis), (4) acceleration, and (5) follow-through. All rotator cuff muscles fire maximally preventing cephalad movement of the humerus when arm is maximally overhead.

Lyons AR, Tomlinson JE. Clinical diagnosis of tears of the rotator cuff. ***J Bone Joint Surg*** **1992;74B:414–415.**
Involves 42 patients in the shoulder clinic. Examination alone rotator cuff tear; gold standard, surgical exploration; sensitivity, 91%; specificity, 75%.

Moseley HF. Ruptures of the rotator cuff. ***Br J Surg*** **1951;38:340–369.**
An excellent discussion of the clinical manifestations of rotator cuff tears, in general, from authors who had to diagnose these entities before the development of magnetic resonance imaging (MRI). Dr. Moseley was an accomplished author, surgeon, and master of the diagnosis and management shoulder problems.

Wolin PM. Rotator cuff injuries. The Physician and Sports Medicine 1997;25:54–74.
Excellent review of the anatomy and pathogenesis of impingement and of cuff tears; some discussion of the physical examination; an excellent discussion on mechanism related to the development of this disorder. Nice review of many of the commonly used tests to evaluate cuff tears: subscapularis lift test of Gerber and Krushell, supraspinatus test, external rotation crank test, internal rotation crank test, Neer impingement sign, and Hawkins impingement sign. Also a nice description and discussion of laxity tests, including anterior apprehension, posterior drawer, and multidirectional (sulcus) test.

Anterior

Adson AW, Coffey JR. Cervical rib. Journal of Western Surgical Association 1926:839–857.
The classic description of this syndrome and its manifestations. Fascinating that the major outcome of Adson's maneuver was not diminished pulses but actually, cyanosis. He used data from the Mayo records: 36 patients with a surgical correction (413/540) seen from January 1, 1910 to October 1, 1926. Sensitivities were based on these 36 patients: cyanosis, 13/36; sensory deficits, 9/36; "darting" pain in the brachial plexus, 26/36.

Allman FL. Fracture and ligament classification of the clavicle and its articulation. ***J Bone Joint Surg*** **1967;99A:774.**
Classification of clavicular fractures is outlined. This is not only of academic interest; medial and lateral fractures, although rare, require a more aggressive imaging and, perhaps, even surgical intervention.

Bach BR, Novak PJ. Chronic AC pain: an overlooked problem. ***The Physician and Sports Medicine*** **1993;21:63–70.**
Nice discussion of this diagnosis of anterior shoulder pain, including- a review of the cross-over test.

Diner, et al. Bicipital tendonitis. ***Clin Orthop*** **1984;164:165–171.**
Small study finding that six of seven patients with bicipital tendonitis indeed had a positive Yergason maneuver: sensitivity, 86%.

Gerber C, Krushell RJ. Isolated rupture of the tendon of the subscapularis muscle. ***J Bone Joint Surg Br*** **1991;73(3):389–394.**
Describes the subscapularis lift test in great detail. Coined term, "Lift-off-test".

Gilcreest EL. Rupture of muscles and tendons, particularly subcutaneous ruture of the biceps brachii. ***JAMA*** **1925;84:1819–1822.**
Classic paper describing manifestations of bicipital tendon rupture and bicipital tendonitis.

Griffths GP, et al. Rupture of the pectoralis major muscles. ***The Physician and Sports Medicine*** **1997;25(8):119–125.**
Excellent review of this uncommon entity. Includes the pathogenesis, manifestations, and a short discussion of treatment. Manifestations include a sudden pop, a change in the size (enlarged) of the anterior axillary fold, in a proximal rupture.

Naviaser RJ. Lesions of the biceps and tendonitis of the shoulder. ***Orthop Clin North Am*** **1980;11:334–340.**
Nice descriptions of manifestations, including Yergason and Speed's signs. Emphasizes that 90% have antecedent or concurrent instability or impingement. Excellent review of the anatomy of the tendons and muscles of the biceps.

Pasteur F. La teno-bursite de la longue portion du biceps. *Gaz d'Hop* 1934;107:477–479.
The classic description of this not uncommon entity.

Yergason RM. Supination sign. *Connecticut Medical Journal,* 1931.
Original description of this sign and its use in the diagnosis of bicipital tendonitis. Of interest is that the paper (paragraph) was based on one patient—"a 45-year-old housewife who developed anterior shoulder pain and a positive supination sign. She was treated with rest, linaments, and electrical treatments"; also, "on inquiry, it was learned that the patient does a large washing daily, wringing all of the clothes by hand and hand hanging them out." "Buying a washer with a wringer and going light on mending with treatment of any other nature, produced recovery in <1 month."

Lateral

Liu, et al. A prospective evaluation of a new physical exam in predicting glenoid labral tears. *Am J Sports Med* 1996;24(6):721–725.
Nice description of glenoid labrum tears, with emphasis on manifestations and the fact that SLAP is the most common type of tear. Describes this novel procedure to diagnosis this often overlooked cause of shoulder pain and laxity. The procedure, Liu's crank test, has a sensitivity of 93% (29/31), a specificity of 91% (28/31), and a positive predictive value (PPV) of 94% and negative predictive value (NPV) of 90%.

Codman EA. Stiff and painful shoulders. *Boston Medical and Surgical Journal,* May 31, 1906.
First description of the upright Codman's maneuver in a supraspinatus tear—active abduction less than passive abduction.

Jobe FW, Jobe CM. Painful athletic injuries of the shoulder. *Clin Orthop* 1983;173:117–124.
Describes Jobe's sign to diagnose supraspinatus tears.

Impingement

Ellenbecker TS. Rehabilitation of overuse injuries. *Clin Sports Med* 1989;8:583–604.
Shoulder overuse, especially overhead overuse, leads to impingement. Nice review of the pathogenesis of impingement and the role of instability in its development. Excellent reviews of the Neer classification of impingement and descriptions of the Neer impingement sign and the Hawkins impingement sign.

Hawkins RJ, Kennedy JC. Impingement syndrome in athletes. *Am J Sports Med* 1980;8(3): 151–158.
Describes this impingement sign; classic.

Neer CS II. Anterior acromioplasty for the chronic impingement syndrome in the shoulder. *J Bone Joint Surg Am* 1972;54(1):41–50.
Describes this impingement sign classic.

Neer CS, Welsh RP. The shoulder in sports. *Orthop Clin North Am* 1977;8:583–591.
Pain with forward flexion at 70 degrees = impingement. Nice review of this classic sign.

Snyder SJ, Kanzel RP, DelPizzo W, et al.: SLAP lesions of the shoulder. *Arthroscopy* 6(4): 274–279, 1990.
Overview of this not uncommon entity of shoulder laxity. SLAP: Superior labrum anterior and posterior was coined in this paper. Reviews that this superior location is common in throwing type athletes (e.g., pitchers) in which it is most often superior and posterior.

Posterior: Scapula

Milch H. Snapping scapula. *Clin Orthop* 1961;20:139–150.
Succinct description of this relatively rare entity.

Dislocation

Neviaser, et al. Concurrent rupture of the rotator cuff and anterior dislocation of the shoulder in the older patient. *J Bone Joint Surg Am* 1988;70:1308–1311.
Older individuals with anterior glenohumeral dislocations and rotator cuffs tears are common; the complication of axillary nerve damage 7.8% incidence.

Ward KR, et al. Posterior dislocation of the shoulder. *Emerg Med* 1988;(Oct):78–82.
Mentions and describes the Napoleon Bonaparte sign and the square-off sign of posterior GH dislocations.

10

Hand, Wrist, and Thumb Examination

PRACTICE AND TEACHING

PALMAR SIDE SURFACE ANATOMY

Wrist (Fig. 10.1)

The **flexor carpi ulnaris** originates near the medial epicondyle of the humerus, inserts on the pisiform, and acts in wrist flexion; its nerve is ulnar. The **ulnar nerve (Box 10.1)** is on the radial side of this tendon; it runs with the ulnar artery through the **ulnar tunnel** and immediately divides into deep and superficial branches. The ulnar tunnel is also known as the "loge de Guyon." The borders of this tunnel include the pisiform, hook of hamate, and the transverse carpal ligament. It contains the ulnar nerve and ulnar artery. The ulnar nerve supplies **sensation** to the ulnar side of the wrist and hand via the palmar branch given off proximal to the ulnar tunnel and to the palmar and dorsal aspects of digits 5 and half of 4 via the superficial ulnar branch. It supplies **motor** to the flexor carpi ulnaris, ulnar nerve proximal to ulnar tunnel,

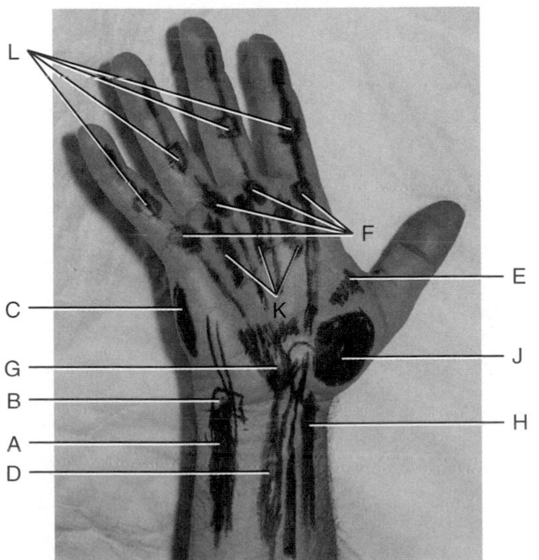

Figure 10.1.

Surface anatomy of the palmar hand and wrist **A.** Flexor carpi ulnaris muscle. **B.** Ulnar tunnel with ulnar artery and nerve. **C.** Hypothenar eminence. **D.** Palmaris longus muscle tendon. **E.** One of the flexor digitorum superficial and deep tendons (digit 2). **F.** Profunda (to DIP) tendon pierces the superficial (to PIP) tendon at the metacarpophalangeal (MCP) joint. **G.** Median nerve, through the carpal tunnel. **H.** Flexor carpi radialis. **I.** Radial artery. **J.** Thenar eminence. **K.** Palmar interossei muscles. **L.** Volar plates over the proximal interphalangeal (PIP) joints.

TIPS

- Flexors of the fingers and wrist: innervated by median AI, and ulnar nerve
- The volar plates cover the palmar aspect of the proximal interphalangeal (PIP) joint
- Palmar interossei muscles adduction of fingers
- Deep flexor tendon pierces the superficial tendon at the heads of the metacarpals
- Thenar eminence: thumb flexion and adduction
- Hypothenar eminence: fifth digit adduction and abduction

Box 10.1.

Innervation of Muscles of Hand and Wrist

Radial and its branch PI

All extensor digitorum (PI)

Extensor pollicis longus (PI)

Extensor pollicis brevis (PI)

Abductor pollicis longus (PI)

Extensor carpi radialis (Radial)

Extensor carpi ulnaris (PI)

Median and its branch AI

Thenar eminence (M)

Flexor carpi radialis (M)

Lumbricals 2, 3 (M)

Flexor digitorum profunda 2, 3 (AI)

Flexor digitorum superficialis (M)

Flexor pollicus longus (AI)

Ulnar

Hypothenar eminence

Flexor carpi ulnaris

Lumbricals 4, 5

Flexor digitorum profunda 4, 5

Interossei palmar and dorsal

PI = posterior interosseous; AI = anterior interosseous; M = median.

and, to the lumbricals of digits 4 and 5, the dorsal and palmar interossei, and the adductor pollicis muscles by the deep ulnar nerve (branch point distal to ulnar tunnel). The superficial ulnar branch specifically provides motor to abductor digiti minimi. The **ulnar artery**, which is immediately radial and posterior to the ulnar nerve, supplies most of blood to the hand and fingers; therefore, its patency must be assessed via the ulnar **Allen test** (Fig. 10.22) before performing any invasive procedure to the radial artery. The **palmaris longus muscle** originates about the medial epicondyle of the humerus; inserts on the palmar, distal aspect of the flexor retinaculum; and acts as a mild wrist flexor; the nerve is median. This muscle is absent in approximately 13% of individuals.

The **median nerve** enters the hand immediately deep to the palmaris longus tendon through the **carpal tunnel**. The carpal tunnel borders are the *roof,* flexor retinaculum; the *floor,* palmar side of carpal bones; *ulnar side,* the pisiform and hook of the hamate; the *radial side,* the tubercle of the scaphoid and the trapezium. The contents of the carpal tunnel include the median nerve and the flexor digitorum tendons. The **palmar aponeurosis** is superficial and distal to the flexor retinaculum; it is triangular shaped and extends into each finger and it covers the flexor tendons in each digit. The **flexor digitorum profunda** (deep) and **flexor digitorum superficial** tendons pass through the carpal tunnel at this point. The flexor tendons are in a common synovial sheath that passes deep to the palmar aponeurosis and the flexor retinaculum. These flexors originate about the medial epicondyle, insert on the base of the middle phalanx (superficial flexor) and the base of distal phalanx (deep flexor). The nerve for the superficial flexor is median; whereas, for the profunda (deep) flexor it is AI* for digits 2 and 3 and ulnar nerve for digits 4 and 5. The deep (distal phalanx) tendon pierces the superficial (proximal phalanx) tendon at the palmar aspect of the metacarpophalangeal joint and, thus, is a site of potential problems. The **flexor carpi radialis** originates about the medial epicondyle, inserts on the base of the second metacarpal bone, and acts in wrist flexion; its nerve is median. The **radial artery** can easily be palpated. The most radial of structures of the palmar wrist are the **scaphoid** bone and the styloid process of the **radius**.

Hand (see Fig. 10.1)

The **hypothenar eminence** is distal to the pisiform and hamate, includes the palmaris brevis, abductor digiti minimi, flexor digiti minimi brevis, and opponens digiti minimi muscles, and acts in digit 5 adduction; its nerve is ulnar, specifically the superficial branch, its branch point being distal to the ulnar tunnel **(Table 10.1)**.

The **thenar eminence** is a group of muscles that comprise the ball of muscles at the base of thumb **(Table 10.2)**. It is composed of three muscles, the abductor pollicis brevis, flexor pollicis brevis, and opponens pollicis, and it acts in thumb flexion and apposition; its nerve is median. The **lumbrical muscles** of digits 2 through 5; their nerve is median for digits 2 and 3 and ulnar for digits 4 and 5. The lumbricales are intrinsic flexors of the digits. The

Table 10.1. Components of the Hypothenar Eminence

Muscle	Nerve	Action
Palmaris brevis	Ulnar nerve	Abduction, flexion
Abductor digiti minimi	Ulnar nerve	Abduction
Flexor digiti minimi brevis	Ulnar nerve	Flexion
Opponens digiti minimi	Ulnar nerve	Apposition

*AI = anterior interosseous.

Table 10.2. Components of the Thenar Eminence

Muscle	Nerve	Action
Abductor pollicis brevis	Recurrent median	Thumb abduction
Flexor pollicis brevis	Recurrent median	Thumb flexion
Opponens pollicis	Recurrent median	Thumb opposition

palmar interossei muscles act in adduction of the digits; the nerve for all is ulnar. The **adductor pollicis** inserts on the medial second phalanx of the thumb, and acts in thumb adduction; its nerve is ulnar, specifically deep ulnar branch, its branch point being distal to the ulnar tunnel.

The **volar plates** are fibrous plates that are contiguous to the flexor tendons located on the palmar side of the proximal interphalangeal (PIP) joint of digits 2, 3, 4, and 5; these prevent inappropriate extension at the PIP joint. When they are damaged, further mischief may occur.

DORSAL SIDE SURFACE ANATOMY (Fig. 10.2)

Wrist and Hand

The **six extensor compartments** on the dorsum of the forearm wrist and hand contain all of the extensors of the wrist, thumb, and fingers and the major thumb abductor **(Table 10.3)**. The *posterior interosseous nerve* as a major branch of radial nerve controls all of these muscles **(Table 10.4)**. The muscle fibers are in the forearm, whereas, the tendons are in the wrist, fingers, hand, and thumb. **Insertion sites** of the extensor tendons are on the dorsum of the digits. The insertion site is a complex of a middle set of fibers that inserts on the base of the distal phalanx and two sets of fibers insert on the ulnar side and radial side of each digit.

Compartment 1, the most radial compartment, contains abductor pollicis longus and extensor pollicis brevis tendons. These are two of three tendons of the anatomic snuffbox. **Compartment 2**, immediately radial to Lister's tubercle, contains the tendons of the extensor carpi radialis longus and the

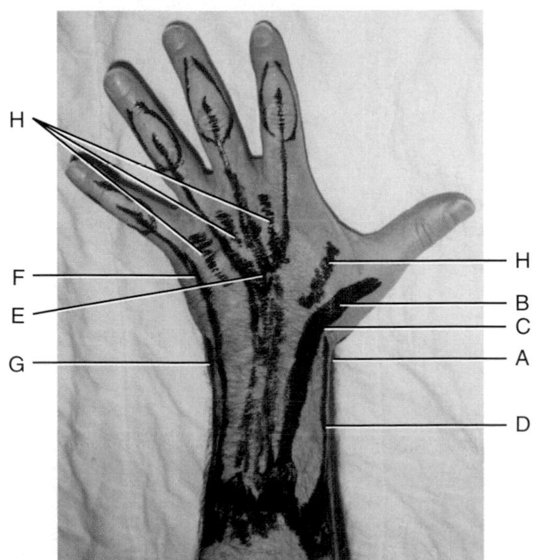

Figure 10.2.

Surface anatomy of the dorsal hand and wrist. **A.** Compartment 1: abductor pollicis longus and extensor pollicis brevis, radial side of snuffbox. **B.** Compartment 3: extensor pollicis longus, ulnar side of snuffbox. **C.** Lister's tubercle on radial styloid. **D.** Compartment 2: extensor carpi radialis longus and extensor carpi radialis brevis. **E.** Compartment 4: extensor digitorum communs and extensor indicis. **F.** Compartment 5: extensor digiti minimi. **G.** Compartment 6: extensor carpi ulnaris. **H.** Dorsal interossei: ulnar nerve.

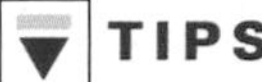

TIPS

- Anatomic snuffbox is bounded by compartments 1 and 3
- Compartment 2: extensor carpi radialis
- Compartment 1: the abductor pollicis longus and extensor pollicis brevis
- Compartment 3: the extensor pollicis longus; hooks about Lister's tubercle
- All extensor compartment muscles: posterior interosseous nerve
- Dorsal interossei: abductors of fingers, ulnar nerve

Table 10.3. Extensor Compartments

Compartment	Contents*
Compartment 1	Abductor pollicis longus muscle Extensor pollicis brevis muscle
Compartment 2	Extensor carpi radialis longus muscle Extensor carpi radialis brevis muscle
Compartment 3	Extensor pollicis longus muscle
Compartment 4	Extensor digitorum communis (digits 2, 3, 4) muscle
Compartment 5	Extensor digiti minimi muscle
Compartment 6	Extensor carpi ulnaris muscle

*Muscle and tendon.

extensor carpi radialis brevis. **Compartment 3** contains the tendon of the extensor pollicis longus, which runs immediately to the ulnar side of Lister's tubercle. This is the third tendon of the snuffbox. **Compartment 4**, slightly ulnar to compartment 3, contains the tendons of the extensor digitorum communis (i.e., tendons to digits 2, 3, and 4). **Compartment 5**, ulnar to compartment 4, contains the tendon of extensor digiti minimi to digit 5. **Compartment 6**, the most ulnar compartment, contains the tendon of the extensor carpi ulnaris; it specifically inserts on the base of the fifth metacarpal bone.

Table 10.4. Neurologic Examination—Selected Procedures

Nerve	Action	Primary muscle
Radial and posterior interosseous	Active extension of hand at wrist	Extensor carpi ulnaris and radialis (compartments 2 and 6)
Posterior interosseous	Active extension third digit at MCP and PIP	Extensor digitorum (compartment 4)
Posterior interosseous	Active abduction of thumb	Abductor pollicis longus (compartment 1)
Superficial radial	Sensation to snuffbox skin	
Anterior interosseous	Active IP thumb flexion	Flexor pollicis longus
Median and anterior interosseous	Active tip-to-tip "OK," against resistance	Flexor pollicis longus (AI) Flexor digitorum profunda 2 (AI) Flexor digitorum superficialis (M)
Median	Active third digit flexion PIP	Flexor digitorum superficialis 3 Lumbrical 3
Median and ulnar	Active flexion of wrist	Flexor carpi radialis (M) Flexor carpi ulnaris (ulnar)
Median, palmar branch	Sensation to thenar skin	
Ulnar	Abduction of digits 2–5	Interossei
Ulnar	Active adduction of the thumb	Adductor pollicis
Ulnar	Active flexion of digit 5 DIP	Flexor digitorum Lumbrical 5
Superficial ulnar	Sensation to hypothenar skin	

IP = interphalangeal; MCP = metacarpophalangeal; PIP = proximal interphalangeal (joints); AI = anterior interosseous; PI = posterior interosseous; M = median.

TEACHING POINTS

PALMAR AND DORSAL SURFACE ANATOMY

Palmar

1. The intrinsic muscles of the hand are predominantly located on the palmar side.
2. The median nerve via the carpal tunnel and the ulnar nerve via the ulnar tunnel enter the hand to provide sensation to the digits.
3. The palmar fascia and flexor retinaculum are superficial to the flexor tendons and intrinsic muscles of the hand.
4. The volar plates at the proximal interphalangeal (PIP) joint of the fingers, the cornerstones of the digits and prevent inappropriate extension.
5. Ulnar nerve: motor nerve for almost all of the hand intrinsics, except for the muscles of thenar eminence and lumbricales 2 and 3, which are median nerve.
6. The furthest domain of the ulnar nerve is the adductor pollicis muscle.
7. Allen test is a great method to assess for ulnar artery patency. Mandatory to assess before performing radial artery procedures.

Dorsal

1. There are six extensor compartments in which all the extensors are located. All innervated by posterior interosseous nerve.
2. Anatomic snuffbox is composed of the tendons from extensor compartments 1 and 3.
3. Compartment 1 has the abductor pollicis longus and the extensor pollicis brevis muscles.
4. The only intrinsic muscles on the dorsal hand are the dorsal interossei (ulnar nerve).

Lister's tubercle, which is on the ulnar side of the radial styloid, is an important landmark. This is a marker for the midaxis line of the wrist and hand. Furthermore, the **extensor pollicis longus** tendon hooks around it. This provides an increased thumb pincer strength to grasp when the wrist is mildly extended (dorsiflexed). The **extensor retinaculum** is a tough, broad ligament over the proximal dorsum of the wrist. This retinaculum covers the extensor compartments. Finally, the **dorsal interossei** muscles are the abductors of the digits. All are innervated by the ulnar nerve, specifically the deep branch.

RANGE OF MOTION: PASSIVE

Two different complementary baseline neutral positions exist for the purpose of assessing hand and thumb ROM. These include a *flat position* in which the thumb is in the same plane as the fingers and the *"C-shaped" position* in which the thumb is perpendicular to the fingers. The range of motion (ROM) should be assessed and documented at all joints using both passive and active procedures **(Tables 10.5 and 10.6)**. Although, when complete, this examination requires a multitude of procedures and data, the examination should be fastidiously appropriate to the patient's problem.

Table 10.5. **Passive Range of Motion**

Movement	Baseline position	Normal (degrees)
Hand flexion at wrist	Forearm pronated	80
Hand extension at wrist	Forearm pronated	70
Wrist radial deviation	Forearm pronated	20
Wrist ulnar deviation	Forearm pronated	30
MCP flexion	Hand neutral	90
MCP extension	Hand neutral	30
MCP abduction	Hand neutral	20
MCP adduction	Hand neutral	20
PIP flexion	Hand and fingers neutral	110
DIP flexion	Hand and fingers neutral	45
PIP extension	Hand and fingers neutral	0
DIP extension	Hand and fingers neutral	20
DIP abduction/adduction	Finger neutral	0
PIP abduction/adduction	Finger neutral	0
Thumb MCP extension	Thumb neutral	0
Thumb MCP flexion	Thumb neutral	20
Thumb MCP adduction	Thumb neutral	0
Thumb MCP abduction	Thumb neutral	0
Thumb IP flexion	Thumb neutral	40
Thumb IP extension	Thumb neutral	0
Thumb IP adduction/abduction	Thumb neutral	0
Thumb MCT flexion	Neutral	15–20
Thumb MCT extension	Neutral	15–20
Thumb MCT adduction	Neutral	15–20
Thumb MCT abduction	Neutral	15–20

DIP = distal interphalangeal; IP = interphalangeal; MCP = metacarpophalangeal; MCT = metacarpotrapezial; PIP = proximal interphalangeal (joints).

Thumb (see Table 10.5)

Passive ROM is measured at three specific joints: the interphalangeal (IP) joint, the metacarpophalangeal (MCP) joint, and the metacarpotrapezial (MCT) joint. **Thumb IP** joint includes flexion to 35 degrees and extension to 0 degrees; the **metacarpophalangeal** joint includes flexion to 20 degrees and extension to 0 degrees. In addition, the MCP joint has 0 degrees of abduction and adduction when the thumb is fully extended and 10 to 15 degrees of abduction and adduction when thumb is fully flexed.

The **MCT** joint includes flexion to 15 to 20 degrees, extension to 0 degrees, abduction to 20 to 25 degrees, and adduction to 15 to 20 degrees. The MCT also provides for circumduction, i.e., thumb twiddling. This circumduction is 20 to 25 degrees from the axis formed by the thumb in neutral C position.

Hand and Fingers (see Table 10.5)

The finger joint ROM is measured at three specific joints, the distal interphalangeal (DIP), the proximal interphalangeal, and the metacarpophalangeal. The **DIP** joint has flexion to 30 degrees, extension to 0 degrees; the **PIP** joint has flexion to 90 degrees and extension to 0 degrees. The **MCP** joint of the

Table 10.6. Active Range of Motion[1,2]

Action	Baseline position	Joints	Muscles	Nerves
Thumb extension	Forearm midpoint between pronation supination	IP, MCP, MCT	Extensor pollicis longus/brevis	PI
Thumb flexion	Forearm midpoint between pronation and supination	IP	Flexor pollicis longus	AI
Thumb abduction	Hand flat, forearm Midpoint between pronation and supination	MCT	Abductor pollicis longus Abductor pollicis brevis	PI Median
Thumb adduction	Midpoint between pronation and supination	MCT	Adductor pollicis	Ulnar
Finger DIP/PIP extension	Hand flat	PIP	Extensor digitorum	PI
Finger DIP flexion	Forearm supinated supported	DIP	Flexor digitorum Profundus	2 and 3: AI 4 and 5: ulnar
Finger PIP flexion	Forearm supinated supported	PIP	Flexor digitorum superficialis	Median
Finger PIP extension	Fist	PIP	Extensor digitorum Compartment 4	PI
Finger MCP abduction	Forearm pronated hand neutral	MCP	Dorsal interossei	Ulnar
Finger MCP adduction	Forearm pronated, digits abducted	MCP	Palmar interossei	Ulnar
Hand grasp	Hand flat, neutral Actively oppose Thumb and fifth digit	MCP, PIP DIP	Thenar muscles Thumb and digit 5 adductors	Median Ulnar
Hand clench (fist)	Hand flat, neutral Actively make a fist	MCP, PIP DIP	Finger flexors Lumbricales and thumb adductors	Mixture of: Median Ulnar AI
Wrist flexion	Hand neutral	Wrist	Flexor carpi Radialis Flexor carpi ulnaris	Median Ulnar
Wrist extension	Forearm pronated	Wrist	Extensor carpi radialis Extensor carpi ulnaris	Radial PI
Radial deviation	Forearm midpoint between supination and pronation	Wrist	Extensor carpi radialis Flexor carpi radialis	Radial Median
Ulnar deviation	Forearm midpoint between supination and pronation	Wrist	Extensor carpi ulnaris Flexor carpi ulnaris	PI Ulnar

DIP = distal interphalangeal; IP = interphalangeal; MCP = metacarpophalangeal; MCT = metacarpotrapezial; PIP = proximal interphalangeal (joints). AI = anterior interosseous; PI = posterior interosseous.

[1] Isolate out specific joints and tendons; fastidious examination required, especially after trauma

[2] See also Table 10.4, especially for "*OK.*"

fingers has flexion to 100 degrees, extension to 0 degrees, abduction and adduction to 15 to 20 degrees, and circumduction of 10 to 15 degrees.

Wrist (see Table 10.5)

Wrist joint is measured between the carpal bones and the radius and ulna. In this joint, palmarflexion is to 90 degrees, dorsiflexion (extension) is to 70 degrees; ulnar deviation to 20 degrees; radial deviation to 20 degrees; and circumduction of the wrist is to 25 degrees.

RANGE OF MOTION: ACTIVE

Thumb (see Tables 10.4 and 10.6)

Active ROM of the thumb should include extension, flexion, abduction, and adduction (Table 10.6). The thumb is pivotal to the overall examination because all three peripheral nerves of the upper extremity innervate the thumb musculature. The radial nerve and its branch the posterior interosseous innervate abduction and extension; the median nerve and its branch the anterior interosseous thumb flexion; and the ulnar nerve thumb adduction.

Hand and Fingers (see Table 10.6)

Active ROM of the fingers should include extension and flexion, both in total, and isolated to the DIP, PIP, and MCP joints. In addition, abduction and adduction of the fingers should be performed (see Table 10.6 for specifics).

Wrist (see Table 10.6)

Active ROM of the wrist should include flexion, extension, and ulnar and radial deviation (see Table 10.6 for specifics).

PALMAR

Carpal tunnel syndrome (CTS) manifests with tingling and pain in the palmar aspect of fingers 1, 2, and 3. Numbness in CTS is limited to fingers **(Fig. 10.3A)** as skin of the palm is innervated by the palmar branch, which comes off proximal to CTS. Thus if numbness of thenar skin, median nerve damage is proximal. An excellent, but sometimes logistically difficult, method to define and describe CTS is to instruct the patient to draw the location of symptoms on a

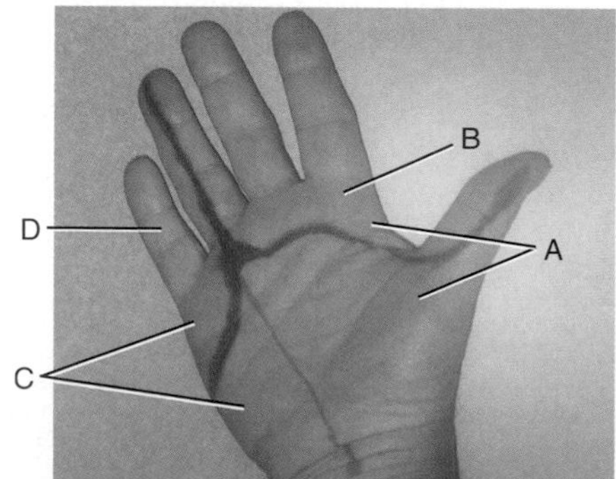

Figure 10.3.

Distribution of numbness in entrapment syndrome. **A.** Proximal median: involves thenar skin. **B.** Carpal tunnel syndrome: limited to fingers of 1, 2, and 3. **C.** Proximal ulnar: involves skin over ulnar wrist and palm. **D.** Ulnar tunnel limited to digits 4 and 5.

 **TIPS**

- If patient is asked to draw or state sites of numbness on a hand diagram, the distribution would be as here
- Ulnar tunnel syndrome: numbness to fingers; if wrist involved, proximal lesion
- Carpal tunnel syndrome: numbness in fingers only; if numb over thenar area, proximal median nerve damage likely

Table 10.7. Evidence Basis for Carpal Tunnel Syndrome

Test	Study	n	Sensitivity (%)	Specificity (%)
Self-reported hand diagram	Katz et al.	60	80	90
	Katz et al.	110	61	71
Tinel's sign	Katz et al.	110	60	67
Phalen's sign	Katz et al.	110	75	47

n = number of patients.

diagram of the hand. Katz reported, in one study, the sensitivity and specificity for this test were better than for any other specific test or maneuver **(Table 10.7)**. Pain and tingling are reproduced in that specific distribution on performing **Tinel's procedure** (test) over the carpal tunnel **(Fig. 10.4)**. In the procedure, the examiner taps up to 10 to 15 times, with reproducible intensity, using the index or middle finger over the carpal tunnel site. The sensitivity for Tinel's sign is 60%, whereas, the specificity is 67%. In addition, findings are reproduced with **Phalen's procedure** (test) in which the patient gently, but maximally, palmar flexes both hands for 30 seconds **(Fig. 10.5)** and with **Worsmer's procedure** (test) in which the patient gently, but maximally, dorsiflexes the hands together for 30 seconds **(Fig. 10.6)**. Phalen's test (palmar flexion) is diagnostically better than Worsmer's procedure; however, dorsiflexion does complement Phalen's test. The sensitivity for Phalen's sign is 75%, whereas the specificity is 47%. Bilić and Pecina have described a novel test, which has, in our view, significant potential. In this test, the examiner places digital compression directly over the CT, the patient then places weight of upper extremity on the hand. Paresthesia that develops in <5 seconds bespeaks severe CTS, in 5 to 60 seconds mild and reversible CTS. **Severe CTS** manifests with atrophy and fasciculations of the thenar muscles **(Fig. 10.7)**, weakness to thumb flexion **(Fig. 10.8)**, and mild weakness to performing a tip-to-tip OK sign **(Fig. 10.9)**. Furthermore, the patient will have mild weakness to flexion of fingers 2

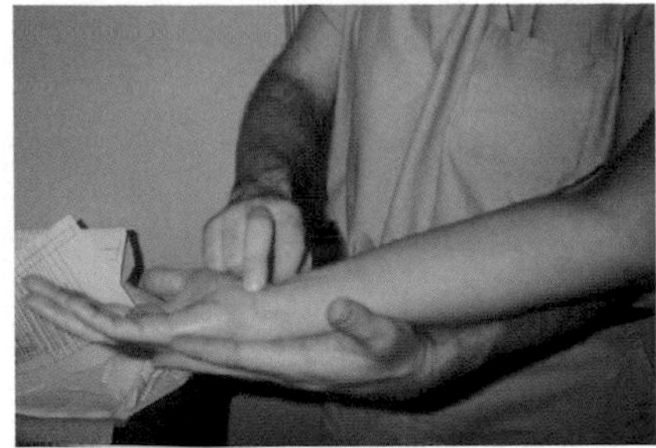

Figure 10.4.

Technique and sites for Tinel's maneuver for Carpal tunnel and Ulnar tunnel.

 **TIPS**

- Use finger or a Queen's square hammer to tap over each site
- Tap briskly with 10 to 15 consecutive reproducible taps
- Carpal tunnel **(A):** midline site
- Ulnar tunnel **(B):** ulnar side site

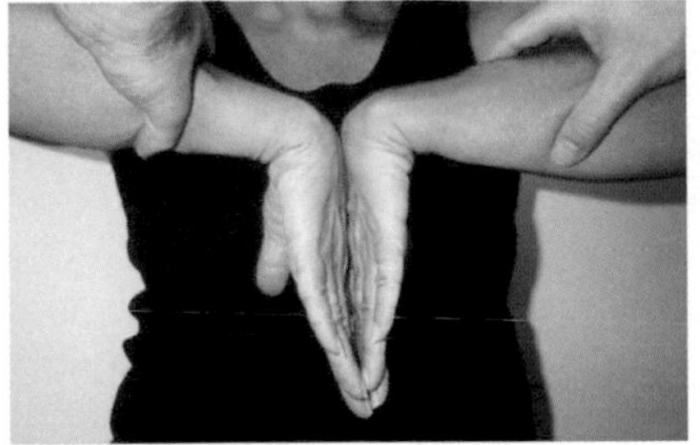

Figure 10.5.

Technique for Phalen's procedure. Excellent in evaluation of carpal or ulnar tunnel syndromes.

 **TIPS**

- The dorsal aspects of hands are placed together and palmar flexed in a reverse prayer fashion position; position held for 30 seconds
- Carpal tunnel syndrome: reproduction of tingling over fingers 1, 2, and 3
- Ulnar tunnel syndrome: reproduction of tingling over fingers 4 and 5

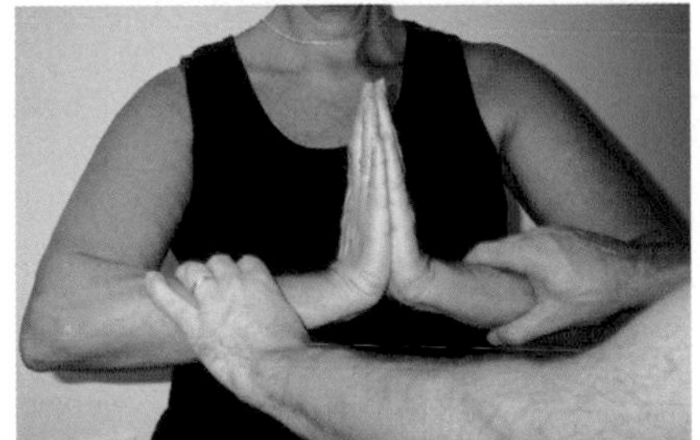

Figure 10.6.

Technique for Worsmer's procedure. Good in evaluation of carpal or ulnar tunnel syndromes.

 **TIPS**

- The palms are placed together and dorsiflexed in a prayer fashion for 30 seconds
- Carpal tunnel syndrome: reproduction of tingling over fingers 1, 2, and 3
- Ulnar tunnel syndrome: reproduction of tingling over fingers 4 and 5

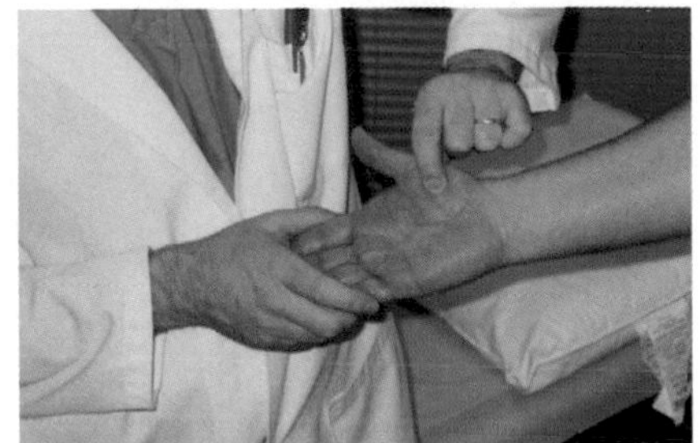

Figure 10.7.

Atrophy of thenar eminence in patient with advanced carpal tunnel syndrome (distal median nerve).

 **TIPS**

- Normal: a ball of muscle at base of thumb in thenar eminence
- Median nerve problem, proximal or distal: atrophy of the thenar eminence
- Anterior interosseous problem: no thenar atrophy

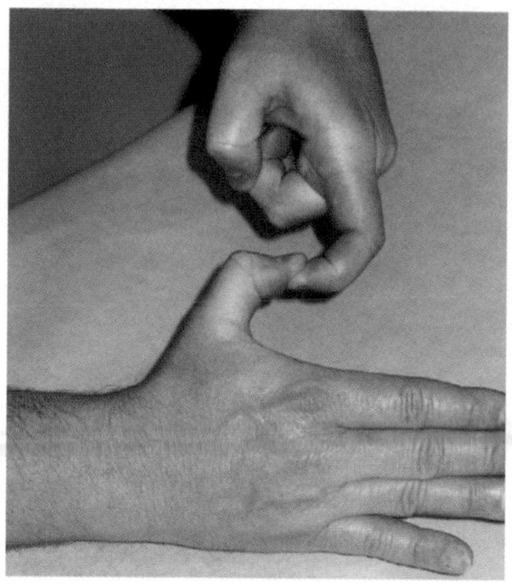

Figure 10.8.

Technique for active thumb interphalangeal (IP) joint flexion to assess the function of the anterior interosseous nerve.

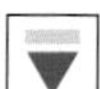 **TIPS**

- Neutral thumb position
- Actively flex the thumb at the interphalangeal (IP) joint; apply resistance to the distal phalanx
- AI or proximal median nerve problem: weakness
- CTS: little if any weakness specific to IP flexion

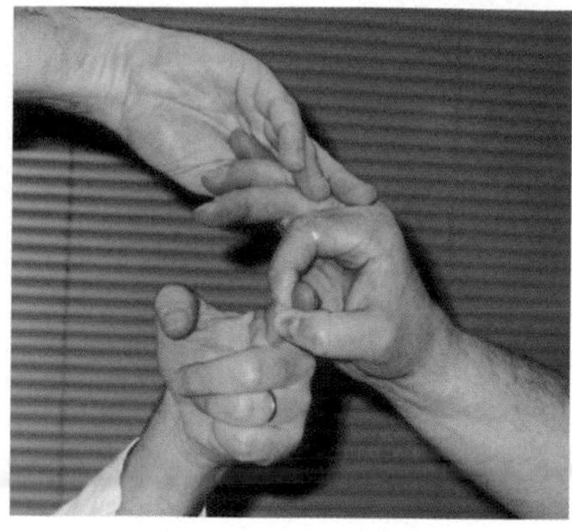

Figure 10.9.

Technique for resisted tip-to-tip "OK" sign.

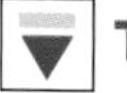 **TIPS**

- Make a tip-to-tip "OK;" tips of thumb and second digit touching
- Specifically apply resistance to the tips
- Normal: able to apply resistance without the tips of thumb and second digit flexion moving apart
- AI or proximal median nerve damage (proximal): weakness to OK, both thumb IP flexion and second digit flexors weak and atrophic; appear in a "pinch-position."
- CTS: little if any weakness to "OK" tip-to-tip

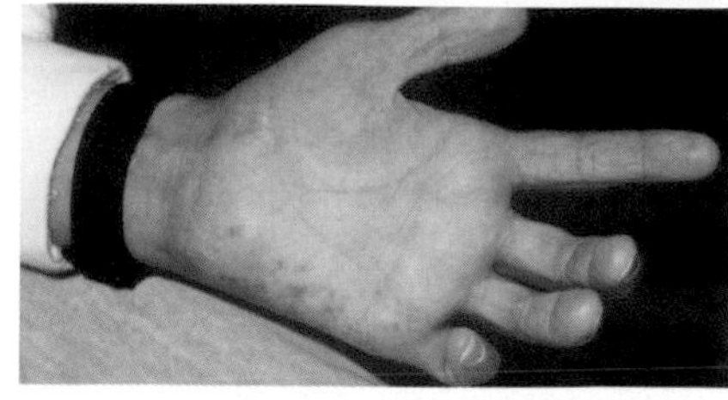

Figure 10.10.

Benediction sign of severe proximal median nerve damage. Patient had been instructed to actively make a fist.

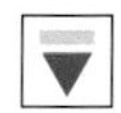 **TIPS**

- Instruct patient to actively flex the digits to make a fist
- Median nerve damage, proximal with blessing or benediction handsign; patient unable to actively flex digits 2 and 3
- CTS: no such finding

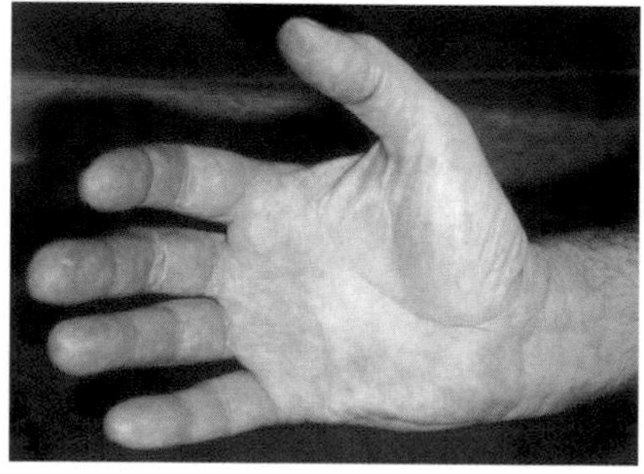

Figure 10.11.

Empty hypothenar sign of atrophy of muscles of the hypothenar eminence in a patient with ulnar nerve damage.

 **TIPS**

- Inspect the hypothenar area
- Ulnar nerve damage: atrophy of the hypothenar eminence, i.e., the empty hypothenar sign

and 3, so mild that if instructed to make a fist, the resulting hand configuration is usually normal. Other sites of proximal entrapment include pronator teres and anterior interosseous syndrome, discussed in Chapter 11.

Ulnar tunnel syndrome (UTS) manifests with tingling and pain in the ulnar aspect of the fingers on the palmar and dorsal aspects of digits 5 and 4 **(Fig. 10.3C)**. Although not studied extensively, the self-reported diagram for manifestations may be an excellent method to define and describe UTS. Pain and tingling are reproduced in that specific distribution on performing **Tinel's procedure** over the ulnar tunnel, in which the examiner taps up to 15 times, with reproducible intensity, using the index finger over the ulnar tunnel site (Fig. 10.4). In addition, findings are reproduced with **Phalen's procedure** (Fig. 10.5) in which the patient gently but maximally palmar flexes both hands for 30 seconds and with **Worsmer's procedure** in which the patient gently but maximally dorsiflexes the hands together for 30 seconds (Fig. 10.6). Phalen's procedure or palmar flexion is diagnostically better than that of Worsmer; however, dorsiflexion does complement Phalen's sign. **Severe UTS** manifests with atrophy and fasciculations of the hypothenar muscles. This atrophy is demonstrated by the empty hypothenar sign **(Fig. 10.11)** and is specific to superficial ulnar nerve damage. Weakness is noted to finger abduction and adduction and to flexion of digits 4 and 5 **(Fig. 10.12)**. Furthermore, there is decreased sensation over the skin of the hypothenar area and atrophy of the dorsal interossei **(Fig. 10.13)**. Finally, weakness to holding a piece of paper

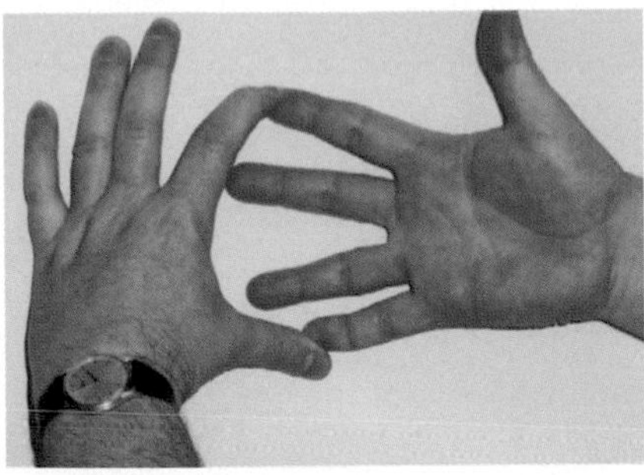

Figure 10.12.

Technique for active finger metacarpo-phalangeal (MCP) joint abduction—digits 2 through 5. Effective method to measure dorsal interossei muscle function and, thus, the ulnar nerve.

 **TIPS**

- Forearm pronated and supported
- Hand neutral, digits adjacent to each other
- Place pressure on the radial side of digit 2 and ulnar side of digit 5; patient actively spreads fingers apart
- Ulnar nerve problem: weakness. Fasciculations or atrophy of dorsal interossei, if severe

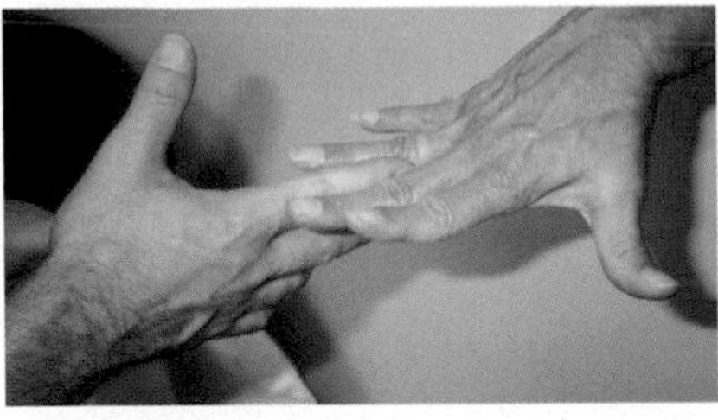

Figure 10.13.

Technique for active finger metacarpophalangeal (MCP) joint adduction. An effective method to measure the palmar interossei muscles and, thus, the ulnar nerve.

 **TIPS**

- Hand neutral, digits apart
- Patient actively adducts fingers against resistance
- Ulnar nerve problem: weakness. Fasciculations or atrophy of palmar interossei, if severe

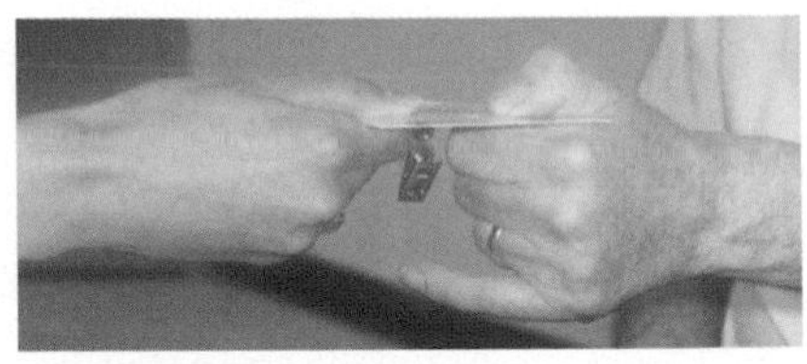

Figure 10.14.

Resisted adduction of the thumb (Froment's sign). Effectively measures the ulnar nerve and the adductor pollicis muscle. Note patient's hand in a mild fist position; note also flexion of IP of thumb to hold paper.

 **TIPS**

- Patient adducts thumb against resistance by holding fast to a piece of paper between the thumb and second digit
- Pull on the piece of paper
- Normal: able to hold fast to the paper
- Ulnar nerve problem: weakness to adduction, unable to hold fast to piece of paper and patient "cheats" by using thumb IP, i.e., the anterior interosseous nerve

fast between the thumb and the second digit and/or the patient flexing thumb at IP to keep paper, i.e., a positive Froment's sign, is noted **(Fig. 10.14)**. **UTS** is caused by repetitive use, overuse, hypothenar hammer syndrome, fracture of the fifth metacarpal bone, or the presence of a ganglion cyst.

Dupuytren's contracture manifests with flexion contractures of the fingers, particularly digits 5 and 4 **(Fig. 10.15)**. Fingers 2 and 3 may be involved; if so, they are concurrent to fingers 4 and 5. There are palpable fibronodular structures noted in the palmaris fascia of the hand and pleats in the skin of the palm. The underlying cause is not completely clear, although there has been some association with excessive alcohol ingestion. In our view, it more likely results from recurrent trauma to the area, e.g., hypothenar hammer.

Other problems include **Golfer's wrist**, a fracture of the hook of the hamate, which manifests with swelling and tenderness over the hook of the hamate, i.e., the hamulus. This is caused by the use of a golf club that is too long and hits the wrist while swinging the club. **Sprain or tear of one or more of the flexor tendons** manifests with pain and swelling at site of laceration or tear, weakness to flexion of the digits involved, which can be the DIP, PIP, MCP, or all three joints. Causes include active synovitis and deep lacerations. Thus a fastidious examination is needed on any patient with a laceration. **Trigger or locking finger** manifests with **triggering**, the acquired inability to extend from a flexed or **locking**, the inability to flex from an extended digit, and an audible click over the palmar head of the digit. Palpable swelling and mild tenderness are often noted on the palmar aspect of the MCP. This is often caused by overuse or compression from the use of a jackhammer, bicycling without gloves, or the incorrect use of crutches.

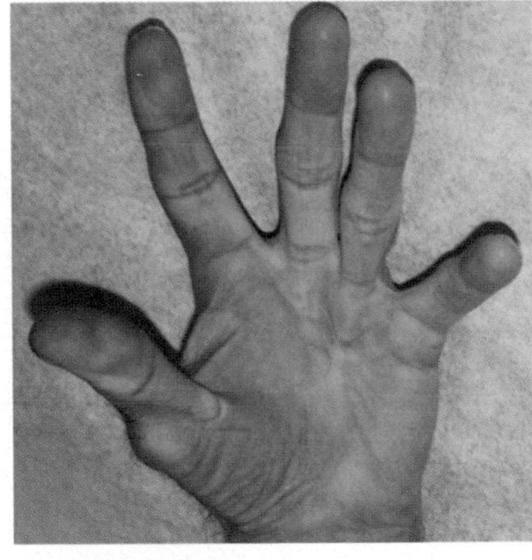

Figure 10.15.

Dupuytren's contracture: Note the flexion contractures of fingers 5, 4, and 3.

 **TIPS**

- Dupuytren's contracture: flexion contractures of digits
- Palpable fibronodular structures in the palmaris fascia and pleating of the overlying skin

TEACHING POINTS

PALMAR HAND AND FINGERS

1. The flexor tendons insert on the bases of the middle (superficial tendon) and the distal (profunda tendon) phalanx.
2. The profunda flexor tendon pierces the superficial flexor tendon over the metacarpophalangeal (MCP).
3. The flexors of the hand, wrist, and fingers are innervated by the median, anterior interosseous, and ulnar nerves.
4. The intrinsic muscles of the hand and digits are innervated by the ulnar and, to a lesser extent, the median nerve.
5. Benediction hand: make a fist, weak digits 2 and 3; proximal median nerve dysfunction, not carpal tunnel.
6. Numbness to thenar: proximal median, not carpal tunnel.
7. “OK” and handwriting require proximal median nerve and AI nerve.

THUMB BASE SNUFFBOX AND DORSAL

Scaphoid fracture manifests with discomfort in anatomic snuffbox that radiates into the *palmar, radial base* of the wrist. Recall, the snuffbox is bordered by extensor compartment 1 (abductor pollicus longus) and 3 (extensor pollicis longus); its base is the scaphoid bone. Pain is increased and localized to the snuffbox with the forearm squeeze test, in which the examiner gently squeezes the radius and ulna together at a site 10 cm proximal to the wrist **(Fig. 10.16)**. Often, the tenderness is most pronounced at the palmar aspect of the radial wrist. This is due to a fall on an outstretched arm. **Scapholunate dislocation** manifests with discomfort in the ulnar side of the base of the anatomic snuffbox. The patient relates that the discomfort worsens with repetitive rotatory movement of wrist, e.g., when using a screwdriver. A palpable dorsal displacement of the lunate and tenderness on the dorsal wrist are often noted. Finally, a click with pain is elicited with *Watson's stress test* in which the examiner's thumb is on the dorsal scaphoid and the tip of the second finger is on the palmar proximal carpal row **(Fig. 10.17)**. Then, the examiner radially and ulnarly deviates the wrist. Scapholunate dissociation is often caused by a fall on an outstretched arm.

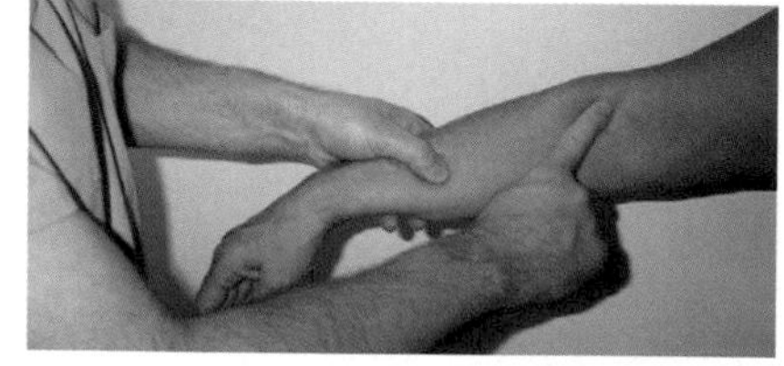

Figure 10.16.

The forearm squeeze is an excellent method to look for concurrent problems in primary wrist or elbow pain syndromes.

 **TIPS**

- Forearm neutral position
- Perform a squeeze in the mid forearm
- Radial head fracture: pain localized to elbow
- Scaphoid fracture: pain localized to the snuffbox

Skier's thumb manifests with pain and tenderness at the palmar, ulnar side of the thumb MCP joint **(Fig. 10.18)**. A cardinal feature is an abnormal laxity to abduction at the thumb MCP when the thumb is in full extension. This is a sprain or tear of the ulnar collateral ligament, most often caused by a fall while skiing and forcibly hyperabducting thumb on the ski pole. It can also develop as the result of an occupation, that of gamekeeper. This occupational injury is due to twisting the necks of rabbits or geese or ducks. In this case, our British colleagues refer to the problem as “Gamekeeper's thumb.”

Colles' fracture manifests with trauma-induced discomfort in the distal forearm, with a visible and palpable deformity of the distal forearm **(Fig. 10.19)**. This deformity, which is the distal radius displaced dorsally, is known as a “dinner fork deformity.” This fracture of the distal radius and ulna is caused by a fall on a forward-placed outstretched hand. Complications include a **saluting hand,**

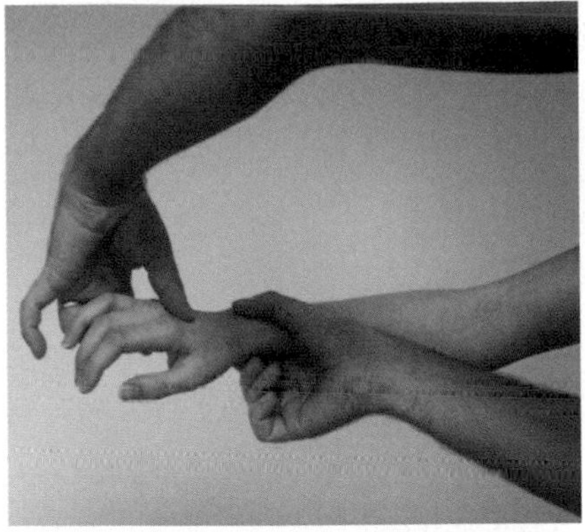
A

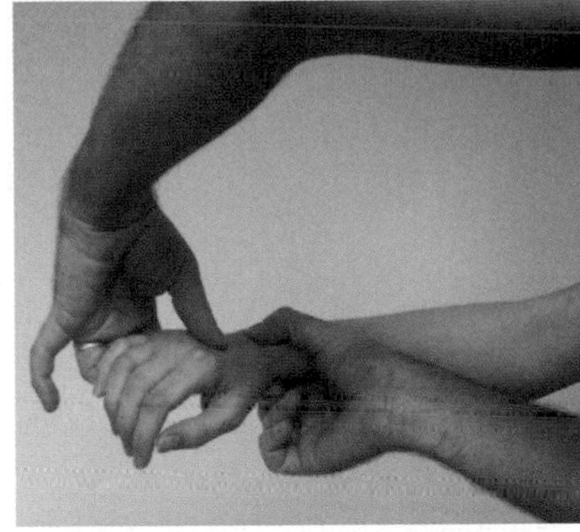
B

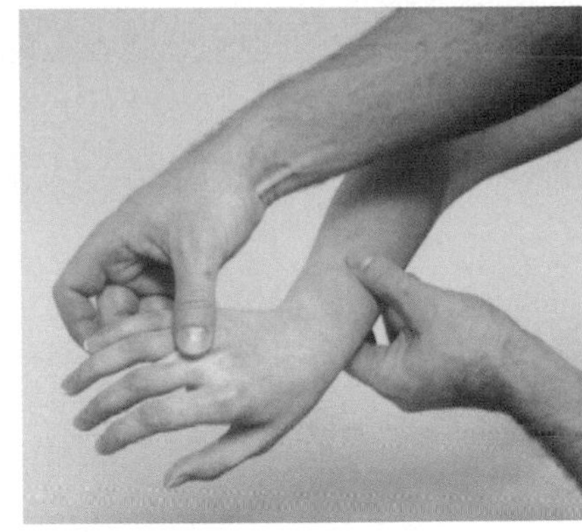
C

Figure 10.17.

Technique for Watson's stress test. Excellent to define a scapholunate dissociation. **A.** Neutral baseline position. **B.** Passive radial deviation. **C.** Passive ulnar deviation.

 **TIPS**

- Place thumb over the patient's dorsal scaphoid, the tip of second finger over the mid-palmar wrist; press firmly
- Passively deviate wrist radially, then ulnarly; repeat
- Scapholunate dissociation: palpable or audible click at snuffbox

which is a flexion contracture of the thumb IP caused by damage to the flexor pollicis tendon.

Intersection syndrome manifests with tenderness and pain over the mid distal radial extensor surface of the forearm, specifically at the intersection of extensor compartments 1 and 2 (Fig. 10.2). The discomfort is reproduced and there is a palpable or even audible squeak present with the *Finkelstein maneuver* **(Fig. 10.20)**. This maneuver consists of the patient making a fist

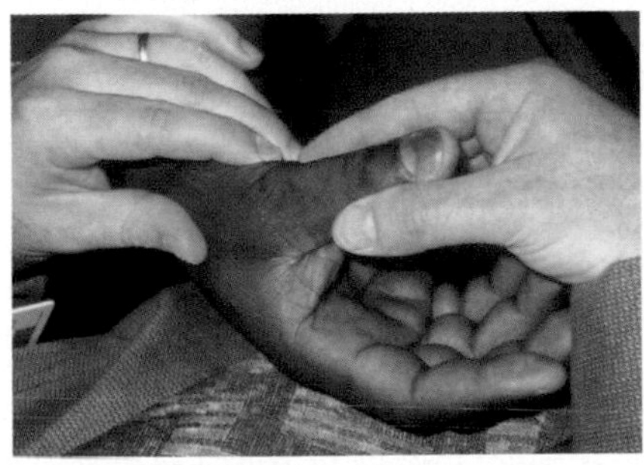

Figure 10.18.

Technique for passive abduction at thumb metacarpophalangeal (MCP) with thumb in extension. Test for ulnar collateral ligament sprain or laxity, also known as "skier's thumb."

 **TIPS**

- Thumb in full extension, passively abduct the thumb at the MCP joint
- Normal: minimal to no abduction
- Ulnar collateral ligament damage (Skier's thumb): abnormal abduction present at MCP

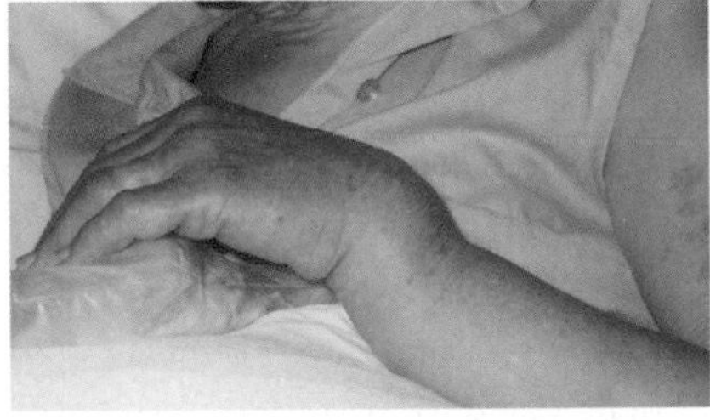

Figure 10.19.

Colles' fracture: This visible deformity at wrist, in which the distal radius is dorsally displaced.

 **TIPS**

- Colles' fracture: visible deformity, known as a "dinner fork" deformity (tongs down)
- Distal radius dorsally displaced

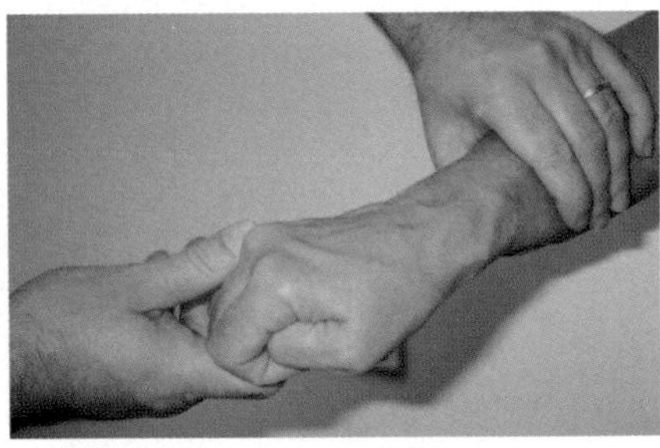

Figure 10.20.

Technique for the Finkelstein maneuver. Excellent test to define deQuervain's and intersection syndromes.

 **TIPS**

- Patient makes a fist with thumb in the fist
- Passively, ulnarly deviate the patient's wrist
- deQuervain's syndrome: tenderness in tendons of snuffbox (sheaths 1 and 3)
- Intersection syndrome: tender proximal to the anatomic snuffbox at extensor compartments 1 and 2

TEACHING POINTS

SNUFFBOX AND DORSAL HAND

1. The radial nerve and its branch posterior interosseous nerve innervates all of the extrinsic muscles involving the hand dorsum.
2. The tendons of the extensors are located in the six compartments of extensor muscles.
3. The only intrinsic muscles located on the dorsal hand are the dorsal interossei.
4. Abduction of thumb, and all extensors of thumb, fingers, hand, and wrist involve the posterior interosseous nerve.
5. Boutonièrre deformity is damage of the finger extensor over the proximal interphalangeal (PIP) joint, with a flexion contracture of PIP joint and extension contracture of the distal interphalangeal (DIP) joint.

with the thumb enclosed and the examiner placing mild to moderate passive ulnar deviation at the wrist. This syndrome is often caused by repetitive rowing or crewing. **deQuervain's tenosynovitis** manifests with tenderness in or near one, two, or all three of the tendons of the anatomic snuffbox, i.e., the tendons of extensor compartments 1 and 3 (Fig. 10.2). The discomfort is reproduced with a Finkelstein maneuver. deQuervain's tenosynovitis is caused by repetitive use of hand and wrist in crocheting, knitting, peeling potatoes, tying sutures, and so on.

Superficial radial nerve entrapment (**Wartenberg's syndrome**) manifests with tingling and pain over the radial dorsal side of the forearm and radiating into the snuffbox: Tingling and pain can be reproduced with Tinel's procedure in the proximal brachioradialis muscle. **Radial head fracture** can manifest with pain in the elbow radiating into the snuffbox. The elbow pain is reproduced by the forearm squeeze maneuver (Fig. 10.16). In addition, a marked decrease in passive and active supination and pronation is noted at the elbow.

Tenosynovitis of extensor compartments manifests with pain on the dorsal forearm. The pain is exacerbated by active wrist dorsiflexion or passive wrist palmar flexion. There may be swelling on the hand dorsum. The pain and swelling may be discrete to one or more of the extensor compartments. An **acute tear** of one of these tendons manifests with acute pain, swelling, and a marked decrease in active dorsiflexion at the fingers (**Fig. 10.21**). This is caused by tendon rupture due to severe synovitis, e.g., rheumatoid arthritis, or a deep laceration.

Figure 10.21.

Acute tear of the extensor tendons, here tendons to digits 5 and 4 (compartments 5 and part of 4) caused by significant inflammatory arthritis.

 **TIPS**

- Baseline fist
- Actively extend the digits from fist position
- Tenosynovitis: pain in one or more of the extensor compartments
- Tear of extensor tendons: swelling and an acute decreased ability to extend the digit

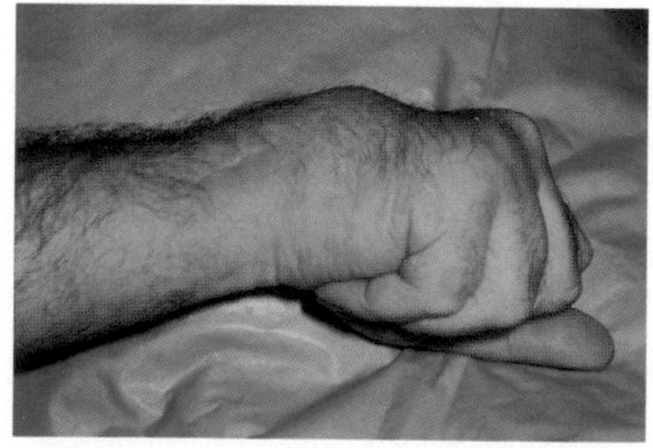

A

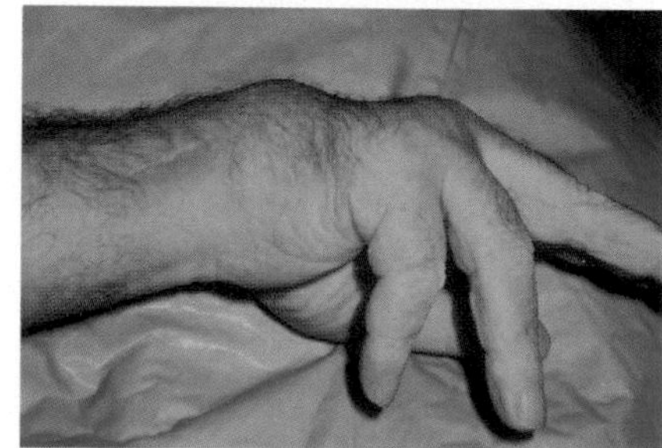

B

ULNAR SIDE

Hypothenar hammer syndrome manifests with recurrent tingling over the ulnar hand and dorsal and palmar aspect of the fifth digit. If severe, there is swelling over the site, weakness to finger abduction and adduction, and decreased active flexion in digits 4 and 5. The company it keeps includes a delayed ulnar Allen test **(Fig. 10.22)** and even development of blue finger(s) **(Fig. 10.30)**.

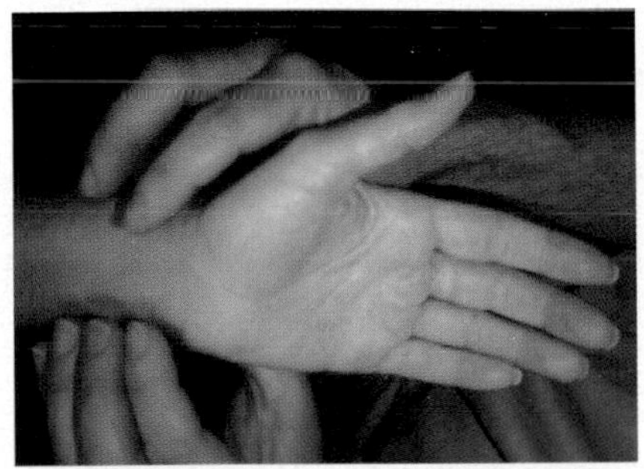

A

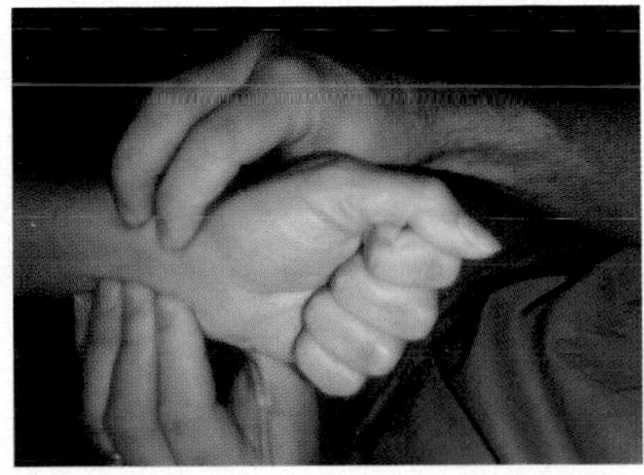

B

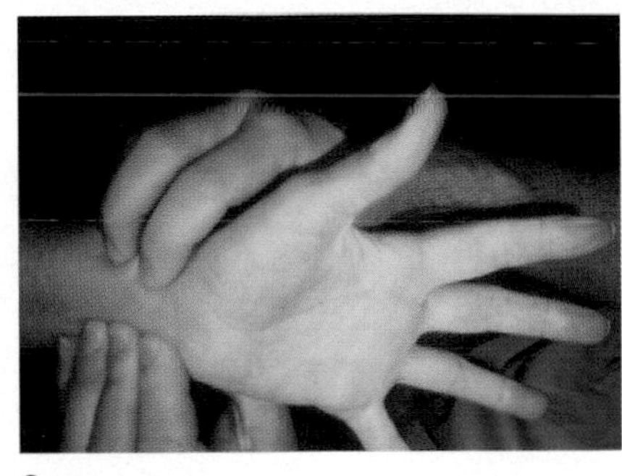

C

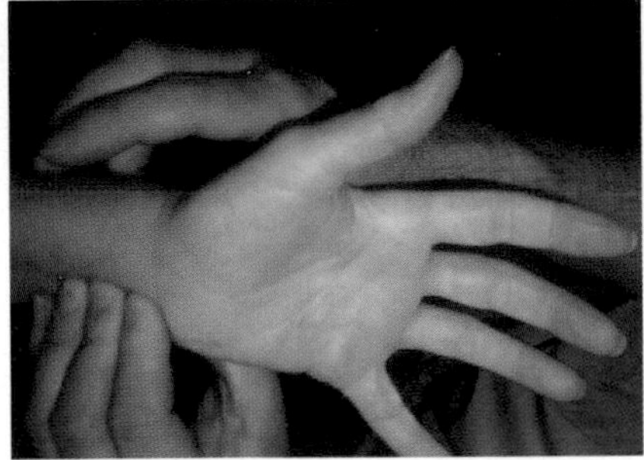

D

Figure 10.22.

Normal Ulnar Allen test. **A.** Step 1: Examiner places index fingers over the radial and ulnar arteries. **B.** Step 2: Patient actively makes a closed fist for 15 seconds, while the examiner maintains pressure on both radial and ulnar arteries. **C.** Step 3: Patient actively opens up the hand. **D.** Step 4: The examiner releases the ulnar artery side only. Normal: a pink flush returns, from ulnar to radial side, in less than 6 seconds.

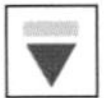

TIPS

- Hand neutral position
- Step 1: Place index fingers over the patient's radial and ulnar arteries **(A)**
- Step 2: Patient actively makes a closed fist for 15 seconds, while the examiner maintains pressure on both radial and ulnar arteries **(B)**
- Step 3: Patient actively opens up the hand (**C**)
- Step 4: Release the patient's ulnar artery side only (**D**)
- Normal: a pink flush returns, from ulnar to radial side, in <6 seconds
- Ulnar artery dysfunction: pink returns but takes >6 seconds
- Complete ulnar artery obstruction: no pink return

TEACHING POINTS

ULNAR SIDE OF HAND, WRIST, AND FINGERS

1. Boxer's fracture is a not uncommon trauma-related fracture of the hand. It involves the fifth metacarpal.
2. Assess the ulnar artery via the ulnar Allen test in cases of any trauma to the ulnar hand.
3. The ulnar artery supplies most of the blood flow to the hand and digits.
4. The ulnar nerve provides motor supply to most of the intrinsic muscles of hand.
5. Hypothenar hammer syndrome, in which the patient uses the fist as a hammer, causes damage to the ulnar artery or nerve, especially the superficial ulnar nerve.

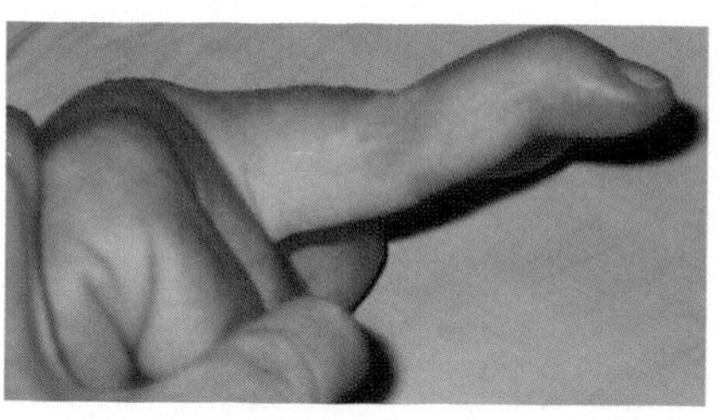

Figure 10.23.

Swan neck contracture.

 TIPS

- Swan neck: contracture of hyperextension at the PIP joint and flexion at the DIP joint in affected finger
- Caused by volar plate tear: trauma or rheumatoid arthritis related

This syndrome can be caused by recurrent use of the ulnar aspect of a closed fist as a hammer, e.g., hitting the top of a dashboard or the top of a TV set. **Boxer's fracture** manifests with acute trauma-related swelling and tenderness of the ulnar side of hand. The trauma is usually self-inflicted, pugilistic activity. This is specifically a fracture of the diaphysis of the fifth metacarpal bone.

FINGERS

Inflammatory arthritis, e.g., rheumatoid arthritis, manifests with a palpable *palmar subluxation* of the proximal phalanx on the metacarpal bone and ulnar deviations of the fingers. The subluxations lead to significant functional embarrassment. The company it keeps includes one or more **swan neck** contractures may be noted, in which there is contracture of hyperextension at the PIP joint and of flexion at the DIP joint **(Fig. 10.23)**. This is caused by damage to the volar plate, either from an inflammatory arthritis or trauma. Swan neck that is isolated to one finger and has no other symptoms is usually trauma-related. Furthermore, one or more **Boutonnière's contractures** may be seen, in which a contracture is noted of hyperextension at the DIP joint and to flexion at the PIP joint. This is due to damage to the extensor tendon, either from an inflammatory arthritis or a laceration. Boutonnière's contracture that is isolated to one finger and has no other symptoms is usually trauma-related. **Typewriter contracture** manifests with a flexion contracture isolated to the PIP joint **(Fig. 10.24)**. This early form of Boutonnière contracture has the same pathogenesis as Boutonnière's contracture.

Fracture of the middle or proximal phalanx manifests with pain, swelling, and marked decreased function over the site of injury. Assess the finger for any abnormal angulation by inspecting the long axes of the fingers while the patient gently makes an incomplete fist. Mal-angulation is present if the long axis is slightly off **(Fig. 10.25)**. Mal-angulation can result in further complications and, thus, requires referral to a hand specialist. A fracture of the digit is most commonly caused by direct trauma to the digit, e.g., a crush injury or jam injury with a baseball.

Proximal interphalangeal dislocation manifests with acute trauma-related onset of severe pain and visible deformity at the PIP. The middle phalanx is dislocated palmarly or dorsally on the proximal phalanx **(Fig. 10.26)**. It is most commonly caused by jamming the finger while catching a ball. The company a dorsal dislocation keeps includes an extensor tendon sprain or

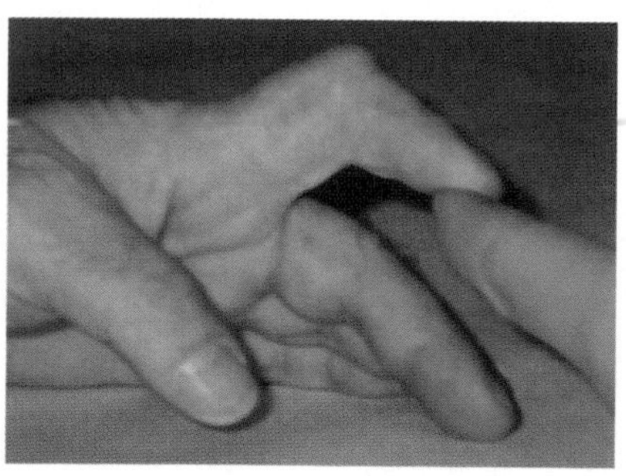

Figure 10.24.

Typewriter finger: flexion contracture of proximal interphalangeal (PIP) joint.

 TIPS

- Boutonnière's contracture: hyperextension contracture of the distal interphalangeal (DIP) joint and flexion contracture of proximal interphalangeal (PIP) joint
- Typewriter finger: flexion contracture of PIP joint, an early Boutonnière's contracture
- Caused by extensor tendon laceration or dorsal PIP joint dislocation: trauma or rheumatoid arthritis related

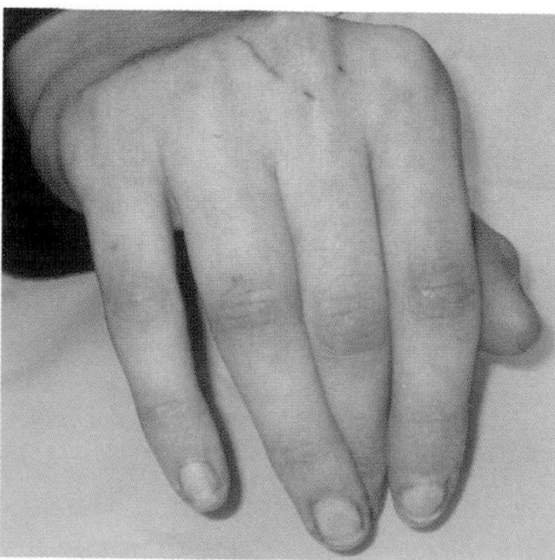

Figure 10.25.

Malaligned finger fracture: on minimal flexion of the digit, significant malalignment is present. A significant finding that requires referral to a hand specialist.

 TIPS

- Inspect the long axes of the digits when an incomplete fist is made
- Normal: long axes of digits point toward the scaphoid
- Mal-angulated fracture: long axis of digit is off
- Malalignment is a significant finding that requires referral to a hand specialist

rupture and, thus, the potential complications of either a typewriter (Fig. 10.24) or Boutonnière's contracture. The company a palmar dislocation keeps includes a volar plate sprain or rupture and, thus, the potential complication of a swan neck contracture.

Degenerative joint (osteoarthritis) disease (DJD) of the fingers and thumbs manifests with Bouchard's nodes, which are painless papules on the PIP joints, and Heberden's nodes, which are painless papules on the DIP joints **(Fig. 10.27)**. An easy method to remember and teach the eponyms here is "BP, British petroleum, Bouchard's proximal." Often, there is concurrent **thumb base osteoarthritis**. This manifests with pain, stiffness, and mild swelling at the base of the thumb MCT joint. DJD is more common in the dominant hand, but can be bilateral. Decreased active and passive ROM is noted, especially prominent in thumb circumduction, e.g. twiddling, and abduction. Often, significant crepitus, which is isolated to the thumb base, is brought on with thumb movement. In severe degenerative disease, the thenar eminence can atrophy, not as the result of recurrent median nerve mischief, but because of disuse.

Mallet finger manifests with a contracture of flexion at the DIP joint **(Fig. 10.28)**. The contracture is present when the mallet is advanced and severe; however, early on, there is a flexion attitude at the DIP joint, incomplete full active extension, but normal passive extension at the DIP joint to 0 degrees. Mallet finger is caused by jamming the DIP joint in flexion, thus, tearing the distal insertion of the extensor tendon.

Ganglion cyst manifests with a nontender fluctuant nodule that is contiguous with the tendon sheath **(Fig. 10.29)**. This is usually not tender, but with application of a light source it is transilluminable. The cyst moves with the tendon itself, which is a defining feature of the cyst. If it overlies an artery or nerve, it

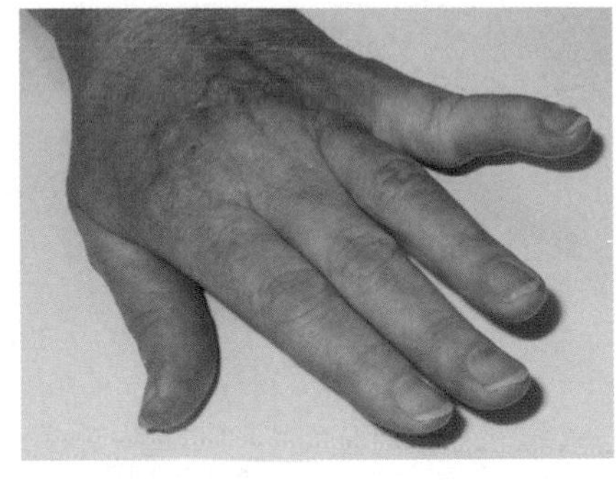

Figure 10.26.

Palmar dislocation of the middle phalanx at PIP.

 **TIPS**

- Middle phalanx dorsal dislocation: extensor tendon damage usually present
- Middle phalanx palmar dislocation: volar plate and, thus, flexor damage usually present
- Either finding is trauma related, e.g., often playing catch or baseball and "jamming" the digit

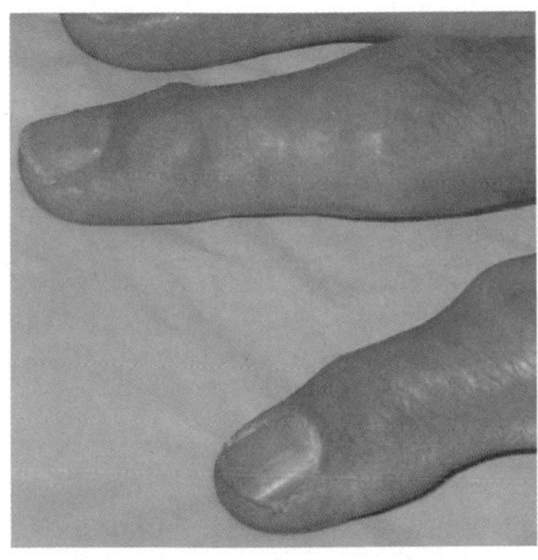

Figure 10.27.

Degenerative joint disease of fingers: Bouchard's nodes on proximal interphalangeal (PIP) joint, Heberden's nodes on distal interphalangeal (DIP) joint. Look for the company of other finger or of thumb osteoarthritis.

 **TIPS**

- Bouchard's nodes: nontender papules on bony surfaces of the PIP joint
- Heberden's nodes: nontender papules on bone surfaces of the DIP joint

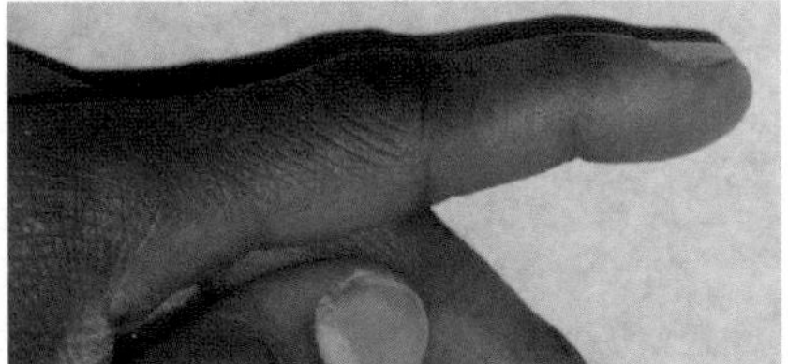

A

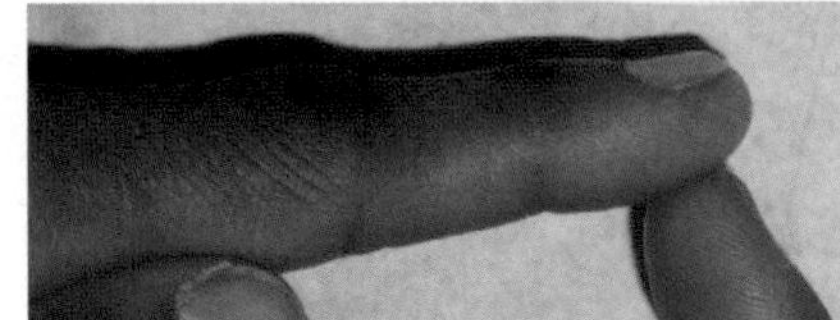

B

Figure 10.28.

Mallet finger: early—unable to actively extend at distal interphalangeal (DIP) joint, but passively can extend fully at the DIP joint.

 **TIPS**

- Inspect the digit from the side, with the digit fully extended
- Normal: 0 degrees of extension at DIP
- Mallet finger: early—unable to actively extend at the DIP joint; passively can extend fully at the DIP joint
- Mallet finger: late—flexion contracture of the DIP joint

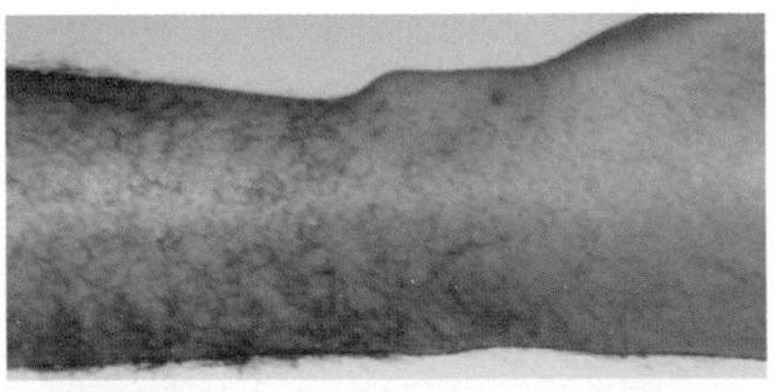

A

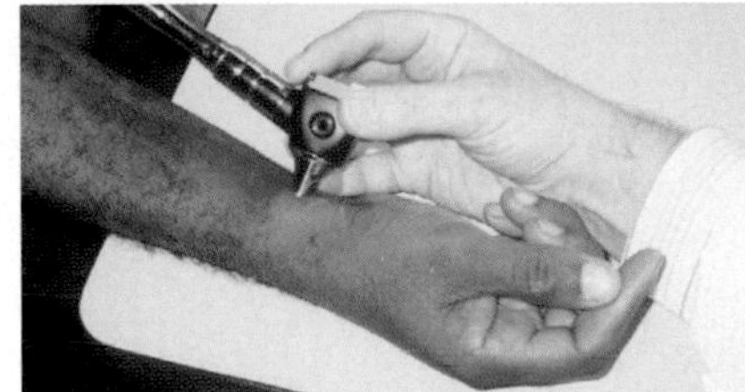

B

Figure 10.29.

Ganglion cyst: nontender, fluctuant nodule contiguous with a tendon sheath. Here, it is the flexor tendon sheath; it moves with the tendon and is transilluminable.

 **TIPS**

- Ganglion cyst: nontender, fluctuant nodule contiguous with a tendon sheath
- Move with tendon
- Transilluminable

TEACHING POINTS

FINGERS

1. Heberden's and Bouchard's nodes are DJD-related bone synovial cysts.
2. Swan neck contracture: related to volar plate damage at the proximal interphalangeal (PIP) joint.
3. Boutonnière's contracture: related to extensor tendon damage at the PIP joint.
4. Anatomically, the volar plate is a foundation of the digit.
5. Finger fracture and dislocation are common.
6. Most common reason for PIP and DIP joint subluxations or dislocations is trauma; inflammatory arthritis can result in similar findings.
7. Most common reason for subluxation of the metacarpophalangeal (MCP) joint is inflammatory; it is extremely rare for trauma-related dislocation at the MCP joint (more common to fracture a bone).
8. PIP or DIP joint subluxation: trauma related is more common than inflammatory related.
9. Felon is a bag of pus in the palmar fingertip.
10. Trauma-related problems involving the fingertip include subungual hematoma and tuft fracture.
11. Tophi of gout can manifest with swelling in the pads of the fingertips.
12. Damage to the extensor tendon via forced hyperflexion of the DIP joint will manifest with mallet finger.

DJD = degenerative joint disease.

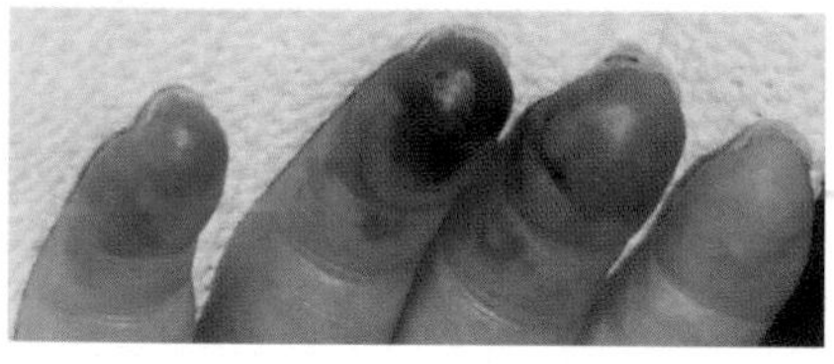

Figure 10.30.

Blue fingers: tender blue to black areas at tips of digits.

 **TIPS**

- Blue fingers: tender blue to black areas at tips of digits
- Look for related symptoms of an underlying cause: the irregularly irregular rhythm of atrial fibrillation or Janeway or Osler's, fever and heart murmur of endocarditis

can cause irritation or entrapment problems. Ganglion cysts, which are caused by outpouching of the sheath, are filled with viscous synovial material.

Blue finger manifests with blue or black areas in the distal digits that are initially extremely painful and tender but, over time, become remarkably painless **(Fig. 10.30)**. The company it keeps is specific to the underlying etiology. Embolic events from atrial fibrillation manifest in a patient who has an irregularly irregular pulse; embolic events from endocarditis manifest with fever, heart murmur, purple papules on the digits (Fig. 14.15) and palms and soles of hands and feet (Janeway and Osler's nodes), and Roth spots on funduscopic examination. Frostbite manifests with a history of exposure to severe cold. Buerger's disease, i.e., thromboangiitis obliterans, manifests with nicotine stains on fingernail plates and a long history of cigarette smoking (Fig. 14.20).

Another diagnosis includes **collar-button abscess**, which manifests with a fluctuant nodule with an overlying callus; however, because severe neuropathy is often present, the area of fluctuance may be remarkably pain free. This is a deep-seated and dangerous abscess that often develops deep to a callus on the plantar aspect of the foot or palmar aspect of the hand. Puncture wounds can contribute to the pathogenesis of these lesions. A **felon**, which is a specific type of collar-button abscess, manifests with an extremely tender swelling on the palmar pad of digit. This deep abscess is caused by a puncture wound to a fingertip, e.g., from a rose thorn or a lancet, especially in a patient with uncontrolled diabetes mellitus. **Tophi** manifest with mildly swollen tender areas on more than one palmar pad. The company it keeps includes papules on the auricles (Fig. 1.4), recurrent polyarticular arthritis, and podagra. **Jersey finger** manifests with a contracture of hyperextension of the DIP joint on the fourth digit. This is found most often on the dominant hand.

This is caused by firmly grasping using the thumb and fourth digit and, thus, tearing the flexor tendon insertion site on the distal phalanx. An example is a football player holding an opponent's jersey while attempting to tackle. **Subungual hematoma** manifests with a tender, purple discrete collection under the nail plate. Often, there is a concurrent tuft fracture. This is caused by a crush injury to the fingertip, e.g., pinching the fingertip in a door jam, freezer door, or car door. **Syndactyly**, which manifests with the congenital absence of one or more digits, can be associated with other congenital manifestations.

Annotated Bibliography

AIDS to the examination of the peripheral nervous system, 4th ed, WB Saunders, Edinburgh, 2000.
The master work. One of the most important references for neurologic examination in existence.

Thumb and Snuffbox

Atkinson LS, Baxley EG. Scapholunate dissociation. *Am Fam Phys* 1994;49(8):1845–1850.
Very good paper on this not common problem. Very good to excellent physical examination, including findings on inspection and description of the Watson stress test. Examination based on anatomy; excellent description of radiographic findings, including Gilula's lines and an angle of >70 degrees between the scaphoid and lunate in lateral view to confirm the clinical diagnosis. Dissociation means sprain, or even dislocation, of this foundation of the wrist.

Carr MM, Freiberg A. Osteoarthritis of the thumb: clinical aspects and management. *Am Fam Phys* 1994;50(5):995–1000.
Overview of this common entity. Limited discussion of the history and physical examination, but good discussion of radiographic and some therapeutic modalities.

Eiff MP. Prevention and treatment of skier's thumb. *Your Patient and Fitness* 1995;10(1): 23–25.
Terse, but satisfactory, overview of a not uncommon entity—sprain of the ulnar collateral ligament of the thumb MCP while skiing. Includes nice description of examination in the acute and subacute settings and a description of Stener lesion.

Finkelstein H. Stenosing tenovaginitis at the radial styloid process. *J Bone Joint Surg* 1930;12:509–540.
Original description of the classic sign: "On grasping the patient's thumb and quickly abducting the hand ulnarward, the pain over the styloid tip is excruciating." The procedure has been modified over time so that the thumb is enclosed in a fist but the original paper remains fascinating and serves as an underpinning of modern physical examination of problems involving the snuffbox and thumb base.

Hankins FM, Smith PA, Braunstein EM. Evaluation of the carpal scaphoid. *Am Fam Phys* 1986;34(2):129–132.
Emphasizes the physical diagnostic and radiographic assessment of the wrist; a nice description of how the scaphoid flexes palmarly with radial deviation.

Husband JB, McPherson SA. Bony skier's thumb injuries. *Clin Orthop* 1996;327:79–84.
Very well-written description of skier's thumb, with emphasis on surgical therapeutic options but good data on physical examination.

O'Dell MJ, Moore JB. Scaphoid (navicular) fracture of the wrist. *Am Fam Phy* 1984;29(4): 189–194.
Good review of the diagnostic assessment of this relatively common fracture. Physical examination includes pain at the snuffbox and with dorsiflexion of the wrist at the snuffbox. The problem of nonunion and when to refer are discussed in addition to a nice, albeit dated, discussion of the surgical techniques available.

Pecina MM, et al: Tunnel Syndromes, 2nd ed, CRC Press, Boca Raton, 1997.
Extraordinary reference for peripheral nerve entrapments.

Schumacher HR, Dorwart BB, Korzeniowski. Occurrence of de Quervain's tendonitis during pregnancy. *Arch Intern Med* 1985;145:2083–2084.
First reported cases of this common entity with pregnancy; in their report of five cases, found the condition was usually unilateral and resolved after delivery.

Servi JT. Wrist pain from overuse. *The Physician and Sports Medicine* 1997;25(12):41–44.
Nice discussion of the intersection syndrome: inflammation of the extensor compartments between 1 and 2. Nice description of physical examination and of synonyms: bugaboo or squeaker wrist.

Wrist

Loder RT, Mayhew HE. Common fractures from a fall on an outstretched hand. 1988;37(2): 327–338.
Instructive paper that describes the most common fractures as the result of a fall on an outstretched hand (Colles', scaphoid, radial neck, posterior elbow dislocation, impacted humeral frac-

ture, and clavicular fracture) as well as some aspects of diagnosis and therapy. Nice description of some of the child-related fractures and the splints required in management of each type.

Ring D, Jupiter JB. Managing fractures of the distal radius. *Journal of Musculoskeletal Medicine* 1995;12(10):59–68.

Satisfactory overview of the most common fractures involving the distal radius, including the Colles', Smith, and Barton. History, physical examination, and radiographic assessment discussed as are potential strategies in the management of such fractures. Radiographic assessment presented in fuller detail than physical examination.

Skolnick AA. Golfer's wrist can be a tough break to diagnose. *JAMA* 1998;279(8):571–572.

Terse description of this fracture of the hamulus of the hamate caused by using the wrong (too long) clubs while golfing.

Ulnar Hand

Rowan LJ. Hand ischemia in active patients. *The Physician and Sports Medicine* 1998;26(1): 57–66.

Nice discussion of hypothenar hammer syndrome (i.e., repetitive blunt trauma resulting in ulnar artery occlusion) especially in athletes. Nice description of the physical examination as well.

Carpal and Ulnar Tunnel

Bracker MD, Ralph LP. The numb arm and hand. *Am Fam Phys* 1995;51(1):103–116.

Complete description of many of the more common entities that cause numbness in the distal upper extremities, including carpal tunnel, ulnar tunnel, pronator syndrome, radial tunnel, cubital tunnel, thoracic outlet, and anterior and posterior interosseous sites; moderately specific on physical examination tests and findings; some discussion on primary care-based therapy. Overall, a highly satisfactory review.

Dawson DM. Entrapment neuropathies of the upper extremities. *N Engl J Med* 1993;329 (27):2013–2018.

Satisfactory review of the various entrapment neuropathies involving the upper extremities; good primary care discussion of assessment and early therapy of carpal tunnel syndrome, ulnar tunnel syndrome, and thoracic outlet syndrome.

Jones JG. Ulnar tunnel syndrome. *Am Fam Phys* 1991;44(2):497–502.

An excellent review and discussion of this often overlooked entrapment neuropathy. Good history and risk factor assessment, including occupational causes and hypothenar hammer. Excellent discussion of the physical examination, based on anatomy, including need for Allen test to assess the ulnar artery, the utility of Tinel's and Phalen's procedures, and the palmaris brevis sign (dimpling of skin over the hypothenar eminence, which indicates sparing of the superficial branch) sensory examination. Tinel's found to be the least effective test. A paper that is required for primary care physicians.

Katz JN, Stirrat CR. A self-administered hand diagram for the diagnosis of carpal tunnel syndrome. *J Hand Surg* 1990;15A:360–363.

Wonderful report of a diagnostic test of a diagram of the palmar and dorsal hand developed by the authors to allow patients to describe the site of maximal symptoms in carpal tunnel syndrome (CTS); used a standardized grading system to interpret the diagrams. In 75 hands with CTS, 60 were positive using the diagrams (sensitivity, 80%); in 10 without CTS, 90% specificity. Interesting small study.

Katz JN, et al. The carpal tunnel syndrome: diagnostic utility of the history and physical examination findings. *Ann Intern Med* 1990;112:321–327.

Well-designed and -written paper using the hand pain diagram rating, Tinel's procedure, and other physical findings to evaluate patients with potential carpal tunnel syndrome (n = 110 patients). Sensitivity and specificity for the tests were, respectively: Tinel, 60%, 67%; Phalen, 75%, 47%; hand diagram rating, 61%, 71%. Excellent attempt to objectify findings and cluster them with symptoms.

Finger

Aronson S. Evacuation of a subungual hematoma. *Hosp Med* 1995;(Nov):17–48.

Extremely practical discussion of the emergent management of an extremely common problem—subungual hematoma.

Bach AW. Finger joint injuries in active patients. *The Physician and Sports Medicine* 1999; 27(3):89–104.

One of the best recent overviews of the common injury-related problems involving the fingers. Physical examination of mallet finger, fractures, dislocations, and collateral ligament sprains are all described in well-written prose.

Chaisson C, McAlindon TE. Osteoarthritis of the hand: clinical features and management. *Journal of Musculoskeletal Medicine* 1997;14(5):66–77.

Nice description of the manifestations of this very common process, including Heberden's and Bouchard's nodes.

Fisk G. The relationship of trauma to Dupuytren's contracture. In: Hueston JT, Tubiana R, eds. *Dupuytren's disease.* Edinburgh: Churchill Livingstone, 1974:43–44.

Interesting discussion of the cause of Dupuytren's disease—genetic predisposition, but recurrent ulnar hand trauma.

Hoffman DF, Schaffer TC. Management of common finger injuries. ***Am Fam Phys*** **1991;43(5):1594–1607.**

Practical review of the assessment and primary care management of many finger problems, including mallet finger; fractures of the digits, including the evaluation for mal-angulation; volar plate and extensor tendon injuries, including swan neck and Boutonnière contracture, respectively. Specific splints for therapy are described in detail. Overall, a highly recommended paper for the primary care physician.

Lairmore JR, Engber WD. Serious, often subtle, finger injuries. ***The Physician and Sports Medicine*** **1998;26(6):57–68.**

Overview of traumatic finger injuries; good discussion of examination and therapy for common dislocations and sprains that involve the digits, including mallet finger. Also describes the thumb injury, skier's thumb, and its treatment.

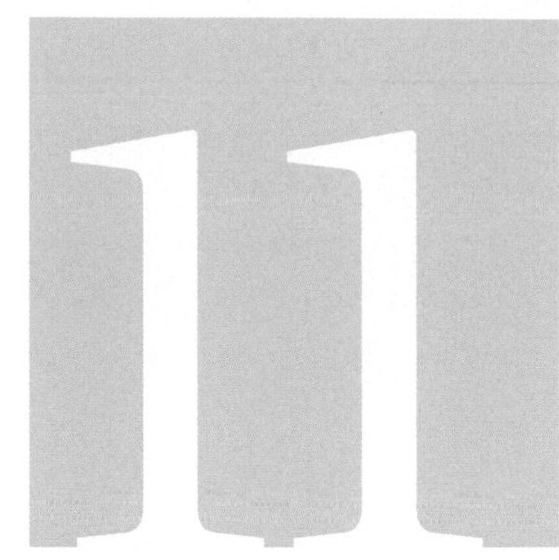

Elbow Examination

PRACTICE AND TEACHING

SURFACE ANATOMY

The surface anatomy of the posterior, anterior, and medial elbow is discussed below. In many ways the elbow is extremely analogous to the knee. See **Table 11.1** for comparisons.

Posterior (Fig. 11.1)

The **triceps muscle**, the largest muscle around the elbow, is proximal and posterior to the joint. It originates on the scapula, inserts on the proximal ulna, and acts to extend the elbow; its nerve radial (C7). The **wrist extensors** originate on the lateral epicondyle area of the humerus, and insert on the dorsal side of the carpals, metacarpals, and phalanges; their nerve is the posterior interosseous (C6 and C7). The **ulnar nerve** runs through the cubital tunnel, then on to the ulnar side of the forearm to the ulnar (Guyon's tunnel) (Fig. 10.1) side of the wrist. **Cubital tunnel** is the sulcus in the posterior medial elbow, between the medial epicondyle and the olecranon process, immediately lateral to the medial epicondyle and the proximal flexor carpi ulnaris (FCU); it is the site through which the ulnar nerve enters the forearm. The **olecranon process** of the ulna is the point

Table 11.1. Comparisons of the Knee and the Elbow

Elbow	Knee
Humeral-ulnar	Femoral-tibial
Ulnar collateral ligament	Medial collateral ligament
Radial collateral ligament	Lateral collateral ligament
Flexion-extension	Flexion-extension
Long head biceps	Semimembranous
Short head biceps	Semitendinous
Triceps	Quadriceps
Olecranon	Patella
Radial/ulnar joint	Fibular/tibial joint
Contrasts	
No cruciate ligaments	Cruciate ligaments present
Supination/pronation	No supination/pronation

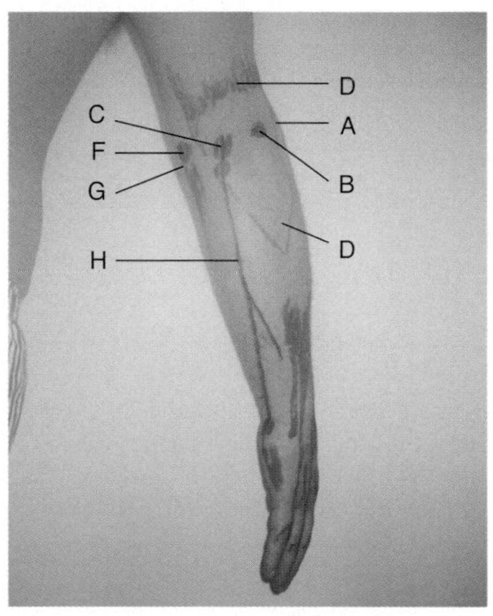

Figure 11.1.

Posterior elbow surface anatomy. **A.** Lateral epicondyle. **B.** Olecranon process. **C.** Cubital tunnel. **D.** Triceps muscle and its aponeurosis. **E.** Olecranon bursa. **F.** Epitrochlear node. **G.** Medial epicondyle. **H.** Ulnar nerve.

 **TIPS**

- Lateral epicondyle: origin of wrist extensors and forearm supinators
- Medial epicondyle: origin of wrist flexors and forearm pronators
- Olecranon process of ulna and its overlying bursa
- Triceps muscle and its aponeurosis: insert on ulna
- Cubital tunnel and groove through which the ulnar nerve runs to enter the forearm
- Epitrochlear lymph node location above medial epicondyle

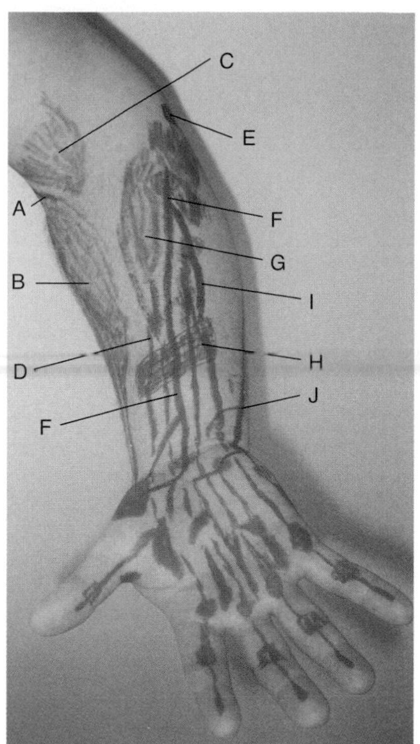

Figure 11.2.

Anterior surface anatomy of elbow and forearm. **A.** Lateral epicondyle. **B.** Brachioradialis. **C.** Biceps brachii. **D.** Flexor tendons (Red). **E.** Medial epicondyle. **F.** Median nerve. **G.** Pronator teres muscle. **H.** Pronator quadratus muscle. **I.** Anterior interosseous nerve. **J.** Ulnar nerve.

TIPS

- Lateral epicondyle: origin of wrist extensors and forearm supinators
- Brachioradialis: supinator of the forearm
- Biceps brachii: flexor of elbow, supinator of forearm
- Brachial artery: adjacent to the biceps insertion site on the ulna; distal to this, it bifurcates into the radial and ulnar artery
- Median nerve: passes through the pronator teres muscle
- Radial nerve: passes through the brachioradialis in the canal of Frohse; gives off superficial radial branch before
- Medial epicondyle: origin of wrist flexors and forearm pronators
- Pronator teres: forearm pronator with arm extended, median nerve; pronator quadratus: forearm pronator with arm at elbow flexed, anterior interosseous nerve

of the elbow; the aponeurosis of the triceps muscle overlies this structure. The **olecranon bursa** is a subcutaneous bursa at the point of the olecranon process deep to the triceps aponeurosis. The **epitrochlear node** is immediately proximal to the medial epicondyle. This node is palpable only if enlarged due to pathology. The **lateral epicondyle** is the origin of the wrist extensors and forearm supinators. The **medial epicondyle** is the origin of the wrist flexors and forearm pronators.

Anterior and Lateral (Figs. 11.2 and 11.3)

The **biceps brachii** muscle originates at the coracoid of the scapula (short head) and the supraglenoid tubercle (long head), inserts on the proximal ulna, and acts to flex arm at the elbow and supinate forearm; its nerve is the musculocutaneous nerve (C5). The **brachioradialis** muscle originates at the lateral epicondyle area of the humerus, inserts on the distal radius, and acts in forearm supination; its nerve is radial (C5, C6). This is the site of entrapment of the *superficial radial nerve,* a purely sensory nerve that branches off prior to the radial tunnel. The posterior interosseous and deep radial branch off after radial tunnel. The **flexors** of the **wrist** and of the **fingers** (long digital flexors) originate on the medial epicondyle area of the humerus, insert on the carpal bones and on the palmar aspect of the phalanges, and act in flexion of the wrist and digits; its nerves are the *median* for flexor carpi radialis and the flexor digitorum superficialis, digits 2–5, *anterior interosseous* (AI) for flexor pollicus longus, flexor digitorum profounda 2 and 3 and pronator quadratus and *ulnar* for flexor carpi ulnaris and the profunda flexors to digits 4 and 5. The **forearm pronators**, specifically the pronator teres muscle, originate on the medial epicondyle of the humerus, insert on the distal radius, and have the median nerve. The more distal pronator quadratus has nerve of anterior interosseous (AI). The nerves that cross the elbow and proximal forearm are the **median**, with its branch the anterior interosseous; the **ulnar**, which enters the forearm through the ulnar sulcus and cubital tunnel; and the **radial** with its specific branches, the posterior interosseous and superficial radial. **Entrapment sites** (see Figs. 11.1, 11.2, 11.3) include the median or specifically its motor branch, anterior interosseous, in the **pronator teres muscle**, ulnar at the **cubital tunnel**, and radial either the superficial radial nerve in the **brachioradialis muscle** proximal to radial tunnel or the deep radial and **posterior interosseous** (PI) as it passes through the **canal of Frohse** in the brachioradialis muscle (radial tunnel = canal of Frohse). The **antecubital fossa** is bounded by the pronator muscle, the brachioradialis muscle, and a line between the lateral and medial epicondyle. It contains the median nerve, the brachial artery, and the insertion tendon of the biceps brachii. The **brachial artery** is adjacent to the insertion site of the biceps on the ulna; distal to this, it bifurcates into the radial and the ulnar artery. The **lateral epicondyle** is the origin of wrist extensors and the forearm supinators. The **medial epicondyle** is the origin of the wrist flexors and the pronator teres.

Medial

The **epitrochlear node** is immediately proximal to the medial epicondyle. This is rarely enlarged, but when so, it is a significant finding that indicates a likely problem. The **ulnar collateral ligament** is on the medial joint line between the medial epicondyle of the humerus and the proximal medial ulna. This ligament prevents inappropriate valgus at the elbow. It is commonly irritated by sidearm throwing or overuse in an adolescent baseball player. The **cubital tunnel** is the sulcus in the ulna, i.e., the posterior elbow, as described on page 277.

TEACHING POINTS

SURFACE ANATOMY

1. Two joints in elbow: hinge-type between the humerus and ulna; rotation-type between the radial head and the ulna.
2. If an isolated decrease in supination or pronation, think radial head problem.
3. Sprain in the ulnar collateral ligament results in medial pain.
4. The olecranon is the point of the elbow and has an overlying bursa.
5. Most of the structures to be examined are easily felt.
6. Three nerves cross the joint, each of which can be entrapped in tissue near the joint: ulnar nerve in cubital tunnel, median nerve in pronator teres muscle, and radial nerve in radial tunnel (canal of Frohse) of brachioradialis.
7. The radial nerve branches into the purely sensory superficial radial and purely motor deep radial and posterior interosseous.
8. The median nerve branches into the purely motor anterior interosseous and mixed sensory and motor median.

The **medial epicondyle** is the distal medial humerus attachment of the ulnar collateral ligament, and the site of origin of the forearm pronators and wrist flexors. **Pronator teres muscle** originates about the medial epicondyle of the humerus and acts in forearm pronation; its nerve is median. The **median nerve** and, its branch, the anterior interosseous, runs through pronator teres muscle and, thus, this is a site of potential entrapment of either nerve. The **ulnar nerve** runs through the ulnar sulcus and flexor carpi ulnaris, i.e., the cubital tunnel, the medial posterior forearm to the ulnar (Guyon's) tunnel. The ulnar nerve can be entrapped at either site.

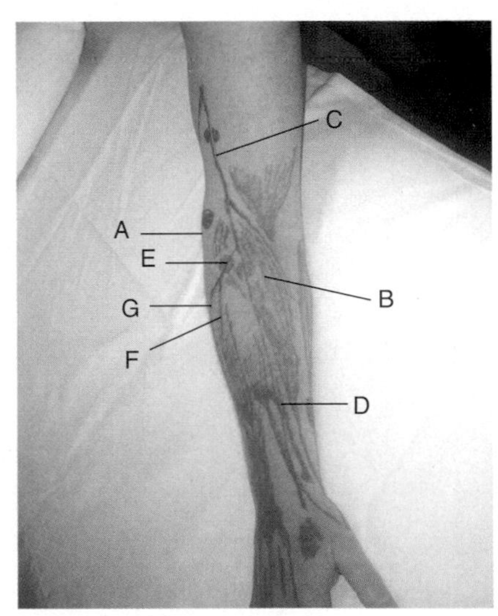

Figure 11.3.

Lateral elbow and forearm landmarks. **A.** Lateral epicondyle. **B.** Brachioradialis muscle. **C.** Radial nerve. **D.** Superficial radial nerve. **E.** Canal of Frohse. **F.** Deep radial nerve. **G.** Posterior interosseous nerve.

RANGE OF MOTION

Passive and active **range of motion** (ROM) of the elbow joint includes **flexion** to 150 degrees, **extension** to 5 degrees at the **humeral ulnar joint, supination** to 70 degrees, and **pronation** to 80 degrees at the **radial–ulnar joint (Tables 11.2 and 11.3)**. The best baseline position to perform ROM is in **Fig. 11.4**. At the outset of the elbow exam and before ROM, determine the **carrying angle** of the elbow. Normally, the elbow is slightly valgus. An old, unhealed fracture of the distal humerus will manifest with a **cubitus varus**, i.e., a gun-stock deformity **(Fig. 11.5)**. There is often concurrent **radial or ulnar nerve** damage.

Table 11.2. Passive Range of Motion (ROM)

Action	Baseline position	Degrees
Flexion	Neutral forearm and hand	150
Extension	Neutral forearm and hand	0 ± 5
Supination	Neutral forearm and hand	70
Pronation	Neutral forearm and hand	85

TIPS

- Lateral epicondyle: origin of wrist extensors and forearm supinators
- Superficial radial nerve purely sensory, goes to skin over snuff box
- Deep radial nerve gives off posterior interosseous, a motor branch

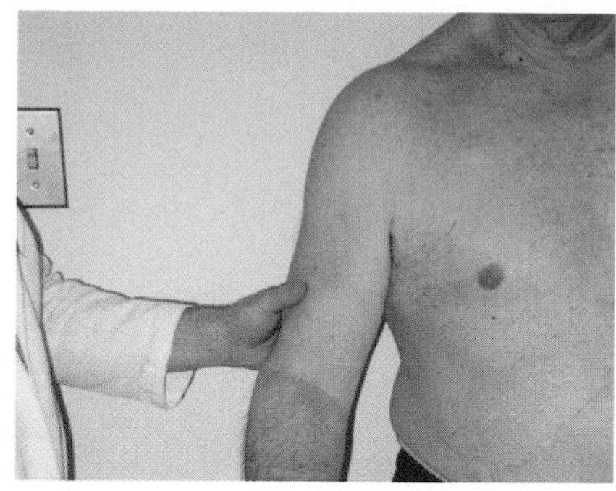
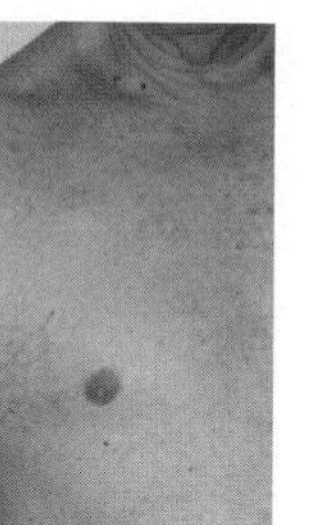

Figure 11.4.

Position of neutral arm and forearm to perform the elbow examination.

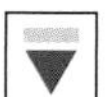

TIPS

- Hand as if in a "handshaking" position
- Forearm and hand parallel to plane of the table or floor

Table 11.3. Active Elbow Range of Motion (ROM)

Action	Muscles	Nerves
Flexion	Biceps brachii	Musculocutaneous (C5 and C6)
Extension	Triceps	Radial (C7)
Supination	Brachioradialis	Radial (C6 and C5)
Pronation	Pronator teres Pronator quadratus*	Median (C7 and C6) Anterior interosseous (C7 and C8)

*Pronator quadratus and thus AI isolated out by pronation with elbow in flexion.

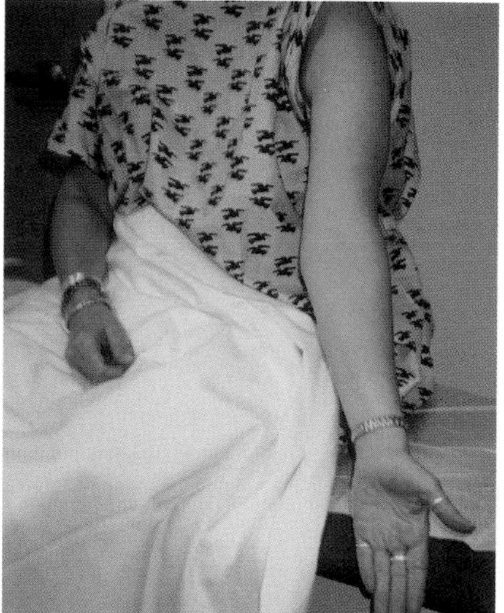

A

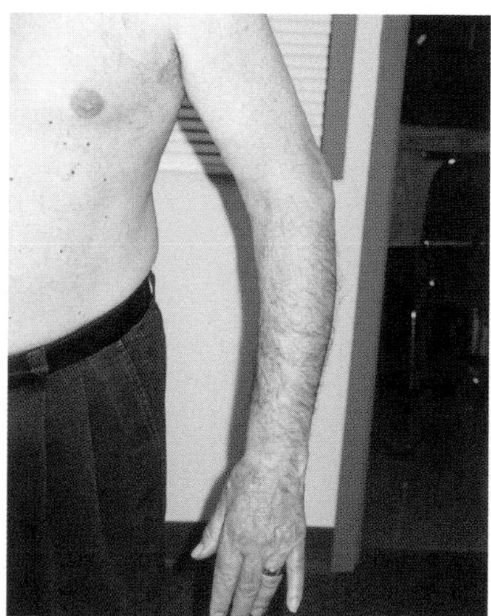

B

Figure 11.5.

Carrying angle of the elbow. **A.** Normal, as here, mildly valgus. **B.** Cubitus varus.

TIPS

- Normal: slight (<5 degrees) cubitus valgus
- Ulnar collateral ligament damage: excessive valgus (>5 degrees)
- Cubitus varus or gunstock deformity: old non-union fracture of the distal humerus

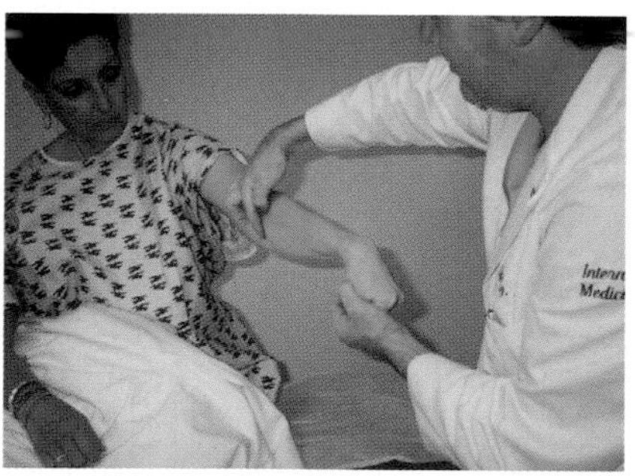

Figure 11.6.

Technique for reverse Cozen's maneuver. Useful in assessment of medial epicondylitis.

TIPS

- Instruct patient to make a fist
- Grasp top and bottom of patient's fist
- Patient actively flexes wrist against resistance
- Medial epicondylitis: tenderness at medial epicondyle

MEDIAL ELBOW

Medial epicondylitis (golfer's elbow) manifests with tenderness at and around the medial epicondyle, especially in the muscle origins adjacent to the site. Tenderness is noted over the site with a **reverse Cozen's maneuver**, i.e., active wrist flexion **(Fig. 11.6)**. This results from overuse in wrist flexion, forearm pronation, or both, usually from golfing, rock climbing, or bowling; usually in dominant upper extremity.

An enlarged **epitrochlear node** manifests with a tender or nontender nodule in the fossa immediately proximal to the medial epicondyle. Epitrochlear

TEACHING POINTS

RANGE OF MOTION: ELBOW

1. Carrying angle: mild valgus; if varus, consider severe distal humerus damage.
2. Extension or flexion: at the humeroulnar joint.
3. Supination or pronation: at the radioulnar joint.
4. Muscle bellies proximal to the elbow are the triceps and biceps (elbow extension and flexion).
5. Muscle bellies distal to the elbow are the brachioradialis and pronators (forearm supination and pronation).
6. C6 root most complex in that it contributes to wrist extension (radial, extensors), forearm supination (radial nerve, the brachioradialis), and forearm pronation (median nerve, the pronator teres and anterior interosseous, the pronator quadratus).

node enlargement is rare today but invariably indicates a problem, most often hand infection, sporotrichosis in fingers, sarcoid, lues, venereum or lymphoma.

An **ulnar collateral ligament sprain** manifests with tenderness at the medial joint line, laxity with the **valgus stress test (Fig. 11.7)**, and a positive *lateral pivot shift test* (**Fig. 11.8**). This is due to overuse in side arm throwing, e.g., in baseball or in tennis. See Figs. 11.7 and 11.8 for specifics on how to perform these tests. **Little leaguer's elbow** manifests with pain and tenderness over the medial joint line, which is caused by traction apophysitis and even sprain of the ulnar collateral ligament in a young pitcher.

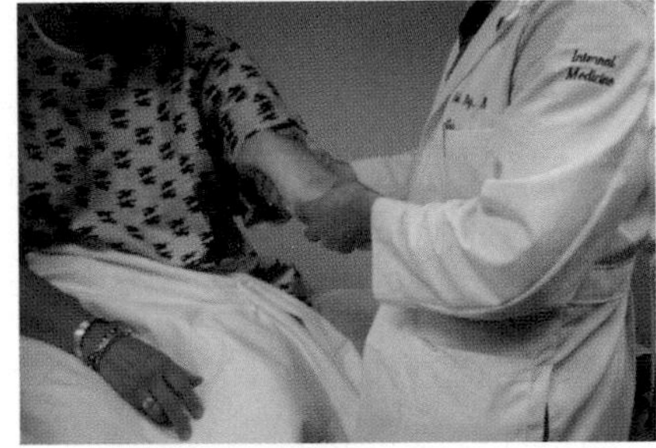

Figure 11.7.

Technique for valgus stress test. Useful to unmask a sprain of the ulnar collateral ligament.

TIPS

- Grasp the distal humerus and the proximal forearm, with patient's elbow slightly flexed at 20 degrees
- Place index finger on medial joint line between medial epicondyle and proximal ulna, i.e., the site of the ulnar collateral ligament
- Place valgus stress on the forearm itself
- Ulnar collateral ligament sprain or "little leaguer" elbow: pain and laxity over the medial joint line

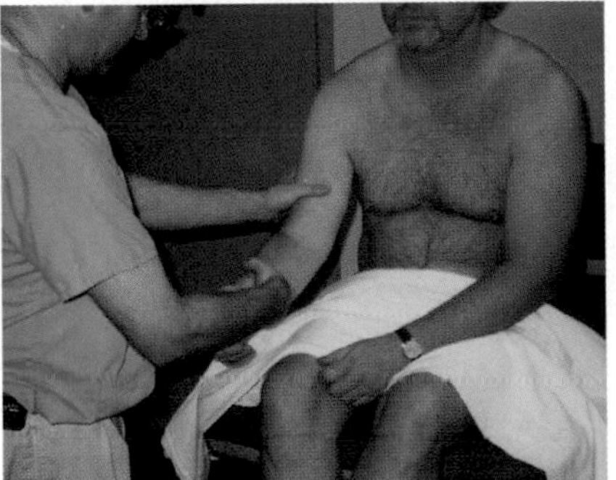

A

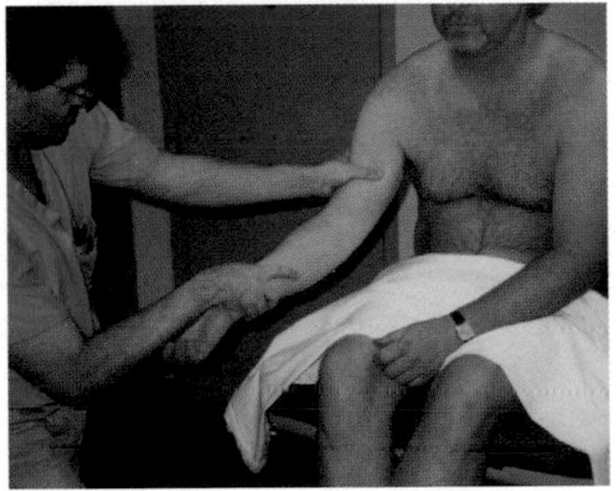

B

Figure 11.8.

Technique for lateral pivot shift. Useful in the assessment of elbow stability, especially the ulnar collateral ligament.

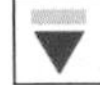

TIPS

- Patient's elbow in a position of 30 degrees of flexion
- Grasp forearm and elbow
- Apply valgus, axial compression, supination, and extension at elbow
- Look at the ulnar side of the elbow
- Normal: no pain, dimpling, or apprehension
- Ulnar collateral ligament (UCL) sprain: prominent radial head with an adjacent dimple

TEACHING POINTS

MEDIAL ELBOW

1. Medial epicondyle of humerus is the site of origin of forearm pronators and wrist flexors.
2. Medial epicondylitis is also known as golfer's or bowler's elbow; also in rock climbers.
3. Tinel's test is an adequate tool for defining entrapments at the cubital tunnel (ulnar nerve) and at the pronator teres (median nerve).
4. Ligamentous damage at the elbow, which is rare in adults, is usually in the ulnar collateral ligament and manifests with medial pain, and laxity with valgus stress.
5. By simple palpation, one can begin to define pronator teres syndrome, cubital tunnel, medial epicondylitis, and ulnar collateral ligament problem.
6. Median nerve may be entrapped at pronator teres or an isolated entrapment of anterior interosseous nerve.
7. As pronation in flexion of elbow is specific for pronator quadratus and the pronator quadratus has the anterior interosseous nerve, this muscle assesses the AI nerve function.

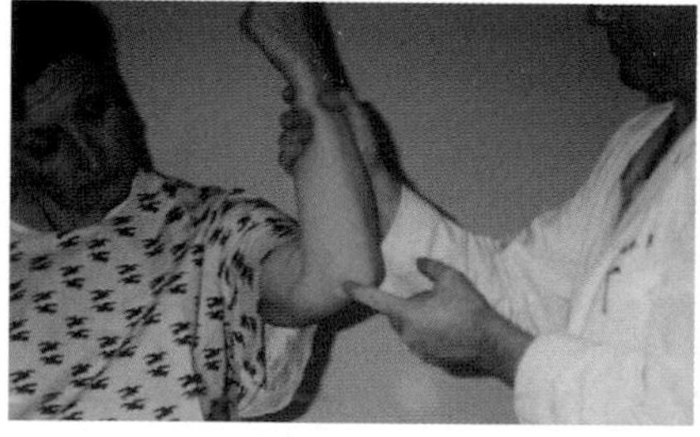

Figure 11.9.

Technique for Tinel's sign for cubital tunnel syndrome. Tingling will be present on the ulnar aspect of the forearm and hand.

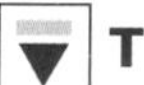 **TIPS**

- Use the finger as a pleximeter
- Tap reproducibly 10 to 15 times over site of cubital tunnel
- Cubital tunnel syndrome: tingling on ulnar aspect of the forearm and hand, including the hypothenar eminence

Pronator teres syndrome manifests with pain and tingling in the palmar side of the wrist and palm, radiating into the palmar side of digits 1, 2, and 3 (Fig. 10.3A) and a positive **Tinel's** test in which tingling occurs in the palmar forearm and wrist with up to 10 to 15 reproducible repetitive taps over the site (Tinel's = tap). This is an entrapment of the proximal median nerve and its branch, the anterior interosseous nerve, in the pronator teres muscle, due to blunt trauma. **Severe proximal median nerve problems** (involving both median and AI), manifests with the patient cannot flex digits 2 and 3 when instructed to actively make a fist. This is called "papal" or "benediction" sign of severe proximal median nerve damage (Fig. 10.10). In addition, there is weakness to thumb IP flexion, forearm pronation, and flexion at PIP of all four digits in this entrapment. The patient is unable to hold a pen and thus can't write. The **anterior interosseous nerve** may be specifically **entrapped**,* which manifests with weakness to holding a pen and pinch to tip-to-tip "OK" (Fig. 10.12) due to the weak flexor pollicus longus and flexor digitus profundus. There are no sensory defects and a negative Tinel's. This is confirmed by weakness of pronator quadratus (all AI), normal pronation strength in elbow extension, but due to the fact pronator quadratus is specific to elbow flexion, weak pronation with elbow flexion.

Cubital tunnel syndrome manifests with pain and tingling on the ulnar forearm and hand and a positive **Tinel's** sign **(Fig. 11.9)**, i.e., reproduction of the tingling on tapping over the sulcus and the proximal flexor carpi ulnaris (Fig. 11.9). There is numbness in ulnar palm, fingers and hypothenar area (Fig. 10.3C). When the ulnar nerve damage is severe or advanced, **weakness** is noted **to finger 2 to 5 abduction** (Fig. 10.12) and **adduction** (Fig. 10.13) and to **flexion** of digits 4 and 5 on making a fist **(Fig. 11.10)**. The company it keeps includes atrophy in the interosseous muscles, hypothenar muscles, and the flexor carpi ulnaris muscle. Finally, an empty hypothenar sign (Fig. 10.11) is seen in the

*The Kiloh-Nevin syndrome.

hypothenar area, which is indicative of hypothenar muscle atrophy. A classic mechanism for bilateral cubital tunnel is a patient who sits in Fowler's position because of chronic severe orthopnea.

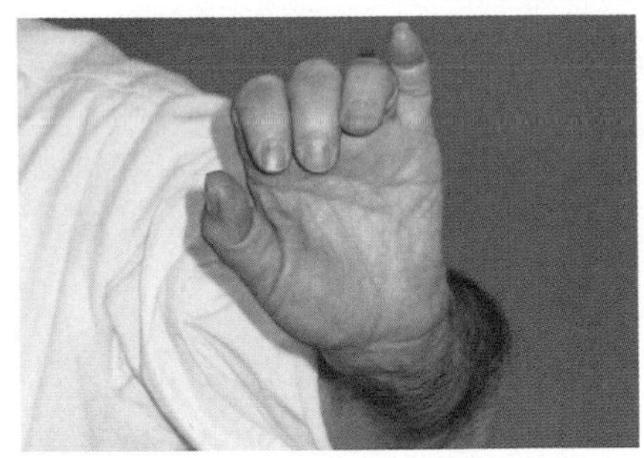

Figure 11.10.

Chronic proximal ulnar neuropathy. Weakness to flexion of fingers 4 and 5 when making a fist. Note the muscle atrophy also.

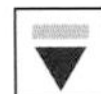

TIPS

- Patient actively makes a fist
- Weak flexion of digits 4 and 5, specifically distal joints, indicates ulnar neuropathy
- Severe proximal ulnar neuropathy: weakness to finger flexion, digits 4 and 5, atrophy of flexor carpi ulnaris, interosseous, and hypothenar muscles

OLECRANON PROCESS AND POSTERIOR ELBOW (Table 11.4)

Olecranon bursitis manifests with a fluctuant swelling over the olecranon process without any significant limitation to elbow or forearm ROM **(Fig. 11.11)**. **Serous olecranon bursitis** manifests with a fluctuant mass that is cool, nonerythematous, and transilluminable. This is due to chronic mild irritation to the area and thus has been called student's elbow, dart thrower's elbow, or miner's elbow. **Infected olecranon bursitis** manifests with a fluctuant mass that is warm, red, tender, and not transilluminable **(Fig. 11.12)**.

Table 11.4. Olecranon Process Diagnoses

Diagnosis	Elbow findings	Company it Keeps
Serous olecranon bursitis	Fluctuant area at point Nontender Not red Transilluminable ROM intact	Minimal
Septic olecranon bursitis	Fluctuant area at point Tender Red Not transilluminable ROM intact	Fevers Immunosuppression of patient
Tophaceous gout	Firm Nontender Not red Not transilluminable	Podagra Gout
Rheumatoid nodule	Hard Nontender Not red Not transilluminable In triceps aponeurosis	Polyarticular arthritis
Triceps strain/ tear	Tender posterior arm Pain and weakness with Active elbow extension Flaccid mass proximal to olecranon	Minimal

ROM = range of motion.

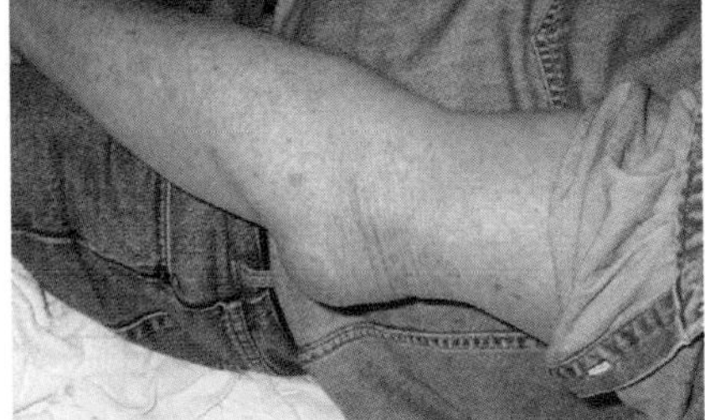

A

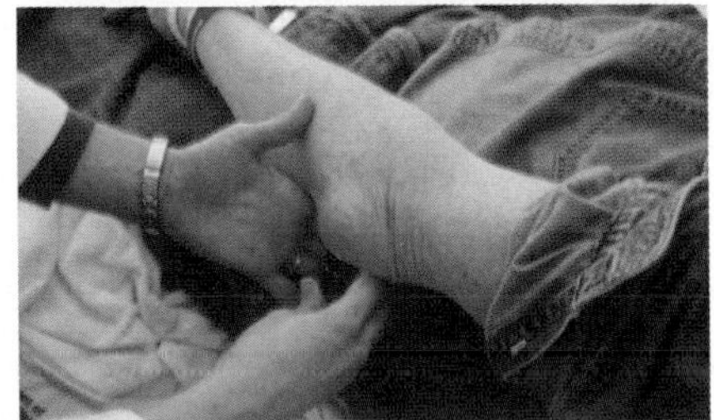

B

Figure 11.11.

Olecranon bursitis. **A.** Fluctuant mass over the olecranon process. **B.** Markedly transilluminable, thus serous in nature.

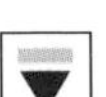

TIPS

- Palpate for any swelling over the olecranon **(A)**
- Nonseptic olecranon bursitis: large fluctuant collection, no decreased ROM of joint
- Shine a light source into the nodule or mass **(B)**

TEACHING POINTS

POSTERIOR ELBOW

1. Entities that cause swellings over the olecranon process include tophi of gout, rheumatoid nodules, and olecranon bursitis.
2. The company elbow tophi keep includes ear tophi and recurrent podagra.
3. The company rheumatoid nodules keep includes polyarticular arthritis, swan-neck deformity, cock-up toes deformity, and metacarpophalangeal (MCP) subluxation deformity with ulnar deviation.

This is due to bacterial infection, usually with staphylococcal or streptococcal species.

Tophi manifest with one or more firm, nontender nodules with a gritty feel to them; the nodules may have yellow-colored papules **(Fig. 11.13)**. The company it keeps includes podagra and tophi elsewhere, including papules on the auricles (Fig. 1.4).

Rheumatoid nodules manifest with subcutaneous, very firm nodules in the aponeurosis of the triceps muscle. The company it keeps includes swan-necking and ulnar deviation **(Fig. 11.14)**. These nodules are clinically identical to those of rheumatic fever. Please refer to Table 14.5 for other features of rheumatic fever. **Strain or tear of the triceps muscle** manifests with painful weakness to elbow extension, and a flaccid mass in the triceps muscle. This is most often trauma-related.

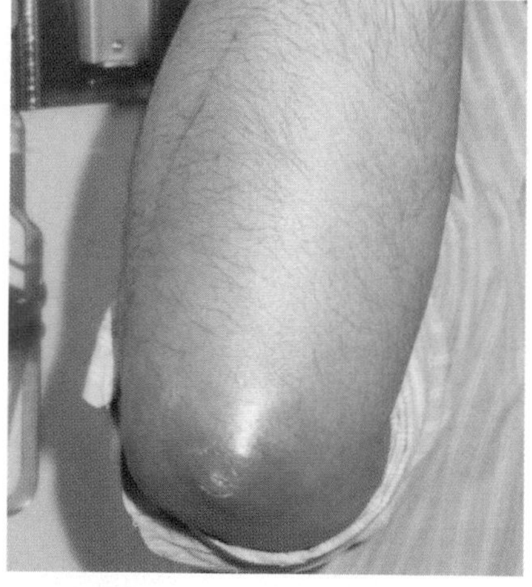

Figure 11.12.

Septic olecranon bursitis. Marked erythema with swelling; here, a draining sinus is seen.

 **TIPS**

- Septic olecranon bursitis: fluctuant swelling with overlying erythema and warmth, not transilluminable
- Bacterial infection, usually staphylococcus or streptococcus organisms

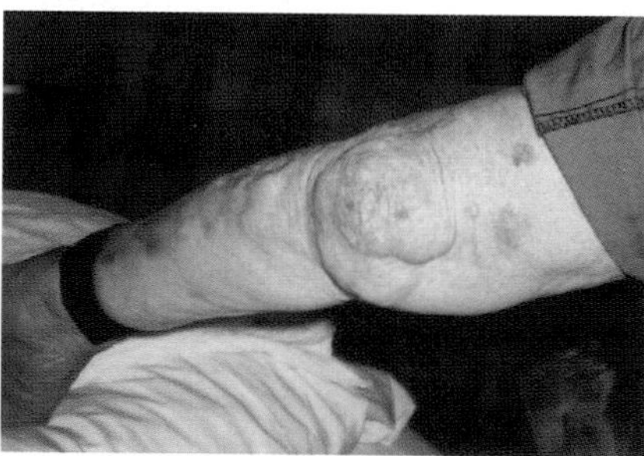

Figure 11.13.

Tophi over the olecranon. Classic firm nodule with gritty feel.

 **TIPS**

- Palpate and inspect the olecranon process and overlying triceps
- Tophi: soft to firm nodule or mass, gritty feel with yellow-colored papules or pustules on surface
- Tophaceous gout

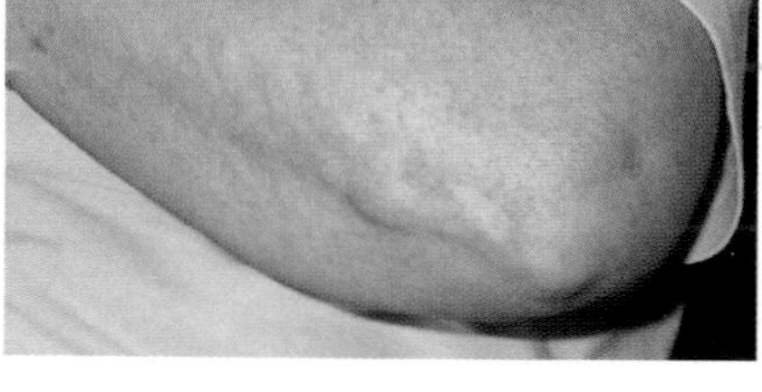

Figure 11.14.

Rheumatoid nodules. Firm, nontender nodules in the aponeurosis of the triceps muscle, often multiple as seen here.

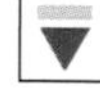 **TIPS**

- Palpate and inspect the olecranon process and triceps muscles aponeurosis
- Rheumatoid nodules: subcutaneous, firm, mobile, multiple in the aponeurosis of the triceps muscle

LATERAL ELBOW

Arthritis specific to the humeral-ulnar joint manifests with a marked decrease in passive and active ROM at the joint and a fluctuant bulge in the lateral elbow **(Fig. 11.15)**, especially at the groove between the olecranon and the lateral epicondyle. This is due to any monoarticular arthritis etiology including infection, crystal-related or trauma-related and mandates arthrocentesis for evaluation.

Lateral epicondylitis, also known as tennis elbow, manifests with significant tenderness and pain in the area adjacent to the lateral epicondyle. The tenderness is in the origins of the muscles of forearm supination and wrist extension. The patient has a pain over the lateral epicondyle with active extension of the wrist against resistance, i.e., **Cozen's maneuver (Fig. 11.16)**. Pain also occurs over the lateral epicondyle with **active supination** against resistance and with **active digital extension of the third digit** against resistance **(Figs. 11.17 and 11.18)**, and over the lateral epicondyle with passive pronation of the forearm, i.e., **Mill's maneuver**. Due to overuse in wrist extension, and forearm supination, e.g., in tennis.

Superficial radial nerve entrapment (Wartenberg's syndrome) manifests with pain and tingling in the dorsal side of the forearm, radiating into the dorsal side of digits 1, 2, and 3, especially in the skin overlying the anatomic snuffbox. A positive **Tinel's** sign is noted over the brachioradialis, proximal to the radial tunnel site; there are no motor deficits **(Fig. 11.19)** due to entrapment of the superficial radial nerve in the brachioradialis muscle as the result of blunt trauma. **Radial tunnel syndrome** manifests with weakness in the hand, starting with the fifth finger and over time progressing to the thumb; there is weakness to extension with atrophy of muscles. No sensory deficits, negative Tinels. Due to entrapment in radial tunnel of brachioradialis; involves deep radial and PI nerve but *not* the superficial radial nerve.

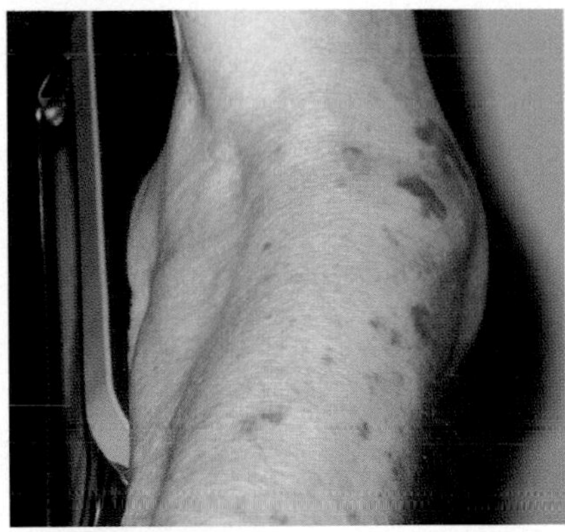

A

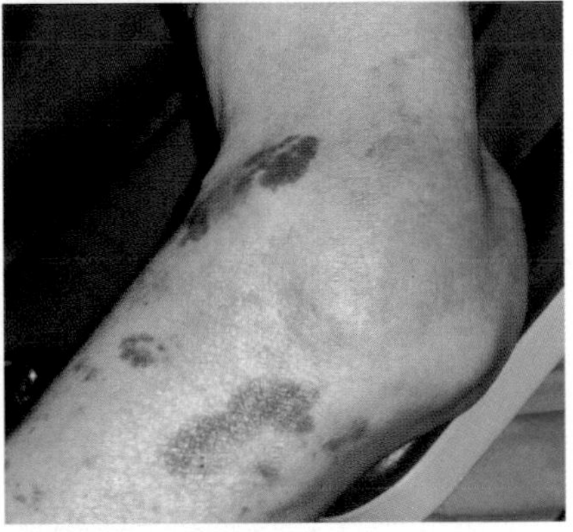

B

Figure 11.15.

Marked effusion of the elbow. Bulging located over the groove between the olecranon and lateral epicondyle.

 **TIPS**

- Inspect the groove between the ulna (olecranon) and the lateral epicondyle
- Effusion: bulge and fluctuant collection at the site, often with a marked decrease ROM

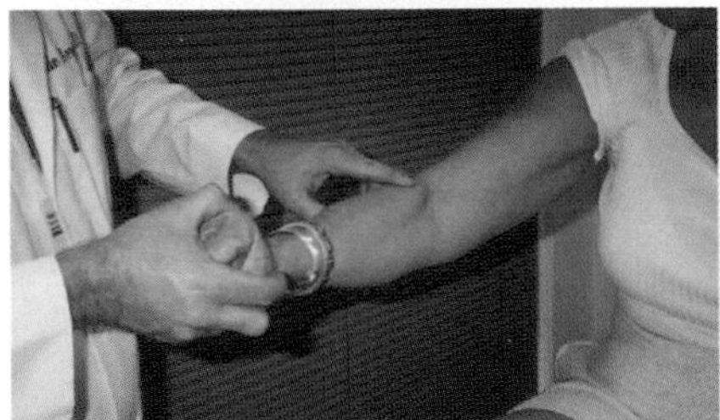

Figure 11.16.

Technique for Cozen's maneuver. Passive dorsiflexion causes tenderness over the lateral epicondyle in lateral epicondylitis.

 **TIPS**

- Patient makes a fist
- Grasp the top and bottom part of the patient's fist
- Instruct patient to actively dorsiflex wrist against resistance
- Lateral epicondylitis: tender over the lateral epicondyle

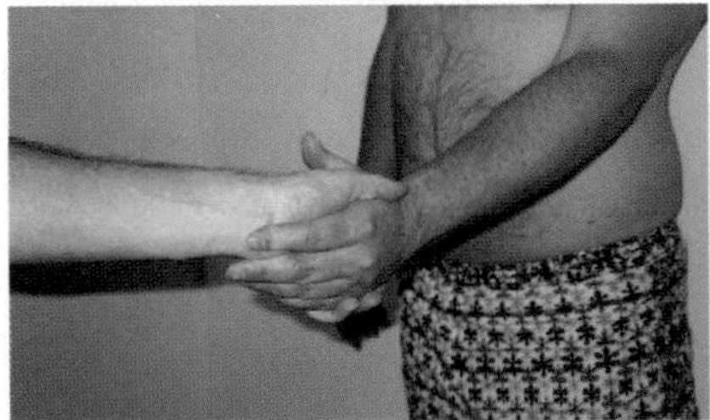

Figure 11.17.

Technique for active supination against resistance. Active supination causes tenderness over the lateral epicondyle in lateral epicondylitis.

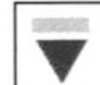 **TIPS**

- Grasp patient's hand as in shaking hands
- Patient places thumb pressure on examiner's thumb, thus supinates against resistance
- Lateral epicondylitis (tennis elbow): pain at lateral epicondyle
- Bicipital tendinitis: pain at the anterior shoulder in the bicipital groove

TEACHING POINTS

LATERAL ELBOW

1. Lateral epicondyle: origin of forearm supinators and wrist extensors.
2. Lateral epicondylitis, also referred to as tennis elbow, is very common.
3. Always check and document supination and pronation to assess the head of the radius in addition to flexion and extension at the elbow.
4. Tinel's sign is an adequate tool for uncovering entrapments in the brachioradialis muscle.
5. Limited supination or pronation: think radial head problems, fracture, or pulled elbow.
6. Superficial radial nerve: no significant motor deficit, all sensory.
7. Radial tunnel syndrome: entraps PI and deep radial nerve, decreased extension of fingers, no sensory defects.
8. Lateral epicondylitis unmasked by active supination or passive pronation of forearm.

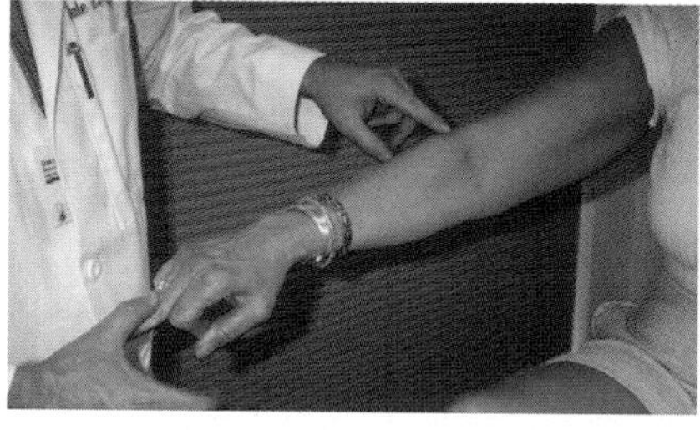

Figure 11.18.

Technique for active extension of middle fingers against resistance. Extension of middle fingers causes tenderness over the lateral epicondyle in lateral epicondylitis.

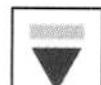 **TIPS**

- Hand neutral, patient actively extends digits 3 or 4 against resistance; uses muscles in extensor compartment 4
- Lateral epicondylitis (tennis elbow): pain at the lateral epicondyle

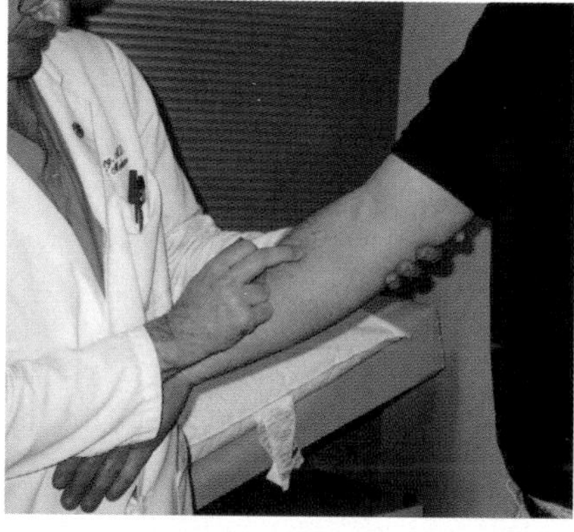

Figure 11.19.

Technique for Tinel's sign in the proximal brachioradialis muscle. This is proximal to radial tunnel site.

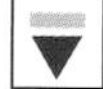 **TIPS**

- Tap 10 to 15 times using standard procedure over the brachioradialis muscle of the forearm at the site through which the radial nerve enters the forearm
- Superficial radial nerve entrapment: tingling in the dorsal forearm and hand, especially over the anatomic snuffbox
- Radial tunnel syndrome: negative Tinel's sign

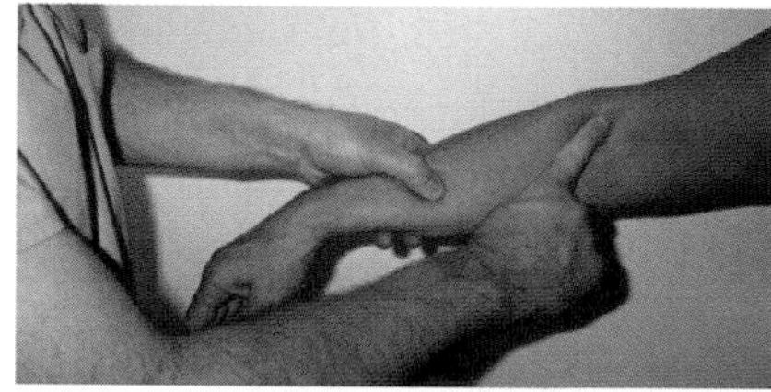

Figure 11.20.

Forearm squeeze test. Good method to evaluate for concurrent problems with a wrist or elbow injury.

 **TIPS**

- Forearm and hand neutral
- Place a squeezing pressure on the patient's midforearm
- Squeeze ulna and radius together
- Scaphoid fracture: tenderness over the snuffbox
- Interosseous damage: tenderness over the entire forearm
- Radial head fracture: tenderness over the elbow

Radial head fracture manifests with trauma-related pain in the lateral elbow and forearm to the anatomic snuffbox, a **squeeze sign (Fig. 11.20)** with pain specific to the lateral, antecubital elbow, i.e., at the radial head and a marked decrease in passive and active supination and pronation. Radial head fracture usually results from a fall on an outstretched hand.

Annotated Bibliography

Buehler MJ, Thayer DT. The elbow flexion test. ***Clin Orthop*** **1988;233:213–216.**
Interesting paper on a sign for cubital tunnel syndrome. On 10 patients with electromyography (EMG)-documented cubital tunnel syndrome, a physical examination test was conducted consisting of the patient actively extending the wrists and extending the elbows for 3 minutes. Tingling or pain occurred in all such individuals. Interesting test that merits analysis for specificity and sensitivity in a larger group of undifferentiated patients with elbow problems.

Dawson DM. Entrapment neuropathies of the upper extremities. ***N Engl J Med*** **1993;329:2013–2018.**
Interesting and educational guide to the types and manifestations of entrapment neuropathies in the upper extremities.

Emery SE, Gifford JF. 100 years of tennis elbow. ***Contemporary Orthopedics*** **1986;12:53–58.**
Review of the history of lateral epicondylitis, including the fact that Runge, a German physician, described this first in 1873 in individuals who did extensive writing; also documents that Mayor first coined the term "tennis elbow" in 1883.

Hannafin JA. How I manage tennis and golfer's elbow. ***The Physician and Sports Medicine*** **1996;24(2):63–68.**
Fair discussion of the pathophysiology and some of the physical examination concepts behind these two entities that cause lateral nod medial elbow problems.

Jobe FW, Ciccootti MG. Lateral and medial epicondylitis of the elbow. ***J Am Acad Orthop Surg*** **1994;2(1):1–8.**
A splendid discussion of the diagnostic features of these entities, written by one of the foremost experts in this joint and endeavor.

Jobe FW, Stark KH, Lombardo SJ. Reconstruction of the ulnar collateral ligament in athletes. ***J Bone Joint Surg*** **1986;68A:1158–1163.**
Treatment of this entity that could have been so devastating to baseball players like Tommy John and Paul Moliter.

Kiloh LG, Nevin S. Anterior interosseous syndrome. ***Br Med J*****, 1952;1:850.**
The original description of AI syndrome.

Kraay MJ. The painful elbow: causes to consider. ***Hosp Med*** **1994;(Jul):25–34.**
Basic overview of the evaluation of common entities of elbow problems: medial epicondylitis, olecranon bursitis, radial tunnel syndrome, and synovitis of the elbow. Nice discussion of posterior elbow pathology and physical diagnostic evaluation.

Leach RE, Wasilewski S. Olecranon bursitis. ***J Sports Med*** **1979;7:299.**
Terse, albeit complete, discussion of manifestations of olecranon bursitis in active individuals.

Major HP. Lawn tennis elbow. ***BMJ*** **1883;2:557.**
Tennis should properly be played on a lawn. Indeed.

Mills GP. The treatment of tennis elbow. ***BMJ*** **1928;1:12–13.**
A classic description of tennis elbow with modest discussion on history and physical examination in such cases.

Nirschl RP. Tennis elbow. ***Orthop Clin North Am*** **1973;4:787–800.**
Excellent review of this common entity.

Nirschl RP, Kraushaar BS. Assessment and treatment guidelines for elbow injuries. ***Phys and Sports Med*** **1996;24(5):43–60.**
Excellent review of anatomy with a robust discussion of nonsurgical intervention for elbow injuries. Excellent description and discussion of the valgus stress test.

Pecina MM, Krmpotic-Nemanic, J, Markiewitz, AD. ***Tunnel Syndrome*****, 2nd ed, CRC Press, Boca Raton, 1997.**
Tremendous and thorough resource detailing tunnel syndrome. A must for primary care physicians.

Pike W. Fracture of the head of the radius. ***J Bone Joint Surg*** **1969;51:198.**
Excellent reminder to primary care physicians to include this entity in their differential diagnosis of elbow pain, especially in cases of limited supination or pronation.

Ritts GD, Wood MB, Linscheid RL. Radial tunnel syndrome. *Clin Orthop* 1987;219:201–205.
Nice review of radial tunnel syndrome. The most common cause of compression of the posterior interosseous nerve branch of the radial nerve is at the canal of Frohse. Reviews therapy and rehabilitation aspects of this disorder.

Romer F. Some observations on "tennis elbow." *Lancet* 1922;(July):67.
Delightfully short discussion of this common entity. Describes other associated causes, including "back-handed play at tennis, while sabre-fencing, fly-fishing, and playing golf."

Sankar NS. Pulled elbow. *J R Soc Med* 1999;92:462–464.
Nice overview on the mechanism, physical examination, and treatment of this relatively common problem. Excellent table on the synonyms of this entity.

Shaffer B, O'Mara J. Common elbow problems. Part 2. Management specifics. *Journal of Musculoskeletal Medicine* 1997;14(4):29–44.
Impressive and well-written paper on the evaluation and management of sports-related elbow problems, Including little league elbow, ulnar collateral ligament sprain, and lateral epicondylitis. Although the physical examination is not robustly described, this is a nice overall paper on these entities.

12

Hip, Back, and Trunk Examination

PRACTICE AND TEACHING

SURFACE ANATOMY (Table 12.1)

Anterior (Fig. 12.1)

The **abdominus rectus** muscle originates on the xiphoid process and the costal cartilages of ribs 5 to 7, inserts on the upper pubis symphysis, acts to forward flex the body, and is innervated by the intercostal nerves derived segmentally from roots T7 to T12. The **external oblique muscle** is the most superficial muscle layer of the abdominal wall; its fibers pass diagonally in an inferomedial direction. It originates on the external surface of ribs 5 to 12, inserts on linea alba and anterior iliac crest, and acts in trunk flexion and rotation; its nerves are the thoracic roots. **Internal oblique muscle**, the middle layer of muscle in the abdominal wall, originates on the anterior two thirds of the anterior iliac crest, inserts on ribs 10 to12, and acts to support the abdominal and trunk wall; its nerves are segmental roots. **Transverse abdominus muscle**, the deepest layer of the wall, originates on the internal surface of ribs 7 to 12 and its insertion, action, and nerves are similar to those of the internal obliquus. **Hesselbach's triangle** is bordered inferiorly by the inguinal ligament, medially by linea alba, and superiorly by the epigastric artery. The **inguinal ligament** extends from the pubis to the *anterior superior iliac spine* (ASIS). The ASIS is an extremely important landmark located on the anterior iliac crest. It is the basis for the Q angle in the knee examination, McBurney's point and line in the abdominal examination, and a defining point of both the femoral triangle and Hesselbach's triangle. The **femoral triangle** is bordered superiorly by the inguinal ligament, medially by the adductor longus

Table 12.1. Landmarks and Levels for Reference

Landmark	Vertebral or other descriptive level
Top iliac crest	L4/L5 interspace
Posterior superior iliac spine	L5/S1 interspace
Sacroiliac joint	S2 and S3
Pubic tubercle	Greater trochanter

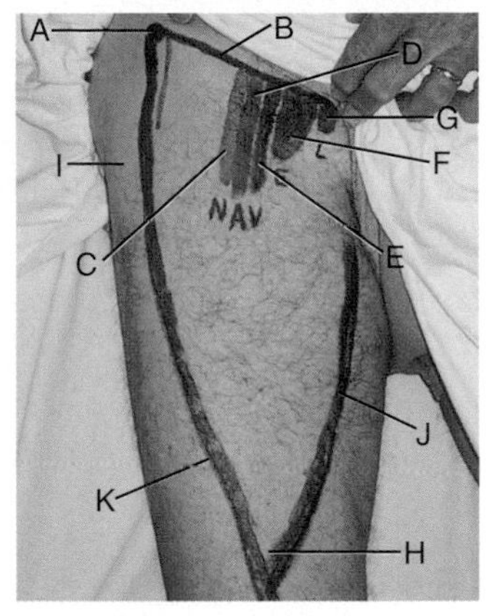

Figure 12.1.

Surface anatomy anterior thigh and femoral triangle. **A.** Anterior superior iliac spine. **B.** Inguinal ligament. **C.** Femoral nerve. **D.** Femoral artery. **E.** Femoral vein. **F.** Femoral canal. **G.** Node of Cloquet. **H.** Adductor canal of Hunter. **I.** Greater trochanter. **J.** Adductor longus, **K.** Sartorius.

TIPS

- Anterior superior iliac spine (ASIS): one of the most important landmarks in the lower half of the body
- Inguinal ligament: between pubic tubercle and ASIS
- Femoral triangle borders, superior: inguinal ligament; medial: adductor longus; lateral: sartorius
- Femoral triangle contents (lateral to medial): femoral nerve, femoral artery, femoral vein, femoral canal, and lymph nodes, specifically the node of Cloquet
- Adductor canal of Hunter: apex of femoral triangle contains the femoral vein and artery and saphenous nerve
- Greater trochanter: iliotibial band (ITB) and gluteal muscles attach here

muscle, and laterally by the sartorius muscle. This triangle contains, most laterally, the lateral cutaneous nerve of the thigh; then, progressing medially, the femoral nerve, artery, vein, canal, and lymph nodes, specifically the node of Cloquet. The femoral artery is midway between the ASIS* and the pubic tubercle. The acronym NAVEL (nerve, artery, vein, canal [empty], and lymph node) is an excellent method to use to remember these structures. The **canal of Hunter** is the inferior apex of the femoral triangle, in which the femoral artery and vein and the saphenous nerve are located. The saphenous nerve is a sensory branch of L4 root that serves the skin overlying the anterior medial malleolus of the ankle. The **lateral cutaneous nerve of the thigh** (L2, L3) is under the extreme lateral inguinal ligament; it is purely sensory to the anterior lateral thigh. The muscles of the anterior thigh include the **sartorius**, which originates from the ASIS, inserts on the pes anserine of proximal tibia, and acts in hip forward flexion, external rotation, and abduction; its nerve is the femoral (L3, L4). The **adductor magnus** originates on the ischial tuberosity, inserts on the distal medial femur, and acts in hip adduction and internal rotation; its nerve is the obturator (L2, L3, L4). The **adductor longus** originates on the pubis, inserts on the mid to distal medial femur, and acts in hip adduction and internal rotation; its nerve is the obturator (L2, L3, L4). The **quadriceps** muscle, which covers most of the anterior thigh, has four bellies: the vastus medialis, vastus intermedialis, vastus lateralis, and rectus femoris. It originates on the inferior aspect of ASIS and the proximal femur; inserts on the anterior tibial tuberosity and acts in knee extension; its nerve is the femoral (L2, L3, L4). The **saphenous hiatus** (fossa ovalis) is the site where the greater saphenous vein, by penetrating the thigh fascia, empties into the femoral vein. This hiatus is several centimeters distal to the inguinal ligament on the extreme medial aspect of the thigh. The **greater trochanter** of the femur is the site of insertion of gluteal muscles; it is the origin of the iliotibial band and has a bursa overlying it. It is at the same level as the pubic tubercles and the midpoint of the gluteal folds. See Table 12.1. The **iliopsoas muscle** originates on vertebra T12 to L5, inserts on the lesser trochanter of the femur, and acts in forward flexion of the hip; its nerves are the roots of L1 to L3. This muscle, along with the quadriceps, forms the floor of the femoral triangle.

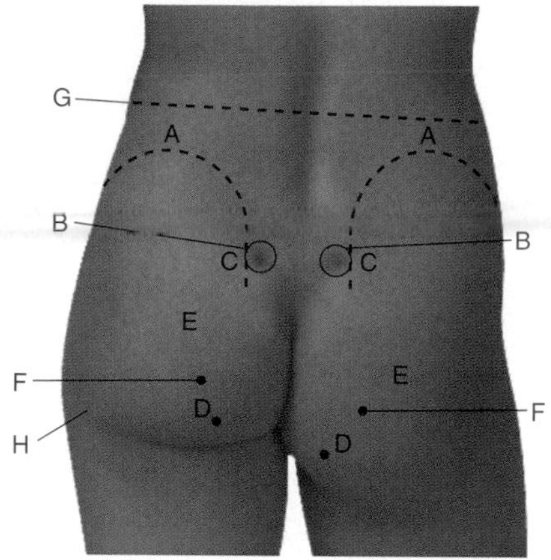

Figure 12.2.

Posterior surface anatomy. **A.** Iliac crest. **B.** Posterior superior iliac spines. **C.** Sacroiliac joints. **D.** Ischial tuberosity. **E.** Gluteal muscles. **F.** Ischiogluteal bursa. **G.** L3, L4 interspace. **H.** Greater trochanteric bursa. (From Moore KL, Dalley AF. *Clinically Oriented Anatomy*, 4th ed. Philadelphia: Lippincott Williams & Wilkins, 1999:566, with permission).

 **TIPS**

- Top of iliac crests **(A)**: level of vertebra L4/L5 interspace
- Posterior superior iliac spine (PSIS): level of vertebra L5/S1 interspace
- Sacroiliac (SI) joints: level of vertebra S2, S3
- Ischial tuberosity: level of midgluteal fold, greater trochanter, and pubic tubercle
- Gluteal muscles, in general, insert on the greater trochanter; they are the major backward flexors, external rotators, and abductors of the hip
- Ischiogluteal bursa **(F)**: between the gluteus maximus and ischial tuberosity
- Greater trochanteric bursa **(H)**: between the gluteus maximus and the greater trochanter
- Sciatic nerve: midway between ischial tuberosity and greater trochanter, adjacent to the ischiogluteal bursa
- Paraspinous muscles: large, longitudinal muscles running between the occiput and sacrum; attach to transverse and spinous processes of vertebral bodies

Posterior (Fig. 12.2)

The **latissimus dorsi** muscle originates on the iliac crest and spinous processes of T7 to T12, inserts on the inferior scapula, and acts in internal rotation, adduction and backward flexion of the shoulder and in trunk rotation; its nerve is the thoracodorsal, from the roots of C6 and C7. The **paraspinous muscles** or the intrinsic back muscles include the iliocostalis (lateral bundle of muscle), the longissimus (intermediate bundle), and the most medial, the spinalis (medial bundle). These very large muscles originate from the posterior iliac crest, posterior sacrum, and sacral and lumbar spinous processes; insert on the transverse processes of the vertebra and act to straighten the spine and keep the spine erect; the nerves are the dorsal segmental roots of the spinal cord. Finally, the **spinous processes** of the vertebrae are palpable in the midline. The **kidneys**, although not specific to the back, are retroperitoneal abdominal structures that can cause back-related problems. Thus, it is important to review the surface anatomy of the kidneys, which are located at the respective costovertebral angles, with the right kidney slightly superior to the left. The paired bones of the pelvis, including the ilium, iliac crests, posterior superior iliac spines, ischia, and the pubis, are important to review and

*ASIS = anterior superior iliac spine.

note. Please see Table 12.1 for specific anatomic levels useful in teaching. The **ischiogluteal bursa** is located between the gluteal muscle and the underlying ischial tuberosity, i.e., the sites upon which one sits. The **gluteus medius** muscle originates on the lateral ilium, inserts on the greater trochanter, and acts in hip internal rotation (anterior muscle), hip external rotation (posterior muscle), hip abduction, and hip backward flexion; its nerve is the superior gluteal (L4, L5, S1). The **gluteus minimus** muscle originates on the mid-ilium, inserts on the greater trochanter, and acts in hip internal rotation, hip abduction, and hip backward flexion; its nerve is the superior gluteal (L4, L5, S1). The **gluteus maximus**, the largest of the muscles, originates on the posterior ilium and the posterior sacrum and coccyx, inserts on and via the iliotibial band to the greater trochanter and onto the lateral proximal tibial at Gerdy's point; acts in hip backward flexion, hip abduction, and hip external rotation; its nerve is inferior gluteal (L5, S1, S2). The **semimembranosus** muscle originates on the ischial tuberosity, inserts on the tibia, and acts in knee flexion and hip backward flexion; its nerve is the sciatic (L5, S1, S2). The **semitendinosus** muscle originates on the ischial tuberosity, inserts at pes anserine over the medial tibia, and acts in knee flexion; its nerve is the sciatic (L5, S1, S2). The **biceps femoris** muscle originates on the ischial tuberosity (long head) and the mid proximal femur (short head), inserts on the lateral fibula, and acts in knee flexion and hip backward flexion; its nerve is the sciatic (L5, S1, S2). The **obturator internus** muscle originates on the posterior medial ischium, inserts on the medial greater trochanter, and acts in external rotation and abduction of the flexed thigh; its nerve is composed of roots L5 through S2. The **obturator externus** muscle originates on the anterior medial ischium, inserts on the greater trochanter, and acts in external rotation; its nerve is the obturator (L3, L4). The **gemelli** muscles originate on the ischium lateral to obturator internus, insert on the medial greater trochanter, and act in external rotation and abduction of the flexed thigh; their nerve is from roots L5 through S1. The **piriformis** muscle originates on the anterior sacrum, inserts on the superior greater trochanter, and acts in external rotation and abduction of the flexed thigh; its nerve is the roots of S1, S2. The **sciatic nerve**, which is derived from roots L4, L5, S1, and S2, passes through the piriformis adjacent to the ischiogluteal bursa, exactly midway between the ischial tuberosity and the greater trochanter, into the posterior lateral thigh. Of further importance in a discussion of landmarks is that the tops of the iliac crests are at the level of the vertebra L4/L5 interspace; those of the posterior superior iliac spine (PSIS) are at the level of the vertebrae L5/S1 interspace, and the sacroiliac joints are at the level of vertebrae S2/S3 interspace (see Table 12.1).

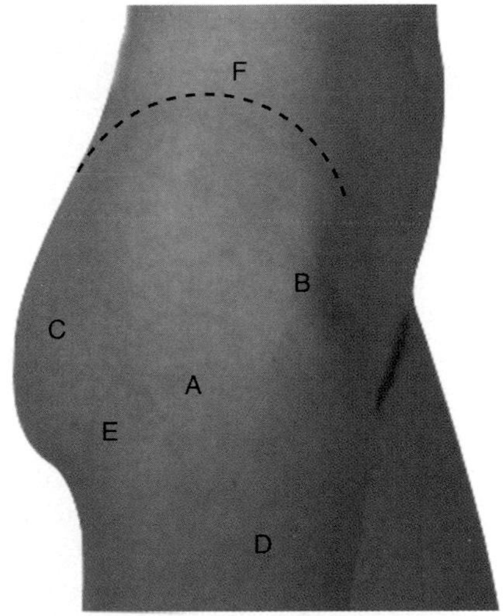

Figure 12.3.

Lateral surface anatomy. **A.** Greater trochanter. **B.** Iliotibial band. **C.** Gluteus maximus. **D.** Lateral quadriceps. **E.** Ischial tuberosity. **F.** Iliac crest. (From Moore KL, Dalley AF. *Clinically Oriented Anatomy*, 4th ed. Philadelphia: Lippincott Williams & Wilkins, 1999: 566, with permission).

Lateral (Fig. 12.3)

The **greater trochanter** of the femur is the insertion site of the gluteal muscles and origin of the iliotibial band (ITB). The **greater trochanteric bursa** is between the gluteal muscles and the greater trochanter. The **iliotibial band** is a broad sheet of tough connective tissue (fascia) from the iliac crest to the proximal lateral tibia, that is Gerdy's tubercle. This is a tension band that improves the mechanical advantage of gluteal muscle actions. The ITB is required for a normal gait. Any inflammation or problem results in a gait disturbance. A loss of the ITB because of an above-the-knee amputation results in severe gait dysfunction. All effort should be made to preserve the knee and, thus, the ITB in any amputation, to minimize such gait disturbance. The **lateral quadriceps muscle**, the vastus lateralis, is a component of that great knee extender. The **biceps femoris** muscle inserts on the proximal fibula and acts in knee flexion; its nerve is the sciatic.

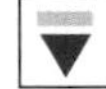 **TIPS**

- Greater trochanter: insertion of gluteus medius, minimus, and the piriformis; origin of the iliotibial band (ITB)
- ITB: greater trochanter to Gerdy's tubercle on the tibia, insertion site of the gluteus maximus muscle
- Lateral quadriceps: knee extensor, femoral nerve (L4)
- Biceps femoris: a knee flexor, sciatic nerve (L5)

Medial

The **medial surface** anatomy of the thigh **adductor longus** muscle originates on the anterior pubis, inserts on the mid to distal medial femur at linea aspera, and acts in adduction and internal rotation of the hip; its nerve is the obturator (L2, L3, L4). The **adductor magnus muscle** originates on the ischial tuberosity, inserts on the distal medial femur, and acts in hip adduction and internal rotation; its nerve is the obturator (L2, L3, L4).* The **semimembranosus** muscle originates on the ischial tuberosity, inserts on the medial tibia, and acts in knee flexion and hip backward flexion; its nerve is the sciatic (L5, S1, S2). The **iliopsoas muscle** originates on the sides of T12 through L5 and the transverse processes of L1 through L5 and the anterior arch of iliac crest, inserts on lesser trochanter, and acts in hip forward flexion; its nerve is composed of the roots of L2 and L3 and the femoral nerve (L4). The **lesser trochanter** of the femur is the insertion site of the iliopsoas muscle. **Gracilis**, the most medial muscle, originates on the pubis, inserts on pes anserine of the tibia, and acts in hip adduction; its nerve is the obturator (L2, L3).

*The component of adductor magnus from ischium has sciatic nerve.

TEACHING POINTS

OVERALL SURFACE ANATOMY

1. Acronym NAVEL (nerve, artery, vein, canal [empty], and lymph node) is an excellent method to remember and teach the contents of the femoral canal as they pass under the inguinal ligament.
2. Femoral triangle borders: adductor longus, sartorius, inguinal ligament.
3. Adductor canal of Hunter: contains the femoral artery and vein and the saphenous nerve which provides sensory to the medial malleolus.
4. Iliotibial band (ITB): the broad band of tendinous extension of the gluteus maximus muscle.
5. Greater trochanter: the origin of the ITB, insertion of gluteal muscles.
6. Sciatic nerve: runs adjacent to ischiogluteal bursa, through the piriformis muscle, either of which are potential sites of complications.
7. Hip joint: analogous to shoulder joint, femur in acetabulum, analogous to humerus, in glenoid; gemelli and obturator muscles analogous to rotator cuff; gluteal muscles analogous to deltoid muscle.
8. The major, if not primary, function of the pelvis is to provide support, and makes biped, upright ambulation possible.
9. The pelvis is fused to the spinal column via very sturdy ligaments.
10. Gluteus maximus acts in external rotation, abduction, and backward flexion.
11. Gluteus medius: external rotation (posterior fibers) and internal rotation (anterior fibers) rotation, abduction, backward flexion.
12. Gluteus minimus acts in internal rotation and abduction.
13. Active external rotation of hip: gluteus maximus, gluteus medius (posterior); obturator externus and internus, piriformis, gemelli, and quadratus femoris.
14. Active internal rotation of hip: gluteus minimus, gluteus medius (anterior fibers).
15. Furthest lateral domain of L4 on surface anatomy: the sartorius muscle.

NEUROLOGIC EXAMINATION

Both the motor and the sensory functions of the nerve roots from L1 to S4 must be assessed in any patient with a hip or back problem **(Table 12.2)**. The sites used to assess function of these roots include the perineum, hip, thigh, knee, and foot. The roots of **L1 and L2** are best assessed by active **forward flexion** of the hip. The patient sits on the edge of the table and actively raises the knee "upward toward head" against resistance; the muscle being tested is the iliopsoas **(Fig. 12.4)**. The roots of **L3 and L4** (femoral nerve) are best assessed by active **extension** of the leg at the knee **(Fig. 12.5)**. The patient sits on the edge of the table and actively straightens the leg at the knee; the muscle being tested is the quadriceps. The root **L5** (common peroneal nerve) is best assessed by **dorsiflexion of the great toe** or by **dorsiflexion of the ankle**. The patient actively dorsiflexes the great toe and then the foot at the tibiotalar joint against resistance; the muscles being tested are from the anterior compartment, specifically the extensor hallucis longus and the tibialis anterior muscles. The root **S1** (tibialis nerve) is best assessed by **great toe flexion** or by **plantarflexion of ankle (Figs. 12.6 and 12.7)**. The patient actively plantar flexes the great toe and then the foot at the tibiotalar joint against resistance; the muscles being tested are from the posterior compartment, specifically the flexor hallucis longus and the gastrocnemius. The root of **S2** (tibialis nerve) is best assessed by **toe adduction and abduction (Fig. 12.8)**. The patient actively adducts the toes against a tongue blade or the examiner's finger is placed between two adjacent toes; the muscles being tested are the intrinsic muscles of the foot. **The roots of S2, S3, S4, and S5** (pudendal nerve) are best assessed by anal sphincter tone and the anal wink. **Anal sphincter tone** is assessed with the patient in lateral decubital position; place a gloved finger into

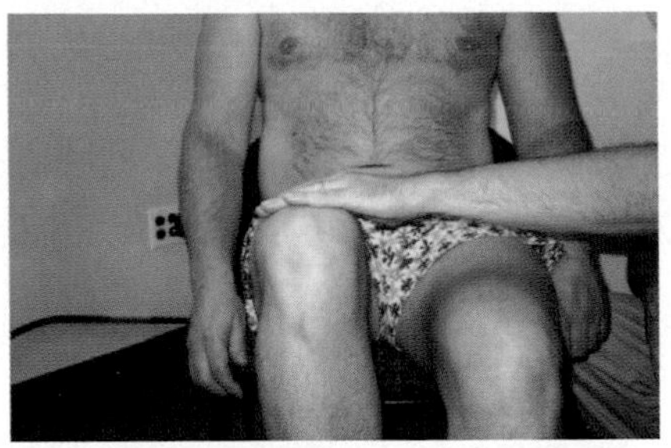

Figure 12.4.

Technique for active forward flexion of the hip. Excellent method to assess roots L1 and L2; and iliopsoas muscle.

TIPS

- Patient sits on table edge, knees bent and legs dangling
- Actively raise knee "toward ceiling" against resistance applied to the top of the knee
- L1 or L2 problems, iliopsoas muscle or proximal muscle problem: weakness
- Lesser trochanter problem: groin discomfort

Table 12.2. Lumbosacral Nerve Roots

Obturator nerve		Femoral nerve		Superior gluteal nerve Sciatic nerve Inferior gluteal nerve		
L1	L2	L3	L4	L5	S1	S2
Hip forward flexion Psoas	*Hip forward flexion* Iliacus	*Knee extension*	*Knee extension*	*Hip backward flexion*	*Hip-* same as	
	Rectus Femoris	Quadriceps	Quadriceps	Gluteus maximus (inferior gluteal nerve)	L5	
	Hip adduction		*Hip abduction*			
	Adductors		Gluteus minimus/ medius (superior gluteal nerve)	*External rotation hip* gluteus maximus (inferior gluteal nerve)	*Foot plantar flexion* (tibialis nerve)	*Foot intrinsic muscles* (plantar branch, tibial nerve)
			Foot dorsi flexion (common peroneal nerve)	*Great toe extension* Common peroneal nerve		
L1	L2	L3	L4	L5	S1	S2

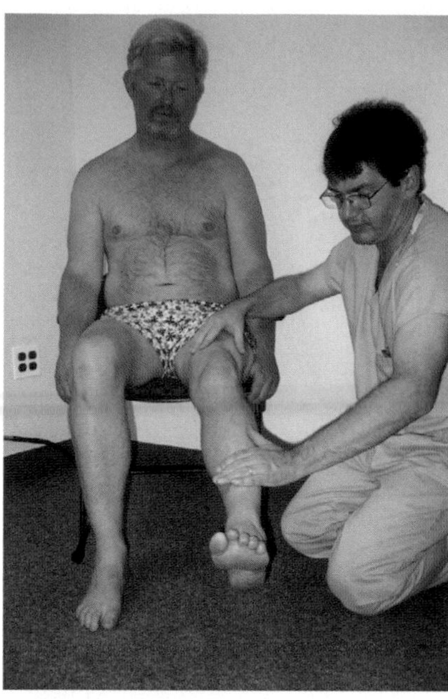

Figure 12.5.

Technique for active extension of knee. Excellent method to assess L3 and L4; quadriceps muscle.

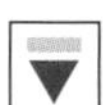

TIPS

- Patient sits on edge of table, knees bent and legs dangling
- Actively extend knee against resistance: apply hand to patient's distal leg
- Quadriceps muscle problem, femoral nerve problem: weakness

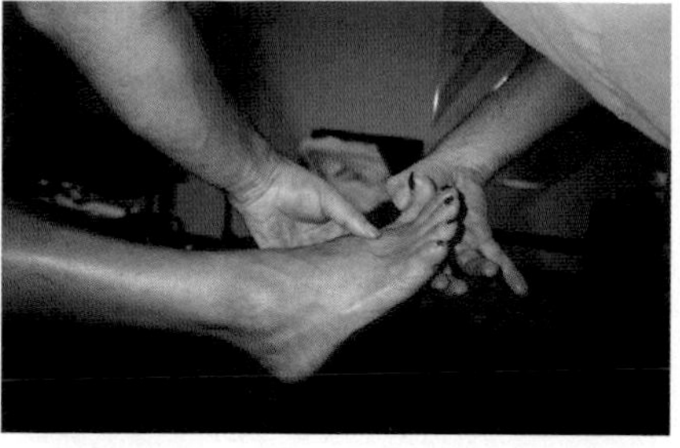

Figure 12.6.

Technique for active dorsiflexion of the great toe. Excellent method to assess L5; anterior leg compartment.

TIPS

- Active dorsiflexion of the great toe against resistance
- Apply thumb to dorsum of patient's great toe
- Extensor hallucis longus muscle, common peroneal nerve, deep peroneal nerve or L5 problem: weakness

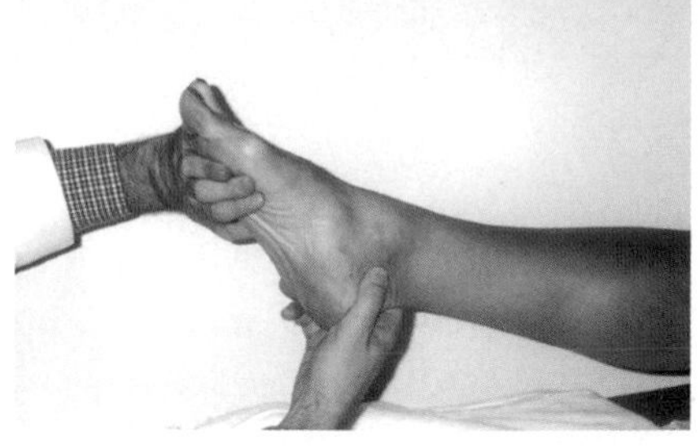

Figure 12.7.

Technique for active plantarflexion at the tibiotalar joint. Excellent method to assess S1; posterior compartment.

TIPS

- Actively plantar flex the foot at the tibiotalar joint against resistance, hand placed on plantar midfoot
- Gastrocnemius muscle, sciatic nerve, tibialis nerve, or S1 complication: weakness

the patient's anus and instruct the patient to squeeze. A normal squeeze indicates a fairly normal pudendal nerve (S3, S4, and S5), whereas a deficit indicates a pudendal nerve or cauda equina or spinal cord problem. The tone assessment is the first-line test; the sensitivity for it is 60% to 80%. Assess the **anal wink** by inserting a gloved finger into the patient's anus and stroke the skin of the proximal medial thigh with a cotton-tipped swab. Note any contraction of the anal sphincter about the finger, which in any spinal cord injury indicates a good prognosis; whereas, in a patient with a nonspecific low back problem **absence** indicates cauda equina syndrome or spinal cord compression. Overall, the anal wink test is best to assess roots S3, S4, and S5. **Cauda equina syndrome** manifests with a sensory deficit in a saddle-type distribution (75% sensitivity), an absent anal wink, and, in severe cases, a deficit in anal and urethral sphincter tone. Thus, in severe cases, the patient has incontinence of urine and even stool. This is due to compression of or damage to the intravertebral column roots distal to the conus medullaris, the most inferior point of the spinal cord itself. Central compression of lumbar spinal cord by herniated disc or tumor manifests in a similar way.

Figure 12.8.

Technique for active adduction of the toes. Excellent method to assess S2.

TIPS

- Place a tongue blade or the tip of a finger between two adjacent toes
- Instruct patient to squeeze adjacent toes together
- S2, tibialis nerve, or intrinsic foot muscle complication: weakness

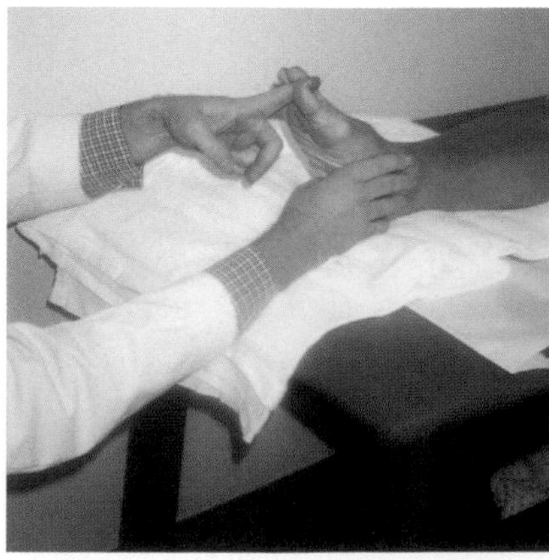

TEACHING POINTS

NEUROLOGIC EXAMINATION

1. Teach, know, and use at least one specific motor function of each nerve root: L1–S4.
2. Knowledge of specific points to touch for sensory examination of L1–S4 nerve roots is requisite to a complete examination.
3. Roots S2–S4: all perineal, although S2 is sensory to popliteal fossa.
4. The best overall reflex for S2–S4: assessment of the anal wink and sphincter tone.
5. S1 and L5: gluteal and sciatic nerves. Gluteal nerve for gluteal muscles and hip movement; whereas, sciatic nerve for foot and ankle movement.
6. Gluteal muscles are not innervated by sciatic nerve.

Sensory

To complement the motor examination, it is important to perform a screening sensory examination using a **cotton-tipped swab** or a **monofilament** to areas specific to roots from T7 to S4. See **Box 12.1** for specific sites.

Box 12.1.

Sensory examination sites for specific roots

Root	Specific site
T4	Areola
T7	Xiphoid process
T10	Umbilicus
T12	Lateral inguinal ligament
L1	Medial inguinal ligament
L2	Anterior medial thigh
L3	Medial patella
L4	Proximal anterior medial malleolus
L5	Dorsal foot
S1	Posterior calf, plantar foot
S2	Popliteal fossa
S3	Outer skin ring of perineum
S4	Skin around the anus
S5	Anal skin

RANGE OF MOTION: HIP, LOWER BACK, AND BONEY PELVIS

Two major joints of mobility are found in the boney pelvis: first, the **hip joint** between the head of the femur and the acetabulum of the pelvis and, second, the **lumbar spine**. The pelvis provides the foundation for standing and walking in a biped—the upright position. The **passive range of motion** (ROM) of the hip **(Table 12.3)** includes **forward flexion**, which is best measured with

Table 12.3. Passive Range of Motion (ROM) at the Hip

Motion	Position of patient	Degrees
Forward flexion	Supine, knee extended	120
Forward flexion	Supine, knee flexed to 90 degrees	150
Backward flexion	Prone, knee extended	30
Abduction	Supine, knee extended	45
Adduction	Supine, contralateral hip abducted	30
Internal rotation	Prone, hip extended, knee flexed to 90 degrees	45
	Supine or sitting, hip flexed to 90 degrees	45
External rotation	Prone, hip extended, knee flexed to 90 degrees	45
	Supine or sitting, hip flexed to 90 degrees	45

the patient supine, normal with patient's knee fully extended is to 120°; whereas, with knee flexed to 90°, it is increased to 160°; **extension (backward flexion)**, which is best measured with patient prone, normal is 30 degrees; **abduction**, which is best measured with the patient supine, normal is 45 degrees; **adduction**, which is best measured with the patient supine, normal is 30 degrees; **internal rotation**, which is best measured with the patient prone or supine, normal is 45 degrees; and **external rotation**, which is best measured with the patient prone or supine, normal is 45 degrees.

ACTIVE HIP AND BACK RANGE OF MOTION

Active **forward flexion** of the hip **(Table 12.4)** involves the iliopsoas muscle; nerve is comprised of roots L1, 2, and 3. Active **backward flexion** (extension) of hip involves the gluteus maximus, medius, minimus, and semimembranosus muscles; nerves are the inferior and superior gluteal and for the semimembranosus, the sciatic. **Active abduction** of the hip to 50 degrees includes

Table 12.4. Active Range of Motion (ROM) at the Hip and Back

Action	Position	Muscle	Nerve
Hip			
Forward flexion	Sits, knee dangling off side of table	Iliopsoas	L1, 2, and 3
Backward flexion	Prone, knee extended; Examiner's hands on midposterior thigh and buttock	Gluteus maximus Gluteus minimus Gluteus medius Semimembranosus	Inferior gluteal Superior gluteal Superior gluteal Sciatic
Backward flexion	Prone, knee flexed to* 90 degrees, examiner's hands on midposterior thigh and buttock	Gluteus maximus	Inferior gluteal
Internal rotation	Sitting, knees flexed to 90 degrees, dangling off table	Gluteus medius Gluteus minimus Abductor magnus Abductor longus	Superior gluteal Superior gluteal Obturator Obturator
External rotation	Sitting, knees flexed to 90 degrees, dangling off table	Piriformis Obturator externus Obturator internus Gemelli Quadratus femoris	Roots S1 and S2 Obturator Roots L5 to S2 Roots L5 and S1 Roots L4 to S1
Abduction	Decubital, side examined up; the leg below is forward flexed to 10 degrees; both fully extended; examiner's hand at mid leg	Gluteus maximus Gluteus medius Gluteus minimus	Inferior gluteal Superior gluteal Superior gluteal
Adduction	Decubital, side examined down; leg down, forward flexed 10 degrees, both knees extended; examiner's hand at mid leg	Adductor magnus Adductor longus Adductor brevis	Obturator Obturator Obturator

*method to isolate out gluteus maximus.

the gluteus maximus, medius, and minimus muscles; nerve is the inferior and superior gluteal. Active **adduction** of the hip uses the adductor longus, adductor magnus, and gracilis muscles, which originate in the pubis and insert on the medial femur and tibia; the nerve is the obturator (L2, L3, L4). Active **external rotation** of the hip involves the gluteus maximus and posterior gluteus medius; and the deeper muscles of the obturator internus, obturator externus, and the piriformis muscles. These last three muscles originate in the lateral sacrum and insert on the superior aspect of the greater trochanter; the nerve is the sciatic. Other external rotators include the gemelli muscle, which originates in the posterior pubis or ilium, inserts on the superior greater trochanter; the nerve is from roots of L4, 5, S1, 2; and the quadratus femoris muscle, which originates in the posterior ilium; inserts in the posterior proximal femur; its nerve is from root of L4, L5, S1, S2. Active **internal rotation** of the hip involves the anterior gluteus medius and gluteus minimus muscles, the nerve is superior gluteal.

Although they act in concert with the hips and pelvis, the **low back and trunk** contribute a different set of actions that allows and supports the individual to be upright and mobile in the upright position. The **lumbar spine**, in the erect position, is lordotic, that is, curved backward, but with forward flexion of the trunk this reverses, i.e., becomes kyphotic, thus affording significant flexibility to the foundation. The ROM, passive and active, of the lumbar

Table 12.4. (continued)

Action	Position	Muscle	Nerve
Adduction	Supine, examiner places fist between knees	Adductor longus Adductor magnus Adductor brevis Gracilis	Obturator Obturator Obturator Obturator
BACK			
Forward flexion to 80 degrees	Standing, arms dangle in front	Abdominus rectus	Segments of TL
Forward flexion	Supine, hands behind head; examiner places pressure on thighs, sit-up	Abdominus rectus Obliquus externus Obliquus internus	Segments of TL Segments of TL Segments of TL
Forward flexion with rotation	Supine, hands behind head; examiner places pressure on thighs, sits up so as to place elbow on other thigh	Obliquus externus Obliquus internus	Segments of TL Segments of TL
Lateral bend to 35 degrees	Standing; bends to one side, "ear to shoulder," hand down the lateral leg	Obliquus muscles Latissimus dorsi	Segments of TL Thoracodorsal
Back rotation to 35 degrees	Standing; examiner places hands on iliac crests, "turn head to right"	Obliquus muscles	Segments of TL
Backward bend to 30 degrees	Standing, patient places palms on each buttock	Paraspinous muscles	Segments of TL
Backward bend	Prone, arms at sides Pillow under abdomen (reverse lumbar lordosis), examiner places arm on pelvis and midback	Paraspinous muscles Erector spinae Longissimus Iliocostalis Spinalis	Segments of TL

TL: thoracolumbar.

TEACHING POINTS

PELVIS, HIP, AND LOW BACK: PASSIVE AND ACTIVE RANGE OF MOTION (ROM)

1. Hip backward flexion: gluteus maximus, medius, and minimus muscles.
2. Hip forward flexion: iliopsoas muscle.
3. Hip internal rotation: gluteus medius (anterior fibers), minimus, gacilus, and adductors.
4. Hip external rotation: gluteus maximus, medius (posterior fibers), piriformis, obturator externus, gemelli, and quadratus femoris muscles.
5. Hip abduction: gluteus maximus, medius, and minimus muscles.
6. Hip adduction: adductor longus and magnus muscles.
7. Pulled groin: strain of adductor muscles, pain is maximal at pubis.
8. ROM specific to low back and trunk: may best be performed in the upright and then the sit-up positions.
9. Abdominus obliquus muscles: assessed by sitting up and rotating trunk.
10. Abdominus rectus muscles: assessed by active sitting up.
11. Gemelli, obturator, piriformis, and quadratus muscles make a rotator cuff of sorts, mainly to effect external rotation of hip.
12. Forward flexion of hip: maximized with concurrent flexion of the knee.
13. Furthest domain of L4 laterally: the sartorius muscle.

spine includes **forward flexion** to 90 degrees, **lateral rotation** left and right to 30 degrees, **lateral bend** left and right to 40 degrees, and **backward flexion** to 30 degrees.

The major forward flexor of the lumbar spine and, therefore, of the trunk is the set of **rectus abdominus** muscles. The **obliquus** muscles contribute to lateral bending of the trunk; whereas, external oblique is specific for trunk rotation; strains of the adductors increase the risk of abdominus obliquus and/or rectus abdominus strains.

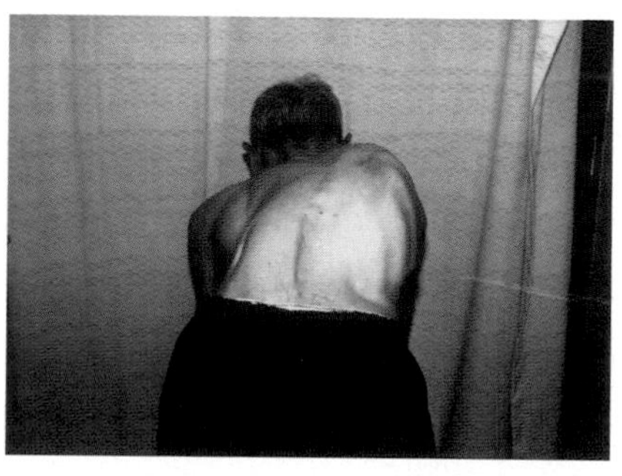

Figure 12.9.

A. Marked thoracic scoliosis. Forward flexion accentuates the finding **(B)**.

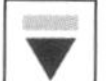

TIPS

- Inspect the back with patient erect and then with patient in forward flexion
- Dextroscoliosis: right deviation of the spine
- Levoscoliosis: left deviation of the spine

INSPECTION OF CURVATURE OF BACK AND SPINE

Inspection of the back for increased or abnormal curves of the lumbar or thoracic spine is basic to the physical examination. Visually inspect the spinal column from behind and from the side; repeat with the patient in bending forward at the trunk. **Scoliosis** is a common finding, with a prevalence of 8%–10%, especially of the thoracic spine **(Fig. 12.9)**. It manifests as **dextroscoliosis**, a right deviation of spinal column or **levoscoliosis**, a left deviation. Scoliosis is often accentuated by forward flexing of the trunk (Adam's test). In this test the asymmetry of the back and a "rib hump" is accentuated in a patient with scoliosis. The potential for restrictive pulmonary disease exists in cases of scoliosis. Accentuation of the **lumbar lordosis**, the presence of straightening, or **kyphosis** at the lumbar spine should also be noted. **Compression fractures** of the thoracic spine manifest, in the acute setting, with severe pain that radiates into dermatomes on both sides and an exacerbation of symptoms on percussion of the affected vertebral body. In addition, over time an accentuation of the thoracic kyphosis develops and a "hump" appears in the upper thoracic spine (a "dowager's" hump). Other names for this often quite remarkable finding include "hunchback" and "humpback." Restrictive pulmonary disease is a potential problem. This is most commonly due to poor posture in youth, but may be osteoporotic in middle-aged to older patients.

LOW BACK PAIN

A physician will see and teach about many patients who present with low back pain. It is a common problem and has a wide differential diagnosis, making it vexing even to master clinicians. The physical examination can and does provide significant information and clues to the underlying diagnosis of the patient's condition. Thus, it is important to be facile with the physical examination techniques, their use, and their limits. One of the first steps in the approach to a patient with low back pain after inspection and neurologic examination, is to perform the FABER maneuver **(Fig. 12.10)**. This term is an acronym for the steps in the procedure, which include: F = forward flexion of the hip, passively, with the patient supine; AB = abduction of the hip, again passively; ER = external rotation of the hip, such that the patient has a configuration of the arabic number 4. This is an excellent first-line test that provides clues to the site of maximal pain and, thus, potential complications. See **Table 12.5** for the different causes of low back and hip pain that the FABER maneuver can help define.

Table 12.5. Low Back Pain

Diagnosis	FABER-pain site	Company it Keeps
L/S1 radiculopathy	Posterior lateral thigh	Positive SLR Positive crossed SLR L5 or S1 motor or sensory findings Classic sciatica
L4 radiculopathy	Anterior thigh	Positive femoral stretch (Dyck)
Paraspinous strain	Paraspinous muscle itself	Spasm Poker gait
Ankylosing spondylitis	Sacroiliac joints	Limited Schober Limited chest wall expansion Erythema nodosum Achilles tendinitis Morning stiffness
Greater trochanter bursitis	Lateral femur, greater trochanter	Lateral buttock pain
Compression fracture	Involved vertebral body	Bilateral symptoms
Hip degenerative joint disease	Inguinal area, medial thigh	Antalgic gait
Ischiogluteal bursitis	Ischial tuberosity	Sciatica
Iliotibial band syndrome	Lateral thigh into Gerdy's tubercle of Lateral tibia	Limp Positive Ober's maneuver

FABER = F = forward flexion of the hip; AB = abduction of the hip, again passively; ER = external rotation of the hip; SLR = straight leg raise.

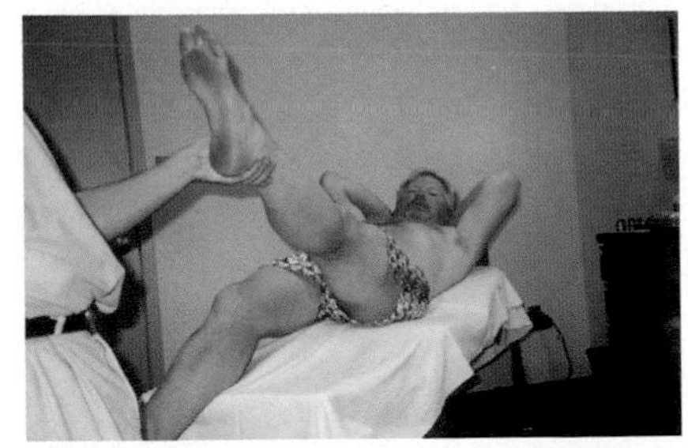

A

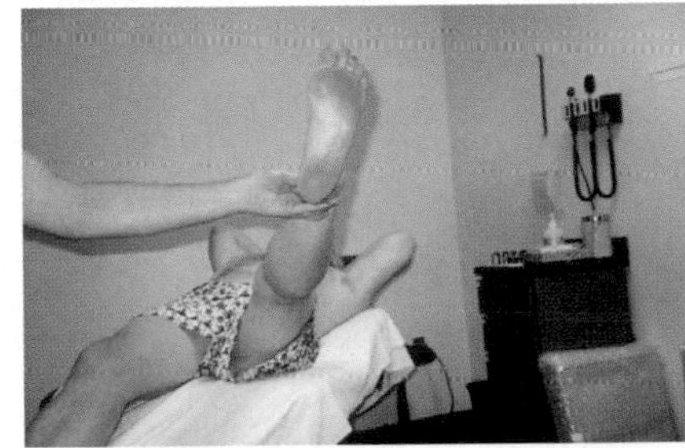

B

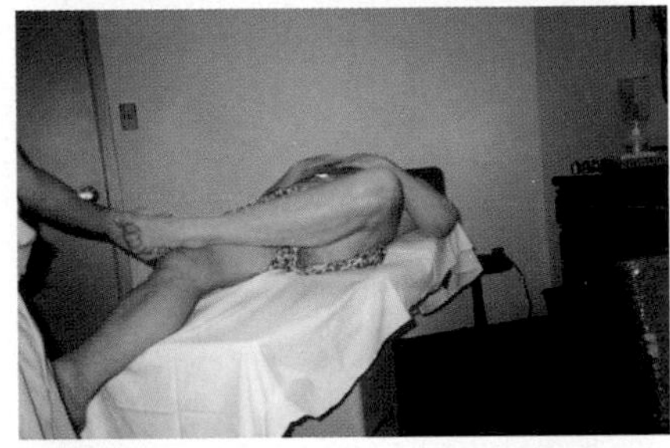

C

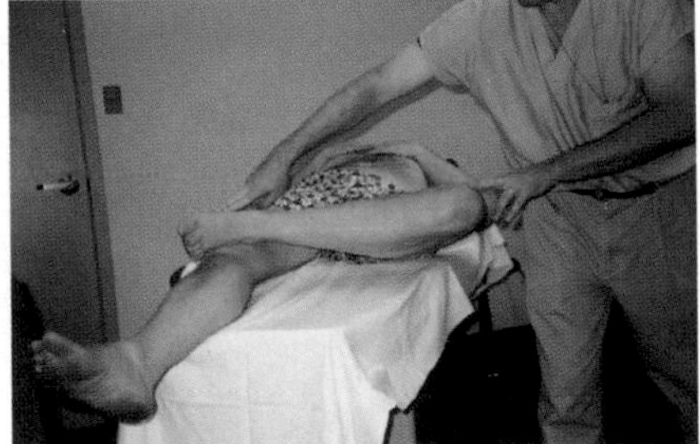

D

Figure 12.10.

Technique for FABER maneuver. **A.** Passive forward flexion of hip. **B.** Abduction of hip. **C.** External rotation at the hip. An excellent first-line screening test to evaluate a patient with low back or hip pain.

TIPS

- Patient supine
- Passively forward flex the patient's leg to 45 degrees **(A)**
- Passively abduct the leg at the hip **(B)**
- Passively externally rotate the leg at the hip **(C)**
- Normal: no pain or discomfort

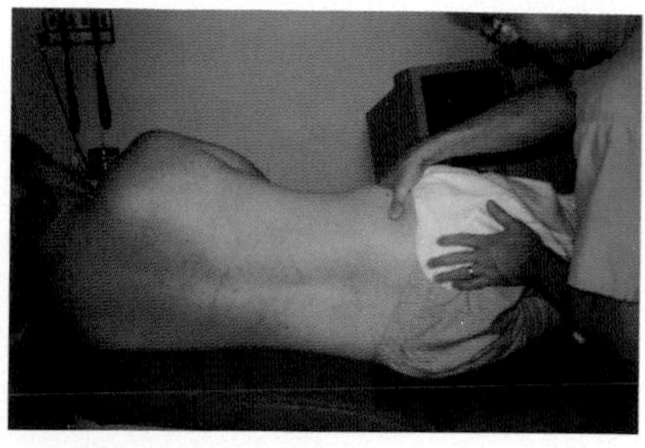

Figure 12.11.

Technique for sacroiliac compression test. Excellent first-line test to assess for ankylosing spondylitis.

 **TIPS**

- Patient in lateral decubital position, side with symptoms superior
- Apply pressure over the iliac crest
- Ankylosing spondylosis: reproducible pain over the SI joint

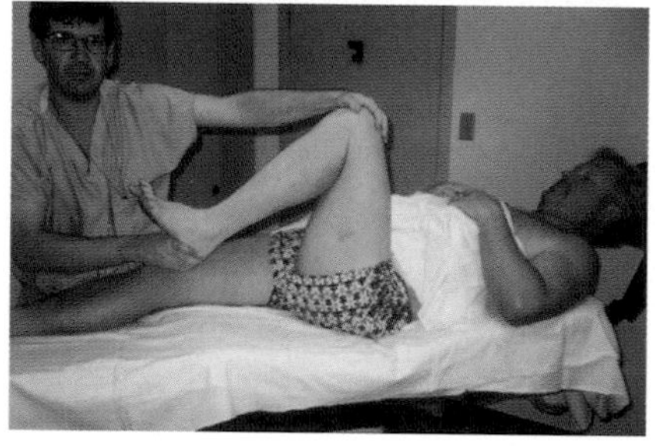

Figure 12.12.

Technique for knee-to-chest position. Excellent first-line test to assess for ankylosing spondylitis.

 **TIPS**

- Patient supine, legs freely flexed over the end of table
- Passively forward flex hip and knee, repeat on other side
- Ankylosing spondylosis: reproducible pain over the SI joint

Ankylosing spondylitis manifests with morning stiffness, large joint involvement, and tenderness at the sacroiliac joints, exacerbated by the FABER maneuver. Pain is also reproduced with the **sacroiliac compression test** in which the patient is in the lateral decubital position with the symptomatic side superior and, with pressure applied to iliac crest, sacroiliac pain is reproduced **(Fig. 12.11)**. In addition, the pain develops with the **knee-to-chest test** in which the patient is supine with legs dangling over the table; with passive flexion of the knee and forward flexion of the hip, sacroiliac pain is reproduced **(Fig. 12.12)**. Furthermore, the patient has a straightened back, with the straightening involving both the thoracic and the lumbar spines, which is particularly evident in the "straight as a poker" gait. Another excellent technique is that of the **Schober maneuver** in which the patient forward bends at the trunk while the examiner notes the lumbar spine **(Fig. 12.13)**. Normally, it becomes arched, that is kyphotic. In ankylosis spondylitis, it remains straight; as such, a stretch of the lumbar spine is <5 cm from erect to forward bend. This maneuver is one of the best methods to define and describe the straightening of the spinal column in ankylosing spondylitis. In severe disease, the company it keeps includes anterior uveitis and erythema nodosum and the development of restrictive pulmonary disease. The **chest wall expansion maneuver**, in which the patient's chest circumference is measured at the area of the areolae (about rib 4) in both full inhalation and exhalation is restricted. The normal increase is >3 cm, if <3 cm it is indicative of restrictive disease. Although the specificity for this test is 99%, the sensitivity is only 9%.

Paraspinous strain manifests with pain, spasm, and tenderness to palpation in the paraspinous muscle, often bilaterally. The patient has a "straight as a poker" gait, which is caused by the severe pain in the lumbar paraspinous area. The paraspinous spasm is objectively demonstrated by a loss of the normal reversal of the lumbar lordotic curve to become kyphotic with forward bend. This paraspinous strain results from lifting or improper lifting of objects, with a resultant stretching or tearing of the paraspinous muscle fibers.

Sciatica manifests with pain in the low back that radiates into the posterolateral thigh and even into the foot. The FABER maneuver reproduces the sciatic distribution of discomfort and focuses on a site of pain origin. In the **straight leg raise** (SLR)test, the pain is reproduced on passively forward flex-

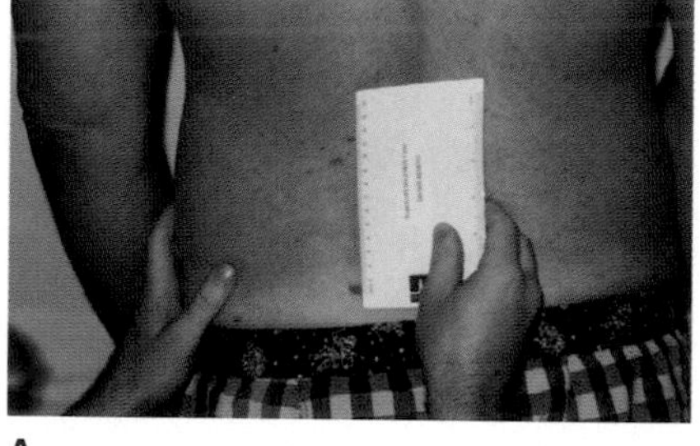

A

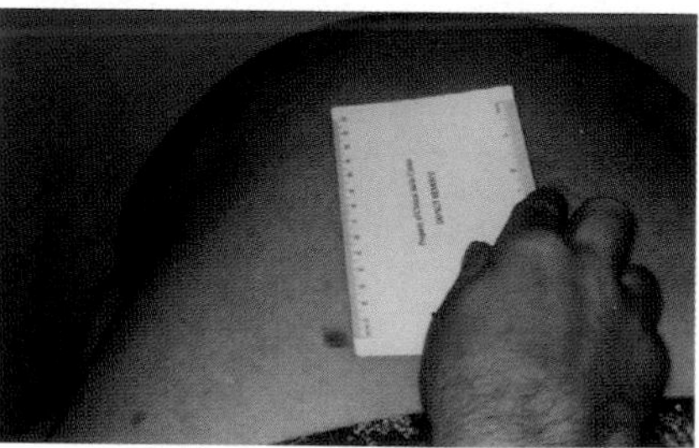

B

Figure 12.13.

Technique for Schober maneuver to define ankylosing spondylitis. **A.** Erect. **B.** Trunk forward flexed.

 **TIPS**

- Patient erect, view from back
- Use mind's eye or a water-soluble marker to mark posterior superior iliac spine and a site 10 cm above
- Instruct the patient to actively fully forward flex at trunk
- Normal: significant increase in the distance (arc is indeed longer straight line)
- Ankylosing spondylitis: distance remains the same (straight line = straight line)

ing the leg at the hip with the patient supine (**Fig. 12.14**). The demonstration of a radicular type pain with the leg forward flexed to <60 degrees, is consistent with sciatica. This maneuver, which was first described by Laguerre in the mid-nineteenth century, is of modest value at best; it has a positive predictive value of 64%, a sensitivity of 80%, and a specificity of 40% (Fig. 12.14). This test has several variants that are useful complements to the original one. The clinician should be able to use and teach these variants. These include the *foot dorsiflexion variant* in which the standard SLR is performed to the point of discomfort, then the angle of forward flexion in the leg is decreased to make the patient asymptomatic, then the foot is passively dorsiflexed to attempt to reproduce the symptoms. Finally, the test with the best evidence to support it is the *crossed straight leg raise* in which manifestations are reproduced with a straight leg raise on the contralateral side. The sensitivity for this test is only 25%; however, the specificity is 90% and it has is a positive predictive value of 97% for sciatica. The sensory examination is of little value in the diagnosis of sciatica; its sensitivity and specificity is only 50%. When severe, weakness may be noted to ankle plantar flexion and dorsiflexion and to great toe flexion and extension; and a diminished or absent plantar reflex (**Table 12.6**). The problem with each of these tests is that they define the features of sciatica, but do not begin to define or describe the underlying diagnosis. Thus, it is important to emphasize and teach the need to diagnose the underlying reason for the sciatica.

The company sciatica keeps defines and helps diagnose the underlying etiology. **Herniated intervertebral disc at L5/S1** interspace is caused most often by the posterior lateral protrusion of the nucleus pulposis of the invertebral

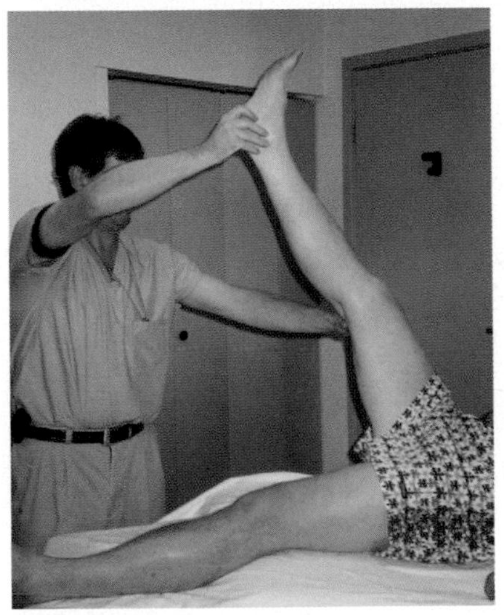
A

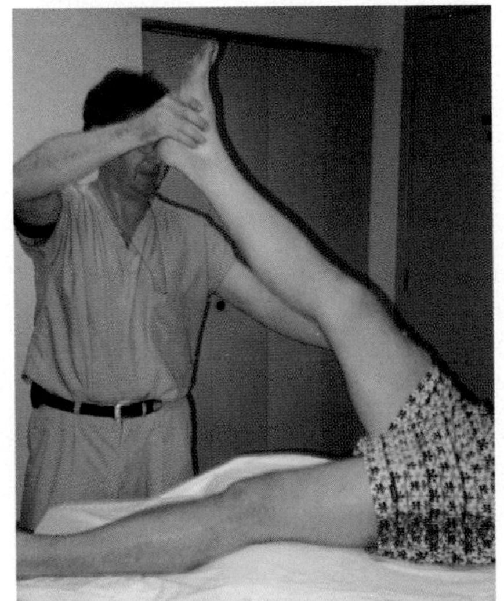
B

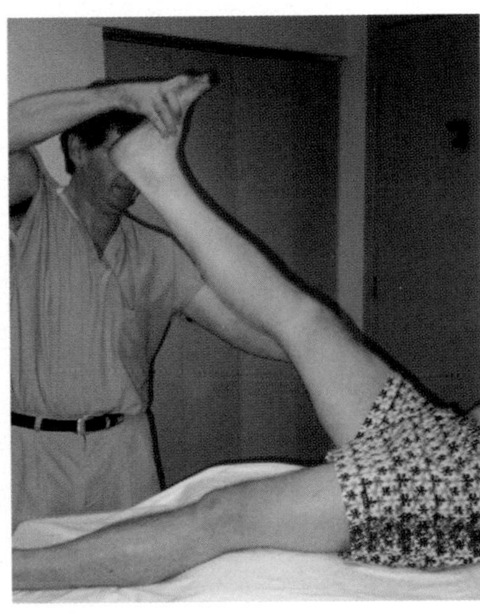
C

Figure 12.14.

Technique for straight leg raise of Laguerre **(A)**. A component of evaluation of patient with potential sciatica. Foot dorsiflexion variant **(B, C)**.

TIPS

- Patient supine
- Place one hand beneath the patient's lower back
- Grasp heel of the ipsilateral lower extremity and passively forward flex the leg at the hip
- Normal: varying degrees of stiffness but no pain to 60 degrees
- Sciatica: pain in posterior lateral thigh with leg at an angle <40 degrees
- Hold the leg at the angle, at which the pain occurs in the straight leg raise, then lower the leg by 5 degrees, and passively dorsiflex the foot at the tibiotalar joint **(B** and **C)**

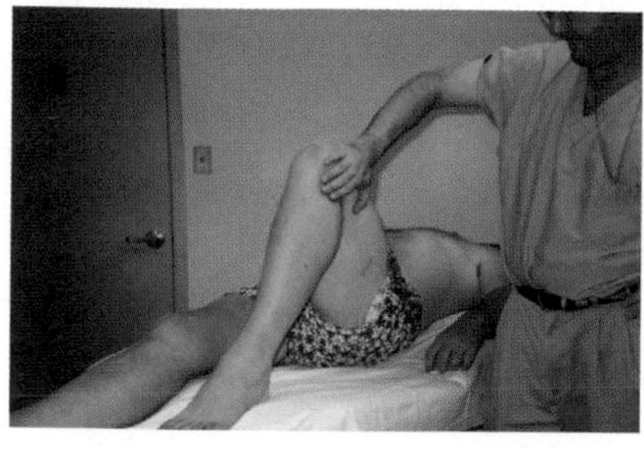

Figure 12.15.

Technique for Pace test for piriformis syndrome. Excellent test to define this specific cause of sciatica.

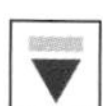 **TIPS**

- Patient supine; knee flexed to 90 degrees, hip flexed to 45 degrees
- Instruct patient to actively externally rotate and abduct the leg at the thigh
- Apply resistance to patient's leg
- Piriformis syndrome or strain: pain in sciatic nerve distribution

Table 12.6. Evidence Basis for Low Back Examination

Diagnosis	Procedure/paper	Sensitivity (%)	Specificity (%)	PPV/NPV (%)
Herniated disc—sciatica	*Straight leg raise*			
	Hudgins			64
	Deyo	80	40	
	Crossed straight leg raise			
	Hudgins			97
	Deyo	25	90	
	Spangfort	25	88	
	Weak dorsiflexors			
	Deyo	35	70	
	Weak great toe extensors			
	Deyo	50	70	
	Decreased Achilles' reflex			
	Deyo	50	60	
	Sensory deficit			
	Deyo	50	50	

PPV = positive predictive value; NPV = negative predictive value.

disc. It manifests with classic features of sciatica, which usually progressively worsen over time and can become associated with motor deficits. Of interest, the L5 roots are thickest, whereas, the foramen of the L5 space is narrowest, thus the greatest risk of entrapment exists here. The discomfort increases when sitting or standing for prolonged periods, decreases when supine with knees flexed; it acutely worsens with cough or valsalva. The patient's stance is listing to side opposite the pain. **Herpes zoster** manifests with pain, cutaneous hyperesthesia, and then clusters of vesicles in L5 or S1 dermatomes. **Piriformis syndrome** manifests with posterior buttock discomfort, dyspareunia in women and sciatica. There is reproduction of the sciatica with the **Pace**

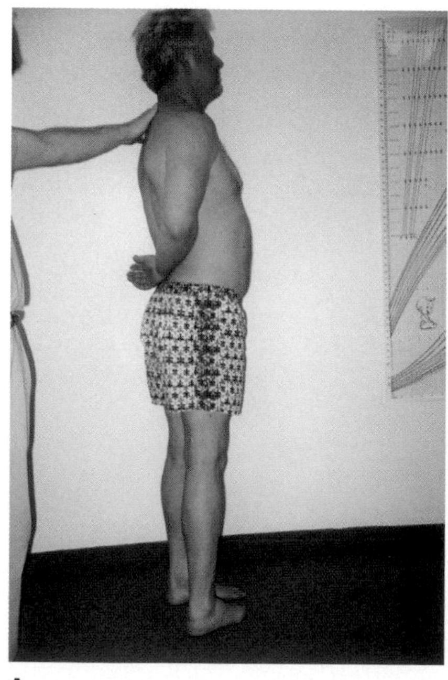

A

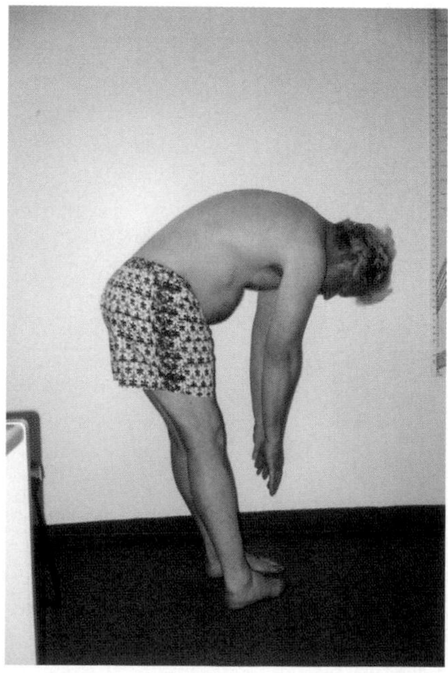

B

Figure 12.16.

Technique for Piriformis test for this cause of sciatica. **A.** Upright position. **B.** Forward trunk flexion.

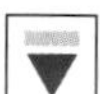 **TIPS**

- Patient standing, symptomatic leg maximally internally rotated
- Patient forward bends the trunk
- Piriformis syndrome or strain: pain in sciatic nerve distribution

test in which the patient is supine, knee flexed to 90 degrees, and hip flexed to 45; patient actively externally rotates and abducts the hip against resistance **(Fig. 12.15)**. Furthermore, the sciatica can be reproduced with the **piriformis test** in which the patient stands, the symptomatic leg is maximally internally rotated, and the patient then bends forward **(Fig. 12.16)**. Piriformis syndrome is irritation of sciatic nerve as it runs under a hypertrophied or inflammed piriformis muscle that often occurs in a "weekend-warrior" soccer player. **Gluteal compartment syndrome** manifests with diffuse swelling and tenderness in the affected buttock(s) due to antecedent blunt trauma, e.g., falling on one's buttocks. It is important to emphasize that blunt trauma to the buttocks can cause this potentially severe syndrome. A **compression fracture** of one of the vertebral bodies manifests with severe, even excruciating, bilateral pain in the affected dermatome. If the dermatome is L5 or S1, bilateral sciatica will likely manifest. In addition, tenderness to percussion is noted over the affected vertebral body. **Ischiogluteal bursitis** manifests with pain and tenderness over the ischial tuberosity, exactly in the midline of the gluteal fold, because the site of the bursa is between the tuberosity and the gluteal muscle. Often concurrent sciatic nerve findings and "sciatica-like" symptoms are noted with the straight leg raise because the sciatic nerve runs adjacent to this structure. This bursitis is caused by irritation to that bursa, such as sitting on a hard surface, e.g., benches at a stadium, or occupation-related "weaver's bottom;" in cyclists, from extensive bicycle riding; or in a patient with a history of sitting with a wallet or chewing tobacco tin in the back pocket. Thus, inspection of the wear and tear in the back pocket of the patient's trousers, e.g., the round marking of a tin of chewing tobacco, may be an important diagnostic clue in a patient with low back pain. **Table 12.7** lists specific causes of sciatica.

Table 12.7. Sciatica: Diagnoses

Diagnosis	Side	History	Company it Keeps
Herniated disc	Unilateral	Recurrent	List to other side Pain increased with cough
Ischiogluteal bursitis	Unilateral	Pain in buttock	Large wallet in back pocket Prolonged sitting on hard surface Tenderness over ischial tuberosity
Piriformis site	Unilateral dominant leg	Soccer player	Tender with Pace sign Tender with piriformis sign
Gluteal compartment syndrome	Bilateral	Recent fall onto buttocks	Ecchymosis Potentially life threatening
Hamstring site	Unilateral	Runners	Pain with hamstring squeeze Limitation of ambulation
Iliotibial band syndrome	Bilateral	Runners	Tender with Ober's maneuver Tender with hyperabduction maneuver
Compression fracture	Bilateral, specific L5 or S1 dermatomes	Severe pain, acute	Recent trauma Osteoporosis risk factors
Herpes zoster	Unilateral L5 or S1	Pain then rash	Clusters of vesicles

TEACHING POINTS

LOW BACK AND HIP PAIN

1. Significant overlap between the hip, the trunk, and the back; either location can result in low back pain.
2. Radicular problems: manifest with dermatomal pain or specific nerve root deficits, usually L5 or S1; less commonly, L4.
3. Compression fracture: manifests with severe bilateral dermatomal pain.
4. Sciatica: a problem, not a diagnosis.
5. Sciatica has a large differential that includes herniated disc, ischiogluteal bursitis, piriformis syndrome, herpes zoster, and gluteal contusion; specific physical diagnostic procedures assist in making the specific diagnosis.
6. Iliotibial band syndrome: lateral pain with ambulation; positive Ober's maneuver.
7. Crossed straight leg raise: the best evidence-based foundation as a provocative test for herniated disc (sciatica).
8. L4 radiculopathy: anterior thigh pain or discomfort; quadriceps assessment.
9. Sciatic nerve evaluation must include foot and ankle exam.

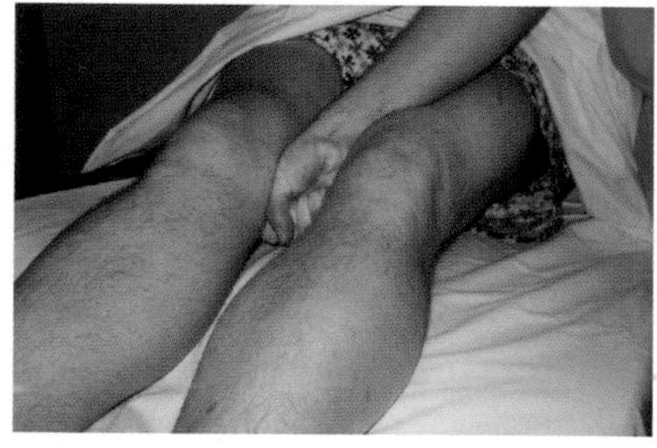

Figure 12.17.

Technique for active adduction of the thighs—excellent method to assess for an adductor muscle strain.

 **TIPS**

- Place fist between the patient's knee
- Instruct patient to actively squeeze the fist (i.e., adduct legs)
- Adductor longus or gracilis strain: pain increased in groin, specifically at pubis (pubalgia)
- Adductor tear: pain at site with a flaccid medial thigh mass
- Look for concurrent abdominus rectus strain

ANTERIOR, MEDIAL HIP, AND THIGH

Adductor muscle strain, which is also known as a "groin pull," manifests with pain in the groin specific to the pubis, i.e., pubalgia. Tenderness is noted in the anterior medial thigh from the pubis to the distal medial femur. The pain is increased with active hip adduction and its opposite, passive hip abduction. One of the best methods to actively adduct the hips is for the examiner to place a fist between the knees of a supine patient and instruct the patient to squeeze (adduct) **(Fig. 12.17)**. This strain is most often caused by recurrent forceful abduction of the thighs and legs, e.g., straddling, and is quite common in soccer players. Often there is company of weak or strained abdominus rectus muscles. A **torn adductor muscle** manifests with a flaccid mass in the medial thigh that becomes more prominent with active adduction. **Horse rider's or rodeo thigh** manifests with bilateral medial thigh pain and tenderness. This is a bilateral adductor muscle strain caused by overuse of the adductors while riding a horse or bull.

Quadriceps muscle strain manifests with pain and tenderness in the anterior thigh, which increases with active knee extension. A **quadriceps muscle tear (Fig. 12.18)** manifests with anterior pain that increases with active extension at the knee. In addition, a *patella baja* is present, i.e., patella is inappropriately distal to the knee and a flaccid mass is noted in the belly of the quadriceps muscle.

Degenerative arthritis of the hip joint or avascular necrosis of the femoral head manifests with the patient having pain in the medial hip and groin. In addition, the patient walks with an *antalgic gait,* that is, one in which the thigh and leg adducted and externally rotated to minimize pain in the groin. There is a decreased ROM to external rotation and internal rotation of the hip often with groin pain. Finally, weakness to thigh abduction is demonstrated using the method described by *Trendelenburg*. In this test, the patient is instructed to place all weight on the symptomatic lower extremity **(Fig. 12.19)**. With this motion, the pelvis inappropriately tilts upward toward the symptomatic side and downward toward the asymptomatic side. Degenerative joint disease of the hip is common. Joints outside of the hip can exacerbate or even be a factor in the development of this degenerative problem. Thus, it is important to examine the back, knee, and foot for contributing lesions and to teach this principle.

Lumbar (L4) radiculopathy manifests with pain radiating into the anterior thigh to the top of the patella. Pain is reproduced with the *femoral traction test* of Dyck **(Fig. 12.20)** in which the patient is in the lateral decubitus position, symptomatic side superior, while the examiner passively extends the knee and passively backward flexes the hip to 15 degrees, then passively flexes the knee. In addition, there is decreased power to knee extension and a decreased or absent patellar reflex develops in severe cases.

Femoral hernia (Fig. 12.21) manifests with a mass or bulge into the anterior thigh, specifically in the proximal medial femoral triangle, inferior to the inguinal ligament. A high risk of incarceration exists because the hernia site has a narrow orifice.

Meralgia paresthetica, which is the entrapment of the lateral cutaneous nerve of the thigh, manifests with tingling and pain in the anterior lateral

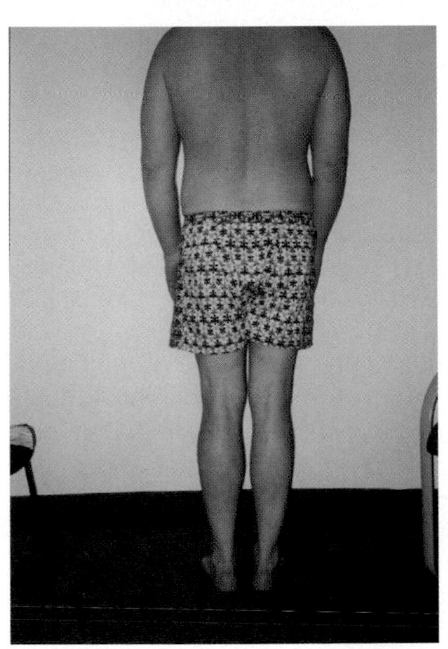

A

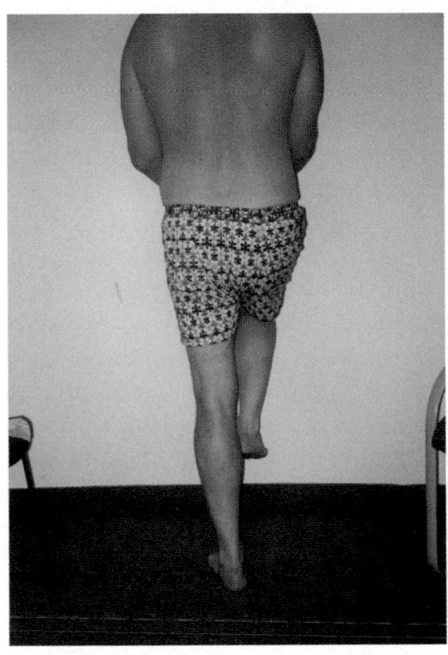

B

Figure 12.19.

Technique for Trendelenburg's test. Method to assess the function of the abductors in a patient with potentially significant unilateral hip degenerative joint disease.

TIPS

- Stand behind the patient, inspect the pelvis
- Patient stands on one leg (the symptomatic side) and raises the foot on the asymptomatic side off the floor
- Normal: pelvis tilts slightly upward toward the non–weight-bearing (asymptomatic) side
- Weak thigh abductors, e.g., in severe unilateral degenerative joint disease: pelvis tilts upward toward the weight-bearing (symptomatic) and downward toward the non–weight-bearing side = positive test

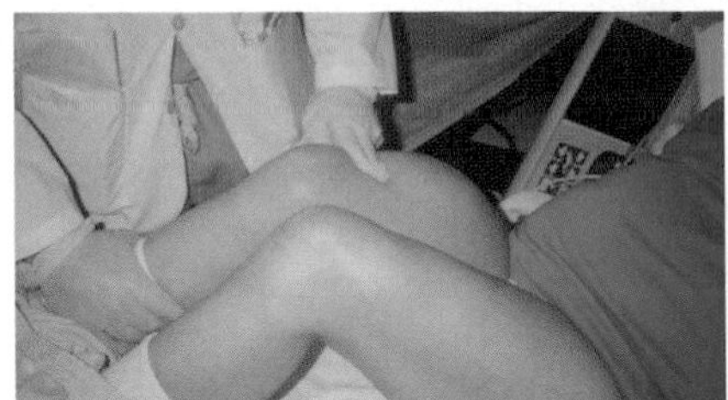

Figure 12.18.

Old quadriceps tear, partial. Note the flaccid mass in the quadriceps muscle and the patella is slightly displaced distally (patella baja).

TIPS

- Inspect the quadriceps muscle when the leg is actively extended at the knee
- Quadriceps tear: flaccid mass in the quadriceps; weakness present with a patella baja
- Tender up to inferior ASIS

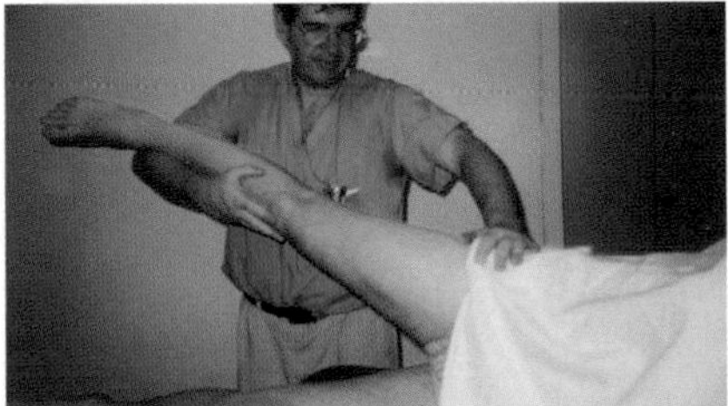

A

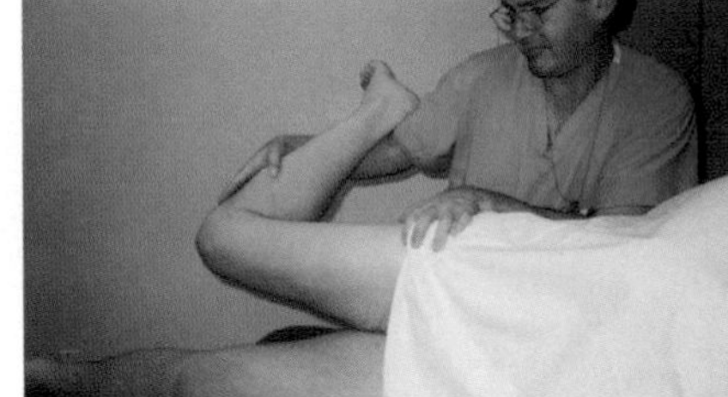

B

Figure 12.20.

Technique for the femoral traction test of Dyck. Excellent method to specifically assess the L4 root.

TIPS

- Patient in lateral decubitus position, symptomatic side superior
- Passively extend the patient's knee and passively backward flex the hip to 15 degrees, then passively flex the knee
- L4 radiculopathy: significant pain in anterior thigh

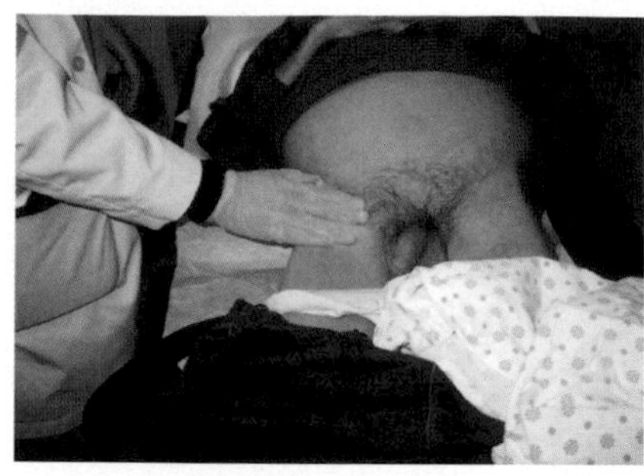

Figure 12.21.

Femoral hernia in the medial anterior thigh passes immediately beneath the inguinal ligament.

 **TIPS**

- Femoral hernia: mass under the inguinal ligament into the femoral triangle
- High risk of incarceration for femoral hernias.

Figure 12.22.

Technique for Tinel's sign using the finger over the lateral inguinal ligament.

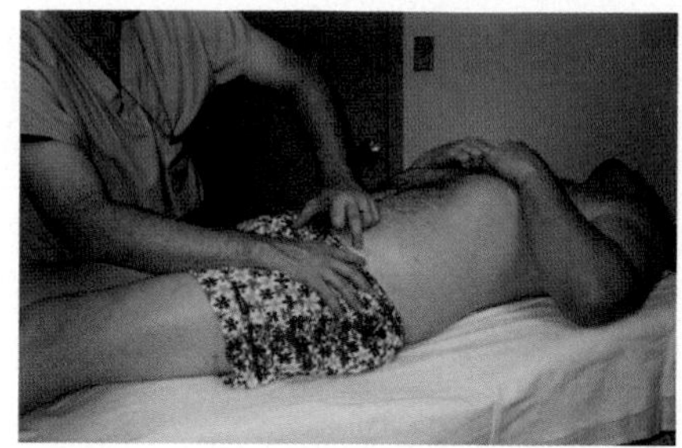

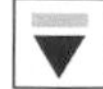 **TIPS**

- Standard procedure of 10 to 15 reproducible taps over extreme lateral inguinal ligament; use finger or Queen square pleximeter
- Meralgia paresthetica: anterolateral thigh paresthesia and pain

thigh, but with no motor deficits. Manifestations can be reproduced with Tinel's **(Fig. 12.22)** sign performed over the lateral inguinal ligament. The patient relates a history that symptoms are increased by wearing tight jeans or by wearing a tight belt. It is also not an uncommon problem during the third trimester of pregnancy.

Other problems include a **fascial hernia** of the thigh, which manifests with a nodule or mass in anterolateral thigh, immediately anterior to the ITB*. The nodule often increases in size with contraction of the quadriceps muscle and decreases in size when the quadriceps is relaxed. This type of hernia is caused by an outpouching of muscle or connective tissue through a defect in this, the thinnest area of fascia in the thigh. The defect can be spontaneous but most often results from an old penetrating injury, e.g., a stab-wound to the lateral anterior thigh. **Inguinal lymphadenopathy** manifests with one or more nodules or masses in the medial anterior thigh, in the area of the inguinal ligament, including the very medially placed node of Cloquet. As with other lymph node enlargement, nodes that are infection-related are tender and enlarged; lymphoma-related are rubbery, not tender, and matted together; whereas, metastatic carcinoma nodes are rock hard, not tender, and fixed to the overlying or underlying fascia. A **femoral artery aneurysm** manifests with a pulsatile mass in the midproximal femoral triangle. Often, a concurrent bruit or even a palpable thrill is noted. This is usually due to trauma. A **hip pointer** manifests with pain, swelling, and tenderness, specifically over the superior ASIS*, that radiates into the sartorius, i.e., the lateral anterior thigh. It is caused by a direct blunt trauma, e.g., hit by the helmeted head of a football player, to the ASIS. **Abdominus rectus muscles strain** manifests with pain and tenderness in the medial anterior abdomen. The pain increases with an active sit-up, often in a soccer player or running back; concurrent adductor sprains are common. **Iliopsoas strain** manifests with anterior medial thigh pain, specific to the lesser trochanter. Often, concurrent ipsilateral lower quadrant abdominal pain is noted. The pain increases with passive external or internal rotation of the hip and with active forward flexion or passive backward flexion of the hip. This strain is common in dancers and gymnasts. **Iliopsoas bursitis** manifests with anterior thigh pain and fullness in the proximal medial anterior thigh, inferior to inguinal ligament. Pain increases with passive backward flexion, adduction, and internal rotation of the hip. **Proximal quadriceps contusion** (charley horse) manifests with anterolateral thigh pain, ecchymosis, and swelling, especially at inferior aspect of the ASIS. The pain is markedly increased on standing erect from a seated position. This contusion most often is caused by a direct blow to the anterior thigh, especially vastus obliquus lateralis and vastus intermedius muscles, i.e., common in American football and thus the need for protective thigh pads. A complication, **myositis ossificans**,

*ASIS = anterior superior iliac spine.

TEACHING POINTS

ANTERIOR AND MEDIAL HIP AND PELVIS

1. Masses in the anterior thigh: old thigh contusion, femoral hernia, femoral artery aneurysm, or inguinal lymphadenopathy.
2. Anterior thigh contusion: can develop the significant sequala of myositis ossificans.
3. Hip degenerative joint disease (DJD) or AVN* of hip: groin pain.
4. Meralgia paresthetica, entrapment of the lateral cutaneous nerve of the thigh at the inguinal ligament: anterior or lateral thigh paresthesia and pain.
5. The structures that pass beneath the inguinal ligament into the femoral triangle lateral to medial: lateral cutaneous nerve of thigh, fat, NAVEL: nerve (femoral), artery (femoral), vein (femoral), and lymphatics.
6. Strain of the abdominus rectus: weak sit-up and anterior lower abdominal pain.
7. Strain of iliopsoas: weak forward flexion of hip and may have nebulous anterior lower abdominal pain.
8. Four common injuries of American football: a hip pointer (ASIS to sartorius), a charley horse (quadriceps contusion), a groin pull (adductor strain) and abdominus rectus strain.
9. Active sit-up test: A good screen for abdominal wall problems.

*AVN = avascular necrosis.

manifests with chronic anterior thigh pain and swelling. This is a chronic manifestation of a contusion caused by heterotopic bone formation that occurs a minimum of 2 to 4 weeks after an injury.

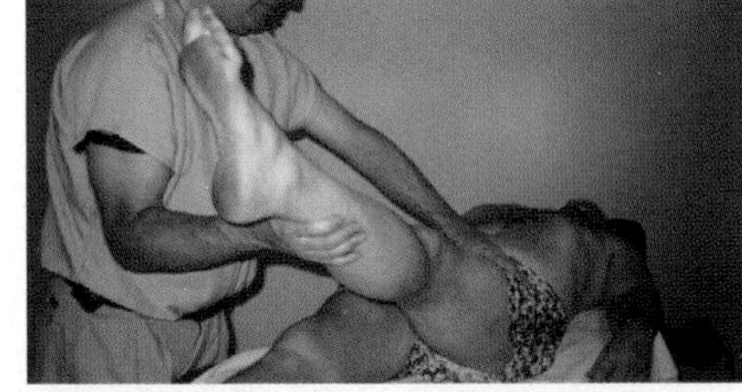

A

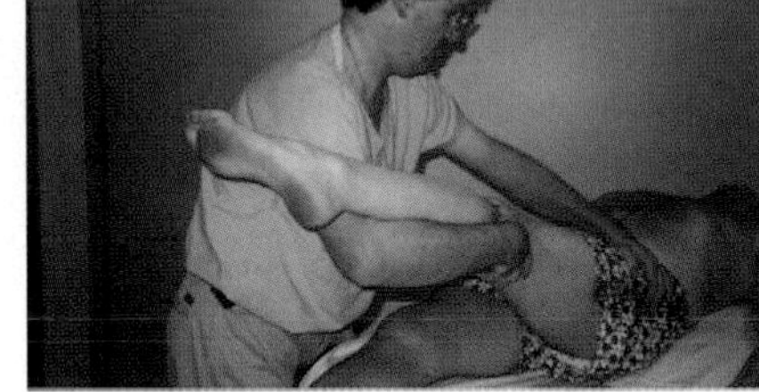

B

Figure 12.23.

Technique for greater trochanteric bursa assessment: passive hip forward flexion and internal rotation.

TIPS

- Patient supine
- Passively forward flex and internally rotate hip
- Greater trochanteric bursitis: increase in tenderness over and behind the greater trochanter

LATERAL HIP AND BONEY PELVIS

Greater trochanter bursitis manifests with pain, tenderness, and swelling between the gluteus maximus muscle and posterior aspect of the lateral greater trochanter of the femur **(Fig. 12.23)**. Discomfort markedly increases when the examiner passively forward flexes and concurrently internally rotates the hip of the affected side.

The **iliotibial band syndrome** manifests with lateral thigh pain that extends to the lateral knee, specifically to Gerdy's tubercle on the proximal lateral tibia and to the ipsilateral buttock. Symptoms are reproduced with the backward flexion and abduction maneuver and with Ober's maneuver **(Fig. 12.24)**. In Ober's maneuver, there is inappropriate pain and stiffness to passive adduction of the affected leg. Sciatica may develop as a component of this syndrome. ITB* syndrome is often caused by running without proper stretching and the use of high arched shoes.

Obliquus externus strain manifests with pain and tenderness in the flank; the pain is markedly increased when the patient performs an active sit-up. This is due to overuse in rotatory trunk movements. **Tear of the obliquus externus and internus aponeuroses** manifests, in the acute scenario, with extreme pain over the lateral flank superior to the lateral iliac crest. The gait is such that the patient cannot stand erect, but has a mild to moderate twist and lists to the side affected. A palpable defect often is noted

*ITB = iliotibial band.

TEACHING POINTS

LATERAL HIP AND PELVIS

1. Pain at the lateral head of the femur: most commonly greater trochanteric bursitis.
2. Greater trochanteric bursa: one of the largest bursa in the body and a common site for problems.
3. Sciatica: manifests with posterior or lateral thigh and leg.
4. Branches of the sciatic nerve: the tibial (sensory: plantar foot) and the peroneal (sensory: dorsal foot).
5. Iliotibial band syndrome: lateral thigh pain and lateral knee pain to Gerdy's tubercle of the lateral tibia.

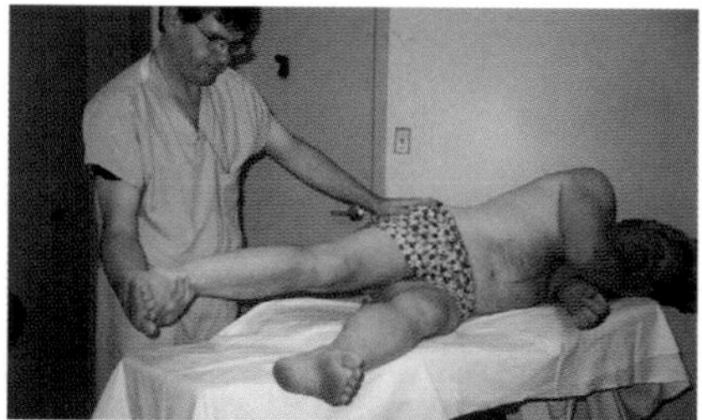

A

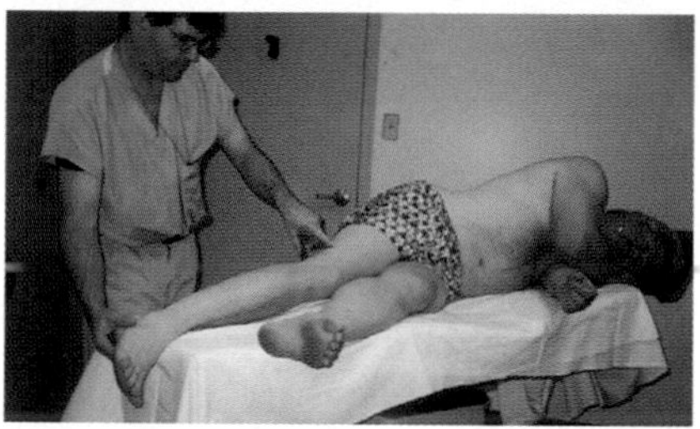

B

Figure 12.24.

Technique for Ober's maneuver useful to assess for tightness in the iliotibial band.

TIPS

- Patient in decubital position, asymptomatic side down
- Leg down is forward flexed at hip and knee
- Leg up is straight at hip and passively flexed at knee
- Passively backward flex the upper leg and then adduct it to attempt to place the leg onto the tabletop
- Normal: able to move leg without pain or stiffness
- Iliotibial band syndrome: pain and stiffness in lateral thigh

in the lateral aponeurosis often with a hernia. This "sausage and spindlelike prominence" is in the lateral aspect of the obliquus internal and external aponeurosis (Malgaigne's sign). The defect or hernia is made more prominent the *active sit-up* test. In this test the patient is supine with hands behind head and the examiner holds the upper anterior thighs in place, then the patient performs an active sit-up so that patient rotates to place the elbow to the other side. This type of tear is caused by a very forceful contraction of the abdominal muscles while the trunk is being rapidly and forcefully pushed to the contralateral side. **Latissimus dorsi strain** manifests with lower and midback discomfort immediately superior to the iliac crest radiating to the ipsilateral shoulder, especially when rotating the trunk, internally rotating and backward flexing the arm, or when performing a sit-up with rotation. This strain is caused by carrying heavy buckets and by bowling. **Gluteal (abductor) muscle strain** manifests with pain and tenderness in the buttock and lateral thigh. The pain often radiates to the greater trochanter and into the lateral knee, as the gluteus maximus and the ITB are usually involved. The pain in the buttock can be reproduced with active hip abduction or active hip backward flexion. Furthermore, a Trendelenburg's sign (Fig. 12.19) is noted, i.e., pelvis tilts upward toward the weight-bearing (symptomatic) side the downward, toward the non–weight-bearing (asymptomatic) side. **Sciatica** and a **hip pointer** also manifest with lateral thigh pain.

POSTERIOR HIP, PELVIS, AND BACK

Hamstring (semimembranous) strain manifests with pain from the groin into the medial knee, specifically on the proximal medial tibia, and with an inability to walk on the affected lower extremity. This is reproduced with FABER maneuver (Fig. 12.19).

In the acute setting, the swelling and ecchymosis are noted in the affected muscles. Pain is reproduced with the **hamstring squeeze sign**, in which the examiner gently palpates or squeezes the semimembranous muscle 10 cm proximal to the knee. In addition, pain and tightness are elicited in the hamstrings with the Wallace stretch test **(Fig. 12.25)**, in which, with the

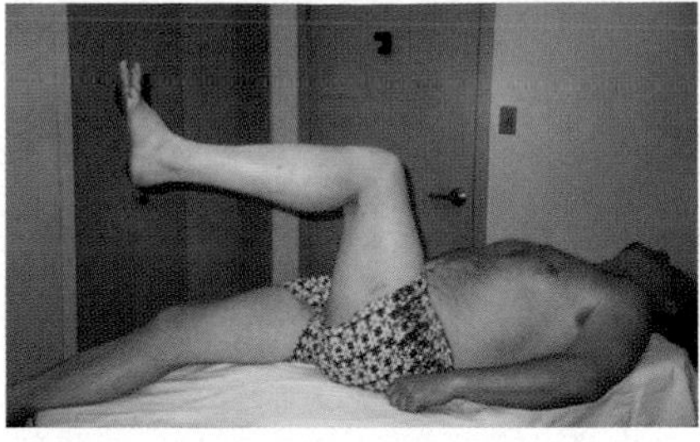

A

B

Figure 12.25.

Technique for Wallace stretch test, an excellent stress test for the assessment of a semimembranosus strain. **A**. Baseline position, **B**. Stretch component.

TIPS

- Patient supine
- Actively forward flex the leg at hip and at knee both to 90 degrees and keep at baseline **(A)**
- Patient actively extends leg at knee **(B)**
- Normal: able to fully extend leg
- Hamstring strain or tightness: unable to extend the leg, degree of tightness measured by angle

patient supine, actively flexes the knee and hip to 90 degrees and maintains that position, then the patient actively extends the leg at the knee. Also, pain is elicited in the hamstrings with the doormat sign of Pecina **(Fig. 12.26)**, in which the patient stands and is instructed to use the leg and foot on the symptomatic side to perform an action akin to wiping the foot on floor or doormat.

Snapping hip manifests with a recurrent, audible, painless snap in the posterior medial hip. This occurs when the patient actively internally rotates and actively adducts the hip. This snap is due to the iliopsoas tendon snapping over the medial hip. A similar snap may occur over the lateral hip with active external rotation or abduction of hip. This snap is caused by the ITB or

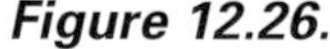

Figure 12.26.

Technique for doormat sign of Pecina. Useful as a confirmatory test for a pulled hamstring specifically, i.e., strain of the semimembranosus muscle.

TIPS

- Patient standing
- Instruct patient to use the leg or foot on symptomatic side to perform action akin to wiping foot on floor or door mat
- Hamstring strain: pain in the medial thigh, especially at the ischial tuberosity

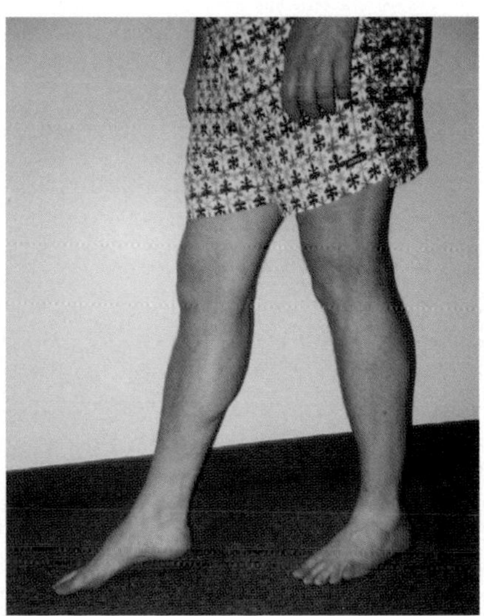

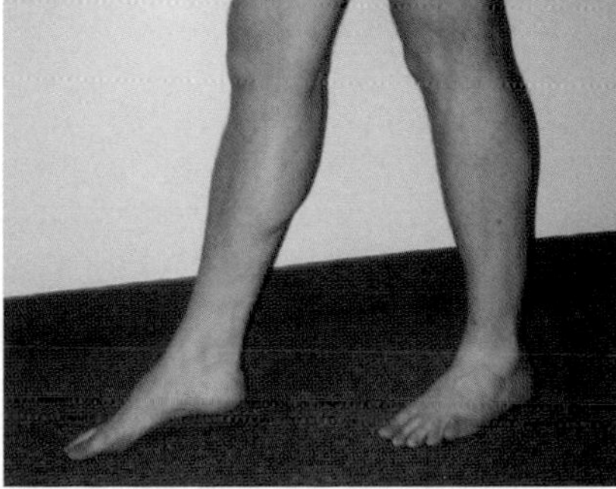

A

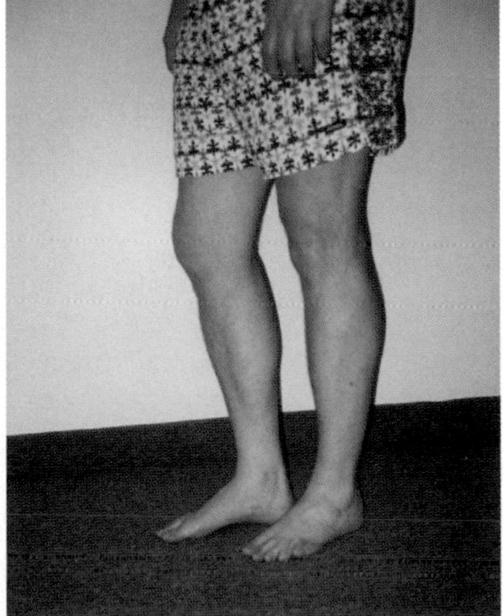

B

the tendon of the gluteus maximus slipping over the greater trochanter, either of which will potentially snap over the lateral aspect of the hip. This is most commonly found in bicyclists. **Ischiogluteal bursitis** manifests with pain in the midbuttock, at the ischial tuberosity, that radiates into the posterior thigh and the hamstring to the medial knee. This is reproduced with a FABER maneuver. The precipitating or exacerbating features include sitting on flat hard surfaces, e.g., a bench or pew, for extended periods without proper padding. Often, concurrent sciatica is present because the sciatic nerve runs adjacent to this bursa. **Gluteus medius strain** manifests with pain in the buttocks that radiates to, but not beyond, the greater trochanter. This is reproduced by the FABER (Fig. 12.19) maneuver. In addition, the pain increases with active abduction or passive adduction of the hip. This strain is caused by overuse and recurrent over backward flexion of the hip, e.g., in cross-country skiing. **Contusion of the sacrum or coccyx** manifests with marked tenderness in the gluteal cleft. On digital rectal examination, severe tenderness is noted in posterior aspect of rectum. Such a contusion is caused by a direct blow to the medial buttocks as the result of a fall, usually on ice. A complication of a coccygeal contusion is **coccydynia**, the severe, chronic, even intractable, posterior pain syndrome in the gluteal cleft. **Spina bifida occulta** manifests with a pigmented patch of hair in the midline of the posterior back. A palpable boney defect is noted in the L5 or S1 spinous process posteriorly. There is no other company in cases of spina bifida occulta; however, if a palpable mass is present overlying the area in a young child, the spina bifida is no longer benign, as this is likely a myelomeningocele. **Compression fracture** of a vertebra manifests with severe, if not excruciating, pain radiating into both sides in a radicular or dermatomal fashion. Pain is reproduced on percussion over the affected spinous process. The company it keeps is a "straight as a poker gait" and a marked decrease ROM of the trunk. If the compression fracture involves the L4 root, pain is in the bilateral anterior thigh; if the compression fracture involves the L5 or S1, bilateral sciatica is noted. **Ankylosing spondylitis, gluteal compartment syndrome, paraspinous muscle strain**, and **unilateral sciatica** are described in detail in the Low Back section.

TEACHING POINTS

POSTERIOR HIP AND PELVIS

1. Significant overlap exists between hip pain and low back pain, especially sciatica, ankylosing spondylitis, and paraspinous strain.
2. Direct trauma to the buttock: can result in coccyx fracture, ischiogluteal bursitis, or a gluteal compartment syndrome.
3. Sciatica: can be caused by a herniated disc, piriformis syndrome, gluteal muscle strain, gluteal compartment syndrome, ischiogluteal bursitis, or herpes zoster.
4. Coccyx fracture: can lead to coccydynia, a chronic pain syndrome of the coccyx.
5. Spina bifida occulta: pigmented patch overlying a palpable defect in spinous processes; may be present undiagnosed into adulthood.
6. Ischiogluteal bursitis: bilateral, usually from sitting on hard surface.

HIP FRACTURES

There are three sites of hip fracture: femoral shaft, the intertrochanteric fracture, and the femoral neck. The femoral neck fracture is also called a femoral intertrochanteric fracture **(Fig. 12.27)**. Either of these fractures manifests with a painful, trauma-related inability to walk or bear any weight on the affected extremity. In addition, either can have an absent note of percussion on auscultation of the pubis while concurrently tapping on the patella (Auenbrugger's sign), Colwill found a sensitivity of 84% and a specificity of 100% for this sign **(Table 12.8)**, and a Grey Turner sign because blood from the fracture often extravasates into the flank subcutaneous tissues. A **femoral shaft** fracture manifests with a leg that is shortened; a **femoral intertrochanteric fracture** manifests with a leg that is shortened and externally rotated. Finally, the clinician must perform and teach students to always assess the patient for concurrent low back, pelvis, and lower extremity fractures, assess the general neurovascular status of the patient and the lower extremities specifically.

Table 12.8. Evidence for Auscultatory Percussion

Diagnosis	Procedure/paper	Sensitivity (%)	Specificity (%)	PPV/NPV (%)
Femur fracture	*Auscultatory percussion*			
	Colwill and Berg	84	100	100/89

PPV = positive predictive value; NPV = negative predictive value.

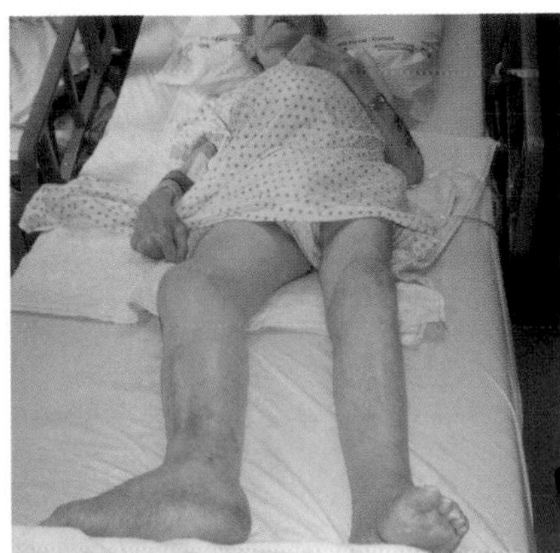

A

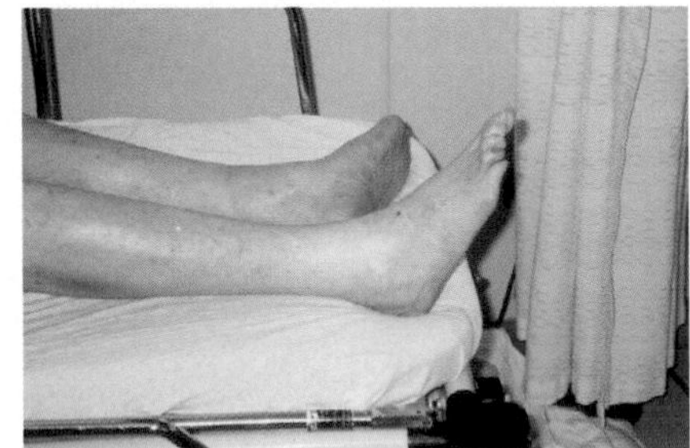

B

Figure 12.27.

Classic intertrochanteric fracture on the left. Note the shortened and externally rotated leg on this individual. **A.** Front view. **B.** Side view.

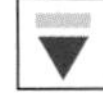

TIPS

- Patient supine, not bearing weight
- Note length of legs, especially the placement of the calcaneus and if foot rotated
- Femoral shaft fracture: leg shortened
- Femoral neck fracture: leg externally rotated and shortened

TEACHING POINTS

HIP FRACTURES

1. Need to assess and document the function of the nerves and vascular system at the time of presentation; also, perform examination with the patient not bearing weight, i.e., supine.
2. Genitourinary complications: not uncommon in pelvic fractures.
3. Intertrochanteric fractures: common, leg shortened and externally rotated.
4. Auenbrugger's sign of auscultatory percussion: good sensitivity and specificity in diagnosing a fracture of the femur. This may be of some use to an ER or primary care physician. Does not replace radiographic imaging.

Annotated Bibliography

Overall

Colwill JC, Berg EH. Auscultation as an important aid to the diagnosis of fractures. *Surgery Gynecology and Obstetrics* 1958;106:713.
In virtually every fracture of a long bone, except impaction fracture of the femur head, the test is excellent. Sensitivity of 84% and a specificity of 100% and a positive predictive value of 100%; negative predictive value of 89%.

Larsson LG, Baum J. The syndromes of bursitis. *Bull Rheum Dis* 1985;36(10):1.
Describes various bursitis syndromes, including ischiogluteal, iliopsoas, and greater trochanter bursitis.

Peltier LF. The diagnosis of fractures of the hip and femur by ausculatory percussion. *Clin Orthop* 1977;123:9–11.
A solid paper detailing the methods involved in bedside diagnosis of hip fractures.

Low Back Pain: Sciatica

Alvarez JA, Hardy RH. Lumbar spine stenosis: a common cause of back and leg pain. *Am Fam Phys* 1998;57(8):1825–1834.
Overview of stenosis of the lumbar spine, including discussion of causes such as epidural disease. Good to very good review of pathoanatomy and history features, including a discussion of claudication versus neuroclaudication. Physical examination discussion is adequate, but not robust; therapeutic interventions are deftly described.

Deyo RA, Loeser JD, Bigos SJ. Herniated lumbar intervertebral disk. *Ann Intern Med* 1990; 112:598–603.
Very good review of an important topic. Some discussion of the physical examination, but a much more robust discussion of diagnostic imaging and therapeutic interventions, including traction and surgery for herniated disc.

Deyo RA, Rainville J, Kent DL. What can the history and physical examination tell us about low back pain? *JAMA* 1992;268(6):760–765.
Excellent review by perhaps the foremost expert on low back pain, Dr. Deyo. Discusses the epidemiology, differential diagnosis, history, and physical examination in the approach to this very common problem. Extremely useful information in terms of historical queries and physical examination techniques, including sensitivities and specificities for each. Emphasizes neurologic examination techniques and the straight leg raise. Reports the following signs to evaluate lumbar disc herniation or sciatica: ipsilateral straight leg raise (SLR), sensitivity, 80%; specificity, 40%; crossed SLR, sensitivity, 25%; specificity, 90%; weakness to ankle dorsiflexion, sensitivity, 35%; specificity, 70%; great toe extension, sensitivity, 50%; specificity, 70%; diminished Achilles' reflex, sensitivity, 50%; specificity, 60%; sensory loss, sensitivity, 50%; specificity, 50%. A valuable paper to read and study.

Frymoyer JW. Back pain and sciatica. *N Engl J Med* 1988;318(5):291–300.
A review of low back pain and sciatica; minimal discussion of history and physical examination, but good differential diagnosis. Good, although dated, therapeutic interventions for this problem.

Hakelius A, Hindmarsh J. The comparative reliability of preoperative diagnostic methods in lumbar disc surgery. *Acta Orthop Scand* 1972;43:234–238.
Nice review of some of the neurologic and stress tests, including the straight leg raise to assess a patient with low back pain looking for sciatica.

Hudgins RW. The crossed straight leg raising test: a diagnostic sign of herniated disc. *Journal of Occupational Medicine* 1979;21:407–408.
Brief overview of this variant of the straight leg raise. Positive predictive value for sciatica, 64% for the straight leg raise, 97% for the crossed straight leg raise.

Mixter WJ, Barr JS. Rupture of the intervertebral disc with involvement of the spinal cord. *N Engl J Med* 1934;211:210.
One of the first descriptions of this now so well-known and recognized cause of low back pain.

Ober FR. Back strain and sciatica. *JAMA* 1935;104:1580.
A great paper in which iliotibial band (ITB) tightness or contracture is described as a cause of significant low back pain. Describes several physical examination techniques to define this cause of low back and hip pain. ITB syndrome tightness was common in his practice as a part of postpoliomyelitis syndrome. Also describes snapping hip in which the causes the snap, and his Ober sign.

Ober FR. The role of the iliotibial band and fascia lata as a factor in the causation of low back disabilities and sciatica. *J Bone Joint Surg* 1935;18:105.
The first description of the iliotibial band being a potential cause of low back pain.

Pecina M. Contribution to the etiological explanation of the piriformis syndrome. *Acta Anat (Basel)* 1979;105:181–187.
Description and physical examination of this relatively uncommon cause of sciatica.

Pecina, M. Tunnel Syndromes, CRC Press, Boca Raton, 1997.
Excellent reference.

Spangfort EV. The lumbar disc herniation: a computer-aided analysis of 2504 operations. *Acta Orthop Scand Suppl* 1972:142:5–95.

Emphasizes the neurologic examination because 95% of lumbar disc herniations occur at levels L4/L5 interspace or L5, S1, thus focus should be on L5 and S1 and a neurologic examination must be performed. The sensitivity for crossed straight leg raise is 25%; the specificity for crossed straight leg raise is 88%.

Van den Hoogen HJ, Koes BW, Deville W, et al. The interobserver reproducibility of Lasegue's sign in patients with low back pain in general practice. *Br J Gen Pract* 1992;46(413):727–730.

Fifteen general practitioners from the Netherlands performed Lasegue's test on patients who presented with low back pain; 50 consecutive patients in which Lasegue's was performed were reexamined within 2 weeks by another clinician. The kappa coefficient for reproducibility was 0.33; the positive agreement was 33% and the negative agreement was 96%.

Wheeler AH. Diagnosis and management of low back pain and sciatica. *Am Fam Phys* 1995;52(5):1333–1341.

Nice overview of low back pain, with a discussion of evaluation and management. Minimal discussion on history and physical examination, but a nice discussion of the imaging techniques and the nonsurgical and surgical options available in the management of this disorder. Interesting algorithms for evaluation and management.

L4: Radiculopathy

Aids to the examination of the peripheral nervous system, 4th Ed, WB Saunders, Edinburgh, 2000.

The masterpiece!

Dyck P. The femoral nerve traction test with lumbar disc protrusions. *Surg Neurol* 1976; 6:163–166.

Describes a specific test to stress the L4 root and thus, differentiate it from other sites of entrapment problems.

Medial: Pulled Hamstring

Pecina M, Bojanic I. Overuse injuries in track and field athletes. Croat. *Sports Med* 1991; 6:24–37.

Describes the "door mat" sign for hamstring assessment. Hamstring injuries can manifest with gluteal pain and even sciatica.

Medial: Adductors

Durey A, Boeda A, Merville L, et al. *Medicine du Football.* Paris: Masson, 1978.

Excellent review of soccer-related groin syndromes, emphasizing the overlap between the abdominus rectus and the adductor muscle problems. Physical examination techniques are nicely described.

Martens MA, Hansen L, Mulier JC. Adductor tendonitis and muscles rectus abdominis tendonopathy. *Am J Sports Med* 1987;15:353–356.

Nice review of groin syndromes, emphasizing that overlap exists between adductor and abdominus rectus problems; emphasis is on athletes, specifically soccer players.

Medial Hip: Degenerative Joint Disease

Johnston RC, Fitzgerald RH, Harris WH, et al. Clinical and radiographic evaluation of total hip replacement. A standard system of terminology for reporting results. *J Bone Joint Surg* 1990;72A:161.

Describes the physical examination features of severe hip degenerative joint disease, including Trendelenburg's sign and other features that make the examination more complete and reproducible.

Khabie V, Sidor ML, Zuckerman JD. The painful hip: narrowing the differential diagnosis. *Hosp Med* 1996;(Jan):13–22.

Nice descriptive paper on the evaluation of hip pain, with emphasis on history, physical examination, and imaging techniques for common causes of hip pain; greatest information regarding degenerative joint disease of hip, rheumatoid arthritis, and avascular necrosis of the hip. Trendelenburg's maneuver is described and demonstrated in the paper.

Lateral Hip

Larsen E, Johansen J. Snapping hip. *Acta Orthop Scand* 1986;57:168–170.

Brief description of this common, usually painless, syndrome.

Anterior: Meralgia Paresthetica

Bernhardt M. Uber isolirt im gebiete des n. cutaneous femoris externus vorkommende parasthesian. *Neurol Zentralbl* 1895;14:242–244.

First description of this syndrome.

Boyce JR. Meralgia paresthetica and tight trousers [Letter]. *JAMA* 1984;12:1553.

A description of this syndrome that is aptly called, "Tight fittin' jeans syndrome."

Deal CL, Canoso JJ. Meralgia paresthetica and large abdomens [Letter]. *Ann Intern Med* 1982;96(6Pt 1):787–788.

Another risk for this entrapment neuropathy.

Roth WK. *Meralgia Paresthetica.* Berlin: S. Karger, 1985.

Coined the term.

Streiffer RH. Meralgia paresthetica. *Am Fam Phys* 1986;33(3):141–144.

Terse, but satisfactory, overview of the pathoanatomy, history, and physical examination of this often overlooked, yet common entrapment neuropathy.

Low Back Pain: Ankylosing Spondylitis

Calin A, Porta J, Fries JF, et al. Clinical history as a screening test for ankylosing spondylitis. *JAMA* 1977;237:2613–2614.

Wonderful paper. Five specific questions developed to screen for ankylosing spondylitis: (1) >3 months of symptoms; (2) morning stiffness; (3) pain before age 40; (4) insidious onset; and (5) discomfort alleviated by exercise. A yes to four of five of the queries has a sensitivity of 95% and specificity of 85%.

Schober P. Leudenvirbelsule und krezchmerzen. *Munchener Med Wochenschr* 1937;84: 336–338.

The classic paper describing this simple, yet profoundly elegant, test.

Schuchmann JA, Cannon CL. Sacroiliac strain syndrome: diagnosis and treatment. *Texas Med* 1986:82(6):33–36.

Overview of the test for low back pain, specifically in the sacroiliac joint. Reported sensitivities of various signs on 19 patients, including FABER: sensitivity, 68%; direct palpation over the sacroiliac joints: sensitivity, 100% (19/19). Nice emphasis on specific physical examination techniques for diagnosis of this relatively uncommon entity. We extrapolate this to other sacroiliac disorders (e.g., sacroiliitis).

13

Foot and Ankle Examination

PRACTICE AND TEACHING

SURFACE ANATOMY

Plantar (Fig. 13.1)

The **calcaneus or heel**, the major bony prominence of the posterior aspect of the foot, is a major site of weightbearing. The medial tubercle of the calcaneus is the origin of the **abductor hallucis muscle**, the **flexor digitorum brevis muscle**, and the **plantar fascia**. The **precalcaneal bursa** is immediately anterior (distal) to the calcaneus. The tendons that run on the plantar surface are the **toe flexors**, including the **flexor digitorum longus**, which originates on the posterior proximal tibia, runs posterior to the medial malleolus, and inserts on the plantar side of toes 2, 3, 4, and 5 via a common tendon sheath; and the **flexor hallucis longus**, which originates on the posterior midfibula, runs posterior to the medial malleolus, and inserts on the plantar aspect of the great

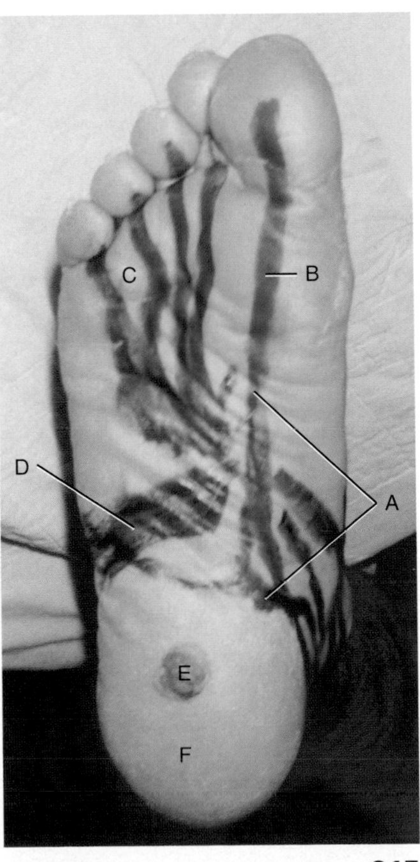

Figure 13.1.

Plantar foot surface anatomy. **A.** Flexor hallucis longus tendon. **B.** Sesamoid bones on plantar hallux. **C.** Flexor digitorum longus tendons. **D.** Peroneus longus tendon. **E.** Precalcaneal bursa. **F.** Calcaneus.

 **TIPS**

- Calcaneus: major weightbearing site of body and foot
- Plantar fascia: originates on the medial calcaneus
- Precalcaneal bursa: immediately distal to calcaneus
- Flexor hallucis brevis: a great toe flexor with two sesamoid bones
- Flexor longus muscles: originate in the posterior leg compartment, toe flexors
- Plantar foot and posterior leg compartment are closely related
- Midaxis of foot: runs through the apex of the arch, middle cuneiform, midline of the second metatarsal and the second toe
- Plantar foot: posterior tibial artery and tibialis nerve.

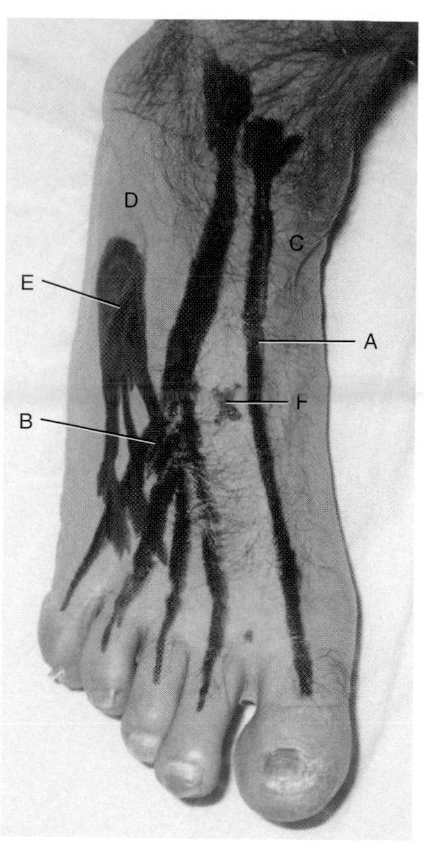

Figure 13.2.

Dorsal foot surface anatomy. **A.** Extensor hallucis longus tendon. **B.** Extensor digitorum longus tendons. **C.** Medial malleolus. **D.** Lateral malleolus. **E.** Extensor digitorum brevis. **F.** Dorsalis pedis pulse site.

TIPS

- Tibialis anterior: most medial, ankle dorsiflexor
- Extensor hallucis longus: middle, great toe extensor
- Extensor digitorum longus: most lateral extensor of toes
- Extensor digitorum brevis: a ball of muscle on the lateral dorsum
- Midaxis of foot: middle of middle cuneiform, second metatarsal, second toe
- Dorsal pedis artery: a branch of popliteal that runs from the anterior leg compartment
- Dorsal foot and anterior leg compartment are closely related
- Dorsal foot: deep peroneal nerve, dorsalis pedis artery

toe. Finally, the **flexor digitorum brevis** originates on the anterior aspect of the calcaneus and runs deep to the plantar fascia to insert on the plantar aspects of the middle phalanges of digits 2, 3, 4, and 5. The **tibialis nerve** innervates each of these flexor muscles. The tibialis nerve branches into the **medial** and **lateral plantar branches** immediately distal to the calcaneus.

Lisfranc's joint is structurally firm, almost rigid, between the metatarsal bases and the distal tarsal bones. It is the foundation of the foot and the key for the longitudinal and transverse foot arches. Anterior (distal) to Lisfranc's joint are the metatarsal bones, the metatarsophalangeal (MTP) joints, and the phalanges of the toes. The tendon of **flexor hallucis brevis** runs over the plantar first MTP. It originates on the plantar midfoot, inserts on the plantar first phalanx, and acts to flex the great toe; its nerve is the medial plantar branch of the tibialis nerve. Two discrete sesamoid bones are located within the substance of this tendon. The **metatarsal heads** of toes 1 through 5 are normal sites of weightbearing while standing or walking. The **peroneus longus** originates in the lateral leg compartment, wraps posterior to the lateral malleolus to cross the plantar foot, inserts on the plantar lateral base of metatarsal 1, and acts to evert the foot; its nerve is the superficial peroneal nerve.

The **midaxis of the foot** runs through the apex of the arch, from the second metatarsal base to the middle cuneiform, down the center of the second metatarsal to the center of the second toe. Adduction and abduction of the toes are defined by this axis. The pyramidal-shaped area on the plantar medial midfoot is formed by the longitudinal and transverse arches.

Dorsal (Fig. 13.2)

The navicular bone is the most medial structure of the foot. It can have a bony protuberance on it, the accessory navicular which can be a potential site of foot problems. The **tibialis anterior muscle** originates in the anterior compartment, inserts on the dorsal bases of metatarsals 2, 3, and 4, and acts in foot dorsiflexion. The **extensor hallucis longus** originates on the medial fibula and inserts on the dorsum of the distal phalanx of the great toe; and the **extensor digitorum longus** originates on the proximal anterior lateral tibia and inserts on the dorsum of middle and distal phalanges of digits 2 through 5; both muscles act in toe extension. The **deep peroneal nerve** innervates all of these muscles. In the group of these three anterior compartment muscles, the tibialis anterior is most medial, the extensor hallucis longus is in the middle, and the extensor digitorum longus is most lateral. **Extensor digitorum brevis** originates on the dorsal foot, specifically the talus and proximal cuboid; it is a ball of muscle on the dorsolateral foot that inserts on the dorsum bases of the proximal phalanges of toes 1 through 4, and acts in toe extension; its nerve is deep peroneal. Note the **phalanges** of the great toe and the four other toes. The **dorsalis pedis artery** is palpable several centimeters proximal to the web space between the first and second toe; this branch of the popliteal artery runs from the anterior compartment.

Medial (Fig. 13.3)

The **deltoid ligament** is a tough triangular-shaped ligament that attaches the medial malleolus of tibia to the tarsal bones. This structure maintains medial ankle stability. The **flexor retinaculum**, a broad band of superficial connective tissue, runs from the medial malleolus to the medial calcaneus. The structures that pass deep to it include, in order, the **tibialis posterior**, which originates on the midproximal posterior fibula, inserts on the dorsal bases of toes 2, 3, and 4, and acts as a foot invertor; the **flexor digitorum longus**, which originates on the posterior proximal tibia, inserts on the plantar aspect of phalanges 2 through 5, and acts as a toe flexor; the nerve is the tibialis. The **posterior tibial**

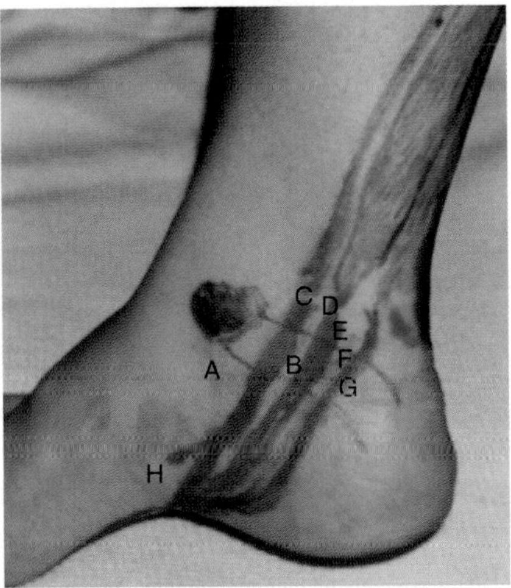

Figure 13.3.

Surface anatomy: medial foot and ankle **A.** Deltoid ligament. **B.** Flexor retinaculum. **C.** Tibialis posterior. **D.** Flexor digitorum longus. **E.** Posterior tibialis artery. **F.** Tibialis nerve. **G.** Flexor hallucis longus. **H.** Navicular bone.

TIPS

- Deltoid ligament: maintains medial stability
- Flexor retinaculum: forms roof of tarsal tunnel, extends from medial malleolus to calcaneus
- Beneath the flexor retinaculum run, listed anterior to posterior are: tibialis posterior tendon, flexor digitorum longus tendon, posterior tibial artery, tibial nerve, and flexor hallucis longus tendon
- Tarsal tunnel: a site of potential entrapment of the tibialis nerve
- Note site of navicular bone, often a site of medial foot pain

artery, which supplies blood to the plantar foot, is a significant medium-sized artery. The **tibialis nerve** innervates all of the muscles of the posterior compartment, the toe flexors, the ankle plantar flexors, and sensation to the entire plantar foot. The **flexor hallucis longus** originates on the posterior midproximal fibula, inserts on the plantar great toe distal phalanx, and acts as a great toe flexor; its nerve is the tibialis. The **tarsal tunnel** is the site through which the tibialis nerve enters the plantar foot beneath the flexor retinaculum to innervate the skin of the plantar aspect of the foot and the intrinsic toe muscles.

Lateral (Fig. 13.4)

The lateral malleolus, i.e., the distal fibula, is smaller and more posterior relative to the medial malleolus. It is attached to the tarsal bones by the three ligaments: **anterior fibulotalar (AFT)**, which runs between anterior lateral malleolus and the neck of the talus; **inferior calcaneofibular (ICF)**, which runs between the lateral malleolus and the lateral calcaneus; and **posterior talofibular (PCF)**, which runs between the posterior fibula and the posterior rim of the talus. This ligament is very deep and never palpable for it is directed in an axis that is medial-lateral, i.e., perpendicular to the other plane of the other two. These ligaments are very tough and maintain lateral stability of the ankle, i.e., they prevent the ankle from rolling laterally (prevents supination). The AFT runs in an anterior-posterior axis, the ICF runs in a superior-inferior axis, and the PTF runs in a medial-lateral axis. The **peroneus longus muscle** originates on the lateral proximal fibula and inserts on the plantar lateral base of the first metatarsal. The **peroneus brevis muscle** originates on the midlateral

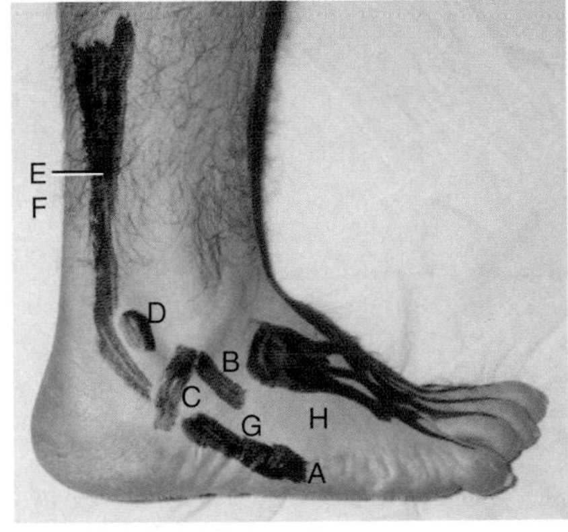

Figure 13.4.

Surface anatomy of lateral foot and ankle. **A.** Base of fifth metatarsal, site of peroneus brevis insertion. **B.** Anterior fibulotalar ligament. **C.** Inferior calcaneofibular ligament. **D.** Posterior talofibular ligament. **E.** Peroneus brevis muscle and tendon. **F.** Peroneus longus muscle and tendon. **G.** Talus. **H.** Cuboid.

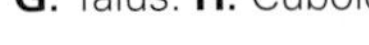

TIPS

- Structures proximal to distal: the lateral calcaneus, talus, cuboid, peroneus longus tendon, fifth metatarsal, and the three phalanges of the fifth toe
- Anterior fibulotalar ligament (AFT): anterior lateral malleolus to the neck of the talus; runs in anterior-posterior axis
- Inferior calcaneofibular ligament (ICF): runs inferior-superior axis
- Posterior talofibular (PTF) ligament: runs from the posterior fibula to the posterior rim of the talus in the medial-lateral axis, i.e., perpendicular to the plane of the ICF and AFT
- Peroneus brevis: inserts on lateral base of the fifth metatarsal; thus a sprain of this can look like a lateral ankle sprain, only posterior to lateral malleolus

Table 13.1. Structures in the Posterior Leg Compartment

Muscle	Nerve	Origin	Insertion
Gastrocnemius	Tibial	Posterior proximal tibia	Calcaneus
Soleus	Tibial	Posterior tibia	Calcaneus
Flexor digitorum longus	Tibial	Posterior proximal tibia	Toes 2–5
Flexor hallucis longus	Tibial	Posterior proximal fibula	Toe 1
Tibialis posterior	Tibial	Posterior proximal fibula	Plantar aspect Toes 2, 3, 4

fibula and inserts on lateral base of fifth metatarsal. Both have a tendon, each of which runs behind the lateral malleolus and acts in foot eversion; the nerve for both muscles is the superficial peroneus.

Posterior Leg

The **posterior leg** structures include the **calcaneus bone** and the **gastrocnemius** muscle, which originates on proximal tibia, inserts on calcaneus via the Achilles tendon, and acts in foot plantarflexion; the **soleus** muscle originates on the proximal tibia, inserts on the proximal calcaneus, and acts in foot plantarflexion (**Table 13.1**). Deep to the foot plantar flexors are the toe flexors. The **flexor digitorum longus** originates on the posterior proximal tibia, runs posterior to the medial malleolus, and inserts on the plantar side of toes 2, 3, 4, and 5 via a common tendon sheath. The **flexor hallucis longus** originates on the posterior midfibula, runs posterior to medial malleolus, and inserts on plantar aspect of the great toe. The **tibialis nerve** innervates all of these muscles. The **tibialis** posterior artery runs through the posterior compartment to supply the plantar foot. Two bursae, the **retrocalcaneal bursa**, which is between the calcaneus and Achilles tendon, and the **supracalcaneal bursa**, which is between the Achilles tendon and the skin, are located adjacent to the insertion of the gastrocnemius muscle to the calcaneus.

Anterior Leg

The anterior leg consists of the tibia and the anterior and lateral leg compartments. The **anterior compartment** includes the **tibialis anterior**, which originates on the anterior fibula, inserts on the dorsal bases of metatarsal 2, 3, 4, and acts to dorsiflex the foot; its nerve is the deep peroneal (**Table 13.2**). The **extensor digitorum longus** originates on the anterior fibula, inserts on dorsal aspects of

Table 13.2. Anterior Compartment Muscles

Muscle	Nerve	Origin	Insertion
Extensor digitorum longus	Deep peroneal	Anterior tibia	Dorsum toes 2–5
Extensor hallucis longus	Deep peroneal	Anterior tibia	Dorsum toe 1
Tibialis anterior	Deep peroneal	Anterior tibia	Dorsal bases of metatarsals

TEACHING POINTS

SURFACE ANATOMY

1. One must emphasize the leg surface anatomy. It is fundamental to the examination of the foot and ankle.
2. Plantar bony structures are the sites of weightbearing. The normal sites are the calcaneus, the lateral foot, and the heads of the metatarsals.
3. Dorsal foot structures, medial to lateral are: tibialis anterior tendon, extensor hallucis longus tendon, dorsalis pedis artery, and extensor digitorum longus tendon.
4. Lateral foot bones, in order posterior to anterior, are: calcaneus, cuboid, fifth metatarsal, fifth toe.
5. Lateral foot and ankle ligaments: anterior talofibular (straight forward), calcaneal fibular (straight downward), and the posterior talofibular (straight medial) ligaments.
6. Medial foot bones, in order posterior to anterior, are: medial malleolus of tibia, talus, navicular, medial cuneiform, first metatarsal, great toe.
7. Structures that pass beneath the flexor retinaculum: tibialis posterior tendon, flexor digitorum longus tendon, tibialis posterior artery, tibialis posterior nerve, flexor hallucis longus tendon.
8. Deltoid ligament: broad, triangular-shaped tough ligament from medial malleolus to talus that prevents abnormal foot eversion.
9. Anterior leg compartment: tibialis anterior muscle, extensor digitorum longus muscle, extensor hallucis longus muscle, deep peroneal nerve, and the dorsalis pedis artery.
10. Lateral leg compartment: peroneus brevis muscle, peroneus longus muscle, and superficial peroneal nerve.
11. Posterior leg compartment: gastrocnemius muscle, Achilles tendon, soleus muscle, flexor digitorum longus, flexor hallucis longus, retrocalcaneal bursa, supracalcaneal bursa, and the tibialis nerve.

toes 2, 3, 4, and 5, and acts in toe extension; its nerve is the deep peroneal. The **extensor hallucis** longus originates on the anterior fibula, inserts on the dorsum of first toe, and acts in great toe extension. The deep peroneal nerve innervates these three anterior compartment muscles. The **lateral compartment** consists of the **peroneus longus**, which originates on the lateral proximal fibula and inserts on the plantar lateral base of the first metatarsal; and the **peroneus brevis**, which originates on the midlateral fibula and inserts on the lateral base of the fifth metatarsal **(Table 13.3)**. Both run immediately posterior to the lateral malleolus and act to evert the foot; their nerve is the superficial peroneal.

Table 13.3. Lateral Compartment Muscles

Muscle	Nerve	Origin	Insertion
Peroneus longus	Superficial peroneal	Midfibula	Base of first metatarsal plantar
Peroneus brevis	Superficial peroneal	Midfibula	Base of fifth metatarsal

NEUROLOGIC EXAMINATION OF FOOT

The neurologic examination of the toes, feet, and ankles is of great importance to the overall examination. The function of the three major nerves of the area the tibialis, deep peroneal, and superficial peroneal are described in **Table 13.4**. The **tibialis nerve** is a branch of the sciatic and is best assessed by active plantarflexion of the foot against resistance, active great toe flexion against resistance, and sensation to the plantar aspect of the foot. Deficits are caused by mischief involving the sciatic nerve or S1 nerve root; or by tibialis nerve damage from an unstable knee, tarsal tunnel syndrome, or posterior compartment syndrome. The **superficial peroneal nerve** is a branch of the common peroneal nerve, which is a branch of the sciatic nerve. This is best assessed by active eversion of the foot against resistance and sensation to the lateral malleolus. Deficits are caused by mischief involving the sciatic nerve or L5 nerve root or fibular head and neck, or by lateral compartment syndrome. The **deep peroneal nerve** is a branch of the common peroneal nerve, which is a branch of the sciatic nerve. This is best assessed by active dorsiflexion of the foot against resistance or active great toe flexion against resistance, and sensation to the dorsum of the foot, specifically the web between toes 1 and 2. Deficits are caused by mischief involving the sciatic nerve or L5 nerve root or fibular head and neck, or by anterior compartment syndrome.

RANGE OF MOTION: PASSIVE

Ankle

It is important to know the range of motion (ROM) at the **ankle**, which includes the **tibiotalar** and the **subtalar** joints (**Table 13.5**). This includes

Table 13.4. Neurologic Examination of Foot and Ankle

Nerve	Action	Primary muscle
Tibialis	Plantar flexor tibiotalar joint	Gastrocnemius soleus
Tibialis	Flexion of great toe	Flexor hallucis longus
Tibialis	Flexion of third toe	Flexor digitorum longus
Tibialis	Sensation to plantar foot	
Superficial peroneal	Eversion	Peroneus longus
Superficial peroneal	Eversion	Peroneus brevis
Superficial peroneal	Sensation overlying the lateral malleolus	
Deep peroneal	Great toe extension	Extensor hallucis longus
Deep peroneal	Toe extension	Extensor digitorum longus
Deep peroneal	Foot extension	Tibialis anterior
Deep peroneal	Sensation on dorsal skin between toes 1 and 2	

Table 13.5. Passive Range of Motion

Movement	Baseline position	Normal
Ankle		
Dorsiflexion	Foot neutral	35
Plantarflexion	Foot neutral	45
Eversion	Foot neutral	15
Inversion	Foot neutral	35
Foot and Toes		
MTP flexion	Foot neutral	40
MTP extension	Foot neutral	30
MTP abduction	Foot neutral	5
MTP adduction	Foot neutral	5
PIP flexion	Foot and toes neutral	70
DIP flexion	Foot and toes neutral	30
PIP extension	Foot and toes neutral	0
DIP extension	Foot and toes neutral	5
Hallux		
IP flexion	Neutral	35
IP extension	Neutral	10
MTP flexion	Neutral	20
MTP extension	Neutral	30

DIP = distal interphalangeal (joint); IP = interphalangeal (joint); MTP = metatarsophalangeal (joint); PIP = proximal interphalangeal (joint).

plantarflexion to 35 degrees, dorsiflexion to 30 degrees, external rotation to 20 degrees, and internal rotation to 20 degrees. In addition, assess passive inversion (supination) to 20 degrees and eversion (pronation) to 20 degrees. **Circumduction** of the ankle is to 20 to 25 degrees.

Foot and Toes

Range of motion at the **foot** is minimal. The two major joints are Lisfranc's (between the metatarsal bases and the distal row of tarsals) and Chopart's (between the proximal and distal rows). These joints are rigid and very strong. ROM of **toes**, other than the hallux, includes flexion at the distal interphalangeal (DIP) joint to 30 degrees and at the proximal interphalangeal (PIP) joint to 60 degrees; extension at the DIP to 10 degrees and extension at the PIP to 0 degrees. The **MTP joints** of the toes include flexion to 40 degrees, extension to 30 degrees, and abduction and adduction to 5 degrees. Toe abduction and adduction are best performed with the toes extended. Passively circumduct each of the toes at the MTP joints 10 to 15 degrees.

Hallux

Range of motion at the **great toe** (hallux) should be performed and documented separately from the other toes. These components should include

IP joint flexion to 35 degrees and extension to 10 degrees. At the MTP joint, include flexion to 20 degrees, extension to 30 degrees, and abduction and adduction with the hallux fully extended 5 to 10 degrees. Perform abduction and adduction with the hallux neutral or flexed to 0 degrees.

RANGE OF MOTION: ACTIVE

In **active plantarflexion** of the foot against resistance **(Table 13.6)**, the major muscle is the gastrocnemius and the nerve is the tibialis; in active **great toe flexion** against resistance, the major muscle is the flexor hallucis longus and the nerve is the tibialis. **Active eversion** of the foot against resistance involves the peroneus longus or brevis muscles and the nerve is the superficial peroneal nerve. In **active dorsiflexion** of the foot against resistance, the major muscle is the tibialis anterior and nerve is deep peroneal nerve; in active **great toe extension** against resistance, the major muscle is the extensor hallucis longus, the nerve is the deep peroneal nerve.

TEACHING POINTS

RANGE OF MOTION

1. The metatarsophalangeal (MTP) joint affords each toe some circumduction.
2. Fused in one position, no movement at that joint = contracture.
3. Eversion and inversion (as well as toe adduction and abduction) are relative to the long axis of the foot.
4. Collateral ligaments of toes prevent abnormal abduction or adduction of the proximal interphalangeal (PIP) and distal interphalangeal (DIP) joints.
5. MTP joints of toes and hallux afford some abduction and adduction, especially with extension.
6. No normal movement at Chopart's or Lisfranc's joint.
7. Dorsiflexion or plantar flexion at tibiotalar joint.
8. Internal and external rotation, supination, pronation, inversion, eversion at subtalar joints.
9. Toe flexors and ankle plantar flexors are in the posterior compartment of leg.
10. Ankle dorsiflexors are in the anterior compartment of the leg.
11. Ankle evertors are in the lateral compartment of the leg.
12. Eversion involves a complex of peroneus longus, peroneus brevis, and flexor hallucis longus muscles.
13. Inversion involves a complex of muscles, the tibialis anterior, tibialis posterior, extensor hallucis longus, and flexor digitorum longus muscles.

Table 13.6. Active Range of Motion

Action	Joints	Muscles	Nerve
Ankle			
Plantar flexion	Tibiotalar	Gastrocnemius Soleus	Tibialis Tibialis
Dorsiflexion	Tibiotalar	Tibialis anterior	Deep peroneal
Inversion	Tibiotalar Subtalar joints	Tibialis posterior	Tibialis
Eversion	Tibiotalar	Peroneus longus	Superficial peroneal
	Subtalar joints	Peroneus brevis	Superficial peroneal
Foot and Toes			
MTP toe flexion	DIP, PIP, MTP	Flexor digitorum longus	Tibialis
MTP toe extension	DIP, PIP, MTP	Extensor digitorum longus	Deep peroneal
MTP adduction	MTP	Plantar interosseous	Tibialis
MTP abduction	MTP	Dorsal interosseous	Tibialis
Hallux flexion	MTP, IP	Flexor hallucis longus Flexor hallucis brevis	Tibialis Tibialis
Hallux extension	MTP, IP	Extensor hallucis longus	Deep peroneal

DIP = distal interphalangeal; IP = interphalangeal; MTP = metatarsophalangeal; PIP = proximal interphalangeal.

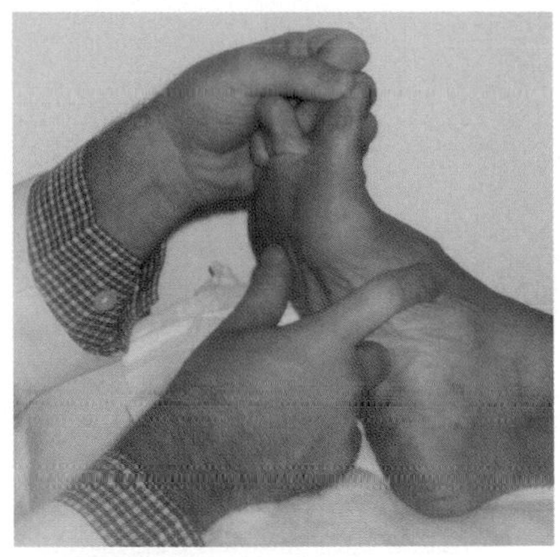

Figure 13.5.

Technique for passive hallux MTP joint extension. This is a good test for flexor hallucis longus tendinitis and plantar fasciitis.

TIPS

- Passively extend the hallux at the MTP
- Flexor hallucis longus tendinitis: increased pain and tenderness over plantar great toe
- Plantar fasciitis: pain and tenderness over the medial anterior calcaneus and midfoot

PLANTAR FOOT

Plantar fasciitis manifests with recurrent discomfort in the medial plantar foot. The discomfort begins immediately distal to the calcaneus, and radiates into the medial plantar foot and into the great toe. The discomfort is reproduced by palpation at that site. Pain is reproduced over the plantar medial foot into the great toe and with passive hallux MTP joint extension **(Fig. 13.5)**. In addition, the patient often has acquired pes planus, i.e., the normal longitudinal arch of the medial foot is flattened **(Fig. 13.6)**. The history often includes a first-step phenomenon, in which the pain is maximal with the first step, then improves with each subsequent step.

Flexor hallucis longus strain manifests with discomfort in the medial foot that extends into the plantar great toe. Pain is increased and reproduced with active great toe flexion against resistance **(Fig. 13.7)** and with passive great toe extension. In addition, the patient may have mild to moderate pes planus. **Sesamoiditis** manifests with significant pain and tenderness on the plantar aspect of the great toe, almost specific to the plantar aspect of the first MTP. Pain and discomfort are increased on bearing weight on the site and with repeated use. Sesamoiditis is caused by a strain of the flexor hallucis brevis and, thus, irritation to the sesamoid bones within, or a direct crush-type injury to, the plantar first MTP of the great toe.

Tarsal tunnel syndrome manifests with tingling and pain in the plantar aspect of the foot. The patient relates that the symptoms worsen with repetitive use. Findings are reproduced on performing Tinel's procedure over the

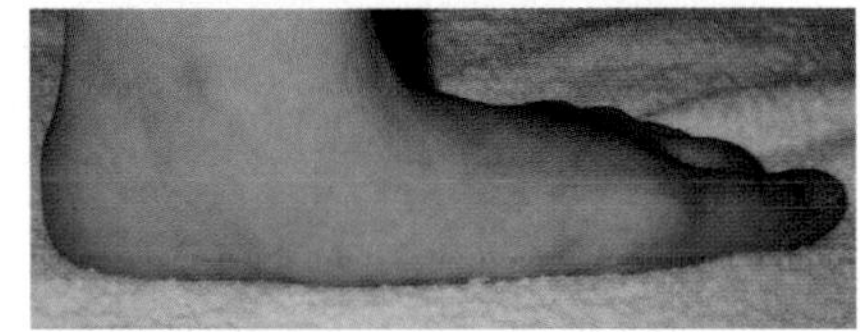

Figure 13.6.

Pes planus. The normal longitudinal arch on medial foot is flattened. May be due to flexor hallucis longus tendinitis, posterior compartment, or plantar fasciitis.

TIPS

- Pes planus: flattened longitudinal and transverse arch of foot, which increases foot pronation
- Increases risk of medial knee mischief

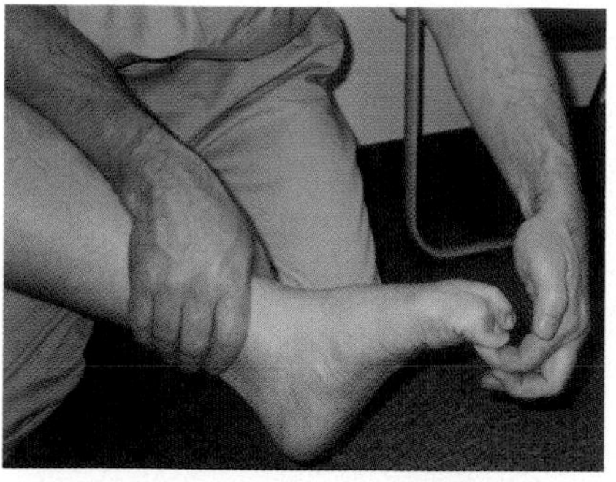

Figure 13.7.

Technique for active great toe flexion. Good test for flexor hallucis longus tendinitis and for sesamoiditis.

TIPS

- Instruct patient to actively flex great toe against resistance, place one finger on plantar aspect of great toe
- Tibialis nerve problem: weakness to flexion
- Flexor hallucis longus tendinitis or sprain: mildly weak flexion with pain in medial plantar foot and posterior compartment

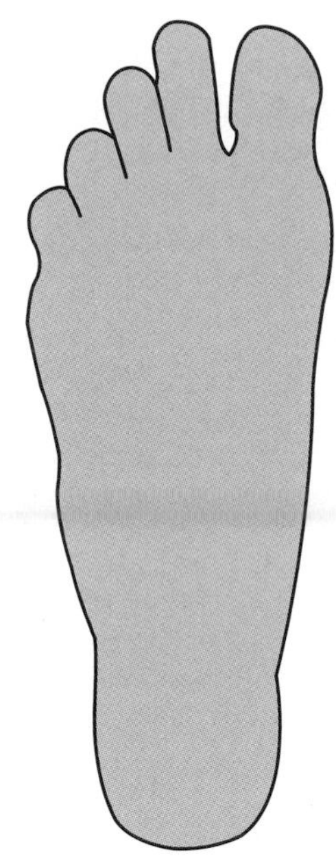

A Tarsal tunnel distribution: Plantar foot, entire surface

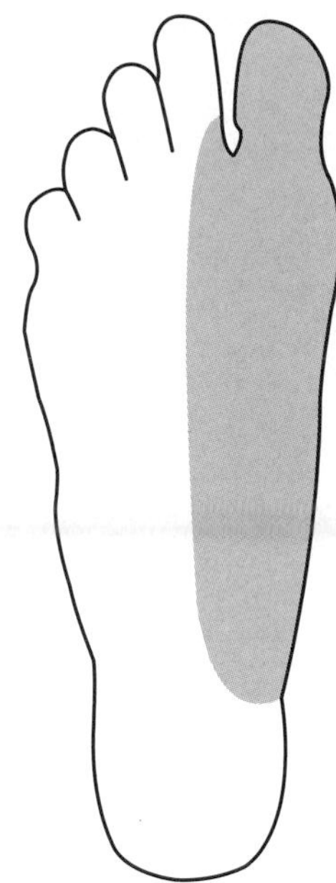

B Jogger's foot: Medial plantar surface, distribution of medial plantar nerve

Figure 13.8.

Distribution of symptoms in tarsal tunnel and jogger's foot. Tarsal tunnel: entire plantar foot involved; jogger's foot: plantar side of great toe involved.

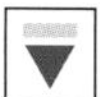

TIPS

- Tarsal tunnel: entire plantar foot involved
- Runner's or jogger's foot: tingling and pain in the medial plantar foot; midfoot and forefoot involved

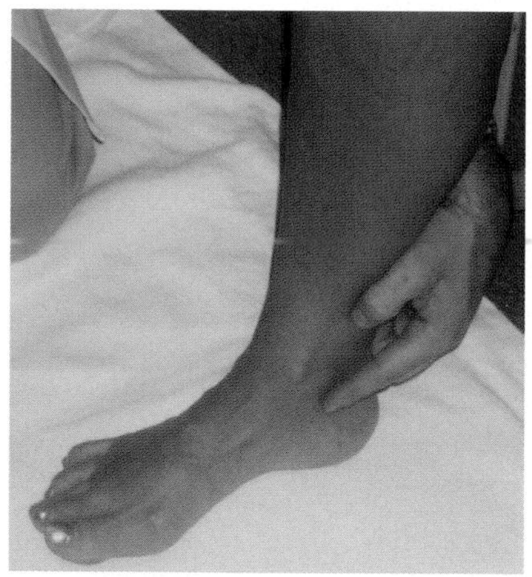

Figure 13.9.

Technique and site of Tinel's sign for tarsal tunnel. Tap with fingertip or plexor over the flexor retinaculum.

TIPS

- Tap reproducibly over the flexor retinaculum immediately posterior to medial malleolus; use finger or a plexor and repeat tap 10 to 12 times
- Tarsal tunnel syndrome: reproduction of tingling, pain, or both on the entire plantar foot
- Jogger's foot: reproduction of pain and tingling on the plantar medial foot

flexor retinaculum immediately posterior to the medial malleolus. If this is severe or long-standing, weakness to, but not an absence of, toe flexion may be noted. In addition, atrophy of the intrinsic muscles of the foot may be present. Normal posterior compartment muscle size and strength to the flexor hallucis longus and gastrocnemius muscles will be noted, however. This syndrome is caused by repetitive use or overuse-type injuries, e.g., ill-fitting shoes. **Runner's or jogger's foot** manifests with tingling and pain specific to the medial plantar foot **(Fig. 13.8)**. This is reproduced or increased on performing Tinel's maneuver over the medial plantar midfoot **(Fig. 13.9)**. The pain increases with repetitive use. Tarsal tunnel syndrome most often is caused by irritation or entrapment of the medial plantar nerve **(Fig. 13.10)**.

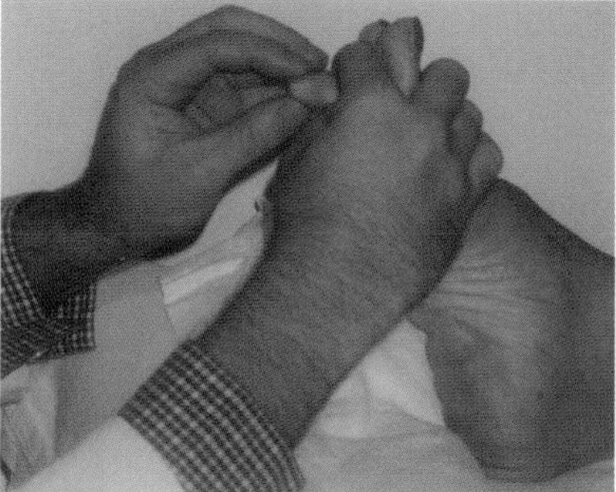

Figure 13.10.

Technique for resisted flexion of toe 3 at the metatarsophalangeal (MTP) joint.

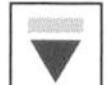

TIPS

- Tarsal tunnel: weak but intact flexion (flexor digitorum longus spared)
- Proximal tibialis nerve problem: very weak or absent toe flexion

Metatarsalgia manifests with pain and tenderness on the plantar aspect of the heads of the metatarsals. Symptoms are reproduced with the forefoot squeeze test (Mulder's maneuver) **(Fig. 13.11)** and with direct palpation of the plantar foot. Often, this results from overuse, e.g., a night of polka dancing while drinking a "few" beers; hence, metatarsalgia is also termed "dancer's foot." **Morton's neuroma** manifests with significant, dysesthetic-type pain and tenderness in the areas of the plantar heads of metatarsals 2 and 3 or 3 and 4. These symptoms are reproduced and often a click develops with the forefoot squeeze maneuver, which accentuates the transverse arch of the foot (Mulder's maneuver). Morton's neuroma is often caused by a severe diabetes mellitus related neuropathy.

Another diagnosis is **precalcaneal bursitis**, which manifests with pain and tenderness, specifically in a discrete area on the plantar aspect of foot, immediately anterior to the calcaneus. Often thought to be plantar fasciitis, it does not radiate into the toes. Often, this is caused by irritation to the fat pad or bursa immediately anterior to the calcaneus and deep to the plantar fascia. **Calcaneal fracture** manifests with widening of, and severe pain and tenderness in, one or both heels. This fracture is caused by a jump from a high place, e.g., often a parachute jumper or, for the romantics, jumping from a second floor bedroom balcony for "Casanova" heel. **Flexor digitorum longus sprain** manifests with pain and tenderness in the posterior compartment radiating into plantar aspect of the foot, toes 2 through 5. An acute tear of the muscle manifests with swelling, pes planus, and a markedly decreased active, and even passive, flexion of the toes. A **Charcot joint** manifests with large swelling in the ankle and plantar foot. It is remarkably painless; there is decreased or increased ROM noted in the tibiotalar and subtalar joints. Because this is caused by severe neuropathy, a severe sensory deficit in a stocking-glove distribution is likely present.

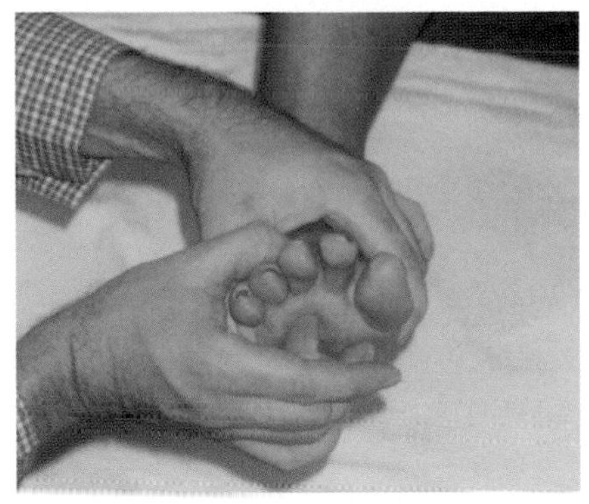

Figure 13.11.

Technique for Mulder's sign. This is a good maneuver for defining metatarsalgia, Morton's neuroma, and avascular necrosis of the metatarsal head.

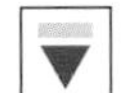

TIPS

- Foot neutral at baseline
- Squeeze the patient's first and fifth metatarsals together
- Morton's neuroma: pain and a click in the interspace between metatarsals 2 and 3 or 3 and 4
- Dancer's foot: increase in pain diffusely on the plantar metatarsal heads
- Stress fracture: increase in pain over foot dorsum.

TEACHING POINTS

PLANTAR FOOT

1. Many entities that manifest with plantar pain are as the result of overuse or ill-fitting shoes.
2. The sesamoid bones of the hallux are in the tendon of the flexor hallucis brevis.
3. The causes of pes planus include flexor hallucis longus tendinitis, plantar fasciitis, Lisfranc's fracture, and diffuse hypotonia.
4. Calluses, i.e., an abnormally hyperkeratotic area, will develop over sites of abnormal wear and tear or irritation on the foot.
5. Morton's neuroma, runner's foot, and tarsal tunnel syndrome are all entrapment neuropathies, usually caused by ill-fitting shoes or is diabetes mellitus-related.
6. Both Morton's neuroma and metatarsalgia manifest with pain on heads of plantar metatarsals.
7. Plantar fasciitis and runner's foot have a similar distribution of pain and discomfort: plantar fasciitis improves with repetitive use, runner's foot worsens with repetitive use.

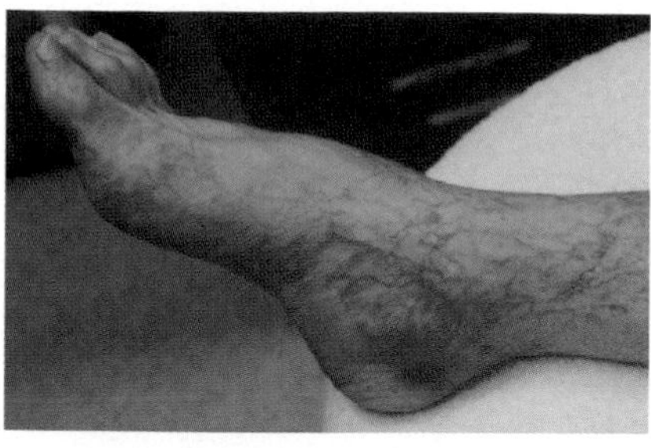

Figure 13.12.

Deltoid ligament, medial ankle sprain. Note the swelling and ecchymosis on the medial aspect of the ankle. If isolated, rare. The most common reason is as the result of a severe lateral sprain.

TIPS

- Always inspect medial foot even if a lateral sprain.
- Deltoid ligament sprain: marked medial swelling and ecchymosis
- Severe lateral sprain: swelling and ecchymosis of medial and even lateral sides indicate an unstable sprain

MEDIAL FOOT AND ANKLE PROBLEMS

Sprain of the deltoid ligament manifests with swelling and tenderness over the medial tibiotalar area (**Fig. 13.12**). The pain is accentuated by passive or active eversion of the foot. This relatively rare entity is caused by either an injury in which the foot is forcibly everted or, more commonly, is the result of a severe lateral sprain. Because the swelling is adjacent to the flexor retinaculum, complications include diminished posterior tibial pulse, tibialis nerve deficits, and/or toe flexor weakness. In the setting of a lateral sprain, medial swelling is a sign of severity. The patient will often have marked tenderness throughout the leg, which can be reproduced with the tibiofibular squeeze test, in which the fibula and the tibia are squeezed together.

Another problem is **Lisfranc's fracture**, which manifests with severe pain and swelling over the medial midfoot. Often, a visible dorsomedial midfoot deformity is noted in which the second metatarsal base is dorsally dislocated. Invariably seen is a flattened foot arch, which is caused by swelling and soft tissue damage. This is an unstable fracture, i.e., the injury will worsen with any use of the area, especially when weight is borne on the joint. The fracture is complex in that it involves the medial or middle cuneiform, often with a dorsal second metatarsal dislocation. There is the potential complication of dorsalis pedis artery damage and a late complication of severe midfoot degenerative joint disease. Lisfranc's fracture is often a rock climbing-related injury.

A **prominent navicular tubercle (accessory navicular)** manifests with pain and callus formation over the medial midfoot, especially when wearing ill-fitting or narrow-fitting shoes. Bilaterally, this is a common reason for medial foot pain; new shoes exacerbate the symptoms. **Tarsal tunnel syndrome**, **flexor hallucis longus strain**, and **plantar fasciitis** are discussed in the section on the plantar foot examination.

TEACHING POINTS

MEDIAL FOOT PROBLEMS

1. Acquired pes planus is caused by Lisfranc's fracture, flexor hallucis longus sprain or tendinitis, or plantar fasciitis.
2. Deltoid ligament sprains are rare, usually concurrent medial swelling is due to severe lateral sprains.
3. Fibula–tibia squeeze test is an important part of the examination of an ankle sprain.
4. Medial sprains require assessment of posterior tibialis artery pulse and tibial nerve, specifically, active toe flexion.
5. Lisfranc's fracture requires assessment of the dorsalis pedis pulse. The fracture is usually caused by rock climbing or hiking.
6. Plantar fasciitis has a classic "first step" pain phenomenon.
7. Pes planus often leads to foot pronation and foot out-toeing.

DORSAL SIDE OF FOOT, ANKLE

Peroneal nerve damage manifests with the patient noting recurrent problems tripping, especially when walking up stairs. Also, mild to moderate numbness is felt in the top of the affected foot. Significant weakness and even atrophy may be present in the anterior (dorsiflexors and toe extensors) and lateral compartments (evertors). The patient will have a classic steppage gait, in which the foot is at baseline plantar flexed and raised off the ground only by knee flexion. The patient's foot is in a baseline position of plantarflexion and out-toeing because of weakness of dorsiflexion and eversion. In addition, sensory deficits are found in the dorsal aspect of the affected foot. **Common peroneal nerve damage (Fig. 13.13)** can be caused by peripheral neuropathy or Charcot-Marie-Tooth disease; in addition, it can be a trauma-related fibular head or neck fracture or caused by anterior compartment syndrome (deep peroneal branch) or lateral compartment syndrome (superficial peroneal branch). **Tibialis anterior sprain or strain** manifests with tenderness and pain in the anterior compartment of the leg radiating into the medial foot **(Fig. 13.14)**. Pain is exacerbated by active dorsiflexion of foot. **Sprain of extensor digitorum longus** manifests with tenderness and pain in the anterior compartment of the leg. The discomfort radiates into the dorsal foot to toes 2, 3, 4, and 5. This is exacerbated by active toe extension, especially against resistance.

Extensor hallucis longus strain (turf toe) manifests with mild to marked recurrent pain and tenderness in the medial dorsal foot, focused maximally at the dorsum of the first MTP. This is reproduced and can be increased with active extension of the hallux and by passive flexion of the great toe (hallux) **(Figs. 13.15 and 13.16)**. This is due to repetitive jumping on tips of great toe and occasionally missing to result in hyperflexion, e.g., in ballet dancing or trampoline use.

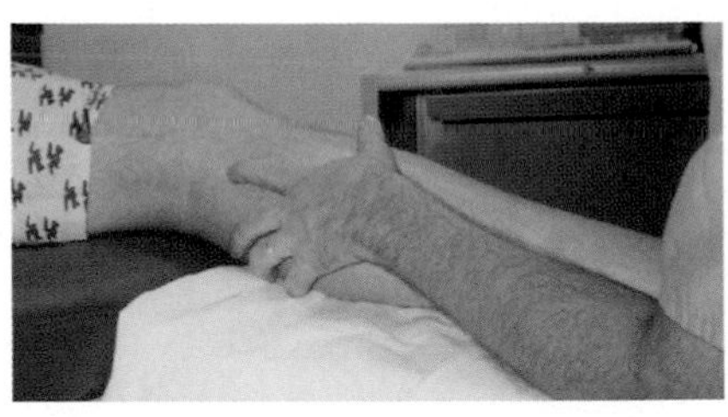

Figure 13.13.

Severe common peroneal nerve damage. Diffuse atrophy of the anterior and lateral compartments and the baseline attitude of the feet—mildly plantar flexed and externally rotated.

TIPS

- Inspect the anterior and lateral compartments of legs
- Severe common peroneal nerve damage: atrophy of the anterior and lateral compartments
- Out-toeing of feet: severe atrophy of anterior compartment

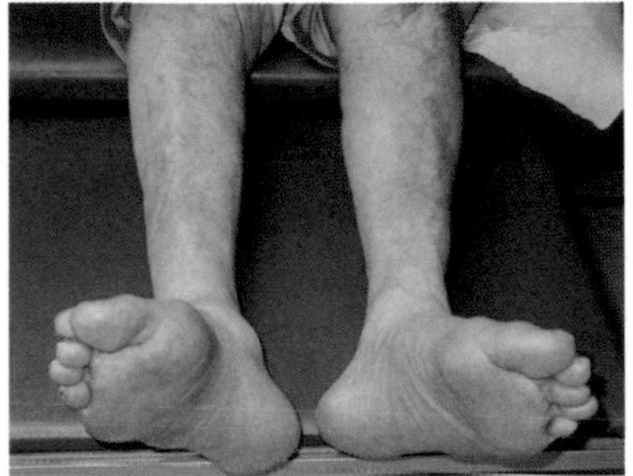

Figure 13.14.

Technique to palpate fibular head and neck. It is important to perform and document this in any lateral ankle sprain or lateral leg trauma.

TIPS

- Palpate fibular neck and head on the lateral knee
- Fracture of fibular head: swelling and tenderness with ecchymosis over site
- Need to assess function of common peroneal nerve

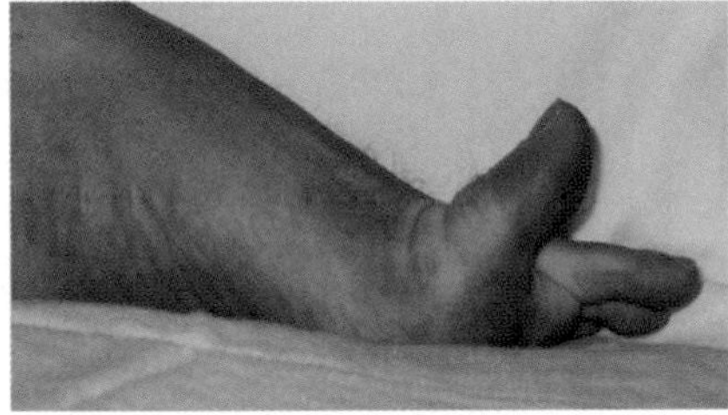

Figure 13.15.

Technique for active first metatarsophalangeal (MTP) toe joint extension. This procedure is useful in defining turf toe and deep peroneal nerve function.

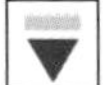

TIPS

- Active dorsiflexion of the great toe; apply resistance on dorsal base
- Deep peroneal nerve or L5 root problem: weak active toe extension
- Anterior compartment syndrome: pain increased in anterior compartment
- Turf toe: increases pain at the dorsum of the MTP-localized to that site

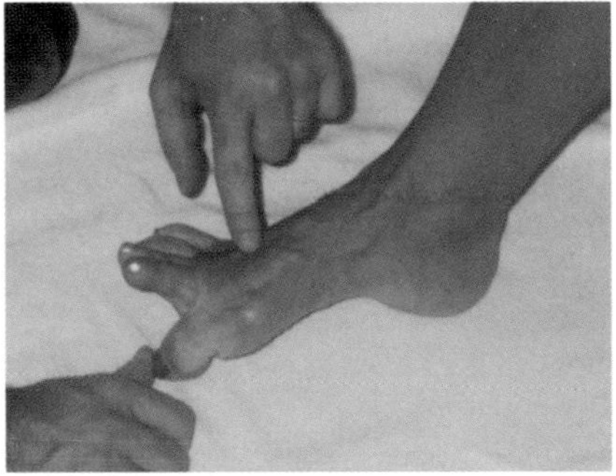

Figure 13.16.

Technique for passive metatarsophalangeal (MTP) joint flexion. This procedure is useful in defining turf toe.

TIPS

- One hand on proximal phalanx, the other on the distal metatarsal
- Passively flex toe at MTP
- Turf toe: increases pain at the dorsum of the first MTP-localized to that site

TEACHING POINTS

DORSAL FOOT PROBLEMS

1. Anterior leg compartment contains the extensors of the toes and the dorsiflexors of the foot.
2. Contusion or cut to the anterior leg compartment will result in mischief in the dorsal foot.
3. The ball of flesh on the lateral dorsal foot is the extensor digitorum brevis, an intrinsic muscle of the foot.
4. Stress fractures of the heads of the metatarsals dorsal forefoot cause pain and tenderness; the symptoms markedly increase with repetitive use.

Another **diagnosis** that involves the foot dorsum is **metatarsal head stress fracture**, which manifests with moderate to severe pain and discomfort over the dorsum of the metatarsal heads of 2, 3, or 4. Pain is reproduced with palpation over the metatarsal heads, and increases with the forefoot squeeze maneuver (Mulder's maneuver) (Fig. 13.11). The pain is progressive in that, with repetitive activity, the duration of such activity decreases each day such that, when severe, prevents this normally active individual from walking. This is a potentially serious injury that can evolve into avascular necrosis. It is most commonly caused by severe repetitive trauma, such as in running in ill-fitting shoes or slapping the ground with the plantar foot when marching in a "goose-step" manner. **Metatarsal exostosis** manifests with one or more bony protuberances. These can be irritated, abraded, or have overlying corns or calluses. **Metatarsal fracture** manifests with marked swelling and pain in the midfoot. Often, there is a history of a heavy object dropped onto the foot. The foot can develop a flattening of the arch or gross bony deformity. **Ganglion cyst** manifests with a fluctuant, nontender nodule adjacent to a tendon. Each cyst is transilluminable. **Corns** manifest with local sites of abnormally thickened skin on the dorsum of the foot or toes. **Charcot joint** and **fifth metatarsal fracture** are discussed elsewhere in this chapter.

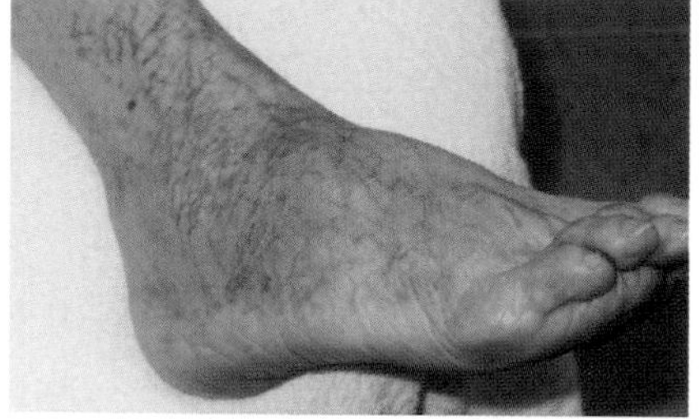

Figure 13.17.

Mild lateral ankle sprain. Note the egg-shaped swelling ecchymosis on lateral ankle, anterior to lateral malleolus.

 **TIPS**

- Lateral ankle sprain: egg-shaped swelling ecchymosis on lateral ankle, anterior to lateral malleolus
- Severe lateral ankle sprain: concurrent medial ecchymosis and swelling present

LATERAL SIDE OF FOOT AND ANKLE

Lateral tibiotalar ankle sprain manifests with swelling and tenderness over the lateral ankle (**Fig. 13.17**). In lateral ankle sprains, which are very common, the most common ligaments damaged are the anterior talofibular and the inferior calcaneofibular. The specific site of swelling and ecchymosis is usually anterior and inferior to the lateral malleolus. This is because the two ligaments most commonly damaged are the anterior fibulotalar and the inferior fibulocalcaneal, which are located anterior and inferior to the lateral malleolus. A sprain of the anterior fibulotalar ligament manifests with pain that is increased, and an anterior laxity of >3 to 5 mm of the calcaneus on the tibia in

TEACHING POINTS

LATERAL FOOT AND ANKLE

1. Lateral ankle sprains are a common injury; due to inversion-type injury.
2. Peroneal tendon sprain is less common, but needs to be considered in the differential diagnosis of lateral ankle pain.
3. Jones fracture and a base or fifth metatarsal tuberosity fracture are remarkably different fractures.
4. Severe lateral sprains can manifest with lateral and medial swelling.
5. The fibula–tibia squeeze test is used to assess for concurrent fibular complications.
6. The anterior drawer maneuver is used to assess the function of the anterior talofibular ligament.
7. The talar tilt test is used to assess the function of the inferior calcaneofibular ligament.

the **anterior drawer maneuver (Fig. 13.18)**. In this maneuver, place the patient's foot in 20 degrees of plantarflexion, so that the anterior talofibular ligament is directly perpendicular to the long axis of the leg. Then, gasp the anterior distal tibia with one hand, the heel with the other hand, and pull anteriorly on the heel (calcaneus). If the sprain is more severe and involves the inferior calcaneofibular ligament, it manifests with increased pain and laxity of >20 degrees of excess inversion, relative to the normal side to the **talar tilt or passive inversion maneuver (Fig. 13.19)**. In this maneuver, place one hand on

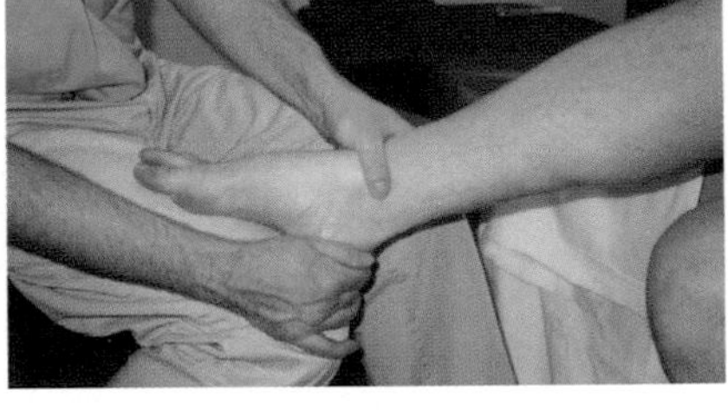

Figure 13.18.

Technique for anterior drawer sign. Excellent test to assess the anterior fibulotalar (AFT) ligament. If AFT is torn, anterior displacement of calcaneus (talus) is present.

TIPS

- Foot is in 20 degrees of plantar flexion (the anterior talofibular ligament is thus perpendicular to the long axis of the leg)
- Grasp the anterior distal anterior tibia with one hand, the calcaneus with the web of the other hand, and pull anteriorly on the calcaneus
- Normal: no or mild movement
- Anterior talofibular ligament damage: anterior movement of calcaneus (talus) on tibia

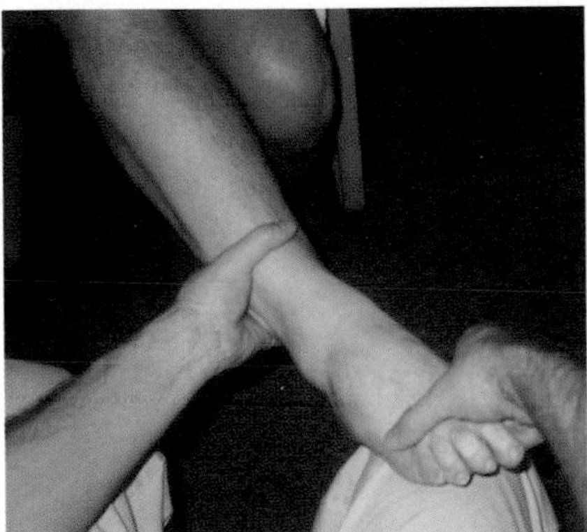

A

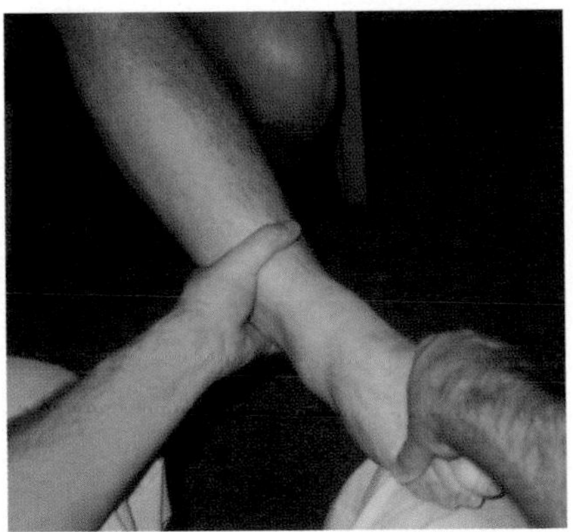

B

Figure 13.19.

Technique for talar tilt (inversion) sign. Excellent test to assess the inferior calcaneofibular (ICF) ligament. If ICF is torn, inversion is excessive.

TIPS

- Place web of hand on calcaneus, passively invert the patient's foot
- Perform after the anterior drawer sign
- Normal: no increase in inversion or pain
- Inferior calcaneofibular ligament damage: excessive inversion present >20 degrees

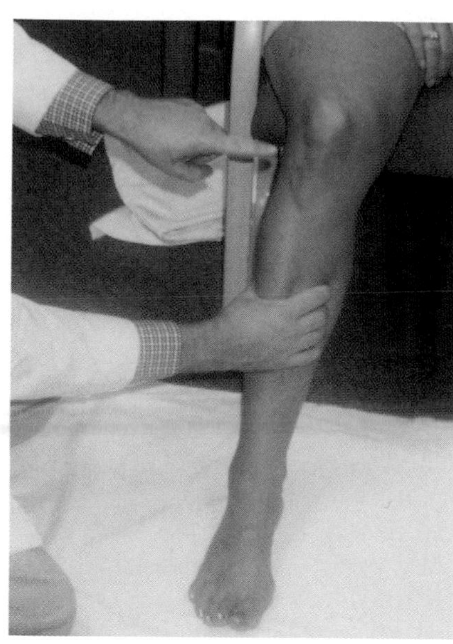

Figure 13.20.

Technique for the fibula–tibial squeeze sign. Highly satisfactory test to assess the leg and knee for concurrent ankle or foot problems.

TIPS

- Foot and ankle neutral
- Grasp the midleg, fingers over the fibula, and squeeze fibula toward tibia
- Fibular head fracture: tenderness in lateral knee
- Lateral ankle sprain: pain and tenderness on lateral and, if severe, medial ankle
- Severe, syndesmotic sprain: tenderness from ankle to knee

heel and passively invert the foot, thus stressing the inferior calcaneofibular ligament. Finally, if the sprain is very severe (3rd Degree sprain), inspection of the medial ankle and foot will reveal medial swelling and tenderness caused by a more severe sprain that involves the posterior talofibular ligament. A lateral ankle sprain is caused by an injury in which the foot rolls over laterally (i.e., it inappropriately inverts).

It is important to look for concurrent injuries such as a fibular head fracture, distal fibular fracture, and a bimalleolar fracture of ankle. A **fibular head or neck fracture** manifests with tenderness over the fibular head and pain is reproduced with the fibular–tibia squeeze maneuver. This maneuver is performed by gently squeezing the fibula into the adjacent tibia at a site in the midleg **(Fig. 13.20)**. **Distal fibular fracture** manifests with lateral swelling, but looks similar to a moderate lateral sprain. A **bimalleolar fracture** manifests with lateral and medial swelling, pain that radiates up to the knee with the fibular–tibia squeeze maneuver, and the inability of the patient to bear any weight on the affected foot. This very serious and unstable fracture was described by Percival Pott in the eighteenth century.

Peroneal tendon sprain manifests with lateral ankle and foot pain that radiates into the lateral leg compartment **(Fig. 13.21)**. The company it keeps

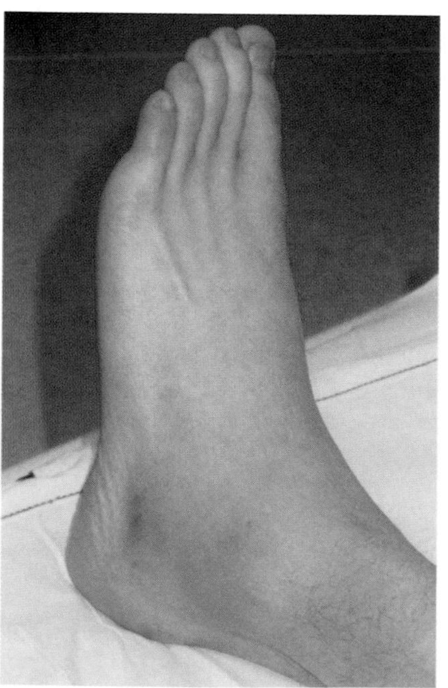
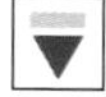

Figure 13.21.

Peroneal tendon sprain. Note the marked swelling and ecchymosis in the area posterior to the lateral malleolus.

TIPS

- Peroneal tendon sprain: pain over the posterior plantar aspect of the foot that radiates into lateral compartment of leg
- Fracture base of fifth metatarsal: swelling and ecchymosis over the base or tuberosity of the fifth metatarsal is a common complication
- Key is location–if swelling posterior to lateral malleolus, consider peroneus longus sprain

includes swelling and ecchymosis that are noted immediately inferior and anterior to the lateral malleolus. Pain increases with passive inversion and active eversion. Concurrent avulsion fracture may be seen in the base of the fifth metatarsal. This common injury can be misdiagnosed as an ankle sprain.

Another diagnosis is **contusion of the extensor digitorum brevis**, which manifests with pain and tenderness over the lateral dorsum of the foot, specific to the ball of muscle located there. The pain is accentuated by active toe extension. Of diagnostic importance is that the pain never radiates into the anterior leg compartment. This often is due to blunt trauma. **Jones fracture** manifests with swelling, tenderness, deformity, and pain over the mid-fifth metatarsal. Often caused by kicking, it is a fracture that has a high incidence of malunion.

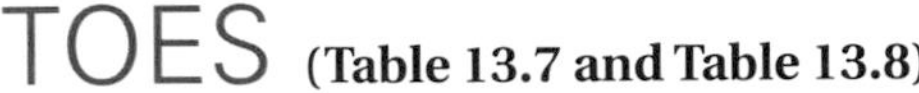

TOES (Table 13.7 and Table 13.8)

Podagra manifests with acute onset of severe pain and swelling on medial aspect of the first metatarsal phalangeal joint **(Fig. 13.22)**. This pain is maximal from the outset; any movement will exacerbate it. Swelling is mild to moderate, at most, and often modest erythema and warmth are present overlying the joint. The company it keeps includes a history of gout and tophi on auricles (Fig. 1.4) and fingers or over the olecranon process (Fig 11.13).

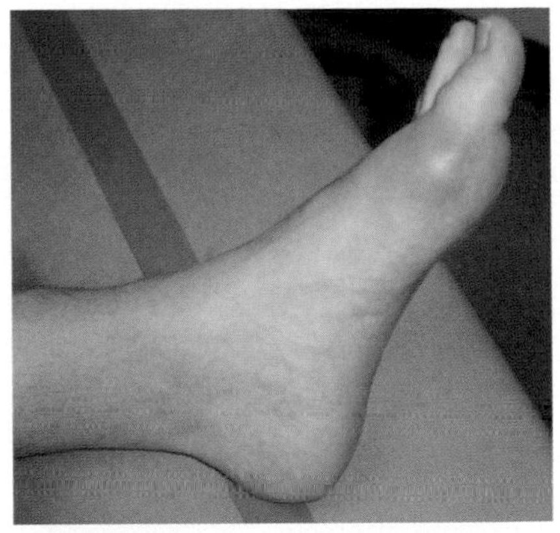

A

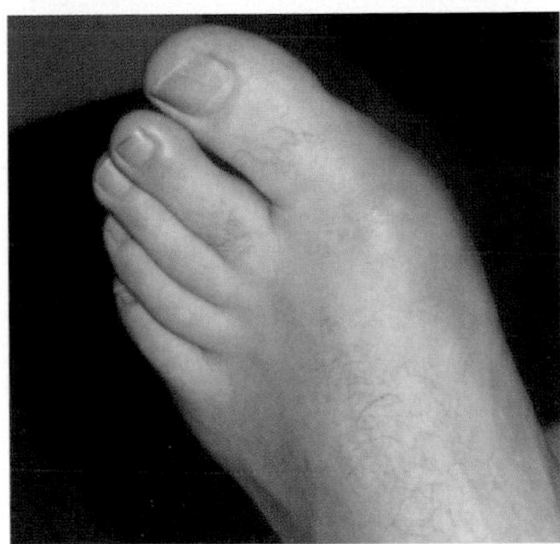

B

Figure 13.22.

Podagra. Acute onset of tenderness and erythema on the medial aspect of the first metatarsophalangeal joint, caused by gout.

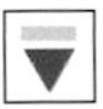

TIPS

- Palpate and inspect medial great toe
- Podagra: severe pain and swelling on the medial aspect of the first MTP joint

Table 13.7. Great Toe Problems

Diagnosis	Site of maximal pain	Company it Keeps
Sesamoiditis	Plantar first MTP	Increased pain with active hallux flexion Increased pain with passive hallux extension
Podagra	Medial first MTP	Auricular tophi Recurrent gout
Bunion	Medial first MTP	Hallux valgus Medial exostosis
Turf toe	Dorsal first MTP	Increased pain with active hallux extension Increased pain with passive hallux flexion

MTP = metatarsophalangeal.

Table 13.8. Toe Problems

Diagnosis	Site of maximal pain	Company It Keeps
Metatarsalgia	Plantar MTP	Increased pain with forefoot squeeze Recent dancing
Stress fracture	Dorsal MTP	Increased pain with forefoot squeeze Goose-step marching or recurrent forefoot trauma
Morton's neuroma	Between MTP 2 and 3, 3 and 4	Increased pain with forefoot squeeze Click present (Mulder's sign) Underlying diabetes mellitus

MTP = metatarsophalangeal.

TEACHING POINTS

TOES

1. The toes are extremely common sites of trauma.
2. To diagnose bunion, the patient must have a hallux valgus at baseline.
3. Ill-fitting shoes contribute to the development of many of the toe contracture problems.
4. Great toe problems include turf toe (pain on dorsal side), podagra (pain on medial side), and sesamoiditis or flexor hallucis tendinitis (pain on plantar side).
5. Sesamoiditis is virtually synonymous with tendinitis of the flexor hallucis brevis.
6. Corns and calluses should be noted, especially in patients with diabetes mellitus or any significant neuropathy.

Bunion manifests with hallux valgus and a swollen bursa over the medial aspect of the first MTP joint **(Fig. 13.23)**. **Hallux valgus** manifests with a deformity in which the axis of the hallux is directed laterally. Most commonly, both of these are caused by wearing ill-fitting very tight shoes.

Cock-up toes manifest with toes in a contracture of hyperextension at the MTP joint and of flexion at the PIP or DIP joint. Furthermore, the toes spread out at the MTP joints. This is usually caused by rheumatoid arthritis. **Claw toes** manifest with toes in a contracture of hyperextension at the MTP joint, flexion only at the DIP joint. **Hammertoes** manifest with toes in contracture of hyperextension at the MTP joint **(Fig. 13.24)** and flexion at the PIP and DIP joints. Often, corns are noted on the dorsal aspects of the toes. **Calluses** manifest with abnormal thickening of highly keratinized skin, i.e., on plantar surfaces, because of irritation to the site. **Corns** manifest with abnormal thickening of lightly keratinized skin, i.e., on dorsal surfaces.

Blue toe often results from embolic events, either in endocarditis or atrial fibrillation or from frostbite **(Fig. 13.25)**. See discussion of evaluation in hand and finger chapter in the section on blue digits.

Another diagnosis is **metatarsalgia (dancer's foot)**, which manifests with pain on the plantar aspect of the metatarsal heads of toes 2, 3, and 4. **Stress fracture of the metatarsal heads** manifests with pain over the dorsum of the metatarsal heads of toes 2, 3, and 4. Pain is progressive, i.e., with repetitive activity, the duration of such activity decreases each day such that, when severe, the patient, who is usually very active, cannot run or walk on the affected

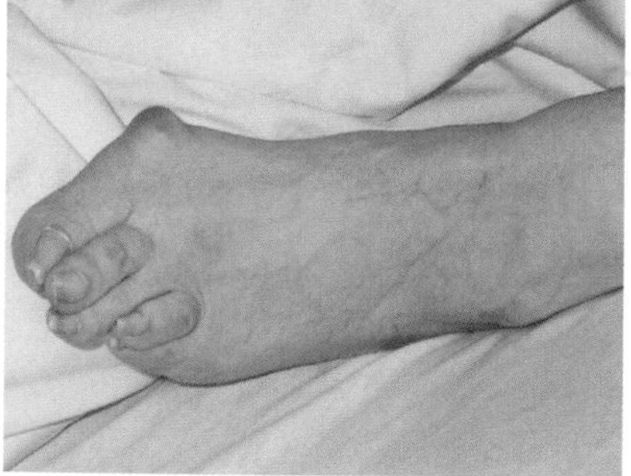

Figure 13.23.

Bunion. The combination of hallux valgus and a swollen bursa over the medial first metatarsophalangeal (MTP) joint.

 **TIPS**

- Inspect and palpate the medial MTP for swelling, exostoses
- Bunion: hallux valgus and swollen bursa over the medial aspect of the first MTP joint
- The medial first MTP area of ten has an exostosis which is boney-hard.

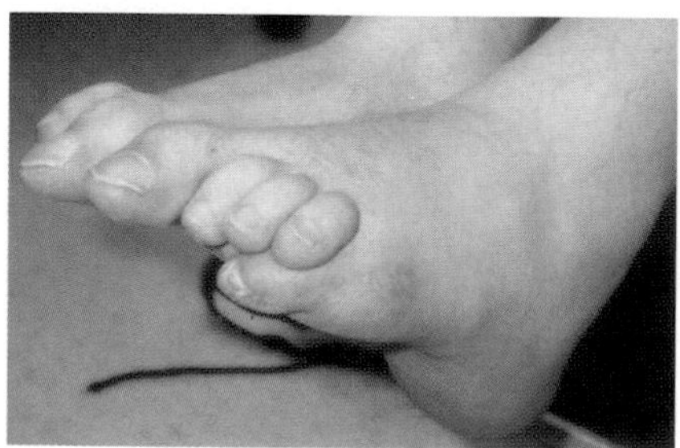

Figure 13.24.

Hammertoes. A contracture of hyperextension at the metatarsophalangeal (MTP) joint, and of flexion at the PIP and DIP joints.

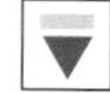 **TIPS**

- Hammertoes: contracture of hyperextension at MTP, and of flexion at PIP and DIP joints
- Usually caused by ill-fitting shoes

foot. **Morton's neuroma** manifests with significant dysesthetic pain and tenderness over the plantar head of metatarsals 2 and 3 or 3 and 4 and pain and a click with the forefoot squeeze sign of Mulder. This is due to the development of a fibrous area in the sheath of a digital nerve; common in diabetes mellitus. **Paronychia** manifests with swelling and fluctuance with exuberant tissue around the lateral or medial nail folds. **Syndactyly** manifests with congenital webbed toes. **Tuft fracture** of distal phalanx manifests with pain and tenderness in distal phalanx with a subungual hematoma, which most often is caused by a crush injury, e.g., tip of toe in door jam. **Tophaceous gout** manifests with papules and swelling around the DIP or PIP joint. The company it keeps includes tophi on the auricle, olecranon process, and podagra. **Subungual hematomas** manifest with an acute, extremely tender, trauma-related collection of blood beneath the nail plate.

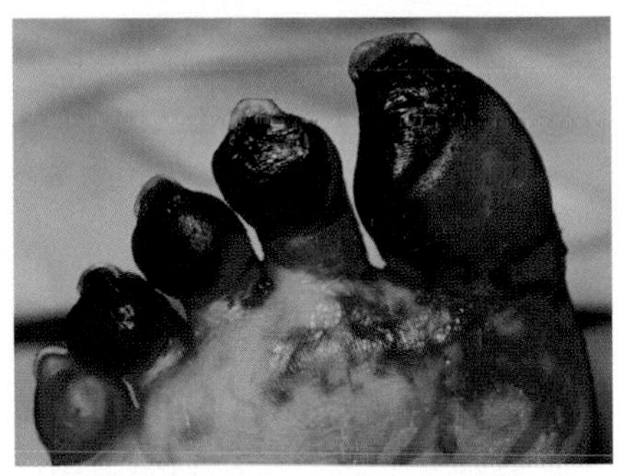

Figure 13.25.

Blue toes. Multiple blue toes as the result of embolic events from atrial fibrillation.

TIPS

- Frostbite or embolic events from endocarditis or from atrial fibrillation: blue toe syndrome

POSTERIOR ANKLE LEG

Retrocalcaneal bursitis manifests with tenderness and swelling immediately deep to the Achilles tendon, proximal to the calcaneus. Pain is exacerbated by active plantarflexion of foot against resistance. **Supracalcaneal bursitis** manifests with tenderness and swelling specific to the area immediately superficial to the Achilles tendon and superior to the calcaneus **(Fig. 13.26)**. Pain is exacerbated by active plantarflexion of the ankle. This is most commonly caused by irritation from shoes. As such, it has been referred to specifically as, "pump-bump." **Achilles tendinitis** manifests with pain and tenderness throughout the Achilles tendon that extends into the muscles of the posterior compartment. Pain increases with active plantarflexion of the foot and passive dorsiflexion of the foot exacerbates the pain. Often bilateral, this tendinitis is usually caused by running without adequate antecedent stretching.

TEACHING POINTS

POSTERIOR LEG

1. Supracalcaneal, retrocalcaneal bursitis, and Achilles tendinitis all present in similar manner: pain above the calcaneus.
2. Posterior compartment syndrome manifests with decreased pulse to the posterior tibial artery and decreased function of tibial nerve.
3. Any compartment syndrome is an emergency; find and treat the underlying cause and protect the neurovascular structures.
4. Acute tear of the Achilles tendon or any posterior compartment syndrome can look like an acute deep venous thrombosis.
5. Long-standing tears of the Achilles tendon manifests with a gap in the tendon and a flaccid mass in the gastrocnemius muscle.
6. Physical examination is poor in the diagnosis of deep venous thrombosis of the lower extremity.

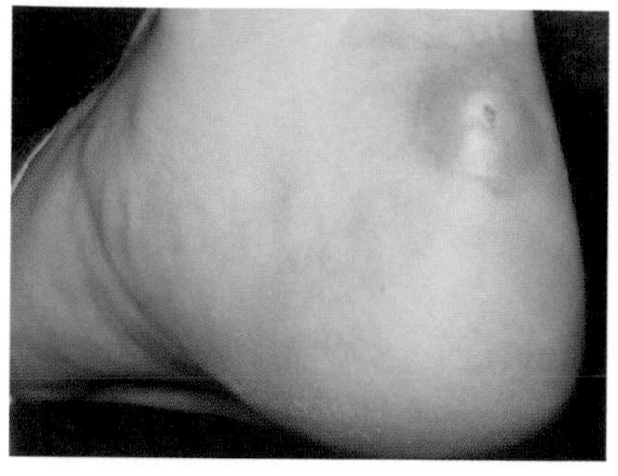

Figure 13.26.

Supracalcaneal bursitis. Note the red, tender area superior to the calcaneus and superficial to the Achilles tendon, caused by ill-fitting shoes.

 TIPS

- Inspect posterior leg and ankle
- Supracalcaneal bursitis: superior to calcaneus, a red, tender, fluctuant bursa superficial to the Achilles tendon
- Achilles tendinitis: tenderness and swelling throughout the Achilles tendon
- Retrocalcalcaneal bursitis: superior to calcaneus, with pain, tenderness, and swelling immediately deep to the Achilles tendon

Tear of the Achilles tendon manifests with acute onset of severe pain, tenderness, and swelling with ecchymosis in the posterior compartment. The patient is acutely unable to effectively walk on the affected leg. A marked decrease is noted in the ability to actively plantar flex the foot. The company it keeps includes an absence of passive plantarflexion of the foot at the ankle on squeezing the gastrocnemius muscle (Thompson's maneuver) and an absence of passive plantarflexion of the foot on pulling upward on the gastrocnemius muscle (Simmond's test) **(Fig. 13.27)**. In the chronic setting, a flaccid mass is often felt in the gastrocnemius muscle and a gap in the tendon itself.

Deep venous thrombosis (DVT) manifests with swelling of the calf and thigh, usually mildly tender, and often with minimal warmth. The classic findings of DVT are both insensitive and nonspecific and, as such, do not merit discussion except that classic physical exam tests for them should not be performed. We recommend thigh and leg circumference measurements for baseline purposes **(Fig. 13.28)**. For this, make an ink mark in the center of the patella; then, measure and mark 15 cm above and below; the circumference at each point on both legs is measured both to compare and to follow size over time. If clinical suspicion is present, one must image with ultrasound. In this disorder imaging is superior to physical examination.

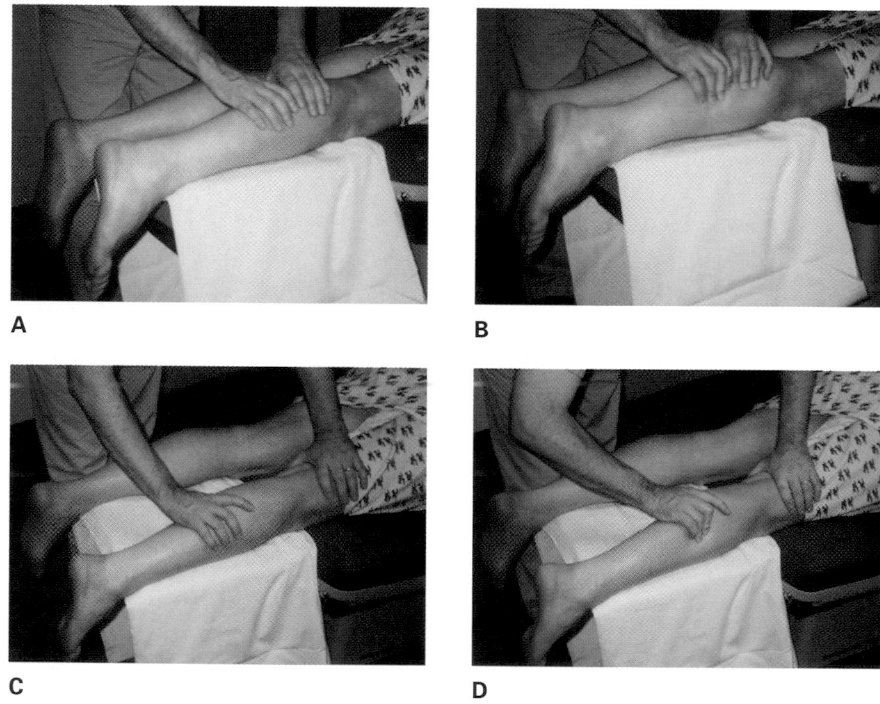

Figure 13.27.

Techniques for Thompson's **(A)** and Simmond's **(B)** stress tests. Excellent tests for chronic tears of the gastrocnemius or the Achilles tendon.

 TIPS

- Patient kneels on a rigid-type chair with foot dangling off the back
- Grasp gastrocnemius muscle and squeeze muscle with hand **(A** and **B)**
- Grasp the midgastrocnemius muscle and pull upward on the muscle with hand **(C** and **D)**
- Normal: passive plantarflexion of the foot with each squeeze
- Acute tears of the gastrocnemius: unable to perform because of pain
- Achilles tendon tear: no passive plantarflexion of the foot with each squeeze

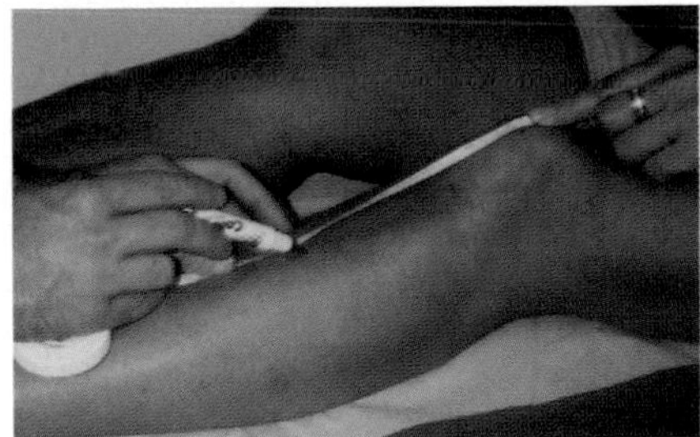

A

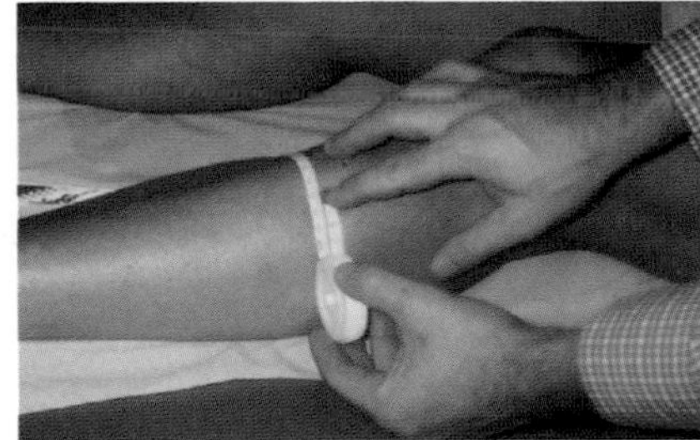

B

Figure 13.28.

Measurement of the lower extremity circumference. Increase in size is consistent with swelling, which might be due to a deep venous thrombosis.

TIPS

- Mark the center of both patellae
- With a flexible tape measure, mark the distance 15 cm **(A)** above and **(B)** below the center of the patella; measure circumference at both sites.
- Normal: no asymmetry; however, does *not* rule out thrombosis

Another diagnosis is **tibial nerve damage**, which manifests with weakness of the muscles of the posterior leg compartment, i.e., the gastrocnemius, as assessed by active foot plantarflexion and the long toe flexors as assessed by active toe flexion against resistance; and the intrinsic flexors of the foot. If the tibial nerve damage is severe or long-standing, concurrent atrophy and fasciculations may be present. Often, sensory deficits involve the entire plantar aspect of the foot. **Posterior compartment syndrome** manifests with swelling and tenderness in the posterior leg compartment. A decrease may be noted in the pulse to the posterior tibialis artery and numbness on the entire plantar foot, i.e., in the tibia nerve distribution. This is usually caused by trauma to the calf, but it can be secondary to leg cellulitis, a severe DVT, a severe ankle sprain, or Pott's bimalleolar fracture. **Calcaneal fracture** is discussed above.

Annotated Bibliography

Overall

Butcher JD, Salzman KL, Lillegard WA. Lower extremity bursitis. *Am Fam Phys* 1996;53(7): 2317–2324.

Overview of the anatomy and pathogenesis of bursitis in the lower extremities, including overall therapy and a description of specific sites. The site-specific evaluation is far from exhaustive, but includes ischiogluteal bursitis (Weaver's bottom); greater trochanteric bursitis pes anserine bursitis, prepatellar bursitis, and for the ankle, retrocalcaneus bursitis.

Dellacorte MP, Birrer RB, Grisafi PJ. The acutely painful foot and ankle: trauma (tic) injuries. *Emerg Med* 1994;(Sept):46–64.

Nice overview of common trauma-related problems involving the foot and ankle. Primary care emphasis on diagnosis using physical examination, radiographic imaging, and management, including types of casts and splints. The problems discussed include lacerations, puncture wounds (98% are stepping on a nail), toenail injuries including subungual hematoma, lacerations, and fractures. The fractures include digits, sesamoids, metatarsals, base of fifth metatarsal (peroneal brevis), and the Jones fracture, a nondisplaced fracture of the proximal diaphysis of the fifth metatarsal bone. Also describes tarsal bone fractures, including the calcaneal fracture (lover's heel). Includes a table describing a grading system for ankle sprains, using the talar tilt test and anterior drawer signs. Emphasizes that a golden period of examination (the first 20–30 minutes) exists in which signs are demonstrable before pain and swelling appears.

Engebretsen L, Bahr R. Foot injuries: office management for the woes of the weekend warrior. *Consultant* 1996;(Feb):209–225.

Nice overview of common overuse problems involving the foot and ankle in patients who intermittently play sports. Highly satisfactory discussion of the epidemiologic and risk factors for such injuries. Primary care emphasis used in the discussion of acquired flat foot, acquired loss of transverse arch, painful heel cushion (precalcaneal bursitis), Haglund's heel (pump-bump), supracalcaneal bursitis, plantar fasciitis; nerve entrapment syndromes, including Morton's neuroma, deep peroneal nerve (deficit in web space between 1 and 2, superficial peroneal numbness on dorsal foot, tarsal tunnel and sural nerve-lateral malleolus); sesamoid (flexor hallucis brevis), and Freiberg's infarction.

Leach RE, Zecher SB. Tennis injuries. *Consultant* 1995;(Nov):1657–1664.

A terse discussion of three types of injuries: ankle sprains, gastrocnemius tear, and Achilles tendon tear. Nice diagrams and a nice image of the procedure for performing an anterior drawer sign.

Mann RA. Entrapment neuropathies of the foot. In: DeLee JC, Drez D Jr. eds. *Orthopedic Sports Medicine.* Philadelphia:WB Saunders,1994:1831–1841.
Excellent discussion of these commonly overlooked, but not infrequent, foot disorders.

Overall: Range of Motion

Kidd JG. The Charcot joint: some pathologic and pathogenic considerations. *South Med J* 1974;67:597–602.
Overview of this relatively uncommon diagnostic finding; describes a somewhat dated, but still appropriate differential diagnosis, including lues venereum and the most common cause today, uncontrolled diabetes mellitus are discussed.

Ankle: Sprains

Bahr R, Engebretsen L. Acute ankle sprains. *Consultant* 1996;(Apri):675–688.
A well-written and practical paper on this extremely common problem. Discusses the epidemiology, functional anatomy, including descriptions of the anterior talofibular, calcaneofibular, and posterior talofibular ligaments; and types of injuries. Defines inversion (supination, internal rotation, plantar flexion) and eversion (pronation, external rotation, dorsiflexion). A useful classification is discussed. ATFL: anterior talofibular ligament; CFL: calcaneofibular ligament. Also discusses syndesmotic sprains. The physical examination is described with satisfactory diagrams: squeeze test and external rotation test, both for syndesmotic disorders; anterior drawer (tests ATFL) and talar tilt (test CFL, abnormal>10 degrees.). Also, an excellent discussion of initial radiographic and therapeutic modalities.

Birrer RB, Bordelon RL, Sammarco GJ. Ankle: don't dismiss a sprain *Patient Care* 1992; 26(4):6–28.
Reviews the importance of the talar tilt test in the evaluation of ankle sprains (talar tilt and calcaneofibular ligament assessment).

Bourne RB, Rorabeck CH. Compartment syndromes of the lower leg. *Clin Orthop* 1988; 240:97–105.
Excellent review of these often overlooked and, therefore, undiagnosed problems. Defines acute (often trauma-related) versus chronic (often exercise-related) syndromes and reviews the manifestations of each compartment. Defines four different compartments: anterior, lateral, and the posterior, which is divided into superficial and deep compartments. Minimal discussion of physical examination; significant discussion on use of slit catheter measurement of intracompartment pressures; if >30–45 mm Hg, diagnostic. Also reviews that chronic (exercise-related) syndromes require measurement during dynamic use (i.e., exertion). Treatment with fasciotomy is also discussed.

Frost HM, Hanson CA. Technique for testing the drawer sign in the ankle. *Clin Orthop* 1977; 123:49–51.
Excellent description of the anterior drawer sign, which is so important in lateral ankle sprain assessment, in general, and the anterior talofibular ligament, specifically.

Rubin A, Sallis R. Evaluation and diagnosis of ankle injuries. *Am Fam Phys* 1996;54(5): 1609–1618.
Excellent review of ankle injuries from a primary care perspective. Reviews anatomy, mechanism for medial and lateral ankle sprains, and manifestations of lateral sprains, including anterior drawer, talar tilt, and the squeeze test (important to evaluate for a syndesmotic sprain injury); also reviews the peroneal sprains that are often overlooked in lateral ankle pain syndromes.

Rubin G, Witten M. The talar tilt angle and the fibular collateral ligament. *J Bone Joint Surg* 1960;42-A:311–342.
The first description of the utility of this sign for the calcaneofibular ligament (i.e., if positive, significant sprain).

Swain RA, Holt WS. Ankle injuries. *Postgrad Med* 1993;93(3):91–100.
A satisfactory review and discussion of common ankle problems, including ankle sprains, with an excellent description of lateral anatomy. Also describes the tests, including anterior drawer, talar tilt, and the squeeze sign. Emphasizes the most common injury—lateral ankle sprain.

Wexler RK. The injured ankle. *Am Fam Phys* 1998;57(3):474–480.
Exceedingly well-written paper that outlines and, with a great degree of practicality and excellence, describes the evaluation of the patient with an injured ankle. Very good discussion of anatomy and grading of sprains, using function as a marker. Reviews the procedure for anterior drawer (hold distal tibia and fibula with one hand, grasp the heel with other, and attempt to move it anteriorly) and defines that >4 mm displacement is indicative of a tear of the anterior talofibular ligament. Also describes the talar tilt test (hold the distal tibia and fibula with one hand, use other hand to invert the foot) to assess the calcaneofibular ligament, a tear of which manifests with a tilt of 5 to 10 degrees greater on affected side. A paper that should be in the files of all primary care physicians.

Foot

Apelquist J, Larsson J, Agardh C. The importance of peripheral pulses, peripheral oedema and local pain for the outcome of diabetic foot ulcers. *Diabetic Med* 1990;7:590–594.
Nice discussion of the importance of factors that clinically can be easily assessed to rate the risk of negative outcome in patients with foot ulcers and diabetes mellitus.

Caputo CM, Cavanagh PR, Ulbrecht JS, et al. Assessment and management of foot disease in patients with diabetes. *N Engl J Med* 1994;331(13):854–860.

Comprehensive review of a topic that is clearly important to primary care physicians, including evaluation and management.

Coady CM, Gow N, Stanish W. Foot problems in middle-aged patients. *The Physician and Sports Medicine* 1998;26(5):31–42.

Overview of common entities that have an impact on the health of the foot, including hallux valgus, hallux rigidus (degenerative joint problems in the first MTP with decreased ROM), hammertoe (extension at MTP, flexed at PIP, extended at DIP), claw toe (MTP hyperextended, PIP/DIP flexed), mallet toe (neutral at MTP and PIP, flexed at DIP), corns, Morton's neuroma (15% bilateral according to this paper), plantar fasciitis (discussion of first step phenomenon), metatarsal stress fractures (discussion of dorsal pain location), posterior tibial tendinitis, acquired pes planus, and tarsal tunnel with a discussion of Tinel's sign and some features of rheumatoid arthritis and diabetes mellitus. The discussion of physical findings is short and not robust, but overall a satisfactory paper.

Edelman D, Hough DM, Glazebrook KN, et al. *JGIM* 1997;12:537–543.

Used features of diabetic ulcers in patients with diabetes mellitus to predict healing; the two features indicating the poorest outcome for these patients with ulcers were the absence of pulses and the absence of pain.

Ferris L, Alexander IJ. Diagnosing and managing persistent medial midfoot pain. *J Musculoskel Med* 1994;11(8):47–59.

A complete and well-written overview of common problems involving the medial midfoot, defined here as between Lisfranc's joint and area that includes the three cuneiforms, the cuboid, and the navicular bones. Diagnoses include Lisfranc's fracture or dislocation, accessory navicular bone, osteoarthritis, tibialis posterior tendon dysfunction, and plantar fasciitis. Includes a discussion of tibialis posterior tendinitis, which manifests with pes planus and foot varus.

Freiberg AH. Infarction of the second metatarsal bone—a typical injury. *Surgery Gynecology Obstetrics* 1914;19:191–193.

A classic; the original description of this AVN process of the second metatarsal head.

Keene JS, Lange RH. Diagnostic dilemma in foot and ankle injuries. *JAMA* 1986; 256(2): 247–251.

Erudite discussion of some of the more vexing foot problems in active individuals: stress fractures of great toe sesamoids, Jones fracture (nondisplaced fracture of the proximal diaphysis), and to the base of the fifth metatarsal bone caused by peroneal tendon sprains. Well-written paper on these common problems.

Leach RE, Schepsis A. When hindfoot pain slows the athlete. *J Musculoskel Med* 1992;9(4):106–124.

Highly satisfactory overview of evaluation and management of Achilles tendinitis, retrocalcaneus bursitis, supracalcaneal bursitis, plantar bursitis, and posterior tibial tendinitis. A satisfactory discussion of these problems.

Mollica MB. Morton's neuroma. *The Physician and Sports Medicine* 1997;25(5):76–82.

Defines the lesion as being a benign, perineural fibrotic lesion of common digital nerve. Reviews the anatomy of the plantar foot innervation, indicts the flexor digitorum brevis as a factor in formation, and reviews the diagnostic features on physical examination, including Mulder's sign (application of manual pressure on the lateral and medial aspects of forefoot—pain and click). Nice review of the nonsurgical and surgical interventions.

O'Keeffe ST, Woods B, Breslin DJ, et al. Blue toe syndrome. *Arch Intern Med* 1992;152: 2197–2202.

An excellent review of this relatively uncommon entity; reviews the manifestations and causes of this problem, including emboli, both thrombotic and cholesterol; vasculitis, hyperviscous states, leukostasis, hypercoagulable states, and medications. Reports that livedo reticularis is common in blue toes related to cryoglobulinemia and cholesterol emboli.

Osler W. Chronic infectious endocarditis. *Q J Med* 1908;2:219–230.

The original description by the master of bedside physical diagnosis. He was correct in his hypothesis: these were truly emboli from the heart valves themselves.

Parkinson RW, Griffin GC. Dermatititis of the feet. *Postgrad Med* 1997; 101(6):95–110.

Excellent overview of common dermatologic entities that primarily involve the feet; tinea and onychomycosis are included in this review.

Pedowitz WJ, Kovatis P. Flatfoot in the adult. *J Am Acad Orthop Surg* 1995; 3(5):293–302.

Excellent review of this common, albeit significant, and underdiagnosed entity.

Youngswick FD. Intermetatarsal neuroma. *Clin Podiatri Med Surg* 1994; 11(4):579–592.

Podiatric review of this common problem, indicating that Mulder's sign is indeed a good sign in the evaluation of this disorder.

Yu WD, Shapiro MS. Fractures of the fifth metatarsal. *The Physician and Sports Medicine* 1998;26(2):47–64.

Practical and very good overview on the features, pathogenesis, potential sequelae, and management of proximal (base of) fifth metatarsal fractures and the Jones fracture.

14

Skin Examination

PRACTICE AND TEACHING

Examination of the skin requires three overall activities: first, a thorough description of the individual lesions; second, defining the pattern of the lesions into a rash; and, third, finding the company the rash keeps. (**Table 14.1**). The **primary lesion descriptors** include **macule** (<1 cm and flat); a **papule** (<1 cm and palpable); a **patch** (>1 cm and flat); and a **plaque** (>1 cm and palpable). A **nodule** is unique in that it is >1 cm, palpable, but subcutaneous. A **vesicle** is <1 cm and filled with a clear fluid; a **bulla** is >1 cm and filled with fluid. A **pustule** is <1 cm and filled with pus. An **ulcer** is a deep loss of skin; an **erosion** is the superficial loss of skin. **Petechia** are purple, nonblanching, 2 to 5 mm in

Table 14.1. Skin Lesion and Finding Descriptors

Descriptor	Definition	Examples
Macule	<1 cm, flat	Nevus
Papule	<1 cm, palpable	Skin tag
Patch	>1 cm, flat	Café au lait
Plaque	>1 cm, palpable	Psoriasis
Nodule	>1 cm, palpable subcutaneous	Lipoma
Vesicle	<1 cm, clear fluid filled	Varicella
Bulla	>1 cm, clear fluid filled	Blister
Pustule	<1 cm, pus filled	Folliculitis
Petechia	2–5 mm, purple, flat	Thrombocytopenia
Purpura	5–10 mm, purple, flat	Coagulopathy
Ecchymosis	>10 mm, purple, flat	Bruise
Hematoma	>10 mm, purple, palpable	Bruise
Urticaria	>5 mm, red, palpable	Insect bite
Excoriation	Linear ulcer or erosion	Pruritus
Scale	Flake or skin	Seborrheic dermatitis
Crust	Ooze, scab	Nonspecific, scab
Crack	Fissure, split of skin	Nonspecific
Herpes	Cluster of lesions	Herpes simplex
Annular	Ring or even target	Tinea corporis Erythema multiforme Urticaria

TEACHING POINTS

BASIC SKIN EXAMINATION

1. A bulla is antecedent to an erosion or an ulcer; flaccid bulla produces an erosion; tense bulla produces an ulcer.
2. Macules and patches are flat, i.e., not palpable.
3. Papules and plaques are raised, i.e., palpable.
4. Knowledge of primary and secondary descriptors of specific lesions is mandatory to a dermatologic examination; these must be memorized.
5. Patterns of lesions provide tremendous clues to the specific rash type.
6. When palpating any rash, always wear gloves.
7. Once the lesions and pattern have been described, look for accompanying findings, i.e., related symptoms of the rash such as murmurs, nail pitting, and so on.

size, and flat; **purpura** are purple, nonblanching, 5 to 20 mm in size, flat or palpable; **ecchymosis** are purple, nonblanching, >2 cm in size, and not palpable. **Urticarial** lesions are palpable, pruritic, red, raised, and solitary or multiple.

Secondary descriptors of lesions are relatively nonspecific, but help define and describe the lesions and, thus, are of importance in diagnosis. **Excoriations** are linear erosions or ulcerations, i.e., scratches often caused by pruritus; **scales** are flakes of superficial skin. **Cracks or fissures** are superficial or deep crevices. The presence of **crust** indicates dried fluid in and around the lesion, also referred to as a "scab." Finally, lesions can be **annular** or ring shaped.

The **pattern** of the lesions to form a rash on a local or body-wide distribution is of diagnostic benefit to the patient. The patterns include **clustering** or grouping of similar lesions. An example of this is herpes simplex. A second pattern is a rash predominantly on the **flexor surfaces**, focused on the antecubital and popliteal fossa. An example of this is atopic dermatitis (eczema). A third pattern is of a rash that is predominantly on the **extensor surfaces**, focused on the knees and elbows. A classic example of this is psoriasis. Another pattern is one in which the rash is predominantly on the **lower extremities**, beginning in the toes and extending proximally. An example of this is stasis dermatitis. A further pattern is of a rash that is in a specific **unilateral dermatome** or two. An example of this is herpes zoster. Another rash pattern is that of predominant involvement in the **intriginous zones**, including the inguinal areas. An example of this rash is tinea or scabies. Finally, **Koebner's phenomenon**, a condition in which lesions of a rash occur in an area of trauma, irritation, or scarring. A classic example of this pattern is psoriasis.

NAILS

Examination of the **skin appendages**, i.e., fingernails, toenails, and hair, is important in the assessment of any rash or in defining and diagnosing any primary skin appendage process. The **normal anatomy** of a fingernail or toenail includes the **lunula**, a white semicircle at the base of the nail bed; the **cuticle**, a superficial and peripheral rim of thin epithelium on the plate; the **nail plate**, a hard keratin structure overlying the bed; the **lateral** or **medial folds** of skin on the sides of the nail plate; and the **proximal fold**, the skin of finger or toe on the proximal aspect of the plate.

Onychomycosis manifests with a thickened, yellow destroyed nail plate **(Fig. 14.1)**. Destruction begins on the distal, lateral, and medial surfaces and progresses proximally. Onychomycosis is caused by poor foot hygiene, recurrent tinea pedis, use of glucocorticoids, or uncontrolled diabetes mellitus. **Psoriatic nails** manifest with multiple superficial pits in the plates of all nails—thickened, yellow destroyed nail plates. The destruction begins proximal and progresses distal. Clinically, it is unusual for onychomycosis to develop in the setting of active psoriasis.

Onychogryphosis manifests with ram's horn configuration of the thickened nails **(Fig. 14.2)**. This is a common problem in which the nails can become so long that specific to toenails the patient effectively walks on them. Often there is a history of poor hygiene, stocking distribution neuropathy, or underlying disability. It is important to stress that an examination is not complete unless the patient removes socks or stockings.

Clubbing manifests with two requisite features, first a flattened (Lovibond's) angle between the plate and the proximal fold **(Fig. 14.3)**. This flattening is further defined by Schamroth's sign in which there is no diamond-shaped space between two juxtaposed finger nail plates **(Fig. 14.4)**. The second feature is on palpation of the proximal nail plate it squishes or floats on the bed. When advanced, the fingertips appear as "lollipops." This is the type of clubbing that Hippocrates probably described 3500 years ago. **Hypertrophic pulmonary osteoarthropathy**, which manifests with small joint polyarticular arthritis and marked clubbing, most commonly is associated with non–small-cell carcinoma.

Beau's lines, which manifest with transverse indentations in the nail plates, is caused by profound acute illness, either a hypercatabolic state or a hypoanabolic state **(Fig. 14.5)**. They occur in each plate at the same distance

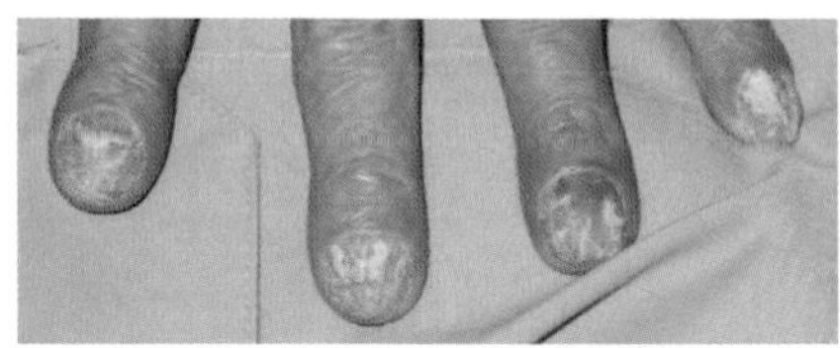

Figure 14.1.

Onychomycosis of nail plates.

 **TIPS**

- Onychomycosis: thickened yellow nails destroyed from distal, lateral, and medial sides; progresses proximally

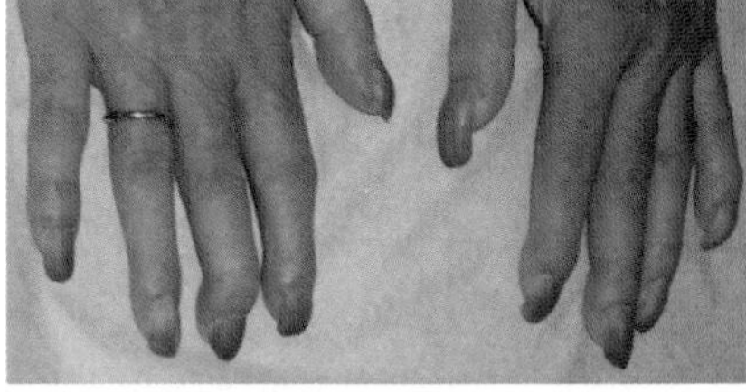

Figure 14.2.

Onychogryphosis of nails.

 **TIPS**

- Ram's horn configuration of the thickened yellow nails
- Can become very long
- Concurrent neuropathy is common

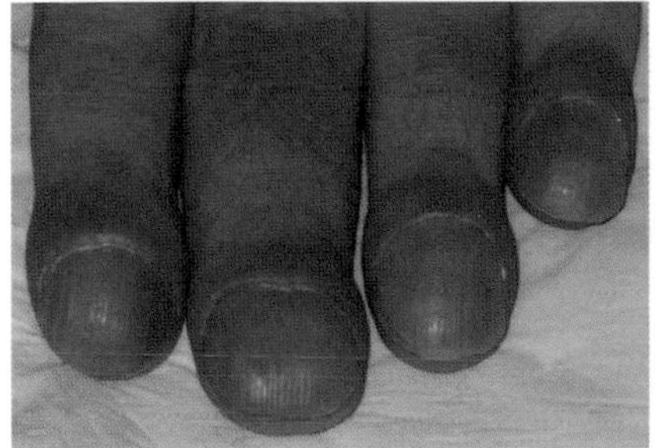

Figure 14.3.

Classic clubbing. Note the "lollipop" configuration of the tips.

 **TIPS**

- Lovibond's angle: formed by the proximal plate and the proximal fold
- Normal: 160 degrees
- Clubbing: 180 degrees

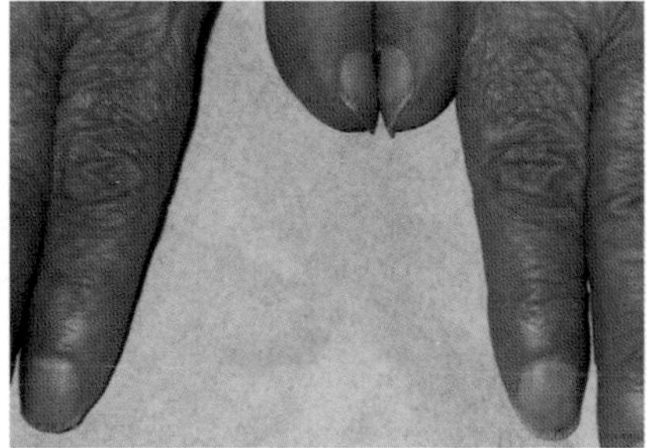

Figure 14.4.

Schamroth's sign indicative of flattening of the plate to fold angle; confirms the flatness of Lovibond's angle.

 **TIPS**

- Place the dorsal aspects of digits together, note the apposition of the proximal folds and plates
- Normal: diamond-shaped slit present
- Clubbing: no such slit present

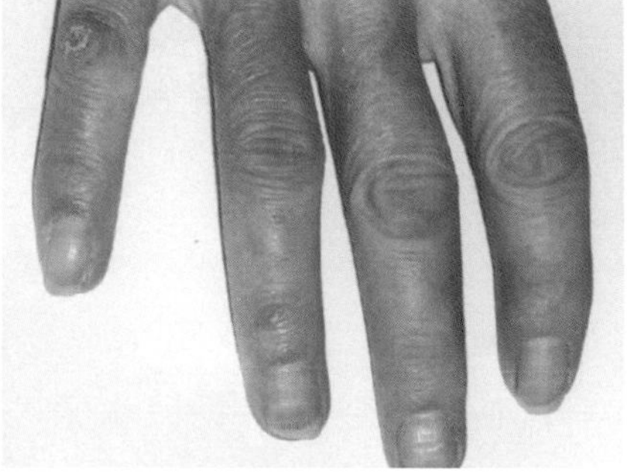

Figure 14.5.

Beau's lines of a severe illness in past. Illness was 5 weeks ago, 5 mm distal to the lunula (plate grows 1 mm/week).

 **TIPS**

- Beau's lines: transverse indentations in the nail plates
- Profound acute illness, either a hypercatabolic state or a hypoanabolic state
- Nail plate grows 1 mm/week

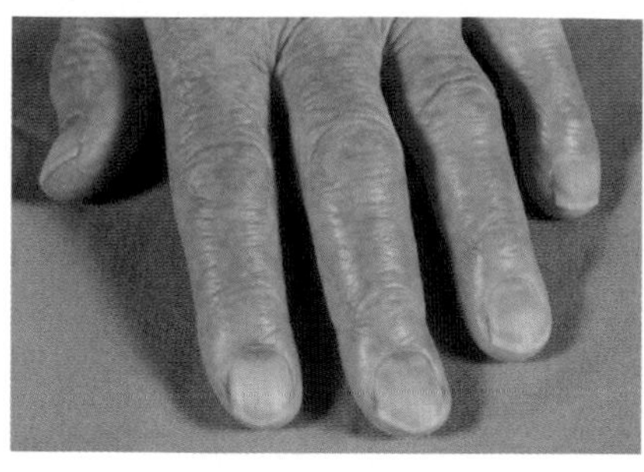

Figure 14.6.

The red lunula of Terry's nails, a related symptom of heart failure.

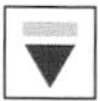 **TIPS**

- Terry's CHF nails: red lunula in all of the nail beds

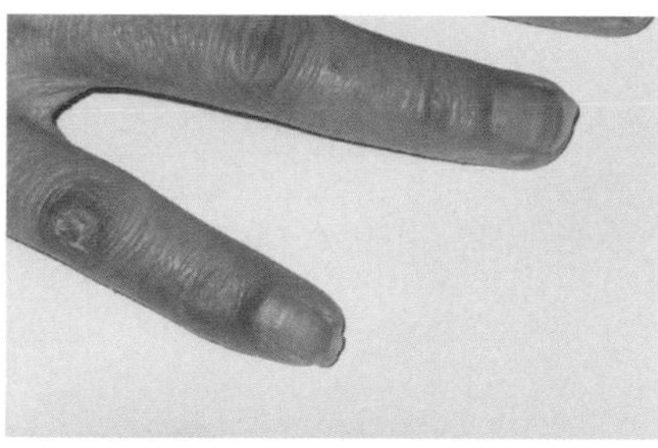

Figure 14.7.

Muercke's lines of profound hypoalbuminemia.

 **TIPS**

- Bands of white in the nail bed, alternating with pink
- Associated with severe hypoalbuminemia, albumin <2 g

from the lunula and, given that fingernail plates grow at a rate of 1 mm/week, one can judge the duration of time since the acute severe event. This is a nonspecific "sick" test that is akin to an erythrocyte sedimentation rate (ESR)—the patient had severe illness but it is nonspecific to etiology.

Severe heart failure can manifest with red lunulae, i.e., **Terry's nails (Fig. 14.6)**. This is a very soft finding, which, at most, is the primary diagnosis. It may be useful in the setting of acute exacerbation of shortness of breath in a patient with congestive heart failure (CHF) and chronic obstructive pulmonary disease (COPD). Terry's nails may be a clue that heart failure is the predominant diagnosis.

Severe liver disease can manifest with proximal pale and distal pigmented nailbeds, i.e., **Lindsey's nails**. **Muercke's lines** manifest as narrow, alternate white and pink bands in the nail bed **(Fig. 14.7)**. These are caused by profound hypoalbuminemia, usually serum <2.0 g of albumin. These are variants of what the classic texts have referred to as the white nails or leukonychia of advanced liver disease.

Malignant melanoma of the nail bed manifests with a linear area of pigment in the nail bed that begins at the germinal matrix, grows outward, and slowly evolves from a very narrow triangle to a triangle with a base that becomes wider over time **(Fig. 14.8)**. Although it appears to be linear, on close inspection, it is triangular shaped; the base is wider than the apex and, over time, it grows outward and the base grows wider. No normal nail bed is seen between the base and the germinal matrix. **Splinter hemorrhages** manifest with one or more narrow purple or black lines in the nail bed. Each of these is parallel to the long axis of the finger. Each hemorrhage, as an entity, grows outward, thus there is always an area of normality proximal to each hemorrhage. Classically, this has been thought to be associated with endocarditis, but splinter hemorrhages more commonly result from mild trauma to the digit or psoriasis. **Longitudinal bands of pigment** manifest with a linear area of pigment in the nail plate itself.

Paronychia manifests with an area of pain, swelling, redness, and fluctuance in the lateral or medial nail fold **(Fig. 14.9)**. Often, there is antecedent or concurrent onychocryptosis, i.e., an ingrown nail. **Eponychium** manifests with an area of pain, swelling, redness, and fluctuance in the proximal nail fold. **Onychia** manifests with painful swelling and fluctuance under the entire nail plate. Eponychia are often caused by nail-biting. This manifests with a loss of the entire nail plate overhang; the plates appear to be chewed off for indeed they are. If there is a relative absence of pain to a paronychia, onychia, or eponychium, assess sensation to look for concurrent peripheral neuropathy.

Koilonychia manifests with spooning of the nail plates upward, i.e., concave up **(Fig. 14.10)**. This process usually affects all of the nail plates. Each plate appears as if a drop of water could be placed and kept on it. These are caused by either profound iron deficiency or significant erythrocytosis. The company koilonychia keeps is specific to the underlying cause. If caused by iron deficiency, there is angular cheilosis (Fig 1.44), fatigue, pale mucous membranes, and pica. Pica includes a craving for non-nutrient containing

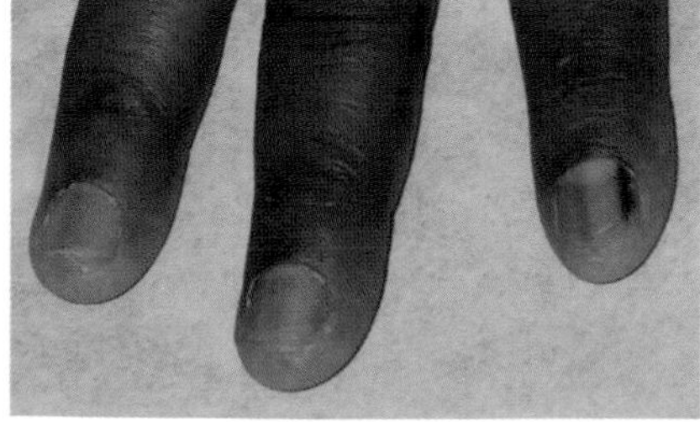

Figure 14.8.

Nail plate: longitudinal black band. Benign.

 **TIPS**

- Splinter hemorrhages: one or more longitudinal black lines; grow out over time, thus, always has a space of normal bed proximal
- Longitudinal bands (normal): increased pigment in a linear pattern in the nail plate
- Malignant melanoma: longitudinal dark line that grows out from the germinal matrix and to the sides so as to be trapezoid shaped

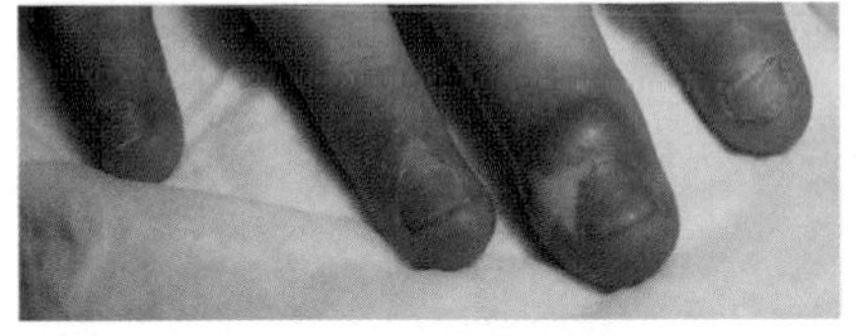

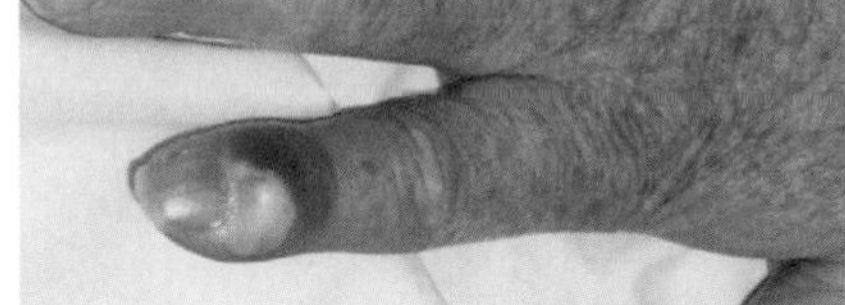

Figure 14.9.

A. Paronychia. **B.** Eponychium. Note the findings of nail-biting.

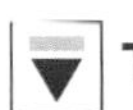 **TIPS**

- Paronychia: pus in lateral or medial fold
- Eponychium: pus in the proximal fold; highly correlated with nail-biting
- Onychia: fluctuant swelling beneath the entire nail plate

material, in this case red clay or ice. The patient need not be anemic to develop koilonychia. If the koilonychia is caused by erythrocytosis, the nail beds are often deep red, each suffused with blood; often, the individual lives at a high elevation. Thus, in the Himalayas, there is a high prevalence of koilonychia not only caused by erythrocytosis, but also iron deficiency from mild chronic blood loss from hookworm infection of the colon.

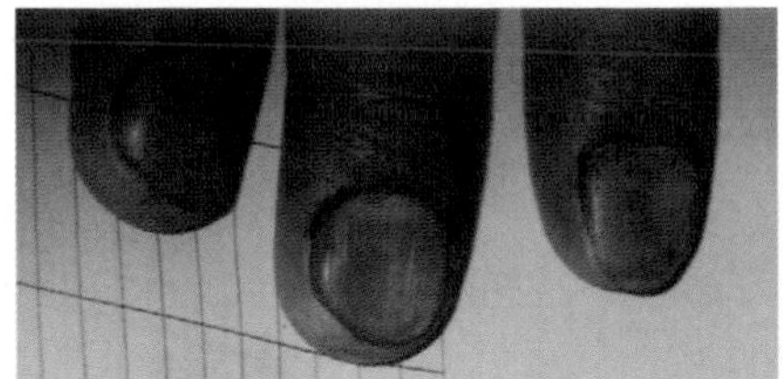

Figure 14.10.

Koilonychia in a patient with iron-deficiency anemia

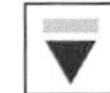 **TIPS**

- Koilonychia: nail plates are spoon-shaped, upward
- A drop of water could be placed in the spoon-shaped structure
- Associated with iron deficiency state or erythrocytosis
- Need not be anemic

TEACHING POINTS

NAILS

1. Primary nail lesions are very common: onychogryphosis, onychocryptosis, and onychomycosis.
2. Onychodystrophy: thickened, brittle nails occur with psoriasis: destruction is proximal to distal; in onychomycosis: destruction is distal to proximal.
3. Thickened nails can result from trauma, onychomycosis, arterial insufficiency, or psoriasis.
4. Onychocryptosis, i.e., ingrown nail, is a risk for paronychia.
5. Nail-biting, i.e., onychophagia, is a risk for eponychium.
6. Splinter hemorrhages are usually caused by trauma, but they may indicate endocarditis.
7. Any "splinter hemorrhage" that starts in the germinal matrix and grows outward without any normal bed between the proximal end and the germinal matrix, think malignant melanoma.
8. White or pale nail beds indicate anemia.
9. White nail plates, think severe liver disease.
10. Koilonychia indicates iron deficiency state or erythrocytosis.
11. Clubbing: specific criteria include flat angle (Lovibond's sign) and sponginess of the plate on the bed.
12. Clubbing affects fingernails, toenails, or both. Systemic disorders manifest with all four extremities involved; coarctation of the aorta manifests with three of the extremities involved, the right hand spared; ASD manifests with clubbing in toes.

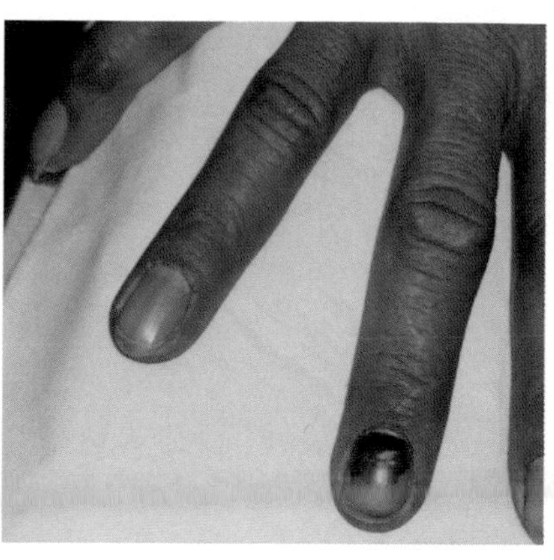

Figure 14.11.

Subungual hematoma.

TIPS

- Subungual hematoma: discrete tender blood collection under the nail plate
- Acute trauma to the fingertip
- Often a concurrent tuft fracture

Subungual hematoma manifests with an intense and specific tender area of purple beneath the nail plate (**Fig. 14.11**), which is a trauma-related collection of blood. These are common entities, most often caused by mild trauma involving the fingertip, such as pinching the fingertip in a door jam or any other crush or pinch-type injury involving the fingertip. The collection of blood increases the pressure and results in the pain. If there is an absence of pain in such a hematoma, consider a peripheral neuropathy.

Other problems include **Plummer's nails** of hyperthyroidism, which manifest with distal onycholysis of all of the nail plates. The nail plates are diffusely thin. Hyperthyroidism manifestations are discussed in Chapter 1, page 31. **Onychocryptosis** manifests with an ingrowth of the nail plate into the skin adjacent to the nail, usually on the medial or the lateral side. This is often caused by a poor nail-cutting technique or chronic trauma. **Anemia**, which manifests with a **pale** color to all of the nail beds, correlates with a hemoglobin level <10 g. The company anemia keeps includes pale mucous membranes, pale palmar, skin creases, fatigue, tachycardia, and signs of high-output heart failure.

HAIR: HEAD AND BODY

Androgen-mediated alopecia manifests with a temporal and occipital loss of hair (**Table 14.2**), more commonly seen in men. If in a woman, ask about other signs of virilization, i.e., increased androgens including hirsutism of facial, chest and abdominal hair, deep voice, and secondary amenorrhea. In women, such manifestations may be caused by polycystic ovary syndrome (PCO); if so, assess also for diabetes mellitus. **Arterial insufficiency alopecia** manifests with a local alopecia in the distribution of the arterial insufficiency. This type is especially evident in the lower extremities. The company it keeps includes the absence of palpable pulses in the area; often, bruits are present in the femoral or aortic areas and the capillary refill is moderately to markedly delayed. **Venous stasis dermatitis alopecia** manifests with local alopecia in the affected areas, especially the lower extremities. The company it keeps includes bilateral brownish-purple pigment, which is hemosiderin-deposited in the skin. There is thinning, atrophy, and mild edema of the affected areas. The pulses are usually present in venous stasis. **Discoid lupus** manifests with destructive alopecia, with concurrent loss of skin pigment and all skin appendages in the affected areas. **Tinea capitis** manifests with patches that may have scales and a destructive alopecia. Hair in the area of alopecia will have broken shafts. On Wood lamp examination, the affected areas are fluorescent. There may be sequelae, including kerion or favus formation. **Kerion** manifests with a nodular or plaquelike lesion on the scalp. This is an area of matted, granulation tissue, skin, hair, fungus, and exudates with an overlying crust. **Favus** manifests with a patch or plaque of granulation tissue at the base of a patch of tinea capitis related alopecia. **Alopecia areata** manifests with patches of hair loss, especially on the head; the skin affected does not fluoresce with Wood lamp examination. If the alopecia areata is caused by thyroid disease, look for other signs of **hyperthyroidism**, specifically thin hair, or **hypothyroidism**, specifically thickened coarse hair and additional alopecia specific to the lateral eyebrows, i.e., Queen Anne's sign. **Trichotillomania** manifests with patchy loss from chronic pulling of hair; concurrent nail-biting is very common. **Secondary lues venereum** manifests with patches of alopecia, classically termed "moth-eaten" appearance. The company it keeps includes antecedent chancre, concurrent manifestations of secondary lues, including an exanthem rash that

Table 14.2. Alopecia

Diagnosis	Hair manifestations	Company it Keeps
Androgen-mediated	Frontal, temporal and occipital loss	Facial hair—beard Chest hair
Arterial insufficiency	Loss in a specific distribution, usually lower extremities	Diminished pulses Delayed capillary refill Cool extremity
Venous stasis	Loss in a specific distribution, usually lower extremities Increased pigmentation in skin, varicosities, and mild edema	Increasing age
Discoid lupus	Destructive alopecia Loss of skin pigment Antecedent malar red rash	Other systemic lupus features
Tinea capitis	Patches with scales with a destructive alopecia Breakage of the hair shafts Fluorescence present	Kerion Favus
Alopecia areata	Patches of hair loss, predominantly on head; regrows	Autoimmune disorders, especially thyroid disease
Queen Anne's sign	Lateral eyebrow alopecia	Hypothyroidism Delayed relaxation phase of reflexes
Trichotillomania	Habitual, obsessive hair-pulling and hair-eating	Nail-biting (onychophagia) Early satiety from a bezoar
Secondary lues venereum	Patches of hair loss Moth-eaten appearance	History of chancre Concurrent papulosquamous rash

TEACHING POINTS

HAIR

1. Localized hair loss on an extremity is usually caused by arterial insufficiency or venous stasis changes.
2. Patchy hair loss can be caused by tinea capitis, discoid lupus, trichotillomania alopecia areata, or thyroid disease.
3. Onychophagia, nail-biting, is common in patients with trichotillomania and trichophagia.
4. Androgen-related alopecia is loss of head hair in temporal and occipital areas.
5. Complications of tinea capitis can include alopecia, favus, or kerion.
6. Areas involved with tinea capitis are fluorescent with a Wood lamp examination.
7. Hypothyroid clues include Queen Anne's sign and thickened strands of hair.
8. Destructive alopecia, i.e., loss of hair and skin substance, can be caused by tinea capitis, burns, discoid lupus, and secondary lues venereum.

involves palms and soles and/or condylomata of skin folds and/or mucous patches in oral mucosa. This is the second (and a systemic) phase of an infection with the spirochete *Treponema pallidum*. **Hirsutism** manifests with the development of hair growth in areas that do not normally bear hair. Most commonly seen in women, it includes hair growth on the face (a beard), and increased hair on chest and abdomen, in a diamond-shaped pattern of hair from the mid-pubis to the umbilicus. Such hirsutism can be caused by polycystic ovary disease (see above). Hirsutism can also manifest with **lanugo** hair, i.e., soft downy-type hair, which may be caused by a paraneoplastic syndrome.

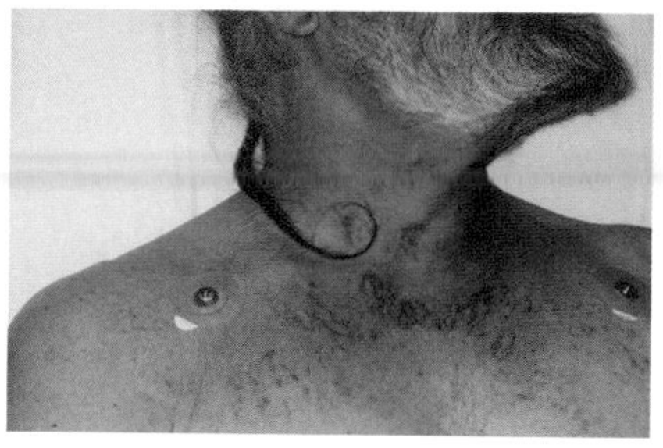

Figure 14.12.

Telangiectasia, here in a patient with superior vena cava (SVC) syndrome.

 **TIPS**

- Dilated vessels in the skin
- Thin in caliber, often multiple
- May or may not blanch with pressure
- Most common reason: atrophy of skin, from solar or actinic changes or use of topical steroids

PURPLE LESIONS

Telangiectasia manifests with dilated vessels in the skin. The vessels are small in caliber and in length (3 to 10 mm) **(Fig. 14.12)**. These are often multiple, but often do not blanch. They are caused by atrophic or thinned skin as the result of topical steroid use or are solar (ultraviolet light) related. Small in size, they are often noted in atrophic or solar-damaged skin. **Spider angioma** manifests with one or more purple spider-shaped lesions **(Fig. 14.13)**. Each lesion has a central pinpoint vessel and vessels radiating outward. The entire structure collapses on placing pressure on the center, and refills with release. These structures, which are located invariably on the shoulders and trunk, are caused most often by elevated estrogen levels. The company spider angiomas keep include end-stage liver disease-related palmar erythema, gynecomastia in males, ascites, asterixis, and abdominal venous collaterals. In addition to end-stage liver disease, spider angiomas may be due to the use of estrogen or estrogen-like agents, e.g., hormonal therapy for prostate carcinoma or may develop during pregnancy. **Coagulopathy** manifests with petechia, purpura, and/or ecchymosis. **Petechiae** are 2 to 5 mm in size and nonblanching; they most often result from quantitative or qualitative problems with platelets. **Purpura** are 5 to 15 mm in size, nonblanching, palpable, or flat. Purpura is due to vasculitis, use of warfarin, liver disease-related, coagulopathy, or typhus. The company purpura keeps helps make the diagnosis. **Ecchymosis** or bruises are >15 mm in size. Primarily nonspecific, they most often result from blunt trauma, i.e., a "black and blue" mark of a healing contusion. Always palpate the area, because there may be a large underlying **hematoma**.

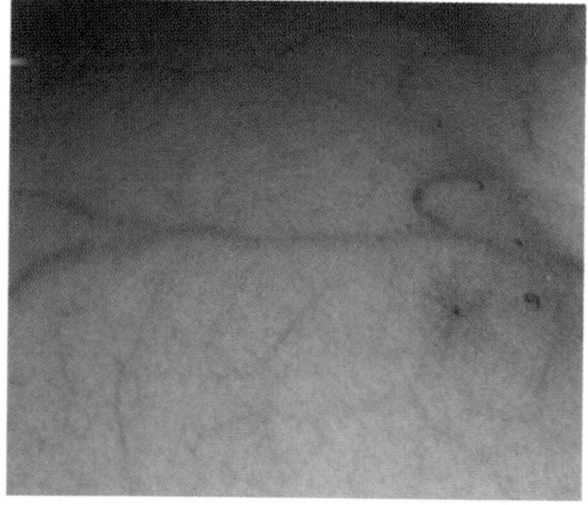

Figure 14.13.

Spider angioma. Lesion collapses on placing pressure on center and refills on release.

 **TIPS**

- Spider angioma: purple spider-shaped lesion; central pinpoint vessel and vessels radiating outward
- Structure collapses when pressure is placed on the center
- Refills with release

Cherry hemangioma manifests with one or more red-purple papule **(Fig. 14.14)**. Nontender and nonblanching, they are invariably benign and increase in prevalence with increasing age.

Port-wine stain, also called nevus flammeus, manifests with a purple, nonblanching patch on the skin. The entity appears to be the purple color of port wine. These patches can be large and, other than of cosmetic concern to the patient, produce little problem. One of the most well-known examples is the port-wine stain on the head of Mikhail Gorbachev. **Sturge-Weber syndrome** manifests with a port-wine stain in the first zone of the trigeminal nerve (V1), with concurrent recurrent seizures, and intracranial calcifications. **Janeway lesions** manifest with one or more purple, nonblanching, purpuric lesions on the plantar aspect of the feet or the palmar aspect of the hands **(Fig. 14.15)**. There is a significant overlap with **Osler's nodes**, which manifest with purple, tender swelling of the pads of the distal digits. Some authors have stated that these are probably manifestations of the same pathophysiology as in endocarditis. Both are caused by endocarditis and the company they keep includes fever, Roth (Litten) spots in the retina on funduscopic examination (Fig 15.29), splinter hemorrhages in the nail beds, and new heart murmur or any diastolic heart murmur. Also, the patient may have evidence of the underlying etiology including severe gingivitis, a history of recent dental work, active intravenous drug abuse, or rheumatic fever. These are pieces of company that need to be looked for in the evaluation of the patient's primary complaint, e.g., fever.

Scurvy manifests with multiple perifollicular hemorrhages **(Fig. 14.16)**. The distribution is classically referred to as being in a saddle pattern, i.e., as if the patient has been riding on a horse. The individual hair strands are dysmorphic, likened to an appearance after having been singed by an open flame. In addition, there are multiple sizes, locations, and ages of ecchymosis and often multiple purpura. Often, severe, even purulent, gingivitis is present. Scurvy is caused by a deficiency of vitamin C, something that remains common in malnourished and alcoholic patients. **Subcutaneous heparin or insulin injections** manifest with purpura and ecchymoses of various ages in the abdominal wall or in the skin of the anterior thigh; each at a site of injection. Concurrent dimpling of the skin may be noted because of adipose atrophy (insulin lipodystrophy).

Kaposi's sarcoma (KS) manifests with one or more nontender, palpable purpura, often in a clustering pattern **(Fig. 14.17)**. The lesions can be fragile

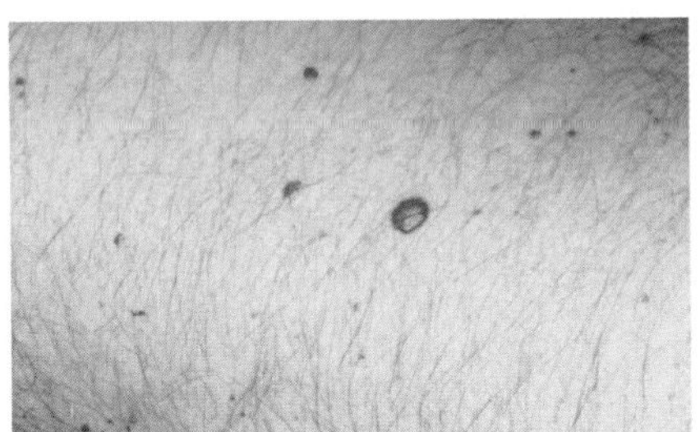

Figure 14.14.

Cherry hemangioma.

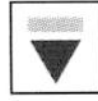 **TIPS**

- Cherry hemangioma: red-purple papules, nontender, nonblanching
- Benign: increasing prevalence with increasing age

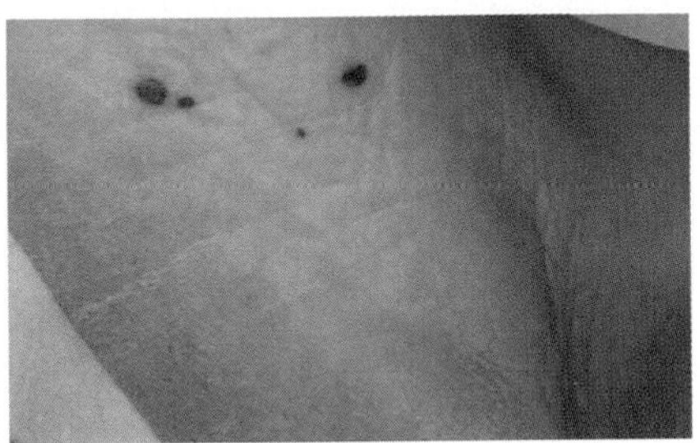

A

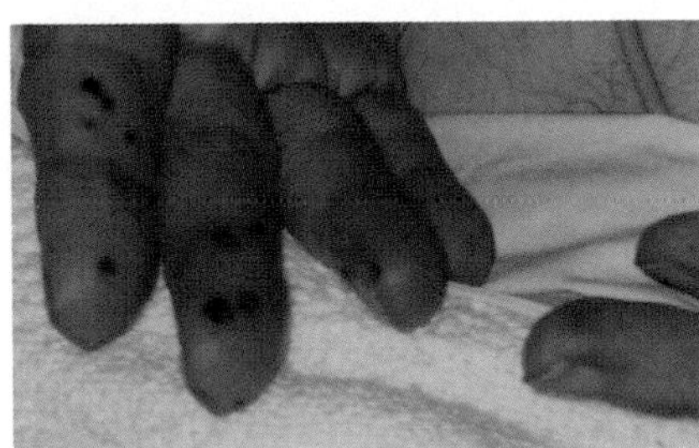

B

Figure 14.15.

Janeway lesions and Osler's nodes in the feet **(A)** and the hands **(B)**.

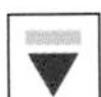 **TIPS**

- Janeway lesions: nonblanching, purpuric lesions on the plantar aspect of the feet or the palms of the hands
- Osler's nodes: tender, blue nodules on finger or toe pads, with a marked overlap between the two
- Concurrent Roth spots, splinter hemorrhages, and fever
- Endocarditis-related
- Most commonly found on the plantar aspect of the feet

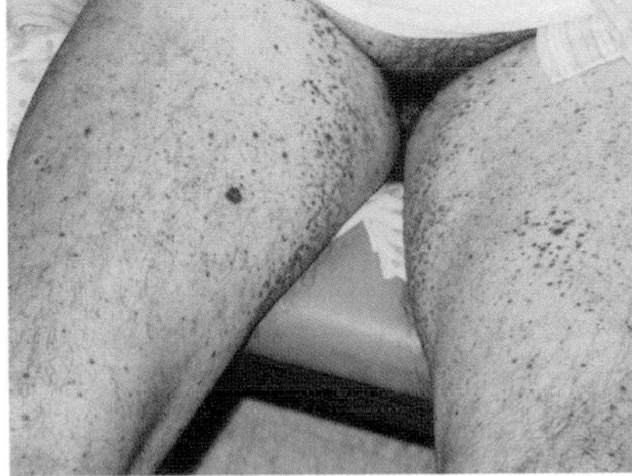

Figure 14.16.

Scurvy.

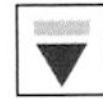 **TIPS**

- Perifollicular hemorrhages and dysmorphic hair
- Multiple ecchymosis in the skin
- Often saddle-distribution of lesions

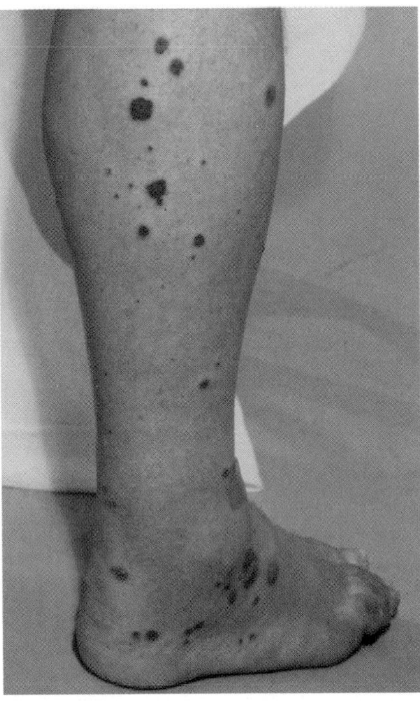

Figure 14.17.

Kaposi's sarcoma in a patient with acquired immunodeficiency syndrome (AIDS).

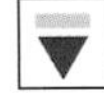 **TIPS**

- Kaposi's sarcoma: nontender, palpable purpura; often in clusters
- Older individuals: limited to the feet and indolent
- Human immunodeficiency virus (HIV)-related: any skin or mucous membrane surface and very aggressive

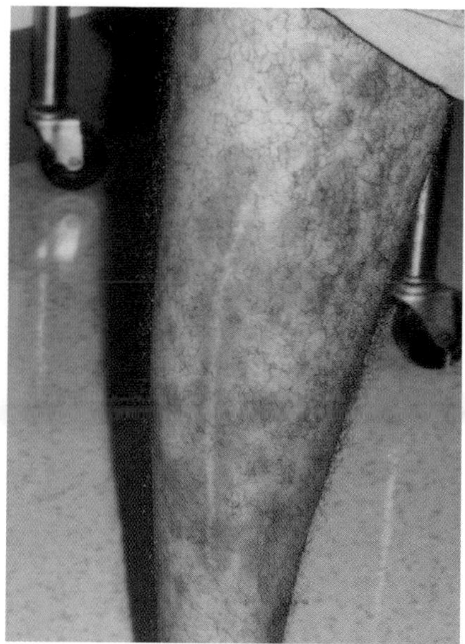

A

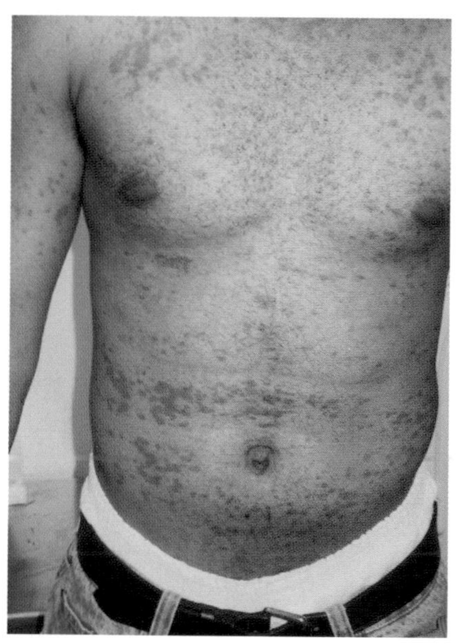

B

Figure 14.18.

Lichen planus

TIPS

- Lichen planus: clusters of severely pruritic papules and plaques; specific lesions pigmented to purple
- Concurrent bullae and mucous membrane involvement are common
- Wickstram's striae: a white, reticulated network on individual lesions
- Koebner's phenomenon is a feature of rash
- Associated with gold therapy and graft-versus-host disease

and bleed easily. In older individuals, they are located on the feet and are relatively indolent; in human immunodeficiency virus (HIV)-related disease, they occur anywhere and have a very aggressive natural history. In patients with HIV disease, its presence is acquired immunodeficiency syndrome (AIDS)-defining. Kaposi's sarcoma is correlated with, and perhaps the result of, infection with herpes simplex type 8. KS has become much less prevalent over the past several years.

Lichen planus manifests with clusters of markedly pruritic papules and plaques **(Fig. 14.18)**. The individual lesions are pigmented to purple in color and have discrete polygonal borders. The rash has a classic **Koebner's phenomenon**, i.e., the lesions occur in areas of scar, areas of irritation, or skin trauma. There may be concurrent bulla formation in the skin and in the mucous membranes. Each lesion may have a discrete white lacy pattern on its surface; this pattern is called **Wickstram's striae**. Today, the most common reason for this rash is related to graft-versus-host disease; in the past, it has been associated with the administration of gold and other therapies for rheumatoid arthritis.

Grey Turner's sign manifests with a nonblanching, nontender ecchymosis on the flank **(Fig. 14.19)**, which can become very large and may be associated with ecchymosis surrounding the umbilicus (Cullen's sign). Although traditionally thought to be a manifestation of hemorrhagic pancreatitis, this is an extremely rare cause of it, one for which we have looked for the past 20 years and yet have not seen. More to the point is that the sign of Grey Turner is a manifestation of any retroperitoneal bleed. Specific causes of retroperitoneal bleeds include coagulopathy, warfarin-related, kidney fracture, ruptured ectopic pregnancy, pelvic or hip fracture, and indeed hemorrhagic pancreatitis.

Blue finger or toe syndrome manifests with blue or black discoloration of the tips of the toes or fingers (Fig 10.30) **(Table 14.3)**. These are often painful and may progress to frank ulceration, infarctions, and dry gangrene. This syndrome is invariably a manifestation of an underlying disorder, if caused by nicotine-related **thromboangiitis obliterans** (Buerger's disease). The company it keeps includes a history of cigarette smoking and nicotine staining of the nail plates and fingertips **(Fig. 14.20)**. If caused by **second-degree frostbite**, there should be a recent history of exposure to extreme cold.

Table 14.3. **Causes of Blue Finger and Toes**

Diagnosis	Local manifestations	Company it Keeps
Raynaud's syndrome	On exposure to cold: Red to white, then to blue of any fingertip of toe tip	Cryoglobulinemia Autoimmune process Sarcoidosis If on nose, lupus pernio
Buerger's disease	Blue to black infarcts, Painful tips of fingers/toes	Smoking Chewing tobacco Nicotine stains
Atrial fibrillation	Blue, painful in distribution of an artery, side of digit	Congestive heart failure Cerebrovascular accidents
Frostbite	Bulla, hemorrhagic Bulla, and blue or black Areas involving distal	Exposure to severe cold
Janeway lesions	Purpuric lesions on palms and soles	Fever Back pain Heart murmur Recent dental work

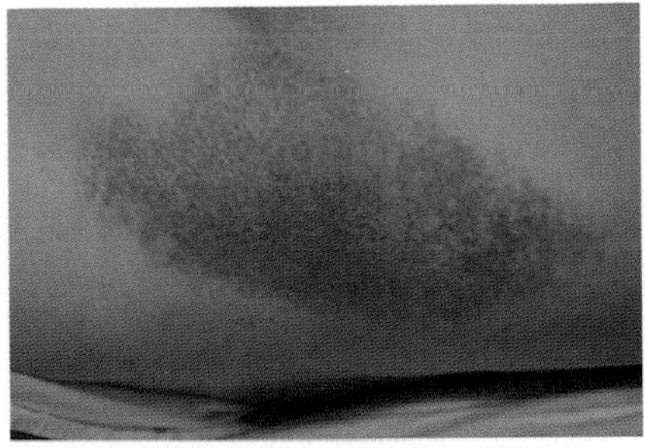

Figure 14.19.

Grey Turner's sign of retroperitoneal blood.

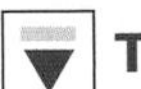

TIPS

- Nonblanching ecchymosis on the flank
- Caused by a retroperitoneal bleed

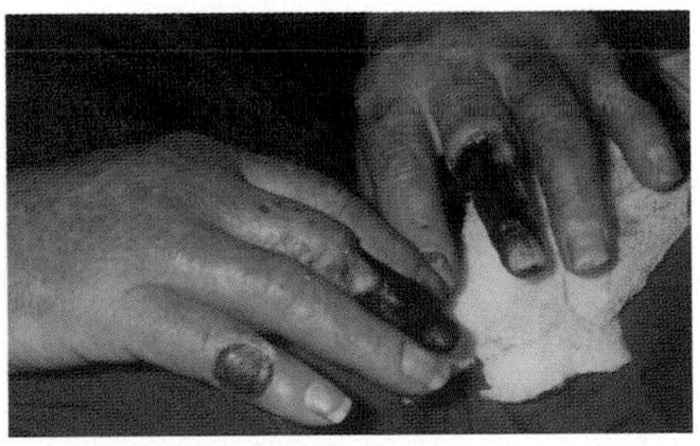

Figure 14.20.

Thromboangiitis obliterans (Buerger's disease)–nicotine-related infarctions of digits.

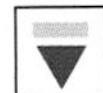

TIPS

- Buerger's disease: bilateral, blue to black fingers and toes
- Caused by nicotine Usually, concurrent nicotine stains on the nail plates

If caused by **Raynaud's syndrome**, related symptoms include a classic history of the normal, baseline pink-*red* colored digits that, on exposure to cold temperature, acutely becomes *white*, with throbbing pain and cold digits, which then develop a profound *blue* color. Raynaud, a French physician, described using the metaphor of the classic tricolor of his native country for this process. This phenomenon can ocur in any digit or appendage exposed to cold temperatures and is, indeed, a cold-mediated vasospasm. The underlying cause of Raynaud's phenomenon may be an autoimmune process, rheumatoid arthritis, or sarcoidosis. If the nose is the specific site, it is called **lupus pernio**. If caused by **embolic** events, it may be from endocarditis or atrial fibrillation. If caused by **endocarditis**, the company it keeps includes fevers, heart murmurs, and Roth spots; if caused by **atrial fibrillation**, the company it keeps includes an irregularly irregular heart rhythm.

Erythema nodosum manifests with one or more, usually multiple tender nodules **(Fig. 14.21)**. These are red or purple in color and often are located on the extensor surfaces of the legs. Although called erythema nodosum, more nodules are actually purple and, thus, the condition is discussed here. The company it keeps is specific to the underlying cause. If caused by **sarcoidosis**, these include Achilles tendonitis, polyarticular arthritis, interstitial lung disease with dry crackles on lung examination, the red-eye of anterior uveitis, Raynaud's phenomenon, and lupus pernio. If caused by **inflammatory bowel disease**, these include pyoderma gangrenosum (Fig. 14.62), bloody diarrhea, sclerosing cholangitis-related tenderness to the right upper quadrant, and a Murphy's sign (Fig 6.18). Finally, injected conjunctiva of anterior uveitis (Fig 15.19) may be noted. If caused by **ankylosing spondylitis**, these include polyarticular large joint arthritis, sacroiliitis, ankylosis with a decreased lumbar stretch with forward bend at the trunk (Schober's maneuver) (Fig 12.13), and restrictive pulmonary disease. In addition, a diastolic murmur of aortic insufficiency (Fig 4.19) may be noted.

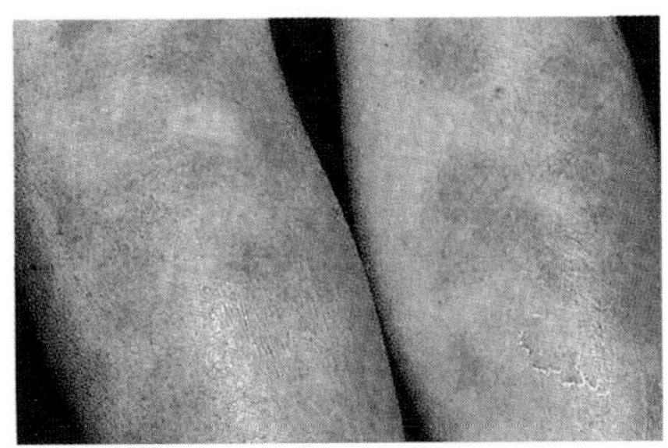

Figure 14.21.

Erythema nodosum.

TIPS

- Erythema nodosum: distinct palpable, purple nodules, each very tender
- Most often on the extensor surfaces
- Caused by sarcoidosis, ulcerative colitis, or ankylosing spondylitis

Heliotropic rash of dermatomyositis manifests with multiple purple macules and patches on or around the eyelids **(Fig. 14.22)**. In point of fact, the periorbital areas appear to be stained purple. The patient often has concurrent proximal muscle weakness of the upper and lower extremities and a waddling-type gait. Often, erythematous plaques and papules are noted on the dorsum of fingers (Gottron's papules). These are especially evident on the

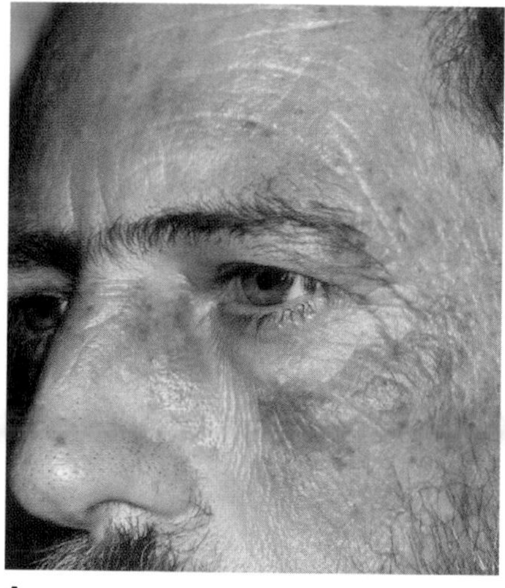

A

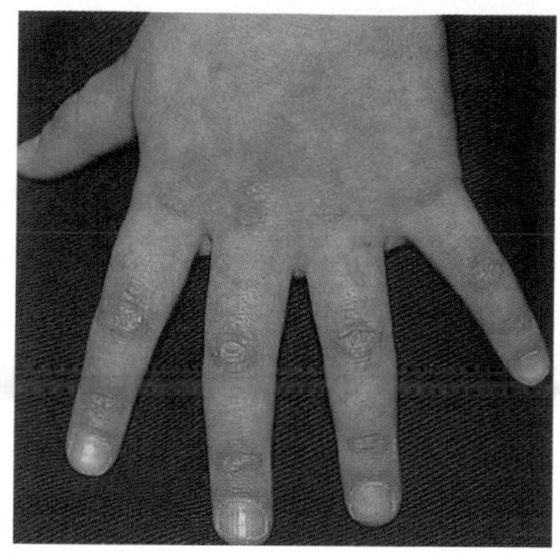

B

Figure 14.22.

A. Heliotropic rash of dermatomyositis. **B.** Gottron's papules of dermatomyositis.

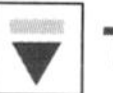 **TIPS**

- Dermatomyositis: purple staining in the eye area; also termed a heliotropic rash **(A)**
- Concurrent Gottron's papules on the dorsum of finger and proximal muscle weakness are likely **(B)**

middle phalanges. This is associated with an underlying autoimmune process or as a paraneoplastic process from an adenocarcinoma.

Scabies manifests with multiple reddish-purple pruritic papules (**Fig. 14.23**). These often appear in lines or "runs." The distribution is such that a greater number of lesions are at skin folds; there is a predilection for the lesions to be in the webs between the fingers and toes, in the axillae, in the inguinal area, under the breasts, and in gluteal folds and cleft. Often seen are concurrent pustules of a secondary bacterial infection. In severe cases or in patients with immunocompromise, the adjacent skin may be hypertrophied with concurrent granulation tissue. This highly infectious variant is called

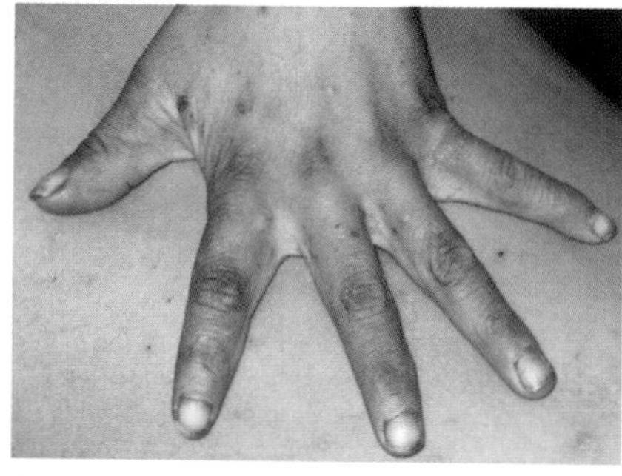

A

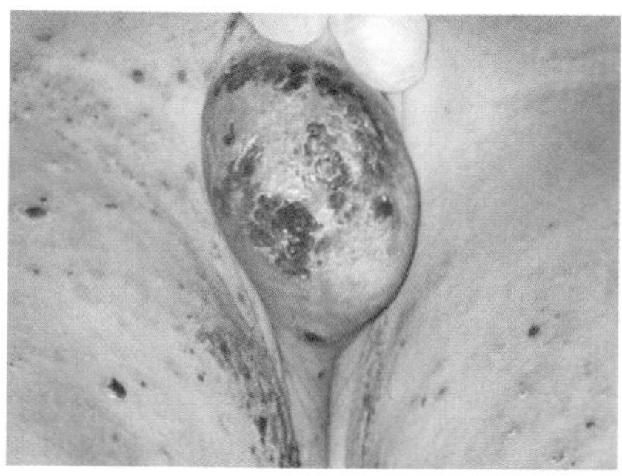

B

Figure 14.23.

Scabies, Norwegian variant; with hypertrophy of skin.

 **TIPS**

- Scabies: multiple, purple-red pruritic papules, often in lines, extremely pruritic
- Increased number in and around the skin folds

TEACHING POINTS

PURPLE LESIONS

1. Spider angiomas are unique vascular structures associated with increased estrogen states.
2. Petechiae, purpura, and ecchymosis are the primary descriptors for purple lesions.
3. Petechiae are the most specific; they are associated with thrombocytopenia and decreased function of platelets.
4. Purpura is associated with inflammatory disease or coagulopathy, but remains relatively nonspecific.
5. Ecchymosis is nonspecific bruising.
6. Endocarditis can manifest with Janeway lesions (purpura) and Osler's nodes (swollen palmar and plantar pad lesions).
7. Blue digits can be caused by emboli, Raynaud's phenomenon, Buerger's disease, or frostbite.
8. Dermatomyositis manifests with proximal muscle weakness, Gottron's papules, and a heliotropic rash in the eye area.
9. Purple-red pruritic papules in lines: must consider scabies.

Norwegian scabies. Because this rash is common and can be nonspecific early in its course, always remember to include it in the differential diagnosis of pruritic purple to red papules or pustules.

PINK AND RED LESIONS

Tinea cruris manifests with a moist, erythematous rash in the groin **(Fig. 14.24)**. Groin is defined as the skin folds between the thigh and scrotum or thigh and labia majora. The rash causes significant problems in that it is intensely pruritic, and can have concurrent papules, vesicles, and even pustules. Tinea cruris is usually caused by infection with *Candida albicans*. Concurrent balanitis, balanoposthitis (Fig 2.4), vulvovaginitis, or onychomycosis (Fig 14.1) are not uncommon.

Tinea corporis manifests as a solitary annular lesion with central clearing and scales on its outer rim **(Fig. 14.25)**. The lesion, which grows centripetally and is moderately pruritic, is usually located on the trunk, back, or thighs. The scales are flakes of epidermis that are infected by the fungus. Classically called "ringworm," akin to the "fairy-ring" pattern of fungi growth in nature, tinea corporis grows outward with central clearing. It may be associated with having a dog with a similar skin infection in the house.

Erythrasma manifests with moderately pruritic, bright red confluent patches in the axillae or groin **(Fig. 14.26)**. A unique feature is that on Wood lamp examination it is fluorescent coral red. This is a rash that looks like tinea cruris, but does not respond to topical or even systemic antifungals. Instead, it is a superficial skin infection with *Corynebacterium* sps.

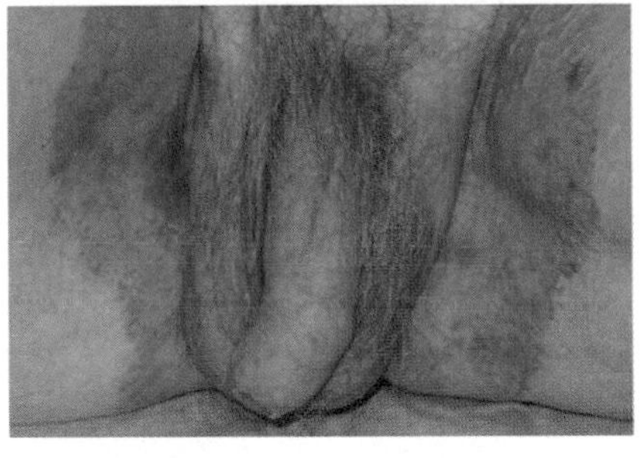

Figure 14.24.

Tinea cruris.

 **TIPS**

- Tinea cruris: moist, erythematous rash on skin of the groin
- Moderate to intense pruritus
- Usually caused by *Candida albicans*
- Concurrent balanitis or vulvovaginitis is common

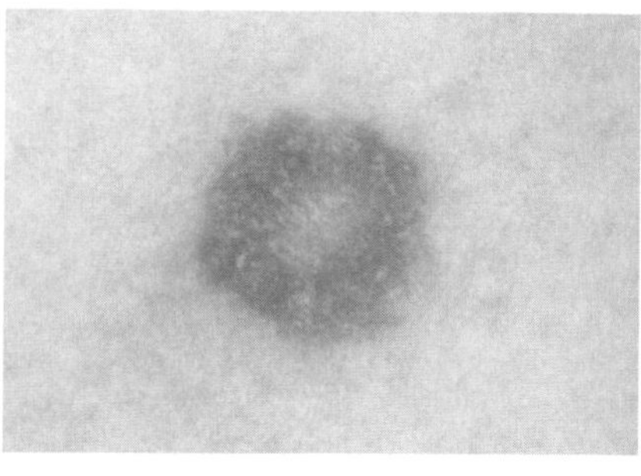

Figure 14.25.

Tinea corporis, ringworm.

 TIPS

- Tinea corporis: solitary, annular lesion, with central clearing, and scales on its outer rim
- Lesion grows centripetally; is moderately pruritic

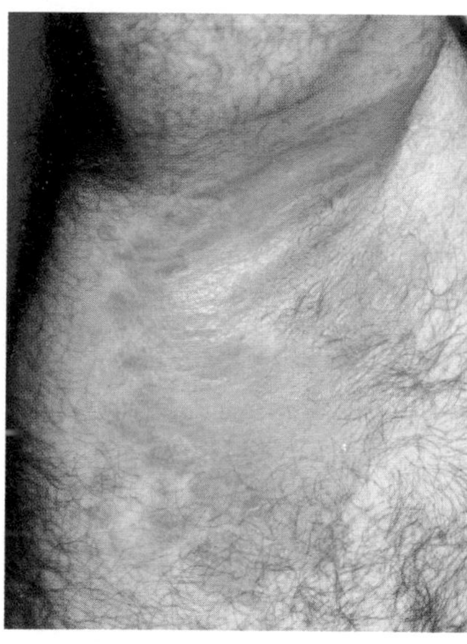

Figure 14.26.

Erythrasma.

 TIPS

- Erythrasma: bright red confluent patches in the axillae or groin
- Moderately pruritic
- Caused by *Corynebacterium* infection
- Wood's lamp reveals coral-red color

Tinea pedis manifests with moderately to markedly pruritic confluent patches of redness in a moccasin distribution on the plantar aspects of both feet **(Fig. 14.27)**. Often, scales, crackles, and even vesicles are noted at the rim of the lesion. This is akin to a large "ringworm" around the plantar foot.

Cellulitis manifests with a warm red rash, confluent patches, or plaques in a relatively discrete topographic area **(Fig. 14.28)**. The areas may be tender and mildly pruritic, but the tenderness is rarely significant. In addition, often mild to moderate nonpitting edema is present, which is a mild form of localized angioedema. Usually, this is associated with a break in the skin. Examples of such breaks in the skin include an animal or insect bite, a scrape, a crack from a fungal infection, or a puncture wound. Uncontrolled diabetes mellitus can worsen the course and increase the risk of development of a cellulitis. The most common organisms are the gram-positives, *Staphylococcus* and *Streptococcus sps.*; however, anaerobes and gram-negative rods may con-

Figure 14.27.

Tinea pedis.

 TIPS

- Erythema in a moccasin distribution on the plantar or side aspect of the feet
- Moderately to markedly pruritic
- Often scales and even a few vesicles may be present at rim

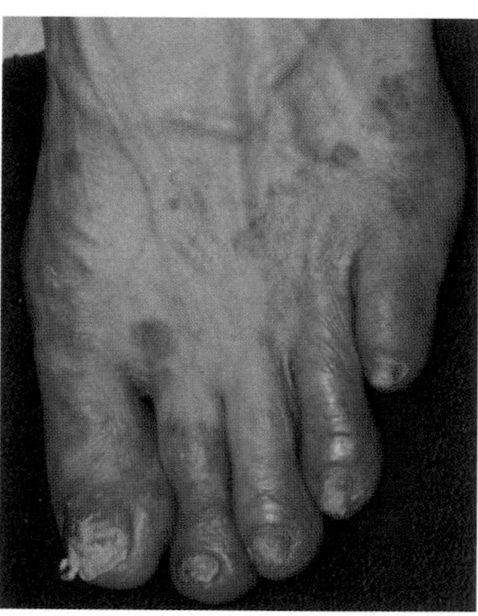

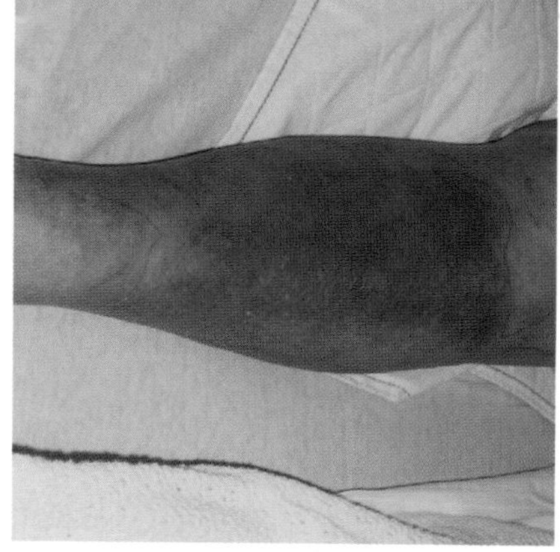

A

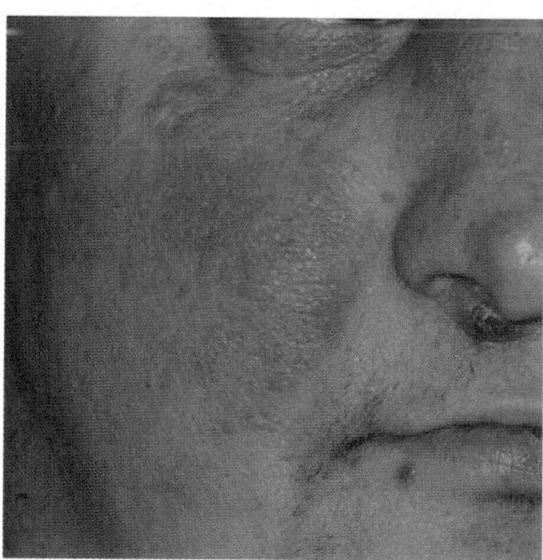

B

Figure 14.28.

A. Cellulitis. **B.** Erysipelas in a patient with Down syndrome.

 TIPS

- Cellulitis: warm red rash, either patch- or plaquelike with discernible edges; may be tender and mildly pruritic, concurrent systemic fever is common
- Erysipelas: superficial, bright red and very warm to hot, nontender, nonpruritic, progressively and rapidly expanding patchlike rash; concurrent high fever very likely

tribute, especially in cellulitis in the *foot* of a patient with diabetes mellitus. **Erysipelas** manifests with a superficial bright red rash. The rash is very warm to hot to the touch and not tender. It has discrete borders and expands rapidly and progressively. It is often on the face, with concurrent fever to 104°F very likely. The infected skin has a superficial thick crust, which appears as a superficial peau d'orange effect in the skin. Erysipelas is most common in immunocompromised patients such as those on high-dose steroids, and those who are neutropenic or who have uncontrolled diabetes mellitus. Untreated, this is a life-threatening infection caused by *Streptococcus sps.* In the preantibiotic era, it was a common reason for mortal streptococcal infections.

Impetigo manifests with an erythematous, well-demarcated patch or plaque with concurrent crust, ooze, and golden yellow discharge. There may be secondary blister or bulla formation, in which case the impetigo is called **bullous impetigo (Fig 14.80)**. This is a superficial infection with *Streptococcus* sps. or, specifically in bullous impetigo, *Staphylococcal* sps. See discussion of bullae below. **Rosacea** manifests with a bilateral diffuse red rash on the face that involves and even focuses on the nose **(Fig. 14.29)**. Noted are concurrent nodules, pustules, and telangiectasia in the skin of the face, and around the auricles and the nose. Concurrent rhinophyma is common (Fig 1.17).

Contact dermatitis manifests with moderately to intensely pruritic plaques and papules of erythema **(Fig. 14.30)**. Often seen are multiple excoriations, and the lesions are weeping and crusting. The lesions are often adjacent to a site of exposure to a detergent, soap, metal, latex, or resin from a plant, e.g., poison ivy or oak. Of interest, nickel-alloy metal often is a cause of dermatitis. Examples of this include inexpensive gold jewelry.

Atopic dermatitis-eczema manifests with moderate to severe pruritus and plaques, patches, and red papules **(Fig. 14.31)**. The pattern is symmetric on the flexor surfaces, i.e., the antecubital and popliteal surfaces, and in distribution. Rarely are there vesicles; there is a history of recurrent flares and excoriations and secondary thickening of the affected skin. When chronic the skin may become woody or lichenified. The company eczema keeps includes a family history of eczema and a personal or family history of asthma.

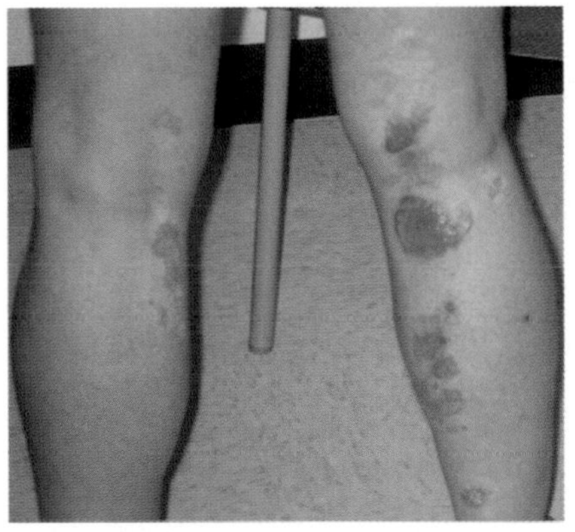

A

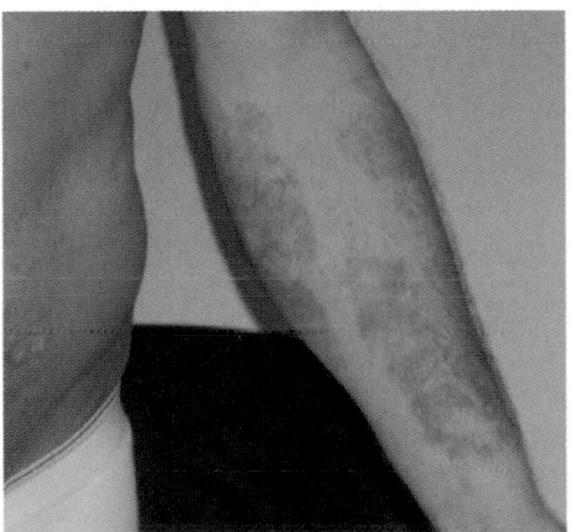

B

Figure 14.31.

Atopic dermatitis.

TIPS

- Atopic dermatitis: red patches and papules; rarely with vesicles
- Moderate pruritus
- Bilateral pattern on flexor surfaces, i.e., antecubital and popliteal surfaces

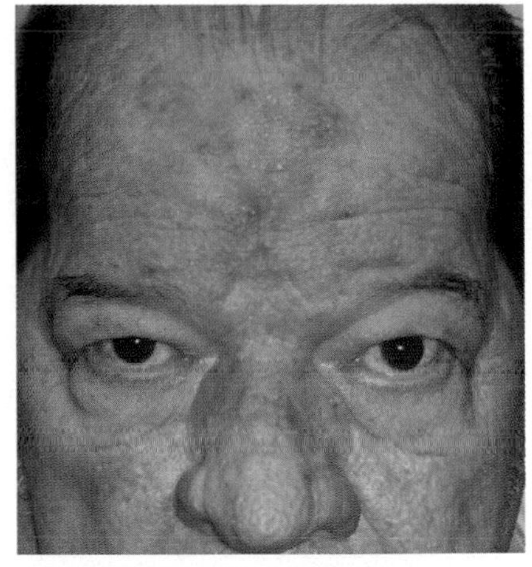

Figure 14.29.

Rosacea.

TIPS

- Rosacea: red papular rash on the face bilaterally focuses on the nose; concurrent telangiectasia
- Concurrent rhinophyma common

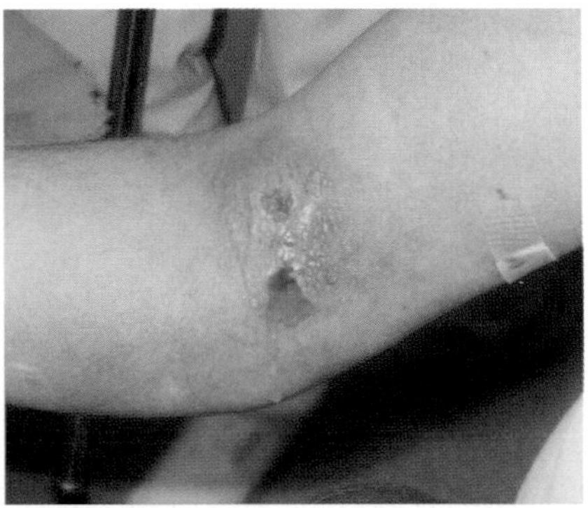

Figure 14.30

Classic contact dermatitis.

TIPS

- Contact dermatitis: intense plaques and papules of erythema, with excoriations
- Weeping and crusting adjacent to the lesions
- May have vesicles or bullae in the mix
- Often adjacent to a site of exposure to a detergent, soap, nickel, latex, or resin from a plant, e.g., poison ivy or poison oak

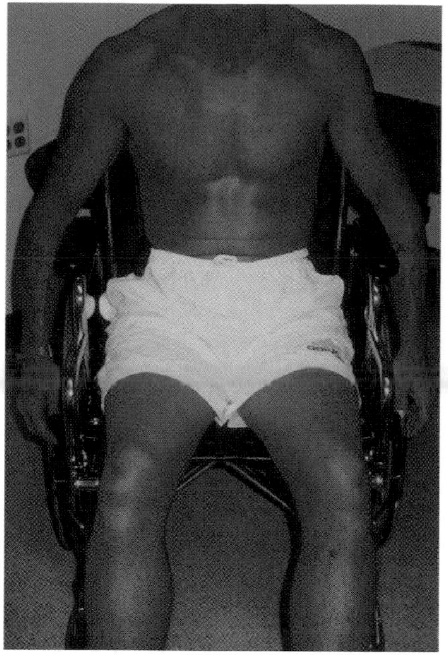

Figure 14.32.

Photodermatitis, i.e. sunburn; here, severe and remarkably diffuse

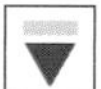 **TIPS**

- Photodermatitis: warm, blanching, nonpruritic red rash
- In and over areas of skin exposed to solar or ultraviolet (UV) light
- Distinct margins are common

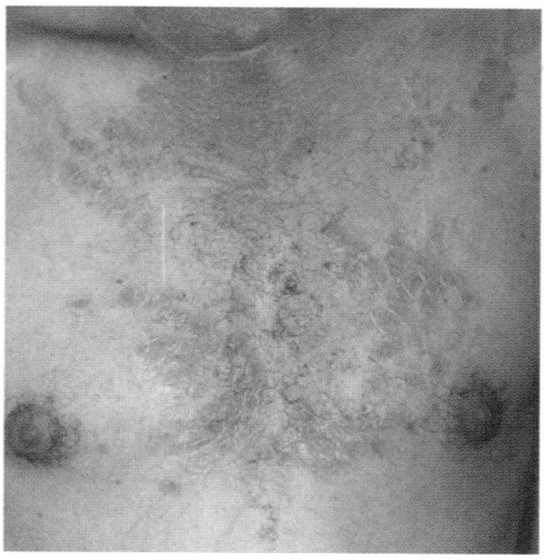

Figure 14.33.

Seborrheic dermatitis.

 **TIPS**

- Seborrheic dermatitis: erythema and scaly rash in and near the eyelashes, the hairline, and the hair of the chest and head; greasy scales, concurrent dandruff
- Often, concurrent blepharitis

Drug-induced dermatitis manifests with a bright red maculopapular rash on the trunk and back. The rash is not warm, has moderate pruritus, begins on the trunk, and spreads peripherally. Early in the course, an agent or drug is associated with rash development.

Photodermatitis-sunburn manifests with a warm, blanching red rash, which is not pruritic, in and over areas of skin exposed to solar or ultraviolet (UV) light **(Fig. 14.32)**. There are distinct margins, e.g., bikini lines, associated with it. In severe cases, bulla formation may be noted. This is an important public health issue in that burns are strongly associated with increased risk for skin cancer. Thus, prevention with sun screen is of extreme importance to all individuals.

Seborrheic dermatitis manifests with a scaly rash of red papules and patches in and near the eyelashes, the hairlines, and the hair of the chest and head **(Fig. 14.33)**. The scales are greasy and have a high concurrence with dandruff and blepharitis.

Nummular eczema manifests with scaly, moderately pruritic, erythematous plaques on the extensor surfaces, especially the legs **(Fig. 14.34)**. The lesions are well-demarcated, classically described as coin-shaped. This is a rash that is particularly exacerbated by dry skin. It can be confused with psoriasis, but does not have the company of nail pitting and arthritis and, unlike psoriasis, readily responds to low-dose topical glucocorticoids.

Venous stasis dermatitis manifests with a diffuse erythematous rash on both feet and lower extremities **(Fig. 14.35)**. Concurrent varicosities and increased skin pigment caused by deposition of hemosiderin are noted. In addition, there is a loss of skin appendages, especially localized hair loss (alopecia) in the affected areas. Furthermore, mild to moderate skin scaling and pruritus may be noted. The company it keeps includes edema, pitting or nonpitting, and the potential development of ulcers in the affected skin. This is a common process caused by chronic stasis of venous blood into a dependent area.

Miliaria, also known as "prickly heat," manifests with multiple tiny pruritic papules on the skin of the arms, legs, and trunk **(Fig. 14.36)**. This is recurrent and flares in summer when the patient sweats more frequently. Of diagnostic importance is that it spares the face. This is due to immature sweat glands; highest incidence of the rash is in preteens.

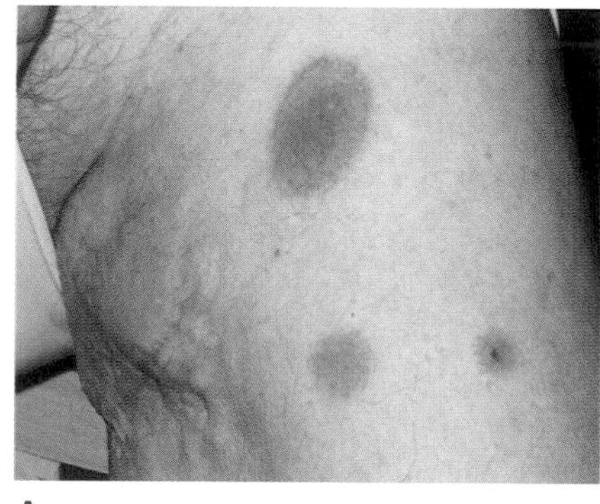

A

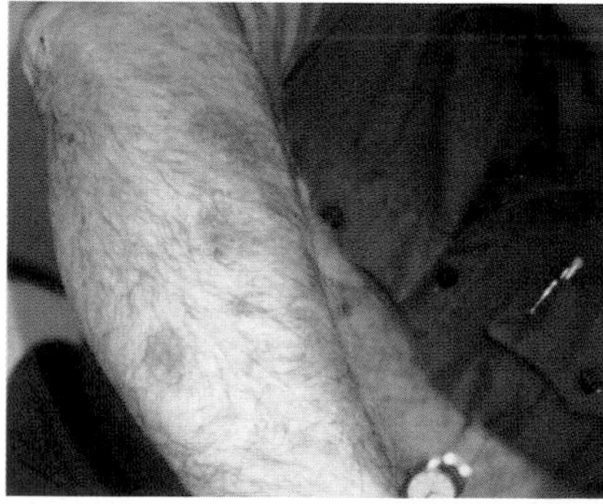

B

Figure 14.34.

Nummular eczema.

 **TIPS**

- Nummular eczema: scaly, moderately pruritic erythematous plaques on extensor surfaces
- Well-demarcated, coin-shaped lesions
- Can be confused with psoriasis

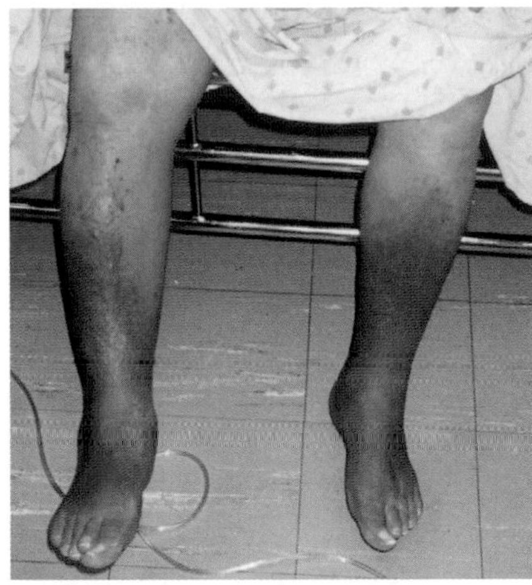

Figure 14.35.

Venous stasis dermatitis.

 **TIPS**

- Venous stasis dermatitis: diffuse, erythematous rash on the feet and lower extremities; concurrent with varicosities
- Increased pigment in the skin, which is hemosiderin
- Localized alopecia is common
- Look for concurrent ulcers in skin

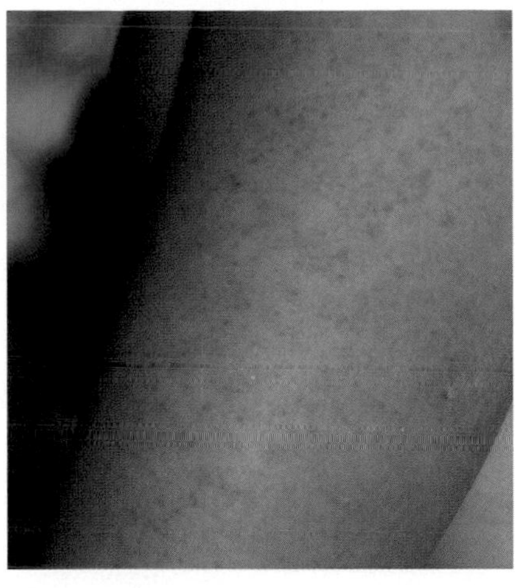

Figure 14.36.

Classic miliaria in a young adolescent; left arm.

 **TIPS**

- Miliaria: multiple small pruritic papules on the skin of arms, legs, and trunk
- Itching is worse in summer when sweating

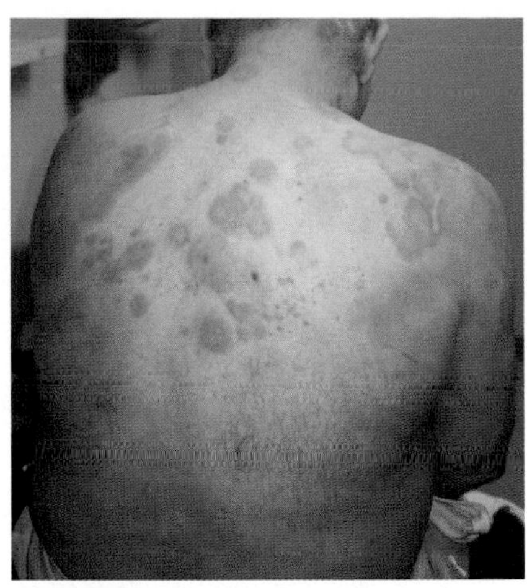

Figure 14.37.

Urticaria.

 **TIPS**

- Urticaria: papules and plaques, often annular-shaped
- Moderate to severe pruritus
- Scratching increases rash, i.e., dermatographism

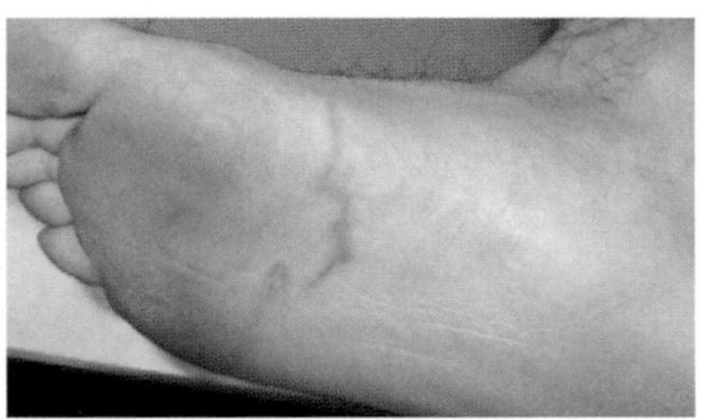

Figure 14.38.

Cutaneous larva migrans.

 **TIPS**

- Cutaneous larva migrans (CLM): serpiginous red entity in skin
- Filiarial larva in skin

Figure 14.39.

Erythema chronicum migrans.

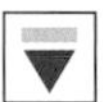 **TIPS**

- Erythema chronica migrans: annular erythematous lesions
- Localized to the site of a recent deer tick bite
- Migrates over time, mildly pruritic, at most
- Develops 10 to 30 days after the original tick bite

Urticaria manifests with one or more red pruritic papules and plaques that are often annular shaped **(Fig. 14.37)**. Often present is concurrent dermatographism, i.e., the development of wheals and flares on stroking the skin with a tongue blade or fingertip. In the acute setting, the company it keeps includes wheezing and stridor caused by angioedema of the lips and airway. The most common local reason for urticaria is a mosquito bite, which is a solitary, classic wheal and flare; the most common generalized reason is also an insect bite, especially a bee or wasp sting.

Cutaneous larva migrans manifests with a solitary, distinct, red serpiginous entity, usually on the plantar foot **(Fig. 14.38)**, that slowly migrates in the skin. It is caused by infection with a filarial larvae primarily found in dogs and is spread by exposure of bare skin to infected dog stool. Although the infection is disturbing to the patient (and physician), the process itself is actually quite benign and self-limited.

Erythema chronicum migrans manifests with an interconnected set of multiple flat annular erythematous lesions **(Fig. 14.39)**. Each lesion has central clearing that is localized to the site of an infected deer tick bite. The set of lesions migrates over time, and can resolve to reappear at a new site. The lesion is mildly pruritic at most and occurs 2 to 3 weeks after the original tick bite. This is primary Lyme disease caused by infection with the organisms

Borrelia burgdorferi. The company it keeps includes concurrent neuropathies, acute Bell's palsy, polyarticular arthritis, and bradycardia from AV-node block.

Erythema ab igne manifests with a reticulated pattern of red patches, which over time become pigmented (**Fig. 14.40**), nontender and nonpruritic; they usually appear on the arms or lower back. Often, the patient reports a history of sitting before an open campfire, fireplace, or radiant heat source as this exposure causes the rash.

Erythema multiforme manifests with one or more raised annular target-type lesions, each with central erythema (**Fig. 14.41**). These do not blanch and are not pruritic. The pattern is such that the palms and soles may be involved. In severe cases, multiple sites and the mucous membranes may be involved as well as formation of concurrent bulla. By definition, erythema multiforme *minor* is one area of involvement; erythema multiforme *major* is two or more areas of involvement; and **Stevens-Johnson syndrome** is major involvement with bullae formation. The company Stevens-Johnson syndrome keeps includes volume depletion and increased risk of infection. Erythema multiforme may be caused by chronic herpes simplex infection, mycoplasma infection, or use of sulfa drugs.

Other erythema include **erythema nodosum**, which manifests with purple-red tender nodules in the skin, especially on the extensor surfaces of legs; it is associated with sarcoidosis, inflammatory bowel syndrome, and rheumatoid arthritis (**Table 14.4**). **Erythema marginatum** manifests with discrete patches of erythema, often with distinct red, raised margins with centers that are pale and flat. This is an erythema that spreads rapidly. The company it keeps includes the features of **rheumatic fever**. These include nontender **subcutaneous nodules**; the wild, involuntary flailing movements of **chorea** (St. Vitus' dance); moderate **polyarticular arthritis**; and **pancarditis**. Pancarditis manifests with pericardial rub caused by inflammation of the pericardium; systolic heart failure caused by inflammation of the myocardium; and murmurs, especially regurgitant murmurs (AI, MR, TR) caused by inflammation of the endocardium (endocarditis). (**See Table 14.5**).

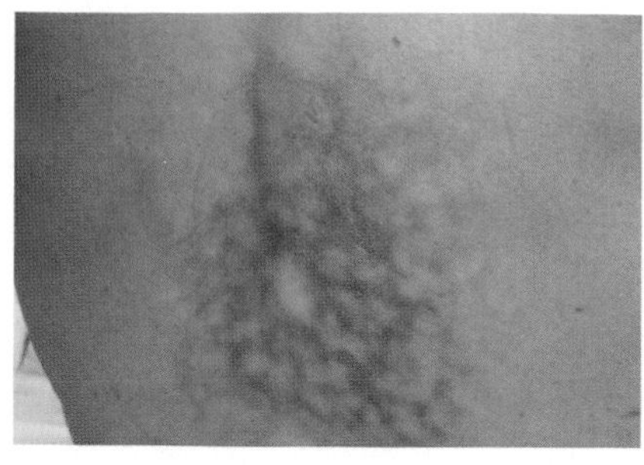

Figure 14.40.

Erythema ab igne.

 **TIPS**

- Erythema ab igne: annular, reticulated set of patches that are red at outset and become pigmented over time, nontender, nonpruritic
- Site of exposure to radiant-type heat, e.g., fireplace, open flame, or heat radiator

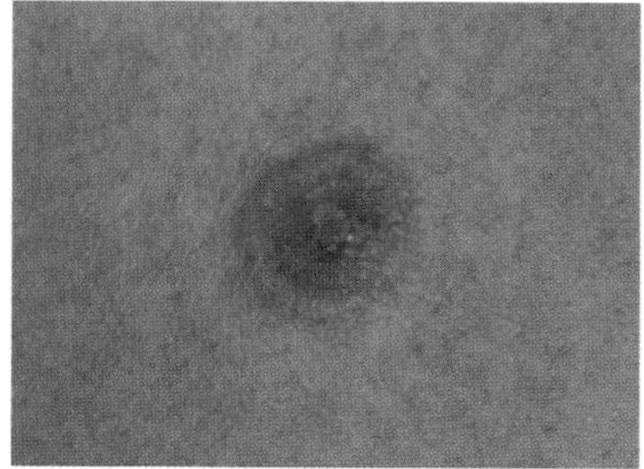

A

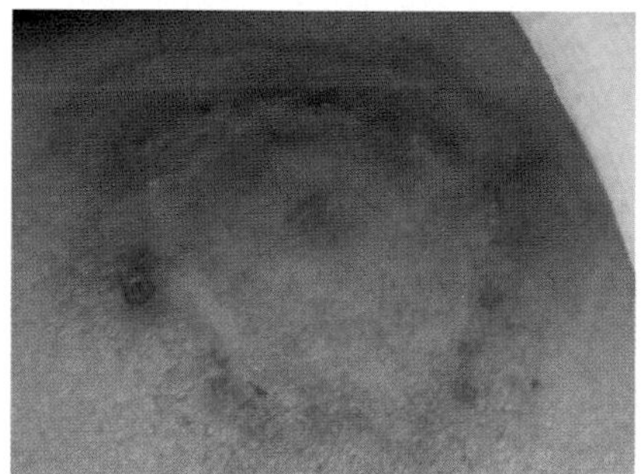

B

Figure 14.41.

Erythema multiforme. **A.** Early. **B.** Late.

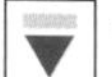 **TIPS**

- Erythema multiforme: annular, target-type lesions, each with central erythema
- Nonpruritic, without blanching
- Can involve mucous membranes and have concurrent bulla formation

Exanthems

Exanthems manifest with a diffuse red rash that is associated with fevers, most commonly, but not exclusively, caused by a viral infection. These rashes

*AI = aortic insufficiency; MR = mitral regurgitation; TR = tricuspid regurgitation.

Table 14.4. Erythemas

Erythema	Specific signs	Underlying cause
Multiforme	Target lesions with red center May have central bulla mucous membrane involvement	Herpes simplex Mycoplasma Drug-related
Ab igne	Reticulated Annular Red, then pigmented	Radiant heat source
Marginatum	Annular patches with raised borders	Rheumatic fever
Chronicum migrans	Interconnected, rings of flat erythema	Lyme disease-related

Table 14.5. Jones' Criteria for Rheumatic Fever

Feature	Descriptors
Erythema marginatum	Annular patches with raised borders
Subcutaneous nodules	Nontender nodules over the extensor surfaces, i.e., the triceps and quadriceps aponeurosis
Polyarticular arthritis	Small joint symmetric arthritis
Chorea or St. Vitus' dance	Large muscle group, automatic, involuntary flailing-type movements
Myocarditis	Displaced PMI, gallop, pulmonary edema
Pericarditis	Pericardial rub
Endocarditis	Regurgitant murmurs

PMI = point of maximal impulse.

are extremely common, especially in children. The company each exanthem keeps includes fevers, cough, sore throat, fatigue, and rhinorrhea. Although these are extremely common and have an extensive differential diagnosis, several unique and specific types merit definition, description, and diagnosis. These include rubeola, scarlet fever, rubella, fifth disease, and roseola. See **Table 14.6** for a summary of each of these. See **Fig. 14.42** for fever curves associated with these specific and definable exanthems.

Table 14.6. Exanthems

Exanthem	Fever	Rash	Desquamates	Company it Keeps	Cause
Rubeola (1st disease)	Antecedent to rash to 104°F	Fine Maculopapular Bright Back, trunk, abdomen, arms	Mild	Cough, nonproductive Severe conjunctivitis Koplik's spots, day before rash	RNA virus
Scarlet fever (2nd disease)	To 103°F during the sore throat	Fine, papular Central to peripheral Trunk and neck to extremities Spares palms and soles Affects skin folds (Pastia's lines)	Yes	Antecedent exudative pharyngitis Strawberry tongue	Group A Streptococcus
Rubella (3rd disease)	Antecedent to rash to 102°F	Fine Maculopapular Light Back, trunk, abdomen, arms	No	Cough, nonproductive Posterior cervical nodes Teratogenic conjunctivitis	RNA virus
Fifth Disease Erythema infectiosum	Antecedent to rash to 103°F	Fine Maculopapular Trunk, back, and face: "slapped-checks"	No	Aplastic anemia	Parvovirus B19
Roseola erythema subitum (6th disease)	Concurrent to 103°F	Diffuse, maculopapular Chest or abdomen	No	Nausea Vomiting	RNA virus

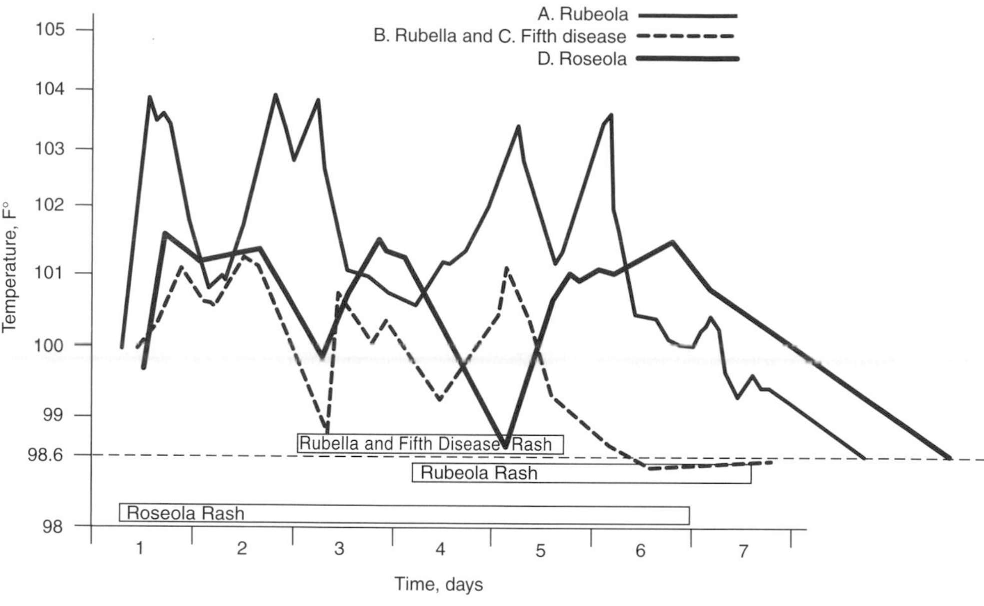

Figure 14.42.

Fever curves for exanthems. **A.** Rubeola. **B.** Rubella. **C.** Fifth disease. **D.** Roseola.

TIPS

- Rubeola has onset of rash after 3 days of high-spiking fever
- Rubella and fifth disease: lower fever and lighter rash
- Rash of roseola early in course of fever

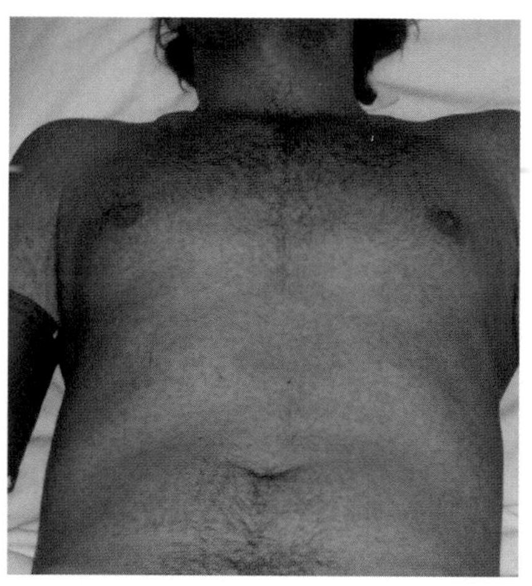

Figure 14.43.

Rash of rubeola (first disease).

TIPS

- Rubeola: diffuse, bright, finely papular rash over the back, trunk, abdomen, and upper extremities
- Often slightly desquamates

Rubeola (first disease) manifests with 3 to 5 days of fevers to 104°F, rhinorrhea, cough, malaise, arthritis, and significant conjunctivitis **(Fig. 14.43)**. On day 3, a cluster of white macules (Koplik's spots) develops in the area of Stensen's duct on the buccal mucosa. On days 4 to 5, a diffuse, bright, finely papular (morbilliform) rash appears over the back, trunk, abdomen, and upper extremities. This rash may desquamate slightly as it heals.

Scarlet fever (second disease) manifests with a diffuse, finely papular red rash on the neck and trunk that progresses to the extremities, but spares the palms and soles. There is significant involvement in skin fold lines, i.e., Pastia's lines. This rash commonly desquamates with healing. A concurrent white then red strawberry tongue is present (see page 27). Often, there is an antecedent exudative pharyngitis from group A streptococcus.

Rubella (third disease) manifests with 2 to 3 days of recurrent fevers to 102°F, rhinorrhea, cough, mild conjunctivitis, and then a mild diffuse, light, finely papular (morbilliform) rash over the back, trunk, abdomen, and upper extremities **(Fig. 14.44)**. This rash never exfoliates or desquamates. Often noted is concurrent posterior cervical lymph node enlargement. Rubella is caused by an RNA virus infection. A major problem exists when a pregnant woman becomes infected, because of a significant risk of damage to her fetus from the virus.

Fifth disease, also known as **erythema infectiosum** manifests with a 2-day history of fevers to 103°F, rhinorrhea, and nonproductive cough; on the third day, a papular rash appears on the trunk, back, and, especially, the face **(Fig. 14.45)**. The facial rash has been described as having what has been described as a "slapped-cheek" appearance. Fifth disease is caused by parvovirus B19 infection.

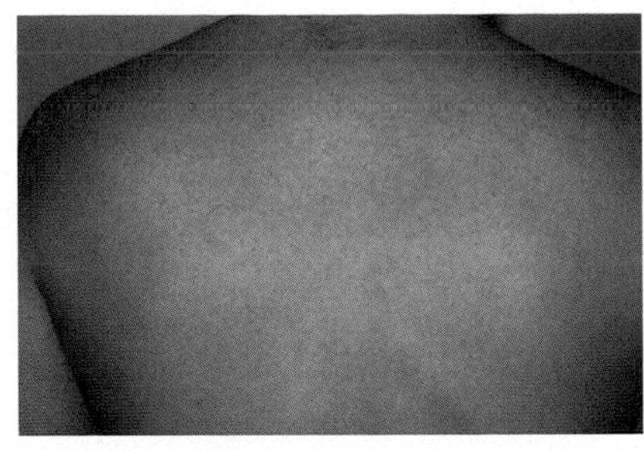

Figure 14.44.

Rash of rubella.

 **TIPS**

- Rubella: mild with a morbilliform, i.e., diffuse, light, finely papular rash over the back, trunk, abdomen, and upper extremities
- Never desquamates

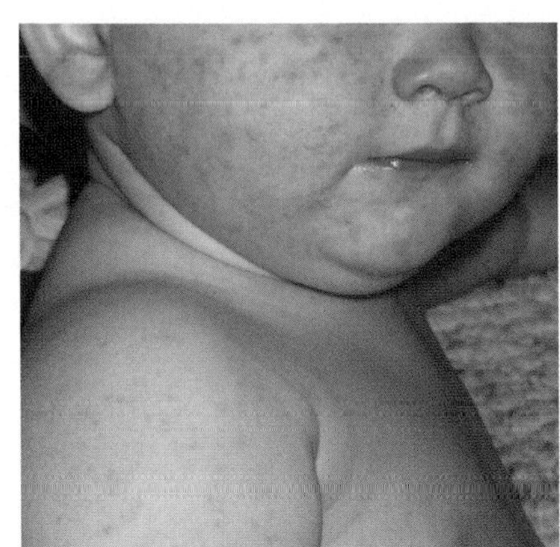

Figure 14.45.

Fifth disease.

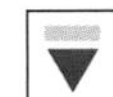 **TIPS**

- Fifth disease: rash on face, trunk, and back
- Especially, face-slapped cheek appearance
- Rash on face, trunk, and back

Roseola (exanthem subitum or **sixth disease)** manifests with a diffuse, maculopapular rash on the chest and abdomen, with concurrent fevers (to 104°F), vomiting, and dehydration; thus, the physical examination for volume status is very important. In classic texts, the term "roseola" was used for the rash of secondary lues; this use is *archaic.*

Other diagnoses with red lesions include **discoid lupus**, which manifests with a malar rash with erythematous papules and patches. It spares the nose; heals with scarring and destructive alopecia (Fig. 14.54). **Gottron's papules** manifest with mildly pruritic red papules and patches on the dorsal aspect of the digits, especially over the middle and proximal phalanges (Fig. 14.22B). Concurrent heliotropic rash appears around the eyes (Fig. 14.22A) and the proximal muscle weakness of dermatomyositis are noted. **Granuloma annulare** manifests with raised annular red lesions with central clearing, rarely more than mildly pruritic, often on the dorsum of hands and feet. Granuloma annulare has been associated with poorly controlled diabetes mellitus.

TEACHING POINTS

RED LESIONS AND ENTITIES

1. Many red lesions that are also pruritic are inflammatory, i.e., dermatitis or urticaria.
2. Any generalized urticaria patient must be emergently assessed for angioedema, stridor, wheezing, and anaphylaxis.
3. Dermatographism is associated with urticaria.
4. Contact dermatitis is one of most common reasons for dermatitis.
5. Nickel in rings or coins is a common cause of contact dermatitis.
6. Moist red rashes in intertringinous areas are usually Candida-related.
7. Warm, red rashes with mild swelling: must consider cellulitis.
8. Erysipelas is a life-threatening, superficial streptococcus infection with a warm, bright red rash.
9. Rashes associated with fevers are called exanthems.
10. The most severe exanthem today is rubeola.
11. Erythema multiforme is usually drug-related; multiple sites or bullae indicate severity.
12. Erythema marginatum is a component of rheumatic fever.
13. Erythema chronicum migrans is the rash of Lyme disease; it occurs 10 to 30 days after the tick bite.
14. The most common cause of a urticaria is an insect or tick bite.

WARTY OR PAPULAR LESIONS

Warty or papular lesions comprise a heterogenous set of entities that have in common the development of papular, nodular, or warty structures in the skin. These may secondarily ulcerate. The warty or papular entity is usually the baseline skin color of the individual. **Molluscum contagiosum** manifests with multiple painless umbilicated papules **(Fig. 14.46)**. Each lesion has a central cheesy core, and some clustering of the lesions may be noted. Most commonly located on the trunk, face, arms, and genitalia, they are caused by a DNA-based poxvirus. Molluscum contagiosum, in fact, is transmitted, i.e., is contagious, by direct contact, including sharing of razors to shave, autoinoculation by "popping" one or more of the papules, and as a sexually transmitted disease.

Common warts (verruca vulgaris) manifest with one or more papules on the skin of the fingers or any skin surface. Each lesion has a rough surface and there often are punctate black spots within each lesion. **Plantar warts** manifest with such a papule on the skin of a toe **(Fig. 14.47)**. These are similar to common warts, but often become larger and, commonly, will ulcerate. The black dots in the wart are small punctate bleeds. Plantar warts are caused by infection with human papilloma virus.

Condylomata acuminata, which manifests with one or more, often multiple warty, moist papules on the perianal, perineal, scrotal, penile, or vulvar skin **(Fig. 14.48)**, has a high correlation with carcinoma development. This is prevalent and is one of the most common sexually transmitted diseases today. The lesions are caused by human papilloma virus. Lesions caused by HPV, types 16 and 18, are at the highest risk for the development of squamous cell carcinoma. **Condylomata lata** manifests with multiple warty lesions in the axilla, inguinal, and groin areas. This uncommon rash is caused by a systemic manifestation of *Treponema pallidum*, which is secondary lues venereum. A history of an antecedent, untreated chancre (Fig 2.3) is not uncommon.

Basal cell carcinoma manifests with a solitary, slowly enlarging papule **(Fig. 14.49)**. The lesion is translucent and has discrete smooth margins; multiple telangiectasia are noted in the lesion, which, when large, can sec-

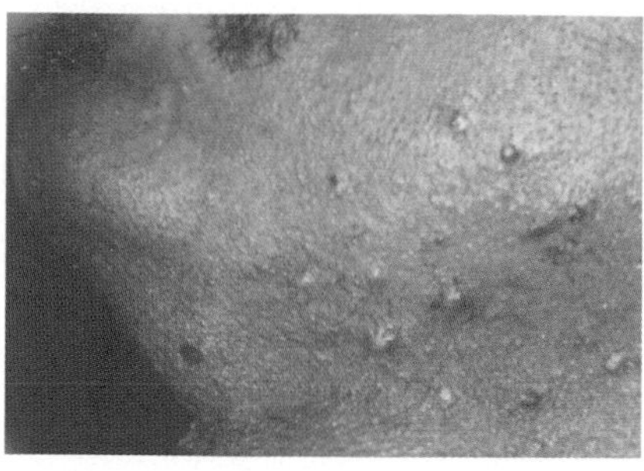

Figure 14.46.

Molluscum contagiosum: face.

 **TIPS**

- Multiple baseline, colored, painless, umbilicated papules, each with central cheesy material
- Located on face, arms, trunk, and genitalia

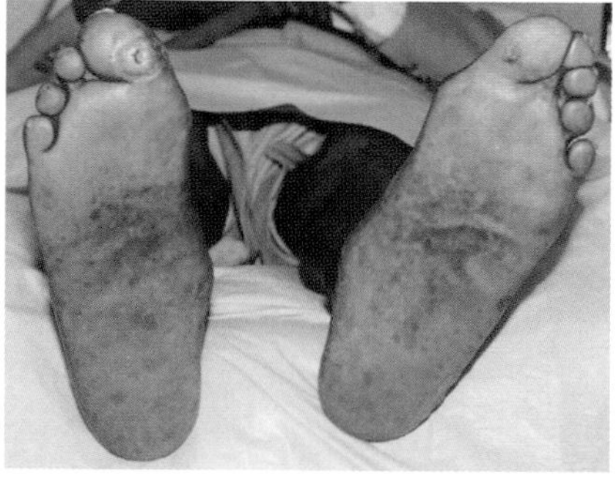

Figure 14.47.

Plantar wart.

 **TIPS**

- Papules on the skin
- Each lesion has a rough surface and multiple punctate black spots in its substance
- Each lesion can erode or ulcerate

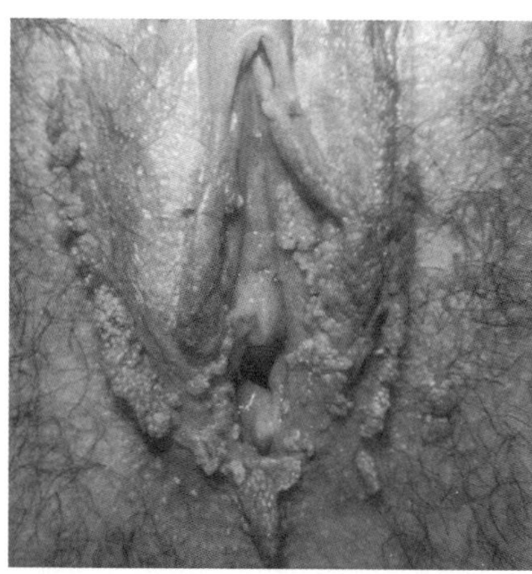

Figure 14.48.

Condylomata acuminata.

 **TIPS**

- Condyloma acuminata: one or more, usually multiple, papules on the perianal, perineal, scrotal, penile, or vulvar skin

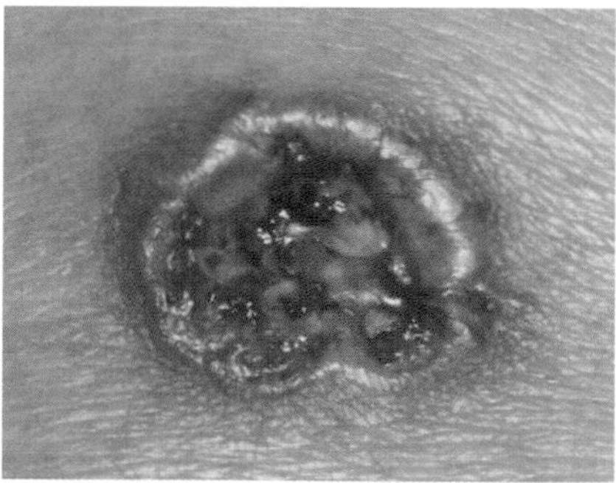

Figure 14.49.

Basal cell carcinoma.

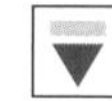 **TIPS**

- Solitary papule; translucent, smooth margins, with telangiectasia
- Can ulcerate, especially when large

ondarily ulcerate. When an ulcer is present, the margins are heaped up and rough and the base of the ulcer is rough. The most common sites for basal cell carcinomas are the face and nose.

Squamous cell carcinoma manifests as a solitary nodule with ulceration or discrete ulcer itself **(Fig. 14.50)**. The ulcer itself is clean, with very distinct borders and minimal debris at the base. The risk factors in the development of squamous cell carcinoma include human papillomavirus infection, especially types 16 and 18, and exposure to UV light, arsenic, and soot. The soot exposure is a fascinating one in that squamous cell carcinoma of the scrotum was common as an occupational hazard in chimney-sweeps. **Keratoacanthoma** (pseudocarcinoma) manifests with a plaque or papule that has central ulceration. These lesions, each of which has a central exophytic plug of keratin, are benign. They are located on the face, dorsal hands, and upper back. We have heard the analogy that a keratoacanthoma looks like a lesion that results from a cigarette burn, which indeed it does. **Actinic keratosis, atrophic or hypertrophic**, manifests with one or more well-demarcated papules or mildly pink macules **(Fig. 14.51)**. Concurrent multiple telangiectasia, which is caused by thinning or atrophy of skin in the atrophic type and cutaneous horns of keratin are noted on the face, arms, neck, and dorsum of hands in the hypertrophic type. These changes are caused by UV exposure and are a clue for squamous cell carcinoma. In point of fact, these discrete actinic lesions are themselves premalignant.

Neurofibromata manifests with one or more nontender nodules on any skin surface **(Fig. 14.52)**. The nodules can be large, umbilicated, and even pendulous and soft in texture. In addition, one or more café au lait spots may be noted; each café au lait spot has a smooth edge, which has been likened to the shape of the coast of California. Furthermore, there are multiple freckles that are invariably present throughout the skin, with multiple pigmented patches, and macules specific to the axillae (Crowe's sign). Finally, clumps of pigment are seen in both of the irises (Lisch nodules). Lisch nodules are one of the most specific findings in neurofibromata-1 (NF-1). Karnes reports a sensitivity of Lisch nodules as 100%. The company NF-1 keeps includes schwannomas, pheochromocytoma, and optic gliomas. **Schwannomas** manifest with radicu-

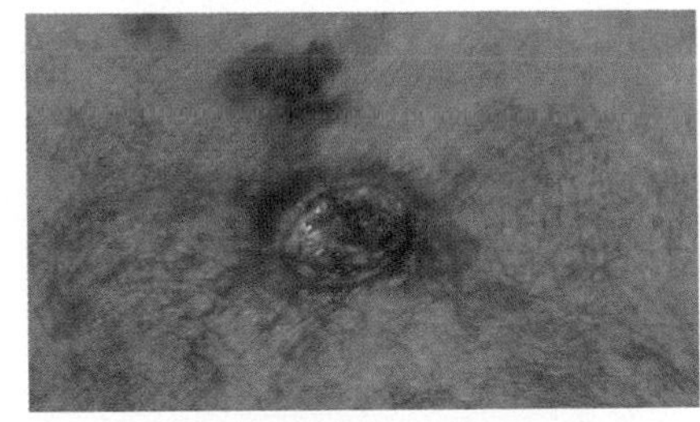

A

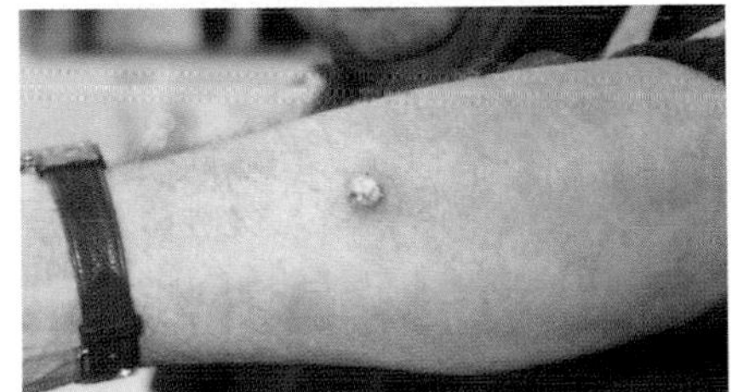

B

Figure 14.50.

A. Squamous cell carcinoma.
B. Keratoacanthoma.

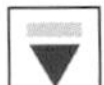 **TIPS**

- Squamous cell carcinoma: solitary nodule with ulceration or an ulcer with surrounding erythema **(A)**
- Located on face, ears, neck, back, or dorsal hand
- Keratoacanthoma: a solitary plaque or papule that has central ulceration and a keratin plug; located on the face, dorsal hands, upper back **(B)**

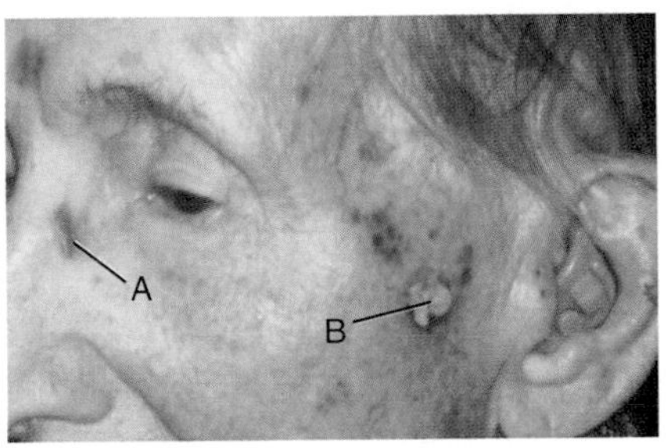

Figure 14.51.

Atrophic **(A)** and hypertrophic **(B)** keratoses.

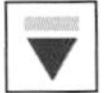 **TIPS**

- Atrophic keratosis **(A):** single to multiple, well-demarcated macules, baseline or pink colored, usually <5 mm in size; concurrent telangiectasia
- Hypertrophic keratosis **(B):** single to multiple well-demarcated macules with cutaneous horns of keratin
- UV light exposure-related

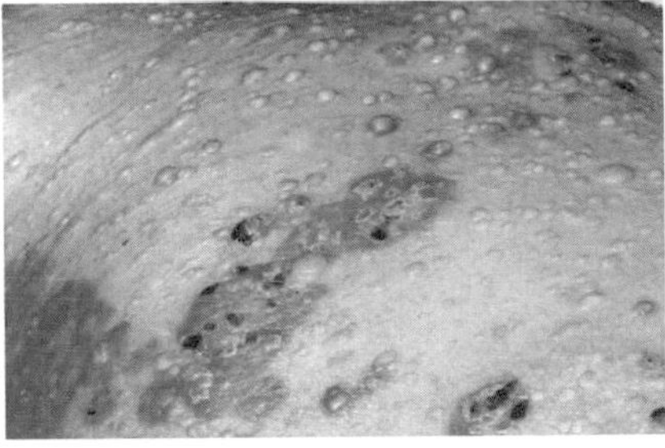

A

B

Figure 14.52.

Neurofibromata and café au lait spots **(A)** and Crowe's sign **(B)** of neurofibromatosis type 1 (NF-1).

 **TIPS**

- Neurofibromata **(A):** nontender nodules, soft in texture with café au lait spots
- Multiple macules and patches in the axilla (Crowe's sign) **(B)**

TEACHING POINTS

FLESH-COLORED WARTY OR PAPULAR LESIONS

1. Verruca vulgaris, a ubiquitous lesion, is a common example of a flesh-colored lesion.
2. Plantar warts are large and can ulcerate.
3. Multiple warts on the genitals are usually HPV-related condyloma acuminatum.
4. Condyloma acuminatum is epidemic as a sexually transmitted disease.
5. Corns are plaques or papules of keratin on the dorsum of the feet.
6. Calluses are plaques or papules of keratin on the plantar aspect of the feet.
7. Umbilicated warty lesions with central cheesy material are consistent with molluscum contagiosum.
8. Flesh-colored nodules, with pigmented patches: consider neurofibromatosis.
9. Recall, NF-1 is associated with pheochromocytomas, schwannoma, and Lisch nodules.

lar pain and weakness specific to that nerve root; **pheochromocytoma** manifests with profound hypertension and tachycardia; **acoustic neuromas** manifest with vertigo, tinnitus, and a unilateral decrease in auditory acuity. NF-1 is due to an autosomal dominant disorder of chromosome 17q.

Other diagnoses include **acrochordons**, which manifests with one or more skin tags. These thin, asymptomatic, pedunculated, flesh-colored papules are most often located on the back, neck, axilla, and inguinal areas. **Keloid formation** manifests with a nodule or plaque that occurs in the site of scar. The tissue is soft and painless, but can be large and disfiguring. One of the most common sites is in the earlobe (Fig 1.8) or any other structure that is pierced. Keloids are caused by exuberant scar tissue in healing. **Callus (tyloma)** manifests with a hyperkeratotic area on the skin that is normally thickly keratinized, e.g., on the plantar foot. **Corn (heloma)** manifests with a hyperkeratotic area that is normally on thinly keratinized skin, e.g., on dorsum of the feet (Fig 14.72). **Nodular** or **cystic acne vulgaris** manifests with one or more tender nodules on the face, neck, upper back, and trunk. Often seen on the facial skin are concurrent or antecedent pustules, also known as open or closed comedones or blackheads. Although the pathophysiology is not clear, acne vulgaris is associated with excessive androgens in puberty and/or the use of steroids.

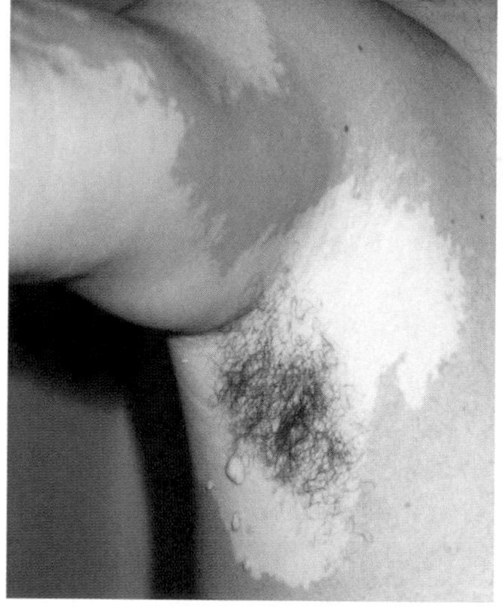

Figure 14.53.

Vitiligo.

 **TIPS**

- Vitiligo: patches of complete loss of pigment, symmetric distribution
- Skin in the area of the mouth, perineum, palms, and soles of the feet
- Progressive, eventually can involve large areas of the skin

HYPOPIGMENTED LESIONS

Vitiligo manifests with patches of complete pigment loss in the affected skin **(Fig. 14.53)**. The patches can be large and multiple and can become confluent. Vitiligo has a symmetric distribution and involves the mouth, perineum, and the palms and soles. It can be idiopathic or autoimmune in etiology. If autoimmune, the company it keeps includes the manifestations of thyroid

TEACHING POINTS

HYPOPIGMENTED LESIONS

1. Tinea versicolor, a common cause of hypopigmented lesions, is especially evident in summer in light-skinned individuals.
2. Tinea versicolor fluoresces golden yellow with Wood lamp illumination.
3. Destructive alopecia with the hypopigmented areas is caused by discoid lupus or full-thickness burns.
4. Vitiligo is symmetric; palms and plantar aspects and the perioral and perineal surfaces are first involved, then it spreads to involve a greater surface area.

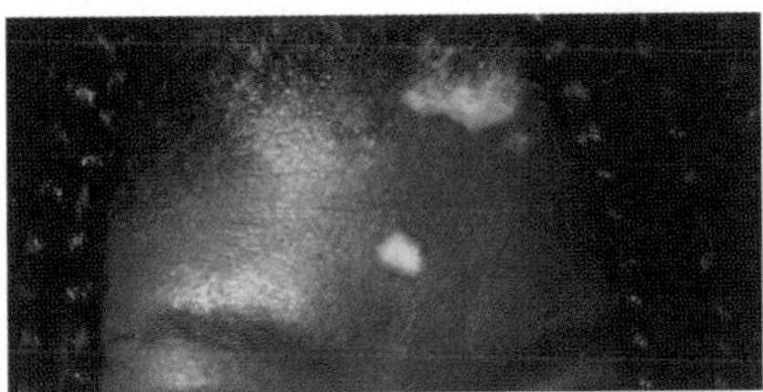

Figure 14.54.

Discoid lupus: old with scarring.

 **TIPS**

- Heals with patches of significant alopecia and loss of pigment
- Destructive form of alopecia

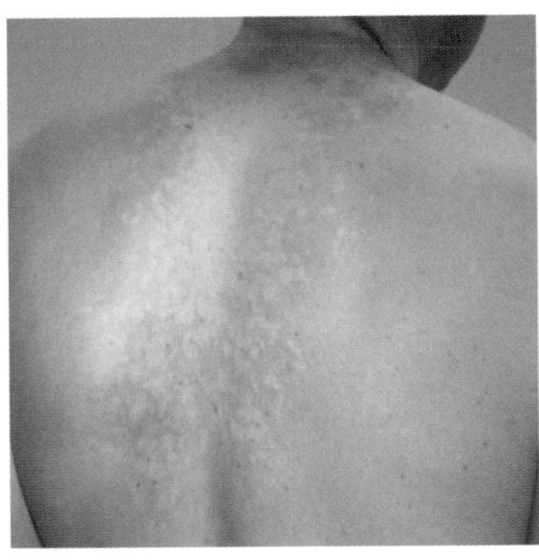

Figure 14.55.

Tinea versicolor.

 **TIPS**

- Macules and patches of hypopigmented areas
- Especially demonstrable in the summer when tanning occurs in the adjacent noninfected skin
- Organism: *Pityrosporum orbiculare,* also known as *Malassezia furfur*

disease. **Discoid lupus-healed** manifests with multiple patches of skin pigment loss **(Fig. 14.54)**, and destructive alopecia in the affected area. The patient often presents with a history of the active lesions of discoid lupus. **Tinea versicolor** manifests with depigmented macules and patches on the shoulders, trunk, and chest **(Fig. 14.55)**. This is especially demonstrable in the summer months when tanning occurs in light-skinned individuals. The areas adjacent to the noninfected skin tan easily. In addition, the affected areas fluoresce golden yellow with illumination from a Wood's lamp. Tinea versicolor is caused by a superficial skin infection with *Pityrosporum orbiculare,* also known as *Malassezia furfur.*

PIGMENTED ENTITIES

Although pigmented entities are ubiquitous, only a very few are malignant or indicate a malignant process. The A, B, C, D, and E method is an excellent paradigm to use in describing pigmented lesions, especially to define benign versus malignant characteristics **(Fig. 14.56)**. In this paradigm, assessment is as follows: **A** = symmetry; **B** = border margins; **C** = color type and quantity in the entity; **D** = diameter of the entity in millimeter; **E** = elevated or flat. A **benign nevus** manifests with **A:** symmetric distribution of pigment; **B:** regular borders; **C:** a single pigment color present in the nevus; **D:** diameter <6 mm; and **E:** not elevated, i.e. flat. Benign nevi are ubiquitous. A **dysplastic nevus** or a **malignant melanoma** manifests with **A:** asymmetry to pigment distribution

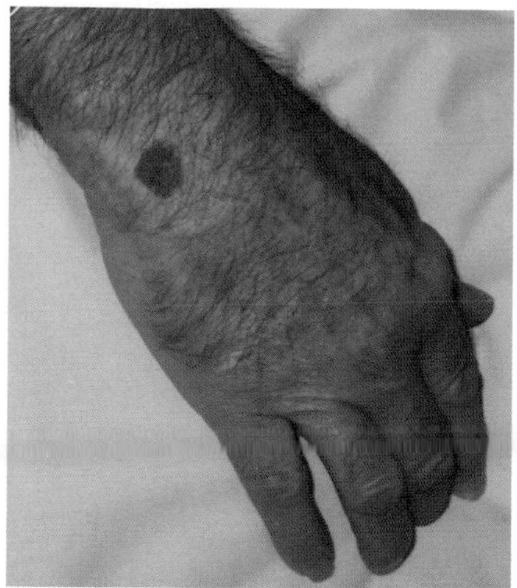

A

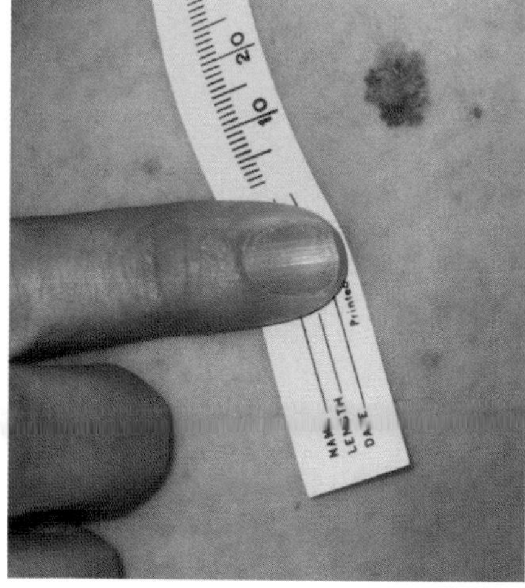

B

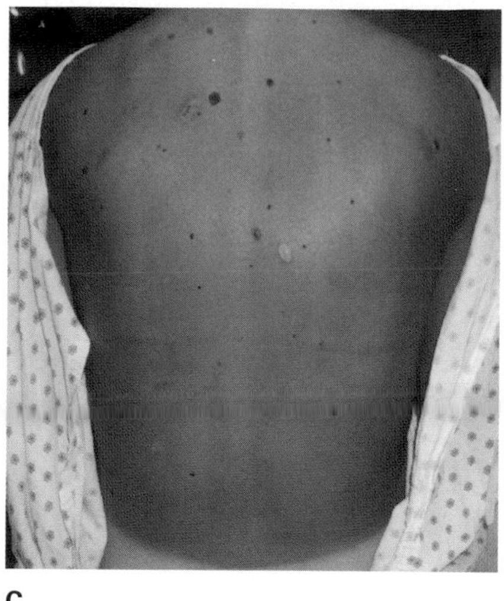

C

Figure 14.56.

A. Benign nevus. **B.** Malignant melanoma. **C.** Nevi in a patient with a suntan.

 TIPS

- Benign nevus **ABCDE** features: **A.** Symmetric. **B.** Regular borders. **C.** Light brown. **D.** <6 mm. **E.** Not elevated. Thus, this is benign
- Malignant melanoma **ABCDE** features: **A.** Asymmetric pigment. **B.** Irregular borders. **C.** Multiple colors of pigment. **D.** Diameter >6 mm. **E.** Elevated lesion

in the entity; **B:** irregular borders; **C:** multiple pigment colors; **D:** diameter >6 mm; and **E:** elevated, i.e., the nevus is palpable. In addition, a melanoma can manifest with secondary ulceration and satellite lesion formation. Whited reported a sensitivity of 100% and, a specificity of 98.4% when using this system. Specific types of nevi include **nevus spilus**, which manifests with a cluster of small benign nevi, usually congenital; and **Sutton's nevus**, which manifests as a nevus with a halo of de- or hypopigment surrounding the nevus **(Fig. 14.57)**. This is may be benign, or a malignant melanoma. A **nodular malignant melanoma** manifests with a palpable jet-black lesion that grows rapidly over time **(Fig. 14.58)**. This is a particularly dangerous type in that it grows deep and, thus, spreads early in its course.

Seborrheic keratosis manifests with one or more, usually multiple, plaques **(Fig. 14.59)**. Each of these is pigmented and present in a symmetric distribution on the back, shoulders, and trunk. Each has a "stuck-on" appearance. The condition is idiopathic; however, an increased number of plaques are seen normally with increasing age. **Leser-Trélat syndrome** manifests with a rapid increase in number, size, and distribution of seborrheic keratosis. Drs. Leser and Trélat each found an association with an internal adenocarcinoma. This association is loose at best; we, however, have seen this in a number of patients with adenocarcinoma of the esophagus or pancreas.

Necrobiosis lipoidica diabeticorum manifests with multiple pigmented patches and plaques on the anterior tibial surfaces **(Fig. 14.60)**. These are invariably red at the outset and evolve with healing to be pigmented. These pretibial changes are highly correlated with poorly controlled diabetes mellitus. The development of secondary ulcers defines the necrobiosis, lipoidica diabeticorum. **Pretibial myxedema** of Graves' disease manifests with red and, then, pigmented skin lesions that are similar to those described in the

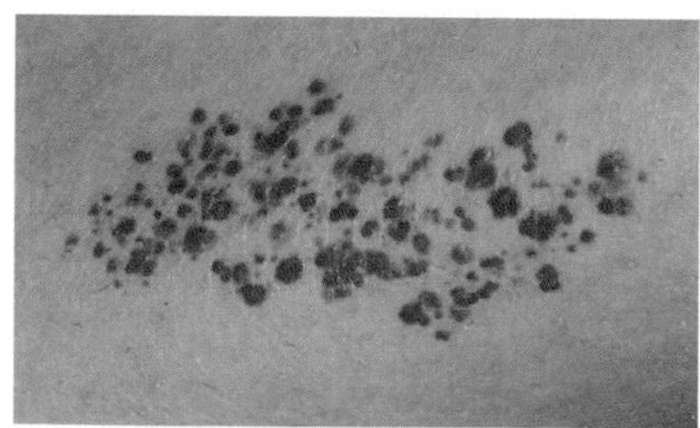

A

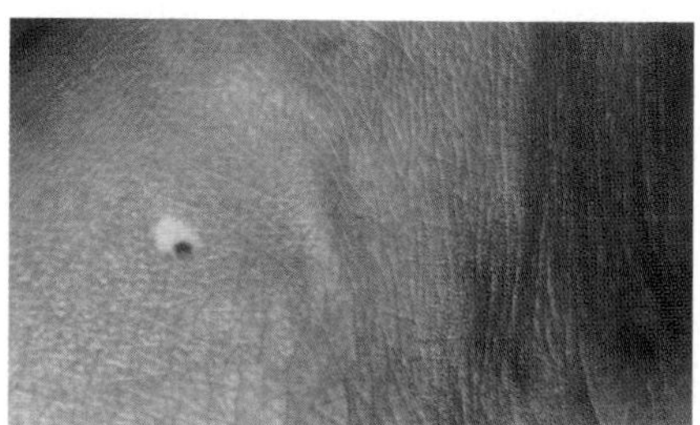

B

Figure 14.57.

A. Nevus spilus. **B.** Sutton's nevus.

 TIPS

- Nevus spilus: cluster of benign nevi
- Sutton's nevus: one nevus with a halo of de- or hypopigment surrounding it

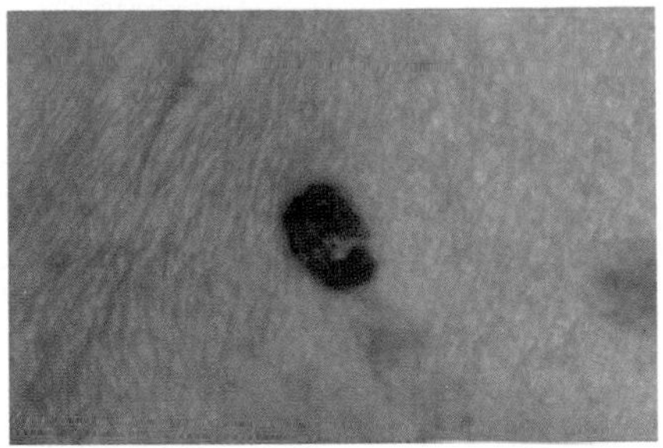

Figure 14.58.

Nodular malignant melanoma: jet-black, a very aggressive form.

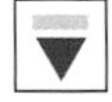
TIPS

- Nodular melanoma: palpable, dark lesion
- Usually advanced at time of diagnosis

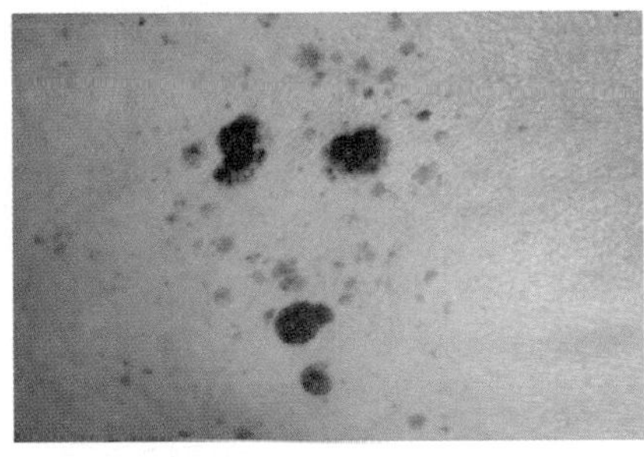

Figure 14.59.

Multiple seborrheic keratoses in this patient with adenocarcinoma of the distal esophagus.

TIPS

- Seborrheic keratosis: multiple pigmented plaques in a symmetric distribution on back, shoulders, and trunk; a stuck-on appearance

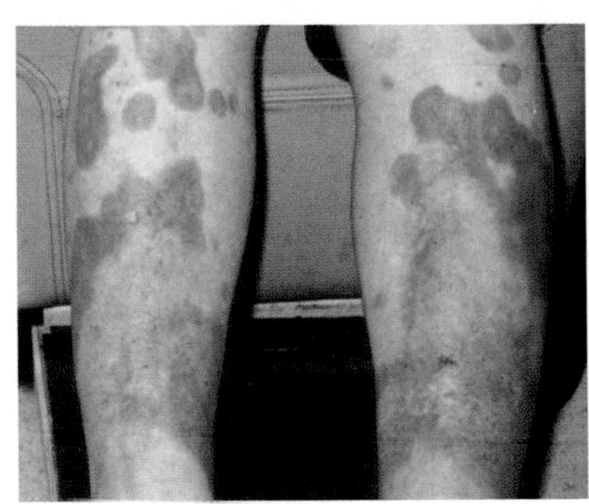

Figure 14.60.

Pretibial diabetic skin changes: necrobiosis lipoidica diabeticorum.

TIPS

- Pigmented patches and plaques on the anterior tibial surfaces
- Antecedent erythematous plaques
- Concurrent uncontrolled diabetes mellitus
- Development of ulcers in the area is indicative of necrobiosis lipoidica diabeticorum
- Similar to pretibial myxedema of Graves' disease

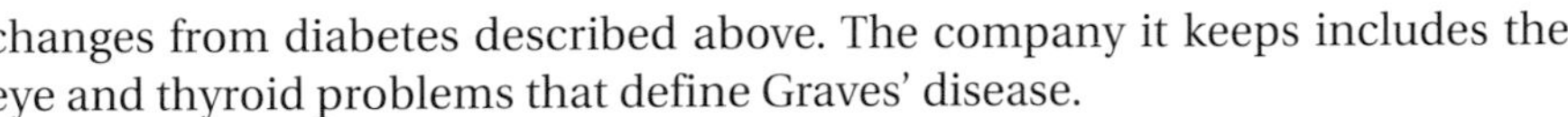
changes from diabetes described above. The company it keeps includes the eye and thyroid problems that define Graves' disease.

Dahl's sign manifests with increased pigment over the elbows and anterior thighs caused by severe COPD or CHF **(Fig. 14.61)**. This is caused by the patient sitting with elbows on thighs and leaning forward to breathe easier (Fowler's position). This is a powerful piece of physical exam company, in that it helps assess the functional severity of the patient's cardiac or lung problem and puts a time frame on it. Dahl's sign clearly bespeaks a chronic and severe condition. Concurrent bilateral cubital tunnel, i.e., entrapment of the ulnar nerve at the elbows, is a common finding in such a patient.

Other pigmented entities include **lentigo**, which manifests with pigmented patches. These are usually on hands and arms in older individuals. They are colloquially referred to as "age-spots" or "liver spots." **Ephelis (freckles)** manifest with multiple small (1–3 mm in size) pigmented entities on the trunk, shoulders, arms, and back. These are variants or normal, usually in individuals of Celtic derivation. **Suntan** manifests with a diffuse, mildly increased pigment to individuals of light skin. Usually, tan lines are seen and a history related of exposure to UV light, either from the sun or a "tanning bed." **Addison's disease** manifests with a diffuse increase in pigment that looks similar to a suntan, but has no tan lines. In addition, there is a marked increase in the pigment in areas of scar, in the perineum and areolae, and in the skin creases, especially the palmar and plantar areas. Addison's disease is primary adrenal insufficiency in which the negative feedback for corticotropin is removed and, thus, corticotropin, with its melanocyte-stimulating effect, causes increased pigment in the skin. **Peutz-Jeghers syndrome** manifests with multiple pigmented macules and patches on the lips, mucous membranes of the mouth and anal area. This is part of a relatively benign polyposis syndrome. **Erythema ab igne** manifests with a set of annular reticulated patches that are red at outset and become pigmented over time. The changes occur in a site of exposure to radiant-type heat, e.g., fireplace, open-flame, or heat radiator (Fig. 14.40). **Acanthosis nigricans** manifests with a large pigmented patch in both axillae. The lesions are deeply and uniformly pigmented and have a velvetlike texture. This finding is strongly correlated with increased insulin states, including severe type II diabetes mellitus and

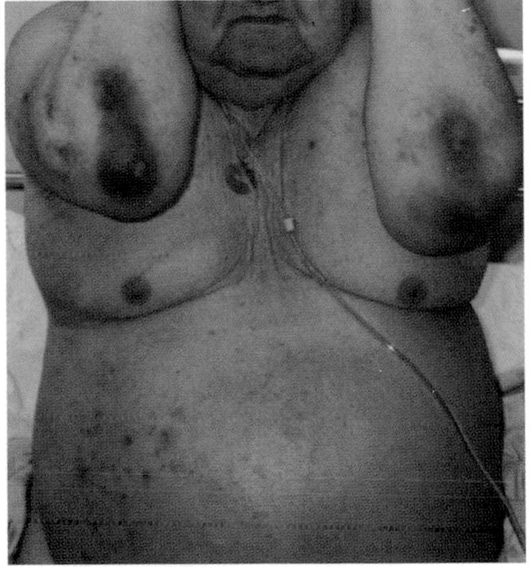

Figure 14.61.

Dahl's sign of increased pigment on elbows and thighs in chronic obstructive pulmonary disease (COPD).

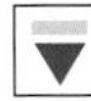
TIPS

- Dahl's sign: inspect the skin overlying the olecranon processes and anterior thighs
- Caused by chronically sitting forward in Fowler's position in patients with severe CHF or COPD

TEACHING POINTS

PIGMENTED LESIONS

1. The ABCDE paradigm is an excellent method to define, describe, and diagnose pigmented skin entities.
2. Seborrheic keratosis is very common in older individuals, but it is benign.
3. Any new nevus on the palm of hand or sole of foot: consider it to be dysplastic or melanoma; any growing or changing nevus, think melanoma.
4. Pigmented lesions with concurrent nontender nodules: consider neurofibromatosis.
5. Anterior tibial pigmented lesions include diabetes mellitus or Graves' disease-related skin changes.

polycystic ovary disease. **Crowe's sign** of neurofibromatosis manifests with multiple pigmented patches and macules in the axillae of a patient with NF-1. The company it keeps includes café au lait spots, neurofibromata (Fig. 14.52), and the Lisch nodules of NF-1. **Dry gangrene** manifests with remarkably painless blackened tissue, usually a digit or distal extremity with mummification of tissue. This is caused by chronic ischemia or infarction of the tissue on the digit, antecedent severe blue toe or finger (Fig. 10.30) (see section on Purple Lesions above), or advanced poorly controlled diabetes mellitus.

ULCERS

An **ulcer** is a lesion in which an actual loss of skin tissue occurs through the epidermis, indeed it can extend into the subdermal tissue. An **erosion** is a superficial ulcer in which the tissue loss is limited to the epidermis. Bullous lesions often precede an ulcer or erosions. Thus, it is important to emphasize this point and make certain to ask a patient what was present before the ulcer or erosion; if a bulla or blister, include this in the differential diagnosis. **Pyoderma gangrenosum** manifests with a deep necrotic ulcer **(Fig. 14.62)**. It is painful, progressively increases in size, and has a necrotic, purulent base. This is associated with inflammatory bowel disease and rheumatoid arthritis.

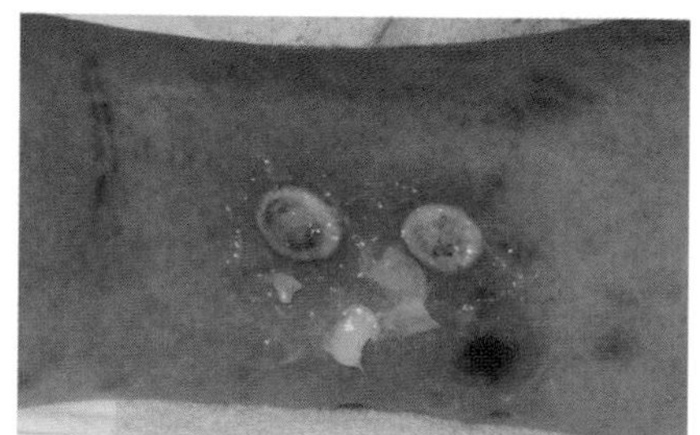

Figure 14.62.

Pyoderma gangrenosum.

TIPS

- Pyoderma gangrenosum: deep ulcer that progressively enlarges and has a necrotic, purulent base
- Associated with inflammatory bowel disease, especially ulcerative colitis

Neurotropic ulcers manifest with one or more painless deep ulcers **(Fig. 14.63)**. These are usually on the plantar aspect of the foot. The company it keeps includes marked sensory deficits to fine touch and vibratory sensation. In addition, there may be amputation of one or more of the toes and the tibiotalar and subtalar joints may have a loose, "bag-of-bones" feel to them when performing a passive ROM. This is a severely damaged, albeit minimally painful, Charcot-type joint. Although the ulcer and its joint do not hurt, that is not good news.

Arterial insufficiency ulcers manifest with deep ulcers **(Fig. 14.64)**. These ulcers are often painful, unless concurrent neuropathy exists. A loss of pulses is noted in the affected area; for example, if a foot ulcer, there is severe

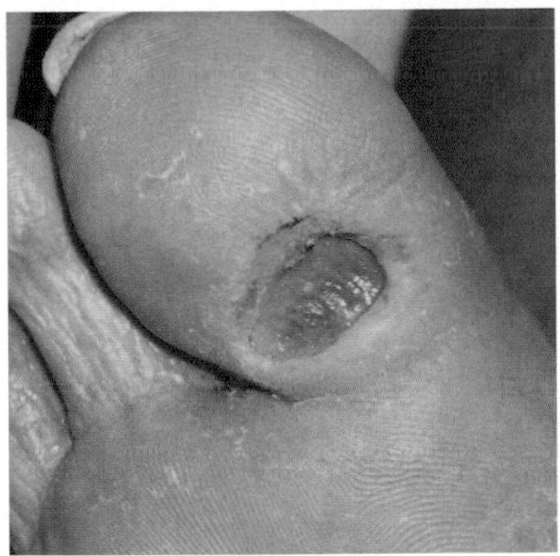

Figure 14.63.

Neurotropic ulcer; note loss of toes 4 and 5.

TIPS

- Neurotropic ulcer: erosion or deep ulcer, usually on the plantar aspect of foot; associated with adjacent callus
- Invariably painless

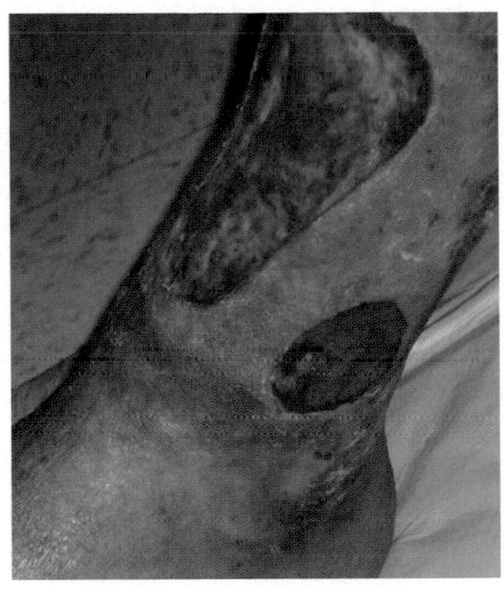

Figure 14.64.

Arterial insufficiency ulcer.

TIPS

- Arterial insufficiency ulcer: painful or painless ulcers that are very deep; concurrent localized alopecia

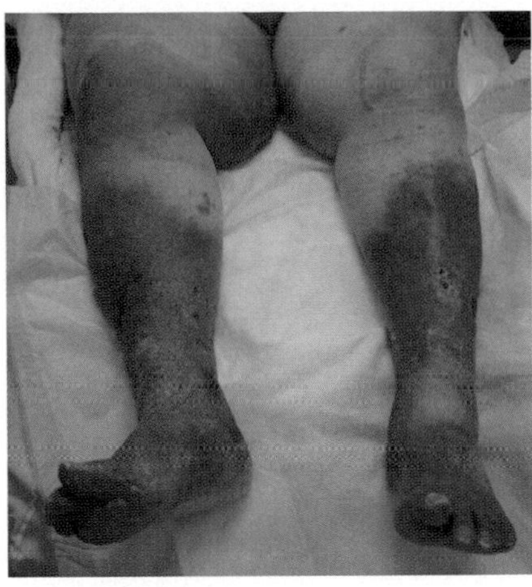

Figure 14.65.

Venous stasis ulcers with dermatitis.

TIPS

- Venous stasis ulcers: superficial or deep ulcers, with loss of hair in appropriate distribution
- Increased pigmentation and varicosities
- Nonpitting edema

diminishment or even absence of dorsalis pedis and posterior tibialis pulses. Often, noted are concurrent localized loss of hair and a prolonged (>6 seconds) capillary refill time. The **capillary refill time** is performed such that the examiner blanches the skin on the great toe and measures the time required for the pink to completely return to the blanched area. Normal is <6 seconds; arterial insufficiency is >6 seconds.

Venous stasis ulcers manifest with superficial or deep ulcers **(Fig. 14.65)**. These are located usually on the lower extremities, but normal pulses are

TEACHING POINTS

ULCERS

1. Relatively painless indurated ulcer on the penis, vulva; chancre of primary lues venereum.
2. Pressure ulcers are decubital ulcers that can be extremely deep and extensive.
3. Lower extremity ulcers can be venous stasis, pigmented, alopecia, varicosities; or arterial insufficiency, pale, alopecia, decreased pulses, and cool skin temperature.
4. Deep non–trauma-related painful ulcers with good pulses and no alopecia: consider pyoderma gangrenosum.
5. Any large blood-filled bulla, once unroofed, is a deep, usually painful, ulcer.
6. Painless lower extremity ulcers usually indicate significant neuropathy.

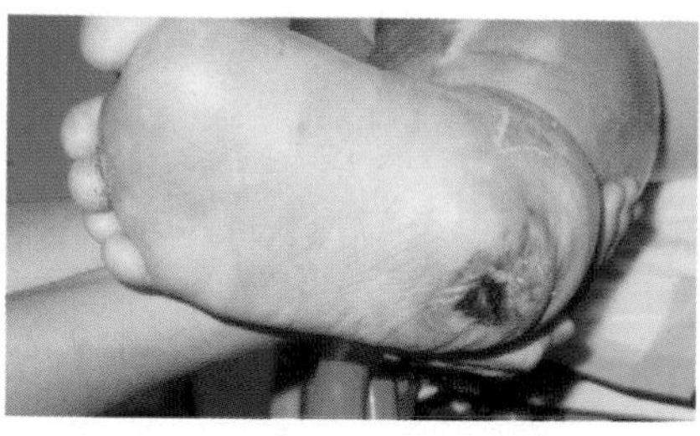

Figure 14.66.

Decubital ulcer over the calcaneus in a patient with clubfoot.

 **TIPS**

- Decubital ulcers: superficial or deep ulcers over sites of pressure, especially buttocks, or calcaneus, e.g., ischial tuberosity or the heels

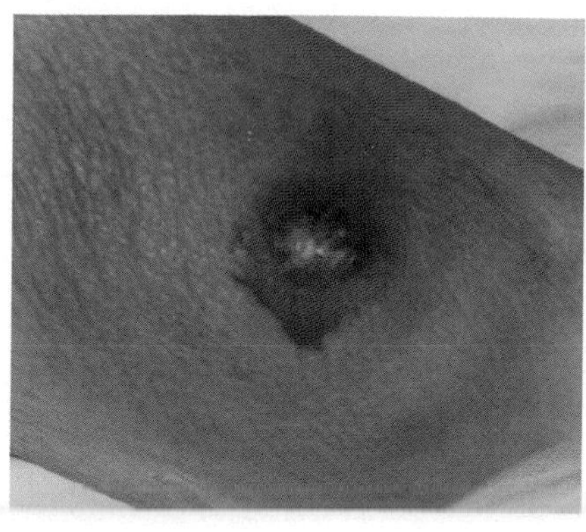

Figure 14.67.

Ecthyma gangrenosum.

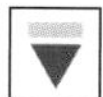 **TIPS**

- Begins as deep, large bullae with surrounding erythema; very tender
- On rupture, a deep ulcer is noted
- *Pseudomonas aeruginosa* bacteremia

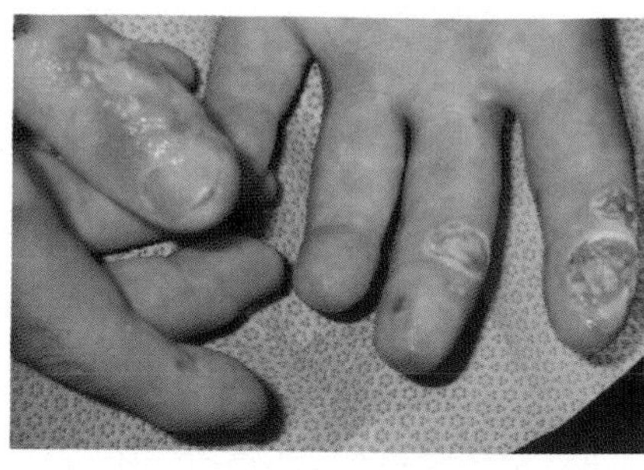

Figure 14.68.

Crack pipe smoker's callus.

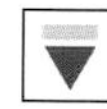 **TIPS**

- Ulcers and calluses on the palmar fingers or on the thumb, usually on the dominant hand
- The metal in the bowl of the pipe is extremely hot—a site-specific burn can occur there

present in the affected areas. A marked localized loss of hair is noted. In addition, there is localized increased pigmentation, which is caused by hemosiderin deposition as the result of stasis of blood in the skin. Often noted are nonpitting edema and multiple varicosities in the affected skin areas.

Decubital ulcers manifest with superficial or deep ulcers over sites of chronic pressure **(Fig. 14.66)**. Several common sites are the ischial tuberosity on the buttocks, over the greater trochanter, or on the malleoli of the ankle. The company it keeps is a history of being immobilized, bedridden, or in a wheelchair. These are simply termed "pressure ulcers." In addition to immobility, malnutrition is a factor in their development. Furthermore, deep ulcers can have underlying adjacent osteomyelitis.

Ecthyma gangrenosum manifests with deep, large, tender black bullae with surrounding erythema; on rupture, a deep painful, necrotic ulcer is seen **(Fig. 14.67)**. This is caused by metastatic deposit of *Pseudomonas aeruginosa*, from a primary infection, most often in the urine or the lung.

Crack pipe smoker's ulcers manifest with ulcers and calluses on the palmar fingertips **(Fig. 14.68)**. The metal in the bowl of the pipe, which is extremely hot, is held by the patient until specific burns occur.

Other diagnoses include **squamous cell carcinoma**, which manifests with a papule or plaque that ulcerates; the ulcer is very clean with smooth edges and borders. **Keratoacanthoma** manifests with an ulcer with a central red firm plug. Certain large **basal cell carcinomas** manifest with ulceration; the ulcer often has debris, is irregular, and has raised, irregular borders. **Chancre** manifests with a relatively painless, most often solitary, ulcer on the mucous membranes of the genitals or oral mucosa. This primary lues venereum is caused by infection with *Treponema pallidum*. **Chancroid**, which manifests with several moderately painful ulcers on the mucous membranes, especially in the genital area, is caused by infection with *Haemophilus ducreyi*. **Full-thickness, second-degree scald** manifests with deep or tense bulla, which on rupture leads to a large ulcer. These can become so tense that, if present on the distal extremities, a risk exists of compartment syndrome. Classic history is exposure to hot water, steam, or heat.

PLAQUES

Psoriasis manifests with one or more pruritic plaques **(Fig. 14.69)**. These plaques have silver-colored scales and a predilection for the extensor surfaces because they develop in areas of mild trauma or irritation (Koebner's phenomenon). In addition, minute, punctate bleeding sites are noted beneath each scale when removed (Auspitz sign). Furthermore, pitting of the nail plates is often seen. Polyarticular arthritis is a related symptom. Recall, little if any relationship exists between the intensity of the arthritis and of the skin rash itself. Today, it is rare to find a patient with classic lesions because many individuals use topical over-the-counter steroids as partial treatment prior to presentation (**Fig. 14.70**).

Kerion manifests with a plaque that is indurated, pustular, and erythematous **(Fig. 14.71)**. It consists of a matted area of pus, granulation tissue, hyphae, and hair. There is concurrent or antecedent tinea capitis. Often found on the occipital scalp, it is commonly seen in football players who wear helmets for extended periods of time; often, the athlete will begin self-therapy by shaving the head hair. Kerion has a high correlation with other dermatologic fungal infections. **Favus** manifests with a matted, crusty area at the base of a site of tinea capitis-related alopecia.

Tyloma, i.e., callus, manifests with a thickened plaque of keratin on normally thickly keratinized skin, e.g., the plantar aspect of the feet. A **heloma i.e., corn,** manifests with a thickened plaque of keratin on normally thinly keratinized skin, e.g., the dorsum of the feet **(Fig. 14.72)**. Any callus in an

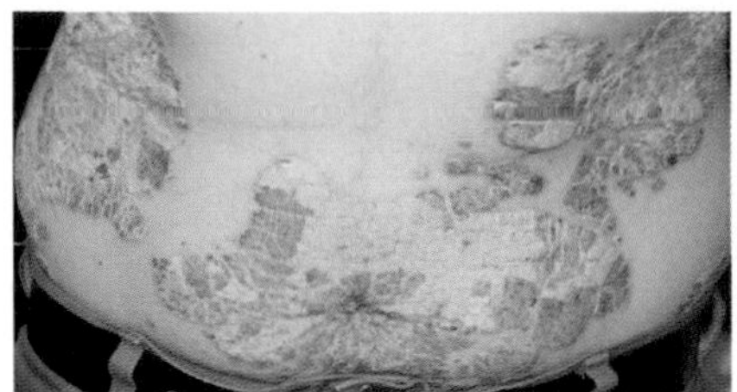

Figure 14.69.

Classic plaque with scales of psoriasis.

 **TIPS**

- Psoriasis: multiple, pruritic plaques with silvery scales
- Usually on extensor surfaces, but can occur in any place of irritation
- Koebner's phenomenon: lesions are in a site of irritation; here, in the belt area, especially under the buckle
- Auspitz sign: punctate bleeds from beneath an unroofed scale

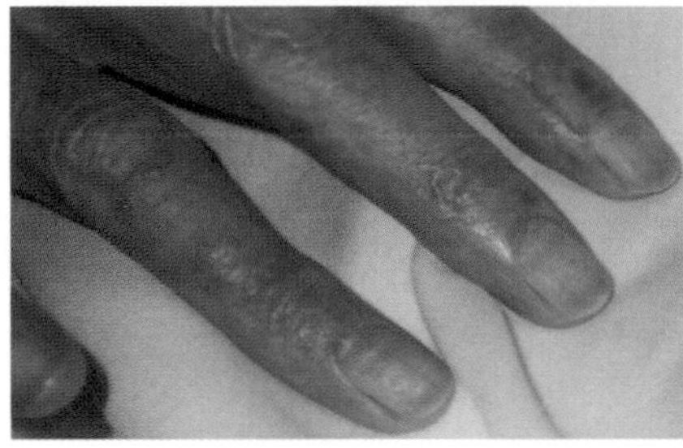

Figure 14.70.

Nail pitting of psoriasis.

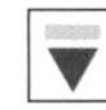 **TIPS**

- Psoriasis: pitting of the nail plates; onychodystrophy is common
- Nummular eczema: no nail pitting

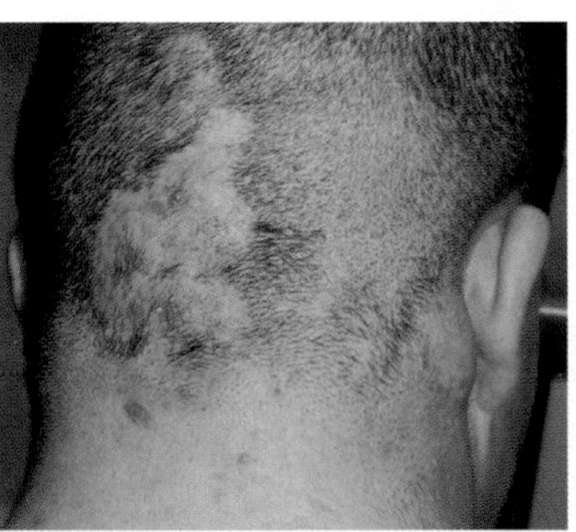

Figure 14.71.

Kerion.

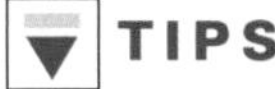 **TIPS**

- Kerion: indurated, pustular, erythematous matted lesion on head
- Concurrent or antecedent tinea capitis

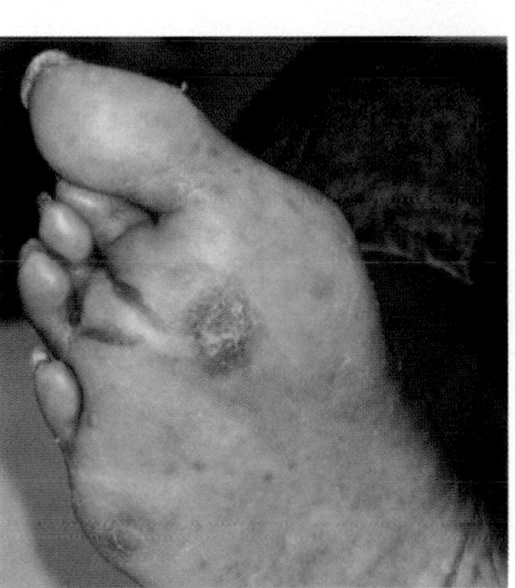

A

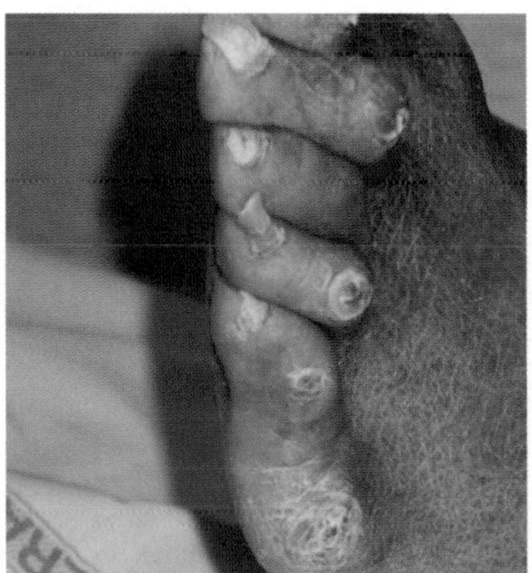

B

Figure 14.72.

A. Callus. **B.** Corn.

 **TIPS**

- Callus (tyloma): plaque of keratin on thickly keratinized skin, e.g., the plantar aspect of the feet **(A)**
- Corn (heloma): plaque of keratin on thinly keratinized skin, e.g., on the dorsum of the feet **(B)**
- Neuropathy: corns or calluses in odd places

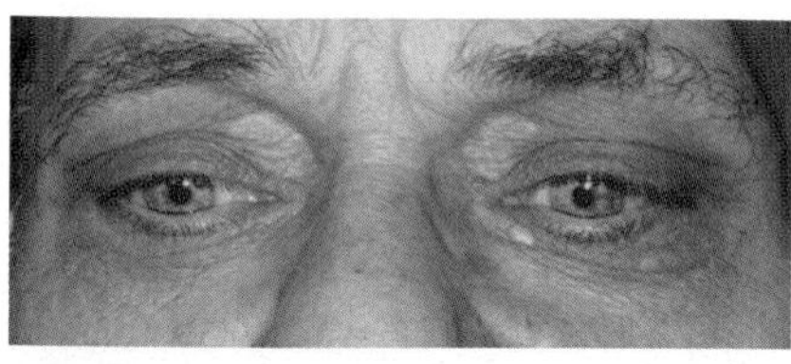

Figure 14.73.

Xanthelasma.

TIPS

- Xanthelasma: superficial cream-colored plaques in periorbital skin
- Look for company of eruptive xanthomas, pancreatitis
- Elevated triglycerides

unusual place or virtually any corn indicates abnormal irritation to the site. Either can be caused by ill-fitting shoes or peripheral neuropathy.

Paget's disease manifests with one or more scaly plaques on the nipple or areola, often with concurrent breast lump or nipple discharge. This is caused by an infiltrating ductal carcinoma. **Xanthelasma** manifests with cream-colored to yellow plaques in the periorbital skin **(Fig. 14.73)**. Asymptomatic, these are associated with hyperlipidemia (type I, IV, or V), elevated chylomicrons and triglycerides. The company it keeps includes eruptive xanthomata on elbows and knees and abdominal pain caused by pancreatitis.

Other problems include **seborrheic keratosis**, which manifests with multiple painless, pigmented papules and plaques on the trunk, legs, back, and shoulders. Found in a symmetric distribution, they are 1 to 1.5 cm in diameter. **Nummular eczema** manifests with one or more coinlike erythematous patches and plaques on the extensor surfaces, which are exacerbated by dry skin, but have no nail pitting. **Pityriasis rosea** manifests with multiple oval reddish scaly patches on the trunk, back, and chest. An antecedent herald patch is seen on the back, which is a larger, but still typical patch. **Tinea corporis** manifests with a ring of erythema with central clearing; it grows outward and has a leading edge of scales. Tinea corporis is caused by a superficial infection of the skin with a dermatophyte. **Atopic dermatitis** (eczema) manifests with one or more patches and plaques on the flexor surfaces of the arms and legs. **Necrobiosis lipoidica diabeticorum** manifests with erythematous papules and plaques on the anterior tibial surfaces, which evolve into pigmented plaques. It is associated with poorly controlled diabetes mellitus. **Pretibial myxedema**, which manifests with Graves' disease-related red plaques on the anterior tibial surfaces, but no scales, can evolve into pigmented areas. **Lichen planus** manifests with multiple purple to pigmented patches, papules, and plaques that are pruritic and may form bulla. Lichen planus have Koebner's phenomenon and often occur after bone marrow transplantation as a component of graft-versus-host disease. **Basal cell carcinoma** manifests with a papule or plaque that is translucent, telangiectasia, and if large, an ulcer.

TEACHING POINTS

PLAQUES

1. Classic psoriasis has nail pitting, polyarticular arthritis, and plaques with silvery scales.
2. Koebner's phenomenon is a feature of psoriasis and lichen planus.
3. Recall, it is more common to irritate the elbow and knee than the other side of arm or leg, thus extensor surfaces are more involved in Koebner's phenomenon.
4. Plaque or papule in the areola needs to be evaluated for Paget's disease and, thus, an underlying infiltrating ductal carcinoma.
5. Nummular eczema looks like psoriasis but no pitting, no Koebner's phenomenon, and no arthritis.
6. Lichen planus is often akin to graft-versus-host disease.

VESICLES

Herpes labialis, also known as a "cold sore," manifests with a small cluster of painful vesicles localized to the lip. These vesicles cross over the vermillion border onto the adjacent skin (Fig 1.42C). The vesicles evolve into pustules, then erosions, and then crust over before they resolve. A recurrence of a primary infection with herpes simplex virus, they can recur with a frequency that is of tremendous irritation to the patient. **Primary herpes labialis** manifests with a larger set of vesicles on the lip, the skin near the lip, and even onto the oral mucosa. Again, a defining feature is that they cross the vermillion border of the lip. Primary herpes labialis is caused by infection with herpes simplex type 1. **Herpes genitalis** manifests with a painful cluster of vesicles on the vulva or penis (Fig 2.2); primary infection is more intense than the recurrent infection, although it can be very frequent. Often the lesions are no longer vesicles but erosions by the time the patient presents for evaluation. As with herpes labialis, these lesions are vesicles that become pustules, then erosions, and then crust over to heal; they are caused by herpes simplex II. See also Chapters 2 and 3.

Herpes zoster manifests with clusters of vesicles in a single unilateral dermatome. A cardinal feature of zoster is that the set does not cross the midline. Pain and dysesthesia are present before the onset of the clusters of vesicles; in point of fact, gentle pinching (Cope's technique) or lightly stroking the skin of the affected dermatome will uncover hyperesthesia. Remember, any dermatome puts the patient at risk; no one dermatomic area is more commonly affected. Thus, sacral or cervical or cranial nerve zoster should be no more surprising than T10 zoster **(Fig. 14.74)**. In addition, zoster can involve more than one dermatome; if it involves more than two or involves dermatomes on both sides of the body, consider immunocompromise.

Varicella, i.e., chickenpox, manifests with the patient developing a set of vesicles on the chest and face, with several days of fevers to 102°F and a nonproductive cough antecedent to the onset of vesicles. The natural history is that of one crop of vesicles, which the next day becomes pustules, the next day crust over, and then resolve. A new crop of vesicles forms daily for 3 to 4 consecutive days (**Fig. 14.75**). The incidence of varicella has markedly decreased over the past decade with the advent of varicella vaccine.

Herpetic whitlow manifests with a cluster of painful vesicles and bulla on the finger (**Fig. 14.76**). The digit can become very swollen and develop ischemia and tingling from a compartment syndrome. This problem is caused by an infection of digits with herpes simplex virus. It is an occupation-related

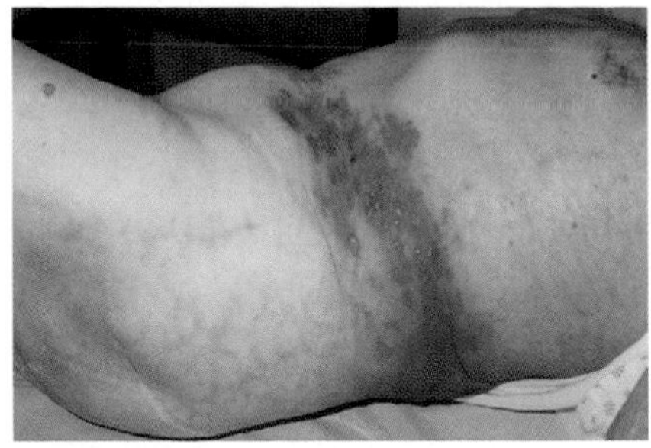

Figure 14.74.

T10 zoster, classic unilateral dermatome.

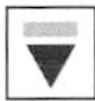 **TIPS**

- Set of painful clusters of vesicles in a single dermatome; does not cross the midline, i.e., T10

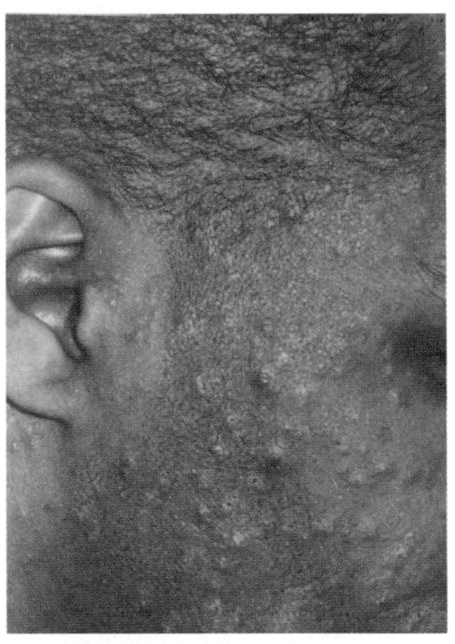

Figure 14.75.

Classic chickenpox (varicella): day 3.

 **TIPS**

- Crop of vesicles, next day become pustules, then crust over; pruritic
- New crops occur each day for 3 to 4 days
- Antecedent fever and dry cough
- Infectious

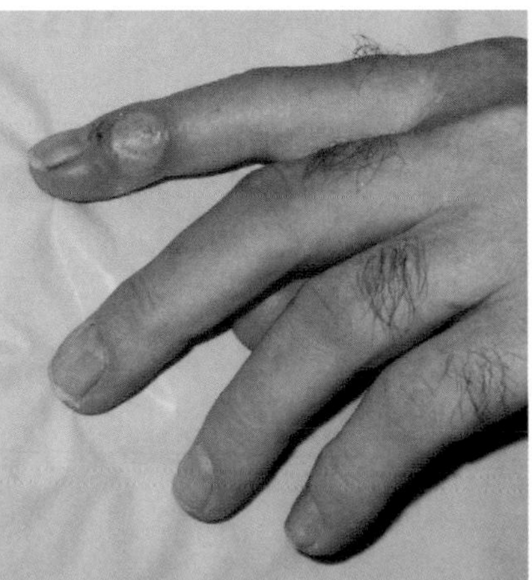

Figure 14.76.

Herpetic whitlow on finger.

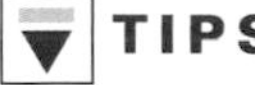 **TIPS**

- Herpetic whitlow cluster of painful vesicles on tip of digit
- Can develop a compartment syndrome in the involved digit

TEACHING POINTS

VESICLES

1. Vesicles are often associated with herpes and with severe dermatitis.
2. Clusters of vesicles are consistent with herpes simplex or herpes zoster.
3. Clusters of vesicles in one dermatome are consistent with herpes zoster.
4. Primary herpes infection is more severe than recurrent.
5. Coxsackie A does not cross the vermillion border of the lip onto the skin; herpes simplex and zoster do cross onto the skin.
6. V_1 zoster requires assessment of ipsilateral conjunctiva and cornea to rule out concurrent herpes keratitis.
7. Poison ivy often will have vesicles in the mix.

process; for instance, a dentist or physician who is not uniformly following universal precautions can inadvertently place an ungloved finger with an abrasion or cut into the mouth of a patient with an active cold sore and develop this problem.

Hand-foot-mouth disease (coxsackie virus A16) manifests with multiple painful vesicles and erosions on the tongue, lips, and posterior pharynx (Fig 1.42A). The lesions do not cross the vermillion border of the lip. The company it keeps includes vesicles on the palms of hands and plantar feet. Caused by the RNA virus made famous in Coxsackie, New York, epidemics occur in child-care centers. The company it keeps includes sore throat and dehydration. **Porphyria cutanea tarda** manifests with vesicles on the hands and on any area of exposure to UV light; it heals with hair formation. **Contact dermatitis** manifests with papules, plaques, and even vesicles at a site adjacent to a chemical substance. The patient relates intense pruritus and mild to moderate deep-seated swelling; often noted are weeping, oozing, and crusting of the rash. A classic example is poison ivy. **Tinea pedis** manifests with erythema and pruritus in a moccasin distribution on the plantar aspect of the feet. Scales and vesicles develop on the periphery.

BULLAE

Bullous or blistering disorders, overall, are extremely common. In point of fact, every human has had bullae. The most common reasons include mechanical or thermal trauma. Although many other causes of bullae exist, these two comprise the vast majority of bullae. **Mechanical trauma**-related bullae manifest with blisters at sites of irritation and recurrent mild trauma, e.g., raking leaves, doing 100 consecutive pull-ups, or running in ill-fitting shoes. Recall, bullae often burst and, if so, they are instead erosions or ulcers.

Bullae can be tense if they have a deep cleavage plane and are hemorrhagic if they are very deep. The term "blood blister" indicates the significant depth of the bulla.

Second-degree burns, especially steam-related scalds, manifest with bullae over the involved site **(Fig. 14.77)**, whereas, **second-degree frostbite** manifests with bullae in areas frozen, most often the fingers and toes, distal to proximal. Thus, steam and frostbite manifest in virtually the same way.

Pemphigus vulgaris manifests with multiple fragile, flaccid bullae **(Fig. 14.78)**. At the time of presentation, they are erosions and often mucous membrane involvement is noted. The bullae of pemphigus vulgaris can be confused with toxic epidermal necrolysis syndrome (TEN) and staphylococcal scalded skin syndrome (SSS) because they are also superficial, diffuse processes. The fragility of the bullae indicates the superficial aspect of the cleavage plane. The lesions will develop with the manual stretch of the skin to attempt a cleavage and bulla, i.e., Nikolsky's sign. Although taught over generations, in our opinion, this maneuver should never be performed. The patient will often, on questioning, relate that mild trauma induces a blister (Nikolsky-like); thus, it is important to know the concept of Nikolsky's sign, which is caused by a superficial cleavage plane formed from IgG against desmosomes in the epidermis.

Bullous pemphigoid manifests with tense clusters of bullae **(Fig. 14.79)**. Each bulla has a base of erythema. The bullae are stable and, thus, at presentation, are demonstrable. **Cicatricial pemphigoid** manifests with clusters of tense bullae and significant involvement of the mucous membranes and the conjunctivae. In point of fact, the defining feature of cicatricial pemphigoid is the severe conjunctivitis.

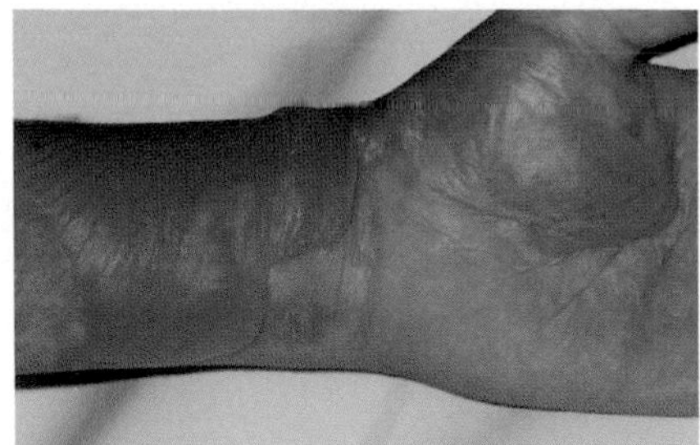

A

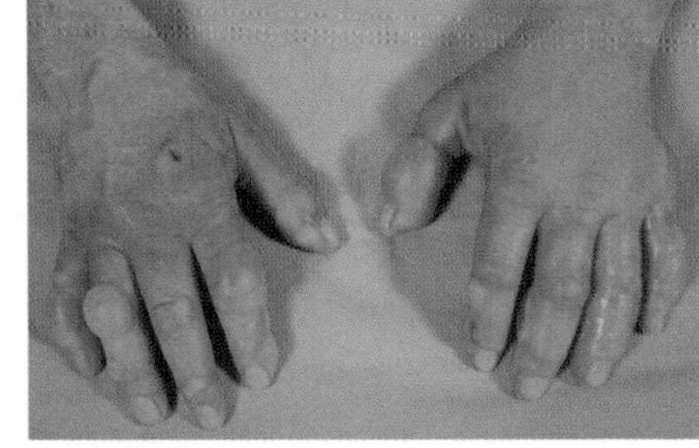

B

Figure 14.77.

A. Scald with bullae. **B.** Frostbite with bullae.

 **TIPS**

- Heat-related **(A):** bullae over the site involved, often the hands
- Steam-related, most risk for scald
- Frostbite **(B):** bullae in areas exposed, often the fingers or toes
- Hemorrhage in the bulla indicates great depth of the damage

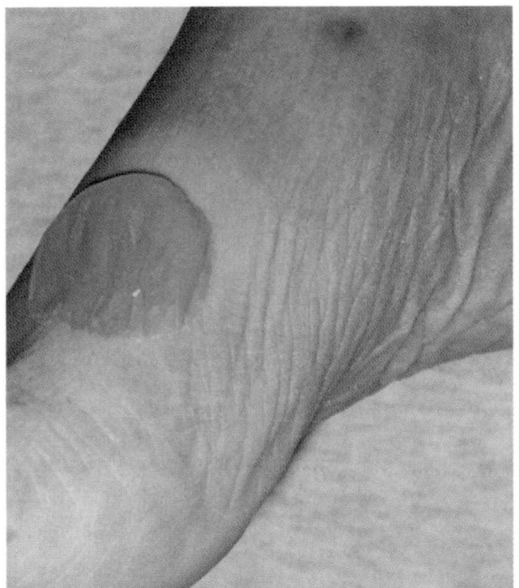

A

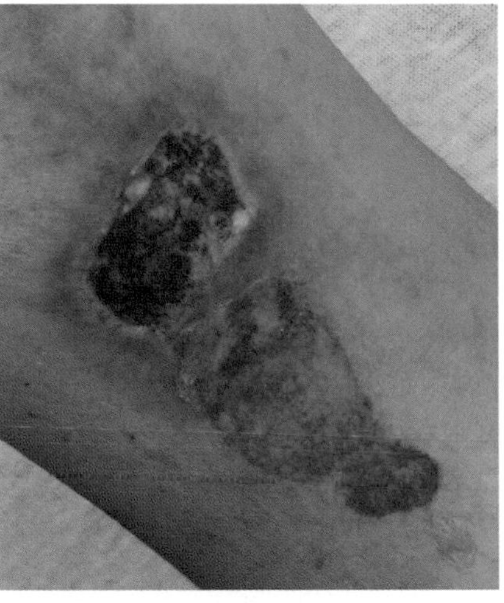

B

Figure 14.78.

Pemphigus vulgaris. **A.** Bulla. **B.** Erosion.

 **TIPS**

- Pemphigus vulgaris: very fragile, flaccid bulla
- Erosions are the predominant feature of the rash
- History of mild trauma inducing a lesion, history-related Nikolsky's sign
- Autoimmune: IgG against desmosomes is pathophysiology

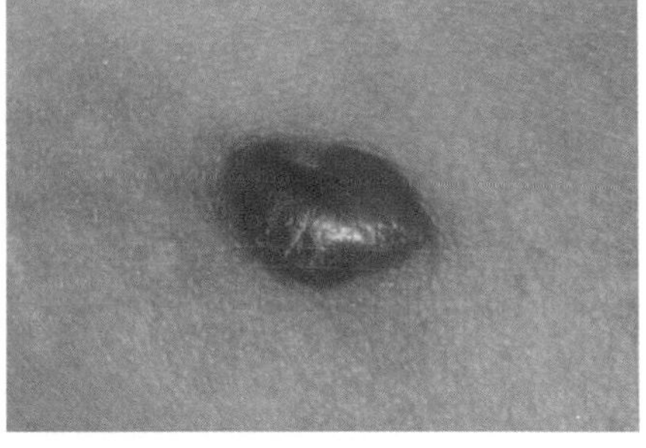

Figure 14.79.

Bullous pemphigoid.

 **TIPS**

- Clusters of tense bullae, with a base of erythema, bullae very stable
- Autoimmune: IgG and complement

TEACHING POINTS

BULLA

1. Most common cause of bulla is mechanical blistering, e.g., from raking.
2. Superficial bulla, fragile ones, easily rupture to form erosions.
3. Deep bulla, tense and stable ones, form ulcers when ruptured.
4. Nikolsky's sign should not be performed; however, the concept should be understood.
5. Autoimmune bullous lesions, although rare, are important to know. Such lesions manifest like a severe burn, and the patient may require burn unit admission.
6. Severe erythema multiforme major, which can cause bulla, is known as the Stevens-Johnson syndrome.

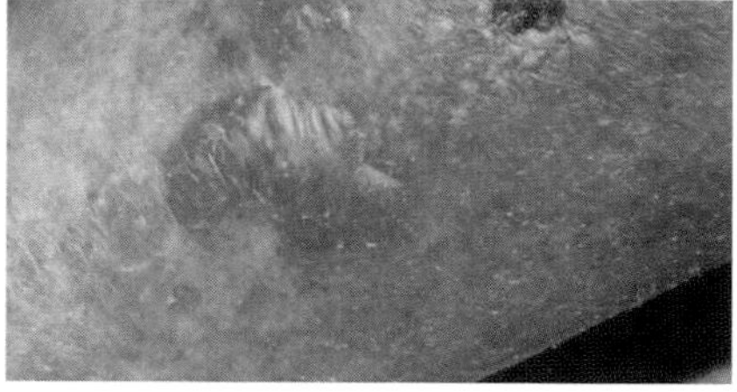

Figure 14.80.

Bullous impetigo.

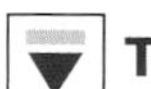

TIPS

- Bullous impetigo: localized area of bullae formation in an area of localized cellulitis
- *Staphylococcus aureus* infection in adjacent skin

Other bulla include **toxic epidermal necrolysis syndrome**, which manifests with diffuse bulla and, therefore, erosion formation. As large swaths of skin can be involved, a great risk exists of volume depletion, protein loss, and infection. A variant of this is the phage-mediated **staphylococcal scalded skin syndrome**. These potentially life-threatening entities can easily be confused with pemphigus vulgaris, but they are caused by the toxin-related damage to the epidermis by a phage-producing epidermolytic toxin. The phage is in the bacterium *Staphylococcus aureus.*

Bullous impetigo manifests with a localized area of bulla formation in an area of localized cellulites **(Fig. 14.80)**. This is caused by *Staphylococcus aureus* infection of the skin; cellulitis is antecedent to the bulla.

Other problems include **dermatitis herpetiformis**, which manifests with clusters of bullae with erythema at their bases. There is often concurrent gluten-sensitive sprue. This is an autoimmune, IgA process, most common in those of Celtic derivation. **Erythema multiforme major** (Stevens-Johnson syndrome) manifests with multiple areas of erythema multiforme and bullous formation. Often noted is mucous membrane involvement and the patient may have diffuse bullae leading to volume depletion, protein depletion, and infections. Erythema multiforme major is caused by a medication side effect, especially due to sulfa drugs.

PUS-CONTAINING STRUCTURES

Furuncle manifests with a tender, fluctuant nodule in the subcutaneous tissue, often with overlying erythema **(Fig. 14.81A)**. A **carbuncle** manifests with multiple furuncles, usually on the posterior neck or buttocks (Fig. 14.81B). Risk factors for carbuncles include uncontrolled diabetes mellitus and high-dose steroid use. Carbuncle is often caused by *Staphylococcus* or *Streptococcus* sps. or by anaerobes. Other antecedent risks include intravenous drug abuse and sebaceous cysts.

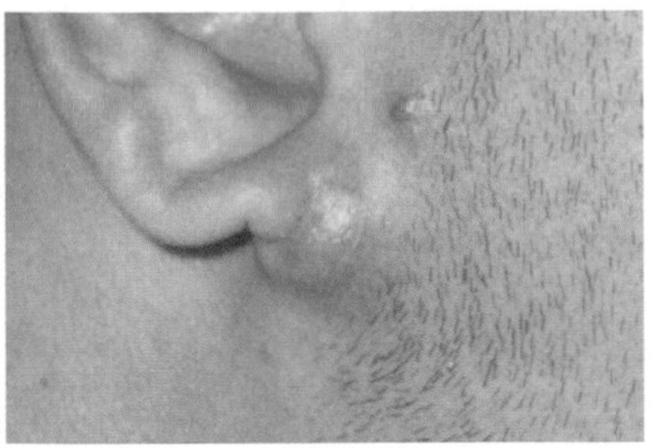
A

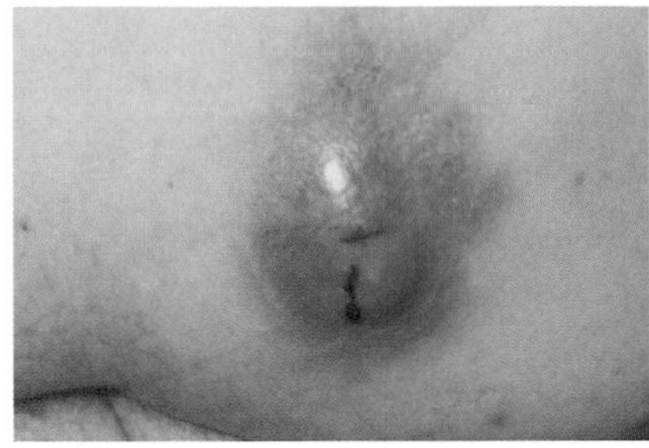
B

Figure 14.81.

A. Furuncle. **B.** Carbuncle.

TIPS

- Furuncle: solitary, tender, fluctuant nodule in subcutaneous tissue, overlying erythema
- Carbuncle: multiple furuncles, usually on the nape of the neck or buttock; lesions are interconnected
- Associated with poorly controlled diabetes mellitus

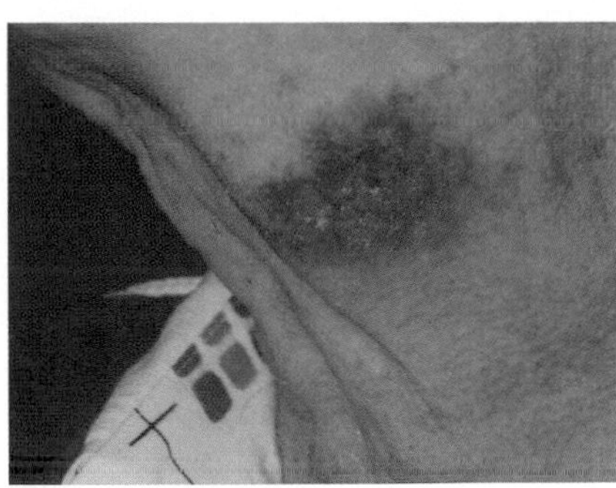

Figure 14.82.

Tinea barbae.

TIPS

- Tinea barbae: multiple, tender or pruritic pustules or nodules in the hair of the face
- Fungal infection of individual follicles

Tinea barbae manifest with one or more tender or pruritic infected pustules or nodules in the hair of the face **(Fig. 14.82)**. This is due to dermatophitic infection of the hair follicles of the beard. Risks include sharing razors and uncontrolled diabetes mellitus.

Other diagnoses include **folliculitis**, which manifests with a pustule in and around individual follicles; **hiradenitis suppurativa**, which manifests with one or more tender, indurated, or fluctuant nodules or masses in the hair-bearing areas of the axilla or pubis; **varicella**, which manifests with several crops of pustules, developed from vesicles, and progresses to crust over and then heal with fevers, and a cough; and **kerion**, which manifests with a plaque that is indurated, pustular, erythematous, matted, and concurrent with tinea capitis.

TEACHING POINTS

PUSTULES

1. Many pustules evolve from vesicles, especially if vesicles are viral-related.
2. Pustules adjacent to hair follicles = folliculitis.
3. Furuncle is a large pustule that is fluctuant, tender, and erythematous.
4. Carbuncle is composed of multiple, interconnected furuncles, and is usually seen on the buttock or posterior neck of a patient with diabetes mellitus.
5. Multiple crops of pustules evolve from vesicles: consider varicella infection.

Annotated Bibliography

Overall

Cherubin CE, Sapira JD. The medical complications of drug addition and the medical assessment of the intravenous drug user: 25 years later. *Ann Intern Med* 1993;119:1044–1046.

The manifestations and sequelae of this common and devastating problem. A must for emergency room and primary care physicians.

Cockerell CJ Nonmalignant dermatologic disorders in HIV disease. *The AIDS Reader* 1994; Jan/Feb:13–27.

A text- and table-rich descriptive set of dermatologic findings in chronic HIV infection. A paucity of images.

Graham BS, Schneiderman H. Physical diagnosis skills: skin signs of systemic disease *Consultant* 1996;(Jun):1193–1218.

A set of 19 different cases in which a thorough physical examination and history held clues that were key to making the diagnosis. Makes the case for a thorough and sophisticated physical examination, in general, and a dermatologic examination, specifically.

Klecz RJ, Schwartz RA. Pruritus. *Am Fam Phys* 1992;45(6):2681–2686.

Excellent review of the pathophysiology and evaluation of this common symptom; discusses the causes, which include primary skin disorders, e.g., atopic dermatitis and scabies; systemic disorders, e.g., malignancy-related, liver disease, HIV-related; and environmental, e.g., very low humidity. Discusses signs that develop as the result of chronic itching, including lichenification, hyperpigmentation, nodule formation (hence prurigo nodularis), and cellulitis. Scabies is included and emphasized in the paper.

Larkin RG. The callus of crack cocaine. *N Engl J Med* 1990;323:685.

Describes a callus on the ulnar aspect of thumb on the dominant side; often, with metallic linear discoloration in the callus.

McDonald CJ, Kelly AP. Diseases of black skin. In: Demis A, ed. *Clinical Dermatology*, 4th ed. New York: Harper and Row, 1987.

Excellent chapter on this extremely important topic for primary care physicians.

McKnight JT, Jones J. Jaundice. *Am Fam Phys* 1992;45(3):1139–1148.

Practical and robust paper describing the manifestations, differential diagnosis, and evaluation of jaundice. An excellent table describes the physical diagnosis of many causes of jaundice, including hemolytic anemia, congestive heart failure, and obstructive jaundice, either neoplastic or stone related.

Phillips TJ, Dover JS. Recent advances in dermatology. *N Engl J Med* 1992;326(3):167–178.

Review of acne vulgaris, psoriasis, warts, skin cancer, mycosis fungoides, HIV-related disease, and impetigo. An erudite discussion of each of those topics. Great bibliography.

Poole S, Fenske NA. Dermatologic clues to cancer. *J Intern Med* 1991;12(11):21–32.

A review of some skin manifestations of systemic malignant disease: Sister Mary Joseph's nodule, Muir-Torre syndrome, Peutz-Jeghers syndrome, acanthosis, Trousseau's sign, amyloidosis, and acanthosis nigricans.

Vinson RP, Harrington AC. Clinical significance and treatment of xanthomas. *Am Fam Phys* 1991;44(4):1206–1210.

Description, evaluation, and therapy of various xanthomas: tendinous xanthomas, xanthelasma, palmar crease xanthomas, tuberous xanthomas, eruptive xanthomas.

Williams DF, Kaplan DL. Common dermatoses of black skin. *Consultant* 1998;(Jan): 189–199.

A limited review of an important and underdescribed part of the physical examination—the approach to dermatology and description of skin entities in patients of color. Normal variants, including melanonychia and palmar and plantar macule, are discussed, followed by descriptions and discussion of entities, including keloids, sarcoidosis, and pseudofolliculitis barbae. Satisfactory discussion is included; however, there is a need for a much more robust review of this topic.

Red Lesions: Cellulitis

Bagdade JD, Segreti J. The infectious emergencies of diabetes. *The Endocrinologist* 1991; 1(3):155–162.

Excellent paper that reviews the infections that can be associated with uncontrolled diabetes mellitus, with emphasis on cellulites and complicated cellulites, including foot infections, necrotizing fasciitis, necrotizing cellulites, and gas-forming infections. Other infections are also described, including mucormycosis, otitis externa maligna, and gallbladder gangrene. The pathophysiology of the increased risk of these infections is detailed.

El-Daher N, Magnussen CR. Skin and soft tissue infections. *Consultant* 1996;(Dec):2563–2570.

Discusses cellulites, erysipelas, necrotizing fasciitis, and myonecrosis (gas gangrene). Also discusses antibiotics and early diagnosis and referral to surgical consultants.

Red Lesions: Exanthem

Cherry JD. Viral exanthems. DM 28(May), 1982.
Solid review of common viral-related red rashes, i.e., exanthems.

Neoplasia: Nonmelanoma

Beacham BE. Common skin tumors in the elderly. *Am Fam Phys* 1992;46(1):163–168.
Nice discussion of common lesions, both benign and malignant, in the geriatric population. Excellent images of the lesions; benign entities, including seborrheic keratosis, keratoacanthoma, epidermal cyst, cherry hemangioma, angiokeratomas of Fordyce, fibroepitheliomas, and skin tags; premalignant entities, including actinic keratoses, Bowen's disease; malignant entities, including basal cell carcinoma, squamous cell carcinoma, lentigo maligna, malignant melanoma, Kaposi's sarcoma, and angiosarcoma of scalp.

English JC, Canchola DR, Finley EM. Axillary basal cell carcinoma: a need for full cutaneous examination. *Am Fam Phys* 1998;57(8):1860–1864.
An atypical site for a basal cell carcinoma is used as an example to perform a thorough skin examination when seeing a patient.

Preston DS, Stern RS. Nonmelanoma cancers of the skin. *N Engl J Med* 1992;327(23):1649–1662.
Erudite review of the epidemiology, pathogenesis, physical examination, natural history, and treatment of these common skin neoplasms. Excellent photographs of various types of basal cell carcinoma and squamous cell carcinoma are included as are photographs of arsenical keratoses and the benign keratoacanthoma. Describes squamous cell precursor lesions, including actinic keratosis and Bowen's disease. A paper of tremendous value and one that should be in the files of any patient provider.

Ulcers

Greene SL, Su WPD, Muller SA. Ecthyma gangrenosum: report of clinical histopathologic and bacteriologic aspects of eight cases. *J Am Acad Derm* 1984;11:781–787.
Excellent review of a rare, but virtually pathognomonic, skin finding of pseudomonas bacteremia; most, if not all, of the patients in these eight cases were immunocompromised.

Rothe MJ, Grant-Kels JM. Dermatologic emergencies. Part 1: Pyoderma gangrenosum. *Consultant* 1997;(Oct):2721–2727.
The manifestations of this serious and even life-threatening ulcer-forming skin lesion are discussed; includes pathogenesis and underlying diagnoses; inflammatory bowel disease, seronegative rheumatoid arthritis, and myeloproliferative disorder all are associated. Therapeutic endeavors, including use of dapsone, are discussed.

Spoelhof GD, Ide K. Pressure ulcers in nursing home patients. *Am Fam Phys* 1993; 47(5): 1207–1215.
A solid discussion of the pathogenesis, evaluation, and management of pressure or decubital ulcers. Nice description of staging (Shea model) for the ulcers and the Braden for risk stratification of pressure sores; satisfactory presentation of various preventive and therapeutic modalities. Very practical and useful.

Red Lesions: Erythema

Alto WA, Gibson R. Acute rheumatic fever: an update. *Am Fam Phys* 1992;45(2):613–620.
A practical review of acute rheumatic fever with appropriate emphasis on the physical examination features of the disease. Reviews the incidence of specific parts of Jones' criteria of carditis: 55%, polyarthritis: 66%, chorea: 15%, erythema marginatum: 9%, and subcutaneous nodules: 3%. The erythema marginatum is annular, transient, nonpruritic, migratory, and on the trunk and upper extremities. Treatment and prevention are discussed in appropriate detail.

Faria DT, Krull EA. Recognizing and managing rosacea. *Hosp Med* 1996;(Feb):35–40.
Nice paper reviewing the clinical features, evaluation, and management of this common entity. Emphasizes that topical steroids chronically placed can cause it. Written by two dermatologists who give some practical tips on treatment. Excellent images of entities in the differential diagnosis: cutaneous lupus, seborrheic dermatitis, photosensitivity dermatitis, and acne vulgaris.

Schutzer SE. Diagnosing lyme disease. *Am Fam Phys* 1992;45(5):2151–2156.
Overview of Lyme disease, including specific manifestations: erythema migrans >50% incidence; 1 to 3 weeks after the tick bite, expanding, red annular lesion with a clear center, or targetlike with alternating red and pale rings that changes over time. The presence of Bell's palsy is common. Laboratory evaluation and specific management interventions are also discussed in detail that is appropriate to primary care physicians.

Stampien TM, Schwartz RA. Erythema multiforme. *Am Fam Phys* 1992:46(4):1171–1176.
Practical review of this relatively common form of erythema: targetlike plaques, erosions, well-demarcated, may have central blisters; found on the trunk, extremities, and the mucous membranes. Minor versus major forms; major can be the life-threatening Stevens-Johnson syndrome. Discusses three of the most common precipitating agents: herpes simplex, mycoplasma, and drugs (e.g., sulfa, penicillin, phenytoin). Appropriately robust discussions of the pathophysiology and therapy.

Tierney LM, Schwartz RA. Erythema nodosum. *Am Fam Phys* 1984;30(4):227–232.

A interesting overview of this erythema, which has painful, red, cutaneous and subcutaneous nodules; lower extremities mostly involved. Reviews the underlying causes, including sarcoidosis, mycobacterial disease, coccidiomycosis, streptococcal infections, drugs, and inflammatory bowel disease, which are all associated. Includes nice color images.

Red Lesions: Dermatitis

Forsman KE. Pediculosis and scabies. *Postgrad Med* 1995;98(6):89–100.

Manifestations, evaluation, and treatment of scabies and lice. Good images of the mites and of nits are included.

Krenek G, Rosen T. Eczema: the nuts and bolts of management. *Consultant* 1996;(Mar): 486–506.

Review rich with color images of many types of dermatitis, including atopic, contact, stasis, nummular, xerotic, seborrheic, dyshidrotic, and neurodermatitis. Reviews many of the common surface allergens that can cause dermatitis, including nickel, poison ivy, and components in rubber gloves. Includes practical points and discussion of therapeutic endeavors.

Sterling GB, Janninger CK, Schwartz RA. Scabies. *Am Fam Phys* 1992;(Oct):1237–1241.

Practical and succinct discussion on manifestations and treatment of scabies. Good for primary care physicians.

Pigmented Lesions

Karnes PS. Neurofibromatosis: a common neurocutaneous disorder. *Mayo Clin Proc* 1998; 73:1071–1076.

Succinct, but very complete review paper on neurofibromatosis, including type 1 and 2. NF-1: more than six café au lait spots, neurofibromas, freckling of axilla, optic nerve glioma, Lisch nodules in iris, first-degree relative with it; NF-2: bilateral cranial nerve VIII nerve mass, first-degree relative with NF-2. Excellent description of physical examination and of specific sequelae, including malignant neoplasia, neurofibrosarcoma, and the risk of pheochromocytoma. NF-1s autosomal-dominant on 17 q(long arm); 100% sensitivity of Lisch nodules for NF-1 by age 60.

Koh HK. Cutaneous melanoma. *N Engl J Med* 1991;325:171–182.

Erudite review of this increasingly common malignant cutaneous disorder.

Pellegrini JR, Wagner RF, Nathanson L. Halo nevi and melanoma. *Am Fam Phys* 1984;30(2): 157–159.

Review of an uncommon pigmented entity—a Sutton's nevus, i.e., a nevus surrounded by a rim of depigmentation. Often benign, but can be malignant or associated with a malignant melanoma at a distant location, including even intraocular.

Riccardi VM. von Recklinghausen neurofibromatosis. *N Engl J Med* 1981;305(27):1617–1627.

A tremendous review; a very scholarly and robust paper regarding this disorder. Splendid bibliography, very comprehensive.

Whited JD, Grichik JM. Does the patient have a mole or a melanoma? *JAMA* 1998;279(9): 696–701.

Reviews in metaanalysis the ABCD examination: A, asymmetry; B, borders irregular; C, irregular colors; D, diameter >6 mm., Quoted numbers for sensitivity of 100%; specificity of 98.4%; positive predictive value (PPV), 0.62; negative predictive value (NPV), 0.

Bullae

Osborn HH, Schiavone FM. Frostbite. *Hosp Med* 1988;(Jan):16–30.

Case-based paper that reviews the manifestations and treatment of acute and chronic frostbite. Also includes a discussion of other cold injuries, including chilblain (pernio), red or violaceous plaques when skin is exposed to cold, and trench foot, wet cold (<50 degrees). Therapeutic modalities and pathophysiology are also described; interesting observation of increased risk of severe frostbite in individuals who have had a previous cold-related injury.

Peate WF. Outpatient management of burns. *Am Fam Phys* 1992;45(3):1321–1331.

Good overview of burn diagnosis and management with a table and images to support the staging and size of burns.

Rothke MJ, Grant-Kels JM. Dermatologic emergencies. Part 5: Drug induced Stevens-Johnson and toxic epidermal necrolysis. *Consultant* 1998;(Apr):889–895.

Brief, but well-written article on these two specific severe entities. Nice images and definitions; describes systemic manifestations of these systemic disorders.

Rothe MJ, Grant-Kels JM. Dermatologic emergencies. Part 6: Pemphigus and bullous pemphigoid. *Consultant* 1998;(May):1109–1126.

Short review of two potentially severe blistering disorders: pemphigus and bullous pemphigoid. Reviews the most common variants of pemphigus (all with flaccid bullae) and states the site of cleavage for each; vulgaris suprabasilar (definite oral involvement); foliaceus stratum granulosum (minimal oral involvement); paraneoplastic (suprabasilar); and the tense bulla of bullous pemphigoid and its variant cicatrical pemphigoid (involves the conjunctivitis). Good skin images; good tables, fair discussion of therapy.

Nails

Holzberg M, Walker HK. Terry's nails: revised definitions and new correlations. *Lancet* 1984; 1:896–899.
Reviews and updates this set of interesting nail findings, red lunula, which is associated with CHF.

Kabongo ML, Bedell AW. Nail signs of systemic conditions. *Am Fam Phys* 1987;(Oct):109–116.
Nail findings of systemic disease are described, including Lindsay's and Terry's nails, splinter hemorrhages, Beau's lines, Mees' lines, koilonychia, and nail clubbing.

Montana JB, Scher RK. Nail tumors: benign and malignant. *Emerg Med* 1994;(Apr):12–32.
Satisfactory review of common tumors involving the finger and toenails, including verruca vulgaris (warts), molluscum contagiosum, myxoid cysts, pyogenic granuloma, glomus tumor; and the malignant, squamous cell carcinoma and subungual melanoma. Treatment modalities are discussed in some detail; quite good images.

Muerhcke RL. The fingernails in chronic hypoalbuminemia: a new physical sign. *BMJ* 1956; 1:1327.
Classic description of this fascinating finding of hypoalbuminemia.

Noronha PA, Zubkov B. Nails and nail disorders in children and adults. *Am Fam Phys* 1997; 55(6):2129–2140.
A good discussion of nail problems, including descriptions of clubbing (Lovibond's angle), Schamroth's sign, koilonychias, Beau's lines, Muercke's lines, subungual hematoma, nail-biting, paronychia, onychomycosis, and nail pitting.

Schneiderman H. Onychogryphosis (ram's horn nails) and onychomycosis. *Consultant* 1992;(Aug)32:61–62.
Short, informative, and with great images from one of the masters of physical diagnosis.

Strobach RS, Anderson SK, Doll DC, Ringenberg S. The value of the physical examination diagnosis of anemia: correlation of the physical findings with the hemoglobin concentration. *Arch Intern Med* 1988;148:831–832.
Pale palmar creases are correlated with a hemoglobin level that is<10 g.

Hypopigmented Lesions

Dunn JF. Vitiligo. *Am Fam Phys* 1986;33(5):137–143.
Satisfactory review of this relatively rare disorder, with very good images included.

Savin R. Diagnosis and treatment of tinea versicolor. *J Fam Pract* 1996;43(2):127–132.
Very good overview of this common entity, Wood lamp and potassium hydroxide examinations, and treatment, including oral and topical agents.

Sweet RD: Vitiligo as a Koebner phenomenon. *Brit J Derm* 1978;99:223–224.
Confirms a clinical observation: that vitiligo occurs in sites of scars.

Weitzner JM. Alopecia areata. *Am Fam Phys* 1990;41(4):1197–1201.
Nice review with excellent images of this form of patchy hair loss, which is associated with autoimmune and thyroid diseases. Describes nail pitting in a grid pattern and that hair that regrows may be pure white. Reviews severe variants, including alopecia totalis, i.e., loss of all head hair.

Purple Lesions

Callen JP. Dermatomyositis. *Lancet* 2000;355:53–57.
A scholarly review of this inflammatory myopathy; skin manifestations include the periorbital edema (heliotropic rash) and the presence of Gottron's plaques periungual telangiectasia, rash over the joints.

Hermans PE The clinical manifestations of infective endocarditis. *Mayo Clin Proc* 1982; 57:15–21.
A comprehensive review of the physical examination manifestations of endocarditis, including dermatologic findings such as splinter hemorrhages, Osler's nodes, and petechiae.

Klippel JH. Raynaud's phenomenon. *Arch Intern Med* 1991;151:2389–2393.
Reviews the classic tricolor of white, blue, and red in digits exposed to cold in the differential diagnosis of blue digits.

Peery WH. Clinical spectrum of hereditary hemorrhagic telangiectasia (Osler-Weber-Rendu). *Am J Med* 1987;82:989–996.
Excellent review of the manifestations and pathogenesis of this autosomal dominant disorder. Includes telangiectasia, arteriovenous malformations, aneurysms, bleeding from the gastrointestinal tract, and strokes.

Wirth FA, Lowitt MH. Diagnosis and treatment of cutaneous vascular lesions. *Am Fam Phys* 1998;57(4):765–777.
Nice review of red and purple vascular entities, including flat salmon patch (nevus simplex, including Unna nevus on nape of neck), port-wine stain (nevus flammeus), and hemangiomas, in-

cluding cherry hemangioma and the more complicated, cavernous hemangioma. Excellent color images of these entities, along with a discussion of some associated congenital syndromes.

Hair

Berfield WF, Helm TN. Hair loss. *Consultant* 1994;(Oct):1390–1400.
Satisfactory review of this common entity, with hair loss syndromes described limited to the head hair. Describes generalized hair loss syndromes in addition to localized entities. Emphasizes the importance of assessing location and concurrent findings to arrive at the underlying cause. Generalized alopecia includes androgenic, which can be exacerbated or accentuated by hypothyroidism; telogen effluvium (rapid, diffuse hair loss on the entire scalp), which is caused by cessation of growth of anagen hairs. Hair loss because of major illness, surgery, childbirth, or nutritional deficiency; anagen effluvium (hair growth abruptly ceases, the hair breaks off because of chemotherapy); trichotillomania, which is related to neurotic, compulsive behavior, also has onychophagia (nail-biting) –patches of various aged hairs; and discoid lupus (alopecia with scarring, tinea capitis; and secondary lues (a moth-eaten appearance). Does not discuss vascular alopecia of extremities.

Slagle DA, Martin TA. Trichotillomania. *Am Fam Phys* 1991;43(6):2019–2024.
Nice review of a common disorder, pulling of hair and even eating thereof (trichophagia). Manifestations, evaluation, and therapy are discussed in appropriate detail for primary care physicians.

Vesicles

Rosen T, Ablon G. Cutaneous herpesvirus infections update: Part 1: Herpes simplex virus types 1 and 2.
A good review of common herpes simplex infections, including herpes gingivostomatitis, herpes labialis, herpes genitalis, and the trauma-related, herpetic whitlow and herpes gladiatorum. Color images of many of these entities are included.

Psoriasis

Rothe MJ. Grant-kels psoriasis. *Consultant* 1997;(May):1171–1185.
Discusses various types of psoriasis. Emphasis is on therapy, less on diagnosis, although some good images of various types of psoriasis are included.

15

Eye Examination

PRACTICE AND TEACHING

ANATOMY

The eye itself consists of an ovoid structure—the globe—that is composed of a wall of tough collagen material called the **sclera**. At the most anterior aspect of the sclera is a circle of transparent tissue—the cornea. The sclera is lined anteriorly with the conjunctiva, a thin membrane that contains vessels. The *conjunctiva* does not cover the cornea. The inside layer of the sclera and thus the globe is lined with a pigmented layer called the **uvea**. The choroid, iris, and retina are derived from and are components of the uvea. Filling the major portion of the interior of the globe is a viscous clear substance, the **vitreous humor**. The **anterior chamber** of the eye contains the lens, iris, and ciliary body. This chamber is immediately posterior to the cornea and anterior to the vitreous. The **cornea** is composed of several layers, which are in order, superficial to deep: the epithelium, also known as Bowman's membrane, the stroma, and Descemet's membrane, which is adjacent to the endothelium. The blood supply to the eye is twofold: the **ophthalmic artery** gives off the central retinal artery, a major branch to the posterior retina, which provides blood from the deep to peripheral side; and second, the diffuse **choroid plexus** in which the blood flows peripheral to deep. The **macula** is the site where all retinal vessels terminate (or originate); thus, the macula and its center, the fovea centralis, receives blood from the choroid plexus alone. The nerves that supply the eye are **cranial nerve II** in the optic disc, which is the sensory nerve for vision; **cranial nerve V**, which provides sensory to the cornea and conjunctiva; and the *sympathetic* and *parasympathetic fibers* in **cranial nerve III** to supply the pupil for constriction (parasympathetic) and dilation (sympathetic); CN III innervates the levator palpebra muscle for eye opening, especially the upper eyelid.*

The *periorbital structures* include the upper and lower eyelid, both of which are lined on the inside by **palpebral conjunctiva**; the **lacrimal gland** in the upper outer part of the eye socket; the **medial canthus**, with the two puncta of the nasolacrimal duct; and the **visceral conjunctiva** overlying the sclera but not the cornea. The six extraocular muscle actions and their nerves are discussed in the neurologic examination (Fig. 15.2). Eyelashes are on the lid margins; each lash is nourished by a gland of Moll or Zeis.

*Superior tarsal muscle (Mueller's) is smooth muscle, sympathetic innervation, complements levator palpebrae.

Visual acuity is assessed using a **Snellen** chart. Both the left eye (**OS** [oculus sinistra]) and right eye (**OD** [oculus dextra]) must be assessed. Each eye is isolated by applying an eye cover to the other side. **Legally blind** is a visual acuity of 20/200 or worse, i.e., inability to see the top letter of the Snellen chart from 20 feet. To document acuity worse than 20/200, perform the Snellen test at 15 and then at 10 feet. If patient is able to see at 15 feet, acuity is 15/300; at 10 feet, 10/400. If the patient remains unable to see the top figure at 10 feet, perform the **count fingers**, from 3, then 2, then 1 foot (CF 3, 2, 1); **hand movement** from 3, then 2, then 1 foot (HM 3, 2, 1); and, finally, use a **light source** to test for perception of any light. **Total blindness** is defined as no light perceived (NLP). Assess the patient both with and without eyeglasses. A refractory condition, e.g., myopia, hypermetropia, or astigmatism, will improve markedly on application of appropriate lenses; however, a nonrefractory defect will not improve. Another method to differentiate a refractory from a nonrefractory defect is to perform the Snellen chart examination with the patient looking through a **pinhole**: refractory problems improve, whereas nonrefractory problems remain unchanged.

Total blindness is proved by performing the **optokinetic drum** or *banner test.* For this test, a rotating drum or banner painted in a black and white alternating pattern is placed 8 inches (20 cm) in front of, and rotated or moved before, the patient. With total blindness, no eye movement occurs, whereas any individual with some vision develops horizontal nystagmus. This normal nystagmus, which all of us have when looking out the side window of a moving train or car, is called, **optokinetic nystagmus**.

The Snellen chart measures the acuity of central vision, but not of the peripheral vision. Peripheral vision is first assessed by **confrontation**, which is a set of tests complementary to the Snellen chart. This is a screening for gross defects only. Normal visual fields are 60 to 70 degrees above and below the horizontal axis and 80 to 85 degrees from the vertical axis. Standing before the patient with one eye covered, move the index finger inward from the periphery in the nasal, temporal, superior, and then inferior axes.

A further measure of central vision is the **Ishihara chart** for color vision. As the fovea centralis is the only part of the retina that contains cones for color vision, processes involving central vision manifest with defects in color perception. Finally, the **Amsler visual grid** test can be of diagnostic benefit (**Table 15.1**). This grid is a method to assess for macular degeneration and gross scotoma, i.e., blind spots. The normal absolute scotoma, i.e., the blind spot, is a circle of 10 degrees diameter located 10 to 15 degrees

Table 15.1. Diagnostic Utility of the Amsler Grid

Diagnosis	Findings
Normal	Grid is seen as not wavy Central point seen throughout the visual fields to about 40 degrees temporal and 30 degrees nasal Absolute scotoma present 10 degrees on the temporal midline, circle-shaped
Chronic glaucoma	Multiple scotomata, especially on periphery Scotoma on an arc extending from blind spot to the superior nasal area: Bjerrum's scotoma
Macular degeneration	Marked decrease in ability to see central dot Central grid is wavy
Optic chiasm tumor	Loss of entire half of temporal field bilaterally

temporal to the midpoint of the visual field. The technique for this is for the patient to maintain a neutral forward gaze, one fixed on a specific distant point. The *Amsler grid* is placed 8 inches (20 cm) before the eyes of the patient. One eye is covered, while the examiner moves the grid to all areas of the visual fields—superior, inferior, temporal, and nasal—and instructs the patient to state when the central black dot cannot be seen. Normal is that the grid lines are not wavy; and the central point is seen throughout the fields to about 40 degrees temporally and 30 degrees nasally, except for the normal blind spot on the temporal midline field. **Open-angle glaucoma** manifests with an arcuate scotoma that extends from the normal blind spot (Bjerrum's scotoma), and peripheral field scotomata. The company it keeps includes increased intraocular pressure (IOP) and increased cup-to-disc ratio on funduscopic examination. **Optic neuritis** or multiple sclerosis manifests with multiple, often randomly placed scotoma. **Age-related macular degeneration** manifests with a wavy pattern of the central Amsler grid, significant drusen on funduscopic examination, and a decrease in color and night vision.

EXTRAOCULAR MUSCLES (EOMI*)

Assessment of the extraocular muscle function is fundamental to the overall and the eye-specific examination **(Box 15.1)**. Extraocular muscle weakness manifests as strabismus, i.e., weakness or paralysis of movement. The patient will often complain of "double vision," headaches, and loss of depth perception. **Two steps** in physical examination are required and should be performed in this order: **baseline assessment of gaze (Fig. 15.1)** and then **active range of movement (ROM) (Fig. 15.2)** of the eyes to all three axes. One method to recall the function of the extraocular muscles is to group them by cranial nerve.

Cranial nerve III (oculomotor nerve) innervates the superior rectus, inferior rectus, inferior oblique, and the medial rectus muscles. A **cranial nerve III deficit** manifests with multiple extraocular motor defects, either paralysis (tropia) or weakness (phoria) to these movements, and often a baseline gaze of a **walleye**, i.e., **exotropia**. A walleye develops in CN III palsy because the

*EOMI = extraocular muscles intact.

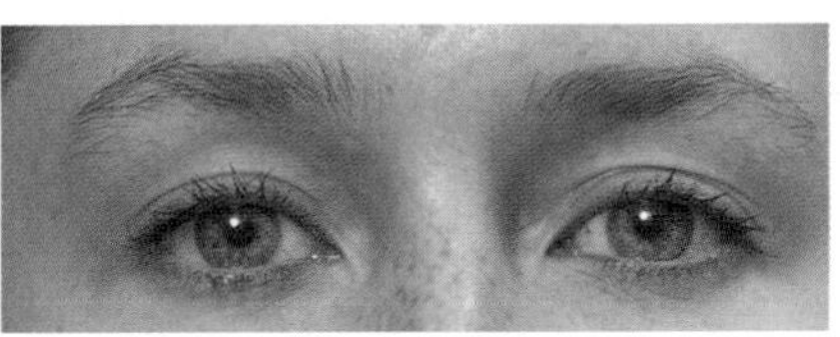

Figure 15.1.

Technique to assess baseline gaze. (From Bickley LS, Szilagyi PG. *Bates' Guide to Physical Examination*, 8th ed. Philadelphia: Lippincott Williams & Wilkins, 2003:121, with permission.)

TIPS

- Starting point for all extraocular examinations
- Instruct patient to gaze naturally at a point of light positioned approximately 2 meters to the front in the horizontal plane
- Note white reflexes from the pupils of both eyes
- Normal: reflexes should be equidistant from the midline, i.e., the tip of the nose and from the upper to lower orbital rims
- Strabismus: pupils not equidistant

Box 15.1.

Rules of Eye Motion Examination

1. All recti muscles move eye outward except, the medial.
2. All oblique muscles move the eye inward, i.e., nasal, but opposite to superior or inferior name.
3. SO4, LR6, all the rest 3 is useful for teaching.
4. Inspect all three axes: superior, inferior, and horizontal.
5. May perform this with eyes closed if photophobic or unable to open eyes.

SO=superior oblique;
LR=lateral rectus.

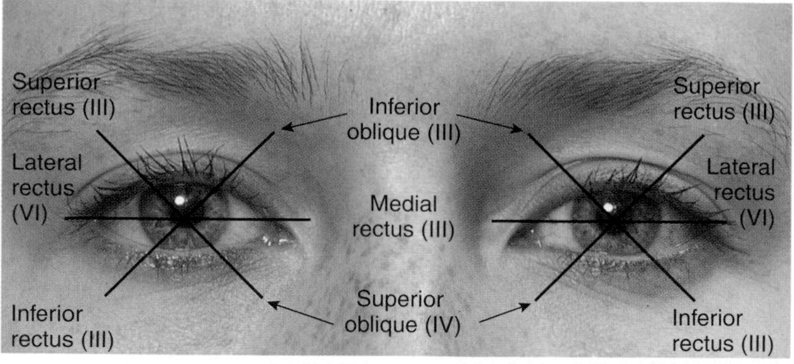

Figure 15.2.

Technique for active range of motion (ROM) in all three axes: horizontal, superior, and inferior. (From Bickley LS, Szilagyi PG. *Bates' Guide to Physical Examination*, 8th ed. Philadelphia: Lippincott Williams & Wilkins, 2003:123, with permission.)

TIPS

- Place one finger in horizontal gaze plane, 20 to 25 cm anterior to the midline of the face
- Place thumb of other hand on patient's chin to stabilize and prevent head movement
- Instruct patient to follow finger with eyes
- Trace the three axes, always returning to the midline

lateral rectus (innervated by CN VI) remains intact and, therefore dominates the eye. **Paresis of CN III** manifests with weakness by the second or third active attempt to medially deviate the affected eye. **Plegia of CN III** manifests with an absolute loss of medial movement in the horizontal axis. This is termed a walleye **(Fig. 15.3)**. The company a CN III deficit keeps includes ipsilateral marked ptosis. CN III deficit is due to trauma or tumor in the orbit. **Cranial nerve IV** (trochlear nerve), the smallest of the cranial nerves, innervates the superior oblique muscle. **Cranial nerve IV deficit** manifests with a paralysis (tropia) or weakness (phoria) to nasal and inferior (down and in) eye movement; thus, a baseline gaze of moderate walleye with a slight upward deviation of the eye. CN IV damage is due to trauma to the orbit or uncal herniation. The reasons for **walleye (Table 15.2)** include damage to cranial nerve III, trauma-related damage to cranial nerve IV, or a retroorbital process. Thus, after any facial trauma, one must, in addition to assessing eye ROM and pupils, assess upper eyelids for ptosis and eye for exophthalmus or endophthalmus by inspection and convergence, as well as inspect and palpate the inferior orbital rim for ecchymosis or any bony step-off.

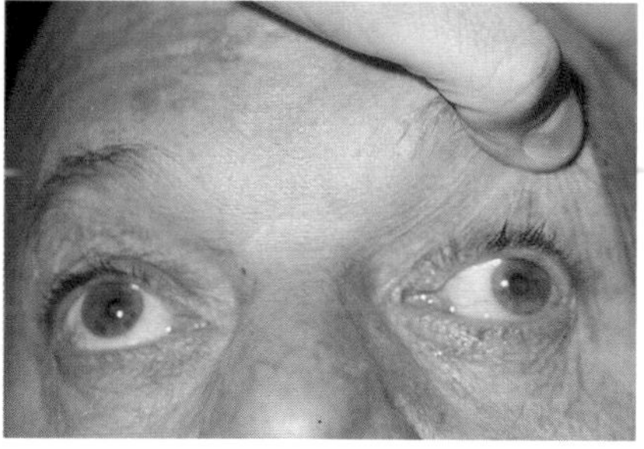

Figure 15.3.

Walleye from cranial nerve III palsy. (From Savino PJ, Danesh-Meyer HV. Neuro-ophthalmology. In: Tasman W, Jaeger EA, eds. *The Wills Eye Hospital Atlas of Clinical Ophthalmology*, 2nd ed. Philadelphia: Lippincott Williams & Wilkins, 2001;351, with permission.)

TIPS

- Baseline gaze of patient
- Cranial nerve III damage: multiple muscle deficits and, therefore, lateral rectus, cranial nerve VI dominates and pulls the eye outward; ptosis often present
- Note asymmetry in light reflex

Table 15.2. **Strabismus: Walleye and Crosseye**

Diagnosis	Mechanism	Company it Keeps
Cranial nerve III	Retroorbital process Orbital fracture Carotid sinus thrombosis	Ptosis Multiple defects Walleye at baseline
Superior oblique entrapment (Brown's syndrome)	Synovitis of trochlea, caused by rheumatoid arthritis	Crosseye at baseline Active polyarticular arthritis
Inferior oblique entrapment, orbital rim fracture	Fracture of the infraorbital rim	Crosseye at baseline Endophthalamus Ecchymosis, specific to medial inferior rim Step-off on bony rim
Cranial nerve IV damage	Basilar skull fracture Weak superior oblique muscle	Walleye at baseline Periorbital ecchymosis Weakness to down and in eye motion Papilledema Dilated pupil from increased intracranial pressure
Cranial nerve VI damage	Congenital trauma	Crosseye at baseline

Cranial nerve VI (abducens nerve) innervates the lateral rectus muscle. **Cranial nerve VI deficit** manifests with paralysis (tropia) or weakness (phoria) to this movement and often a baseline gaze of cross-eye, i.e., esotropia **(Fig. 15.4)**. This is caused by medial rectus and superior or inferior rectus muscles dominating the eye with weakness to, or absence of, lateral movement. This is due to trauma or a congenital LR weakness (see Table 15.2). **Proptosis or exophthalmus** manifests with unilateral or bilateral protrusion of the globe from the orbit, which is caused by retroorbital swelling from Graves' disease, trauma, or an orbital cellulitis. An excellent method to unmask proptosis is to perform convergence (Fig. 1.71). The acquired loss of convergence in one or both eyes is termed "Moebius sign" and indicates exophthalmus.

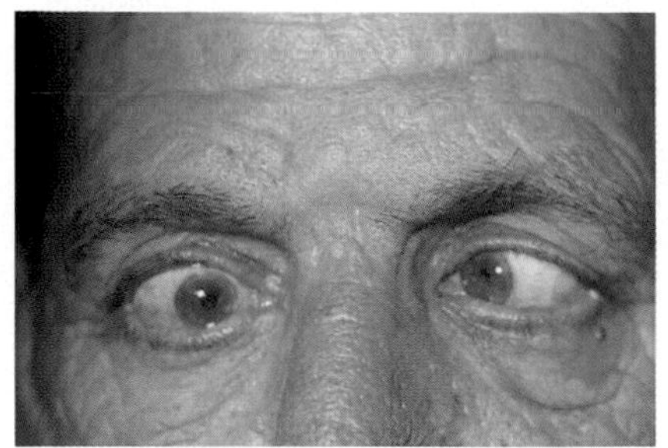

Figure 15.4.

Cross-eye caused by cranial nerve VI palsy. (From Savino PJ, Danesh-Meyer HV. Neuro-ophthalmology. In: Tasman W, Jaeger EA, eds. *The Wills Eye Hospital Atlas of Clinical Ophthalmology*, 2nd ed. Philadelphia: Lippincott Williams & Wilkins, 2001:353, with permission.)

 **TIPS**

- Patient's baseline gaze
- LRVI deficit: Cross-eye caused by other muscle pulling the eye inward (especially III)

PUPILS EQUAL ROUND AND REACTIVE TO LIGHT OR ACCOMMODATION (PERRLA)

Pupil assessment includes looking at size, shape of the pupil and its response to light. The size of the pupils is usually between 1 and 6 mm **(Table 15.3)**. Several reference markers are available at most medical bookstores that allow the clinician easy sizing of the pupils. A small flashlight is an excellent light source; in all cases, the room should be slightly darkened to optimize the examination. **Miosis** (constriction) manifests with one or both pupils that are pinpoint or very small in size. A common example is the use of narcotic agents; **mydriasis** (dilation) manifests with pupils that are very large in size. This is due to either surge of catecholamines, e.g., in fear, or due to death.

Table 15.3. Pupillary Findings

Diagnosis	Darkened room	Direct light	Consensual	Company it Keeps
Normal	Mydriasis, bilateral	Miosis	Miosis	
Uncal herniation	Mydriasis, unilateral	No miosis	No miosis	Decreased LOC Trauma Papilledema
Topical agent	Mydriasis, unilateral	No miosis	No miosis	Scopolamine patch use Mydriatic agent use
Acute angle glaucoma	Modest mydriasis, unilateral	No miosis	No miosis	Red, painful eye Crescent shadow sign in anterior chamber Markedly increased IOP Headache, vomiting
Horner's syndrome	Miosis	No mydriasis	No mydriasis	Ipsilateral ptosis Absent Marcus-Gunn jaw-winking reflex Ipsilateral anhidrosis

IOP = intraocular pressure; LOC = level of consciousness.

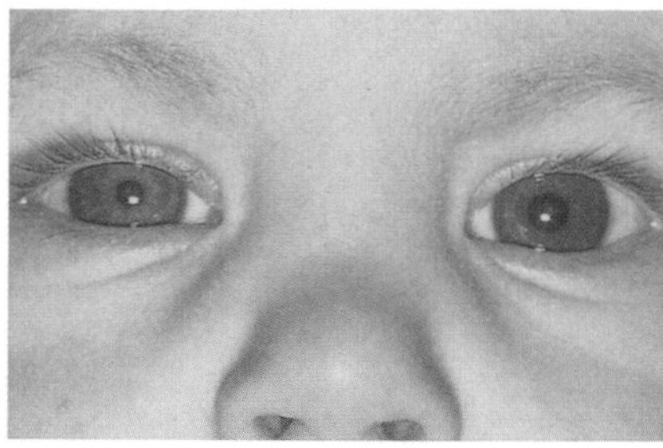

Figure 15.5.

Horner's syndrome: ptosis, anisocoria, and miosis (constriction). (From Zitelli, B. *Atlas of Pediatric Physical Diagnosis*, 2nd. ed.)

TIPS

- Ptosis: eyelid drooped over the upper cornea so that it covers >10% of the cornea
- Ptosis: common but nonspecific finding, the company it keeps makes the diagnosis
- Horner's syndrome: miosis of one pupil on the affected side; concurrent anhidrosis

Anisocoria means pupils that are unequal in size. Anisocoria of <1 mm may be normal; 20% of the population have such anisocoria (i.e., >1 mm difference strongly suggests a problem).

The pupils should be round; if there is a change of shape it is called poikiloscoria. **Adhesions (synechiae)** manifest with poikiloscoria and fibrous bands in the anterior chamber; these are due to healed inflammation.

Normally, pupils should constrict or become miotic when a light is shined into one (direct) or the other (consensual) pupil; repeat in the other eye. **Horner's syndrome (Fig. 15.5)** manifests with a miotic pupil, with an ipsilateral ptosis. The company it keeps includes upward migration of the lower eyelid, and an absent Marcus-Gunn jaw-wink sign **(Fig. 15.6)**. The syndrome is caused by a loss of function of the superior cervical chain, most often due to neoplasia in the lung apex or trauma to neck on ipsilateral side. **Uncal herniation** manifests with a mydriatic ("blown") pupil. The company it keeps includes decreased level of consciousness, often antecedent trauma to head with increased intracranial pressure. **Topical agents**, e.g., the instillation of dialating eye drops, manifest with mydriasis. The company it keeps includes photophobia, and a marked blurring of vision as mydriasis worsens any refractory problem. **Acute angle glaucoma** manifests with a dilated pupil in a painful photophobic red eye (see Fig. 15.12).

Normally, the pupils also constrict to **accommodation**, i.e., instructing patient to follow an object inward so as to internally rotate (converge) both eyes **(Fig. 15.7)**. The **Argyll-Robertson pupil**, which manifests with an inability of the pupil to constrict to direct or consensual light, but does constrict to accommodation, is caused by tertiary *lues venereum*. Accommodation defects are rare. Although it was common in the 1920s when PERRLA was described because *lues* was epidemic, it is now rarely seen. Do not be frustrated if you do not find it. Convergence, however, is an excellent method to assess for early proptosis. The acquired lack of medial eye movement with convergence (Moebius sign) is one of the first signs of proptosis.

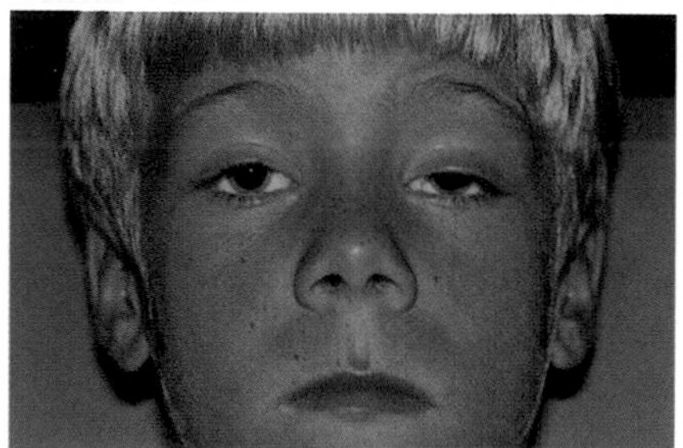

A

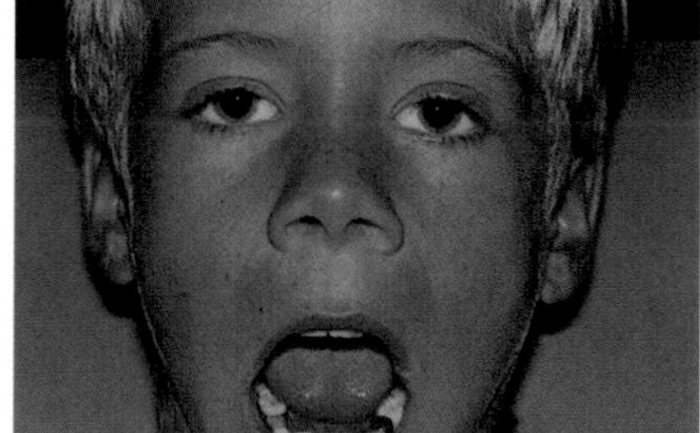

B

Figure 15.6.

Technique for jaw-winking sign—Marcus-Gunn reflex—its absence, as here, confirms Horner's syndrome. (From Bedrossian EH, Penne RB, Stefanyszyn MA. In: Tasman W, Jaeger EA, eds. *The Wills Eye Hospital Atlas of Clinical Ophthalmology*, 2nd ed. Philadelphia: Lippincott Williams & Wilkins, 2001:380, with permission.)

TIPS

- Patient with unilateral ptosis
- Instruct the patient to actively open mouth
- Note location of upper lid of the eye with ptosis
- Congenital ptosis: upper eyelid will open (Marcus-Gunn reflex response)
- Horner's syndrome: no change in the upper eyelid location

ANTERIOR CHAMBER

Inspection of the anterior chamber (Fig. 15.8) with an ophthalmoscope or a slit lamp is of great importance, especially if the patient has a red eye **(Table 15.4)**. The first step in using an ophthalmoscope is to shine the light so as to see a **red reflex**, then move toward the patient's pupil, aiming the light at the center of the red reflex. It is important that the light from the ophthalmoscope be shined both directly into the anterior chamber and also from the side, i.e., tangential light direction. Structures normally present include the **iris**, a pleated, pigmented, circumferential structure in the anterior chamber; the **cornea**, a crystal clear anterior structure; the **anterior chamber** with aqueous humor; and the **lens**, deep to the iris, which is suspended by the small ligaments around its circumference. **Anterior uveitis** manifests with a red eye with significant photophobia, and a decrease in visual acuity. The company it keeps includes cloudiness in the anterior chamber, and, on slit lamp examination, precipitate, synechiae, and even a hypopyon, i.e., a pus level, (Fig. 15.19) in the anterior chamber. **Corneal opacity** manifests with a decrease in visual acuity, partial loss of the red reflex, and a white area in the cornea itself **(Fig. 15.9)**. **Slit lamp** and **ophthalmoscopic examinations** confirm the location of the corneal opacity. **Corneal opacities** are most commonly caused by a corneal ulcer or scar **(Table 15.5)**. **Nuclear cataract** manifests with a decrease in visual acuity, especially at night, and is partial to total loss of red reflex and a white area in the lens itself; slit lamp and ophthalmoscopy confirm the location. **Cortical cataract** manifests with a decrease in visual acuity, especially in bright light, partial to total loss of red reflex, and a white area in the lens; slit lamp and ophthalmoscopy confirm the location. **Lens subluxation** manifests with a marked change in visual acuity and a change in the red reflex so that it is crescent-shaped and a superior or inferior migration of the lens. If subluxation is caused by **Marfan's syndrome**, it is a superior subluxation; if subluxation is caused by **homocystinuria** or Ehlers-Danlos syndrome, it is an inferior subluxation. The company it keeps is specific to the underlying diagnosis (Table 15.4).

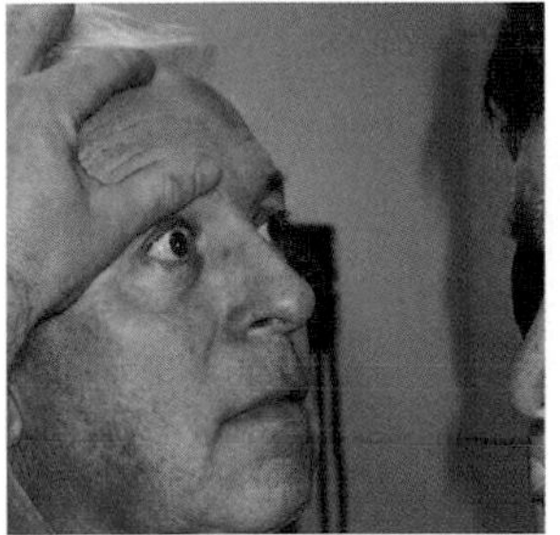

A

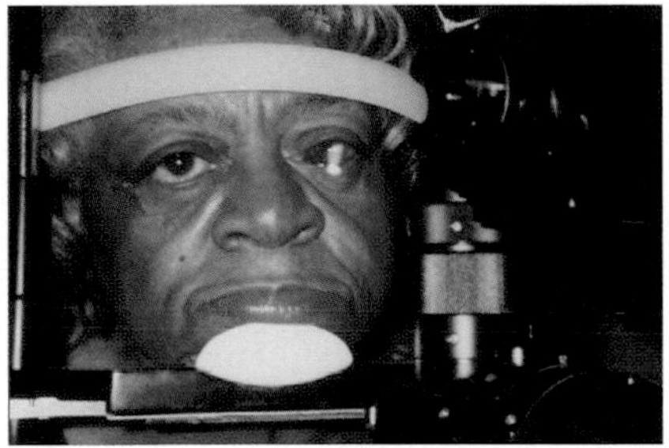

B

Figure 15.8.

Technique for anterior chamber inspection. **A.** Using an ophthalmoscope. **B.** Slit lamp.

 **TIPS**

- Anterior chamber inspection **(A)**
- Patient assumes a baseline horizontal gaze
- Shine the light of an ophthalmoscope into eyes and look through the ophthalmoscope
- Slit lamp **(B)**
- Tangential light: light source shined into anterior chamber from the side
- Normal: round, red reflex in both eyes

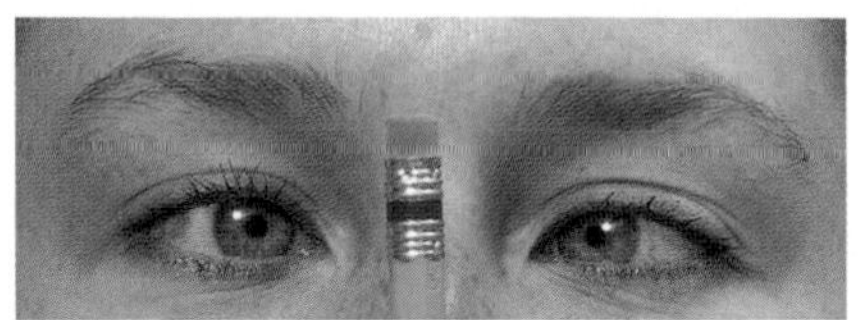

Figure 15.7.

Technique for accommodation: patient actively follows an object in midline so as to converge, i.e., become cross-eyed; observe the pupils with eye movement. (From Bickley LS, Szilagyi PG. *Bates' Guide to Physical Examination*, 8th ed. Philadelphia: Lippincott Williams & Wilkins, 2003:121, with permission.)

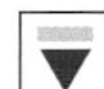 **TIPS**

- Darkened room
- Patient assumes a horizontal gaze
- Place finger 30 cm anterior to patient's eyes
- Move finger toward patient
- Instruct patient to follow finger so as to become cross-eyed, i.e., converge
- Normal: both pupils constrict
- Argyll-Robertson pupil: pupil constriction to convergence but not to light
- Proptosis: unable to symmetrically converge (Moebius' sign)

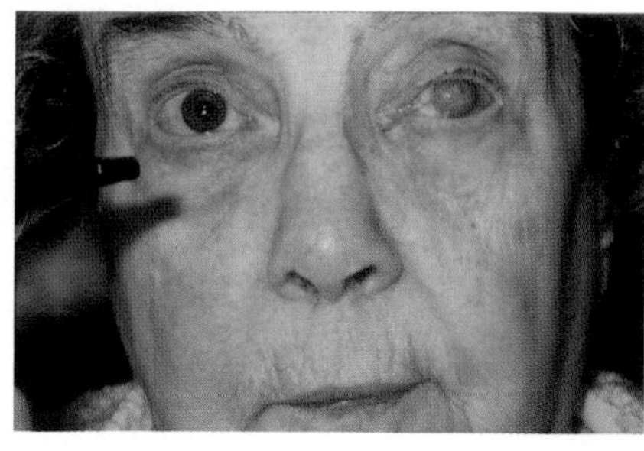

Figure 15.9.

Corneal opacity from old trauma.

TIPS

- Patient seated, baseline horizontal gaze
- Corneal opacity: opacity in the cornea precludes imaging of the anterior chamber structures
- Cataract: opacity in the lens

Table 15.4. Anterior Chamber Findings

Diagnosis	Red reflex	Findings	Company it Keeps
Normal	Red, round		
Marfan's syndrome	Crescent-shaped	Superior lens dislocation 80%	Arachnodactyly Steinberg's thumb sign Aortic insufficiency, Corneamegaly
Trauma	Crescent-shaped	Superior or inferior lens dislocation	Hyphema
Homocyst-inemia	Crescent-shaped	Inferior lens dislocation	Increased laxity of joints
Ehlers-Danlos Syndrome	Crescent-shaped	Inferior dislocation	Increased laxity of joints
Retinoblastoma	Absent, white	Tumor in fundus	Strabismus child
Cataract, nuclear	Absent	Central brown-yellow in lens	Worsens night vision
Cataract, cortical	Absent	Spokelike, in periphery of lens	Worsened symptoms on bright light
Corneal opacity	Absent	On the cornea	
Anterior uveitis	Diffuse	Diffuse anterior Chamber infiltrate	Autoimmune disease Sarcoidosis Inflammatory bowel disease
Corneal perforation	Teardrop	Trauma Red eye	Fluorescein in anterior chamber (Seidel's sign)

Table 15.5. White Pupils

Diagnosis	Signs	Company it Keeps
Nuclear cataract	Brown-yellow opacity in center of the lens	Vision worse at night Exacerbates myopia
Cortical cataract	Spokelike opacities in lens periphery	Worsened in bright light
Mature cataract	White, replacement of entire area Visual acuity worse than 20/200	Markedly decreased visual acuity
Band keratopathy	Fine cover of white on inside of the cornea	Decreased visual acuity
Keratopathy	Opacity in the cornea Unable to image anterior chamber	Decreased vision

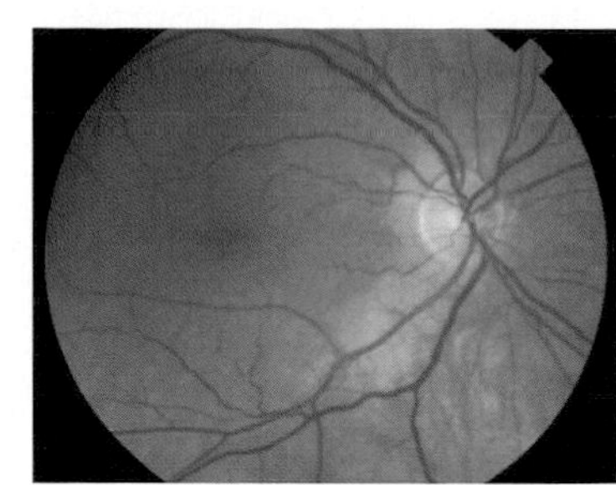

Figure 15.10.

Fundus anatomy. **A.** Optic disc. **B.** Optic cup. **C.** Macule and fovea and centralis. **D.** Paired arteries and veins. (From Moore KL, Dalley AF. *Clinically Oriented Anatomy*, 4th ed. Philadelphia: Lippincott Williams & Wilkins, 1999:906, with permission.)

 **TIPS**

- Optic disc: head of the optic nerve
- Optic cup: central portion of the disc, through which the vessels enter and exit the retina; in most cases, is 40% the size of the disc
- Macule and fovea centralis: site of cones, i.e., seat of color vision
- No vessels overlie the macule: this is the termination or origin of all arteries and veins
- Arteries and veins are paired together

Funduscopic Examination

In a darkened room, apply a mydriatic agent to the inferior conjunctival sac being examined. Funduscopic examination is then performed. Compare one side from the other, note the background color, size of the vessels, the location of the fovea centralis and macula, and the optic cup and disc **(Fig. 15.10)**. The cup is the site where vessels enter and exit and, in most individuals, is approximately 40% of the disc. The disc is the head of the optic nerve itself. Trace the paired arteries or venules outward in four directions; follow some of them to their terminus at the macula and fovea centralis. Any lesions or findings are best described in terms of location and size. One of the best reference tools is that of *optic disc diameters*. This reference is useful to measure size of an entity and its location.

TEACHING POINTS

EYE EXAMINATION

1. All individuals with an eye problem must have a visual acuity test performed at the time of presentation; this should be repeated as necessary.
2. Visual field assessment complements the central visual acuity testing.
3. Scotomata, visual field defects detected only via visual field testing, often indicate severe glaucoma, optic neuritis, or a midline brain tumor.
4. Amsler grid is an excellent screening tool for age-related macular degeneration, but not greatly useful for visual field defects.
5. PERRLA = pupils, equal, round, reactive to light and accommodation; however, convergence remains useful to evaluate for early proptosis.
6. The least useful of the PERRLA is accommodation.
7. EOMI statements are useful for teaching:
   - All the recti muscles move the eye outward, except for the one named medial
   - All the oblique muscles move the eye inward and opposite of superior or inferior names
   - Cranial nerves: SO4, LR6 all the rest are 3
8. Funduscopic examination: describe location and size of lesions in terms of "disc diameters."

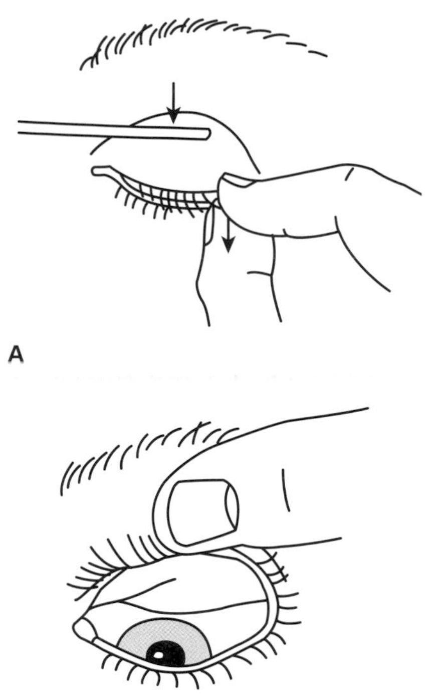

Figure 15.11.

Technique for upper eyelid eversion to inspect for foreign bodies. Must perform to inspect the upper eyelid sulcus for foreign bodies.

TIPS

- Patient looks downward
- Place a cotton-tipped swab longitudinally on the superior side of the lid, above the superior border of the tarsal plate
- Pull the lid margin down and out, while placing inward and downward pressure with the swab so as to flip up the lid

RED EYE

Red eye is a very common problem, one that often is self-limited and benign; but can be a marker for a more severe process. Thus, it is a problem that all physicians must know how to evaluate. As such, it is incumbent to stress the importance of being facile in these techniques and to instruct others to recognize some of the diseases that cause red eye. In addition to the examination described above, one of the first components is inspection of the eye, the periorbital structures, and the conjunctiva. This **conjunctival inspection** must include the lower and upper conjunctival recesses for foreign bodies. The lower lid is easily retracted or everted and, thus, readily inspected; **eversion of the upper eyelid** is somewhat more challenging. This is best performed by placing a cotton-tipped swab handle longitudinally on the outside of the upper lid, immediately superior to the tarsal plate. Then pull the lid margin gently down and out, while placing inward and downward pressure on the lid so as to flip the lid upward (**Fig 15.11**).

The **application of fluorescein dye** to the conjunctiva and assessment of uptake with a cobalt blue light source is important in most cases of a patient with a red eye. The fluorescein is taken up by eroded or ulcerated areas on the surface of the cornea. Either a drop of fluorescein is placed in lower lid recess or better yet, a fluorescein-tipped strip is placed in the lower lid recess for 15–20 seconds; shine a cobalt blue light source, usually on a slit lamp to look for any uptake, which appears as a green color on the cornea. Normally, there is no corneal uptake of fluorescein. In a **corneal abrasion**, there is a patch or linear uptake; in **herpes keratitis**, a dendritic pattern of uptake; in **dry-eye keratitis**, a scattered punctate uptake; and in **actinic or ultraviolet (UV)-related keratitis**, scattered superficial uptake (see **Table 15.6**).

Acute angle glaucoma manifests with an acute onset of marked pain, decreased visual acuity, injection of the vessels, especially about the limbus (perilimbic) **(Fig. 15.12)**, and a pupil that is dilated and unreactive. The company it keeps includes nausea, vomiting, ipsilateral headache, and a crescent-shaped shadow in the anterior chamber best demonstrated with tangential

Table 15.6. Patterns of Fluorescein-Uptake

Normal	Pattern	Company it Keeps
Corneal abrasion	Patch or linear	Severe pain Foreign body
Herpes keratitis simplex	Dendritic pattern ulcers or erosions	Pain Herpes simplex Can be severe
Herpes keratitis zoster	Pseudodendritic	V1 zoster Tip of nose involved
Adenovirus	Superficial punctate	Brilliantly red eye
Actinic keratitis	Superficial punctate	Exposure to ultraviolet light with no eye protection when arc welding Solar eclipse Skiing
Dry eye-related keratitis	Superficial punctate	Bell's palsy

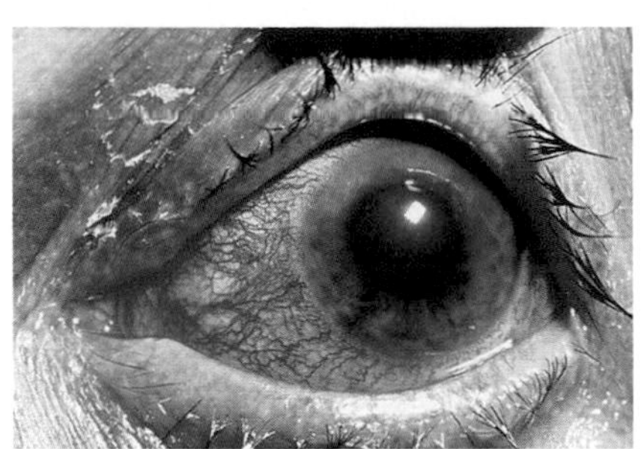

Figure 15.12.

Acute angle glaucoma. (From Azuara-Blanco A, Henderer JD, Katz LJ, et al. Glaucoma. In: Tasman W, Jaeger EA, eds. *The Wills Eye Hospital Atlas of Clinical Ophthalmology*, 2nd ed. Philadelphia: Lippincott Williams & Wilkins, 2001:120, with permission.)

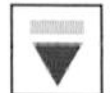

TIPS

- Acute angle glaucoma: injection of vessels about the limbus, pupil is dilated and unreactive
- Intraocular pressure very elevated

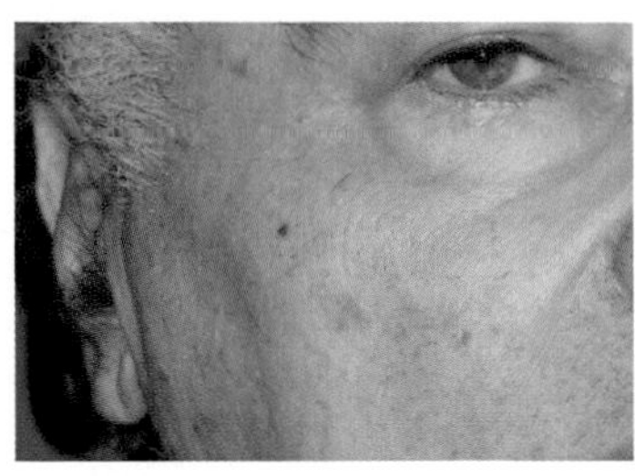

Figure 15.13.

Red eye: Seborrheic blepharitis. Note the concurrent seborrheic dermatitis at hairline.

TIPS

- Edges of eyelids with scales and erythema
- Mild diffuse injection of the conjunctiva: Palpebral conjunctivae involved greater than visceral
- Concurrent seborrheic dermatitis

light, i.e., light source shone from the side. Fluorescein is not taken up by the cornea with this problem. This is a congenital and very often bilateral problem and it is important to assess the asymptomatic eye as well. The IOP in an acute attack can reach 50 to 70 mm Hg* and readily cause retinal damage.

Blepharitis manifests with bilateral itchy eyes, no decrease in visual acuity, mild bilateral diffuse conjunctival injection, and mild erythema and scales at the edges of the eyelids **(Fig. 15.13)**. The company it keeps includes one or more styes or chalazia. If due to seborrhea, there is concurrent eyebrow seborrheic dermatitis.

Stye (Fig. 15.14) manifests with one or more papule(s) or pustule(s) at the eyelid margin, which are caused by inflammation of the eyelash glands of Moll or Zeis. An **internal hordeolum** manifests with a tender papule on the

*Normal IOP: 12–18 mm Hg.

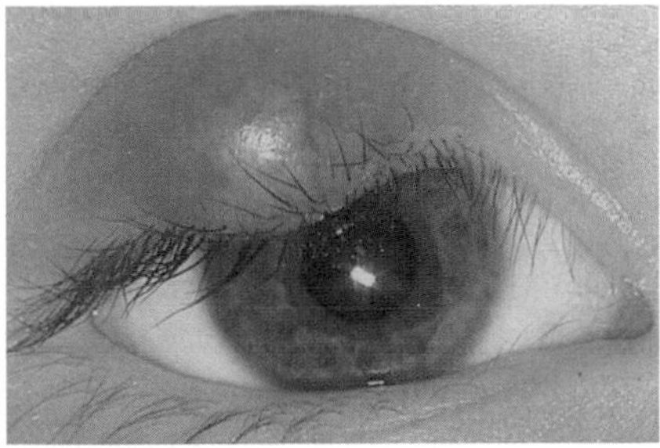

A

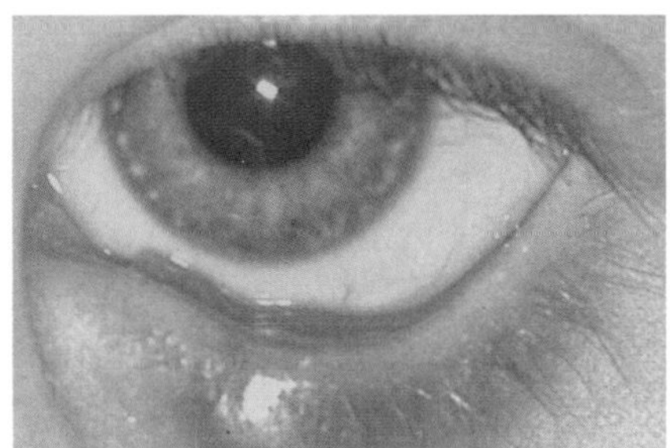

B

Figure 15.14.

Red eye. **A.** Stye located on the lid margin. **B.** A chalazion located deep from the margin.

TIPS

- Stye: tender papule on the eyelid margin **(A)**
- Stye: an inflammation of a gland of Moll or Zeis
- Chalazion: one or more nontender papules or nodules deep from the eyelid margin **(B)**
- Chalazion: chronic inflammation of a meibomian gland

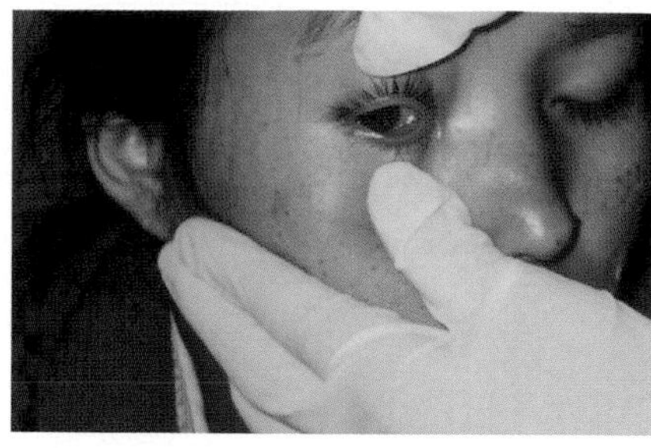

A

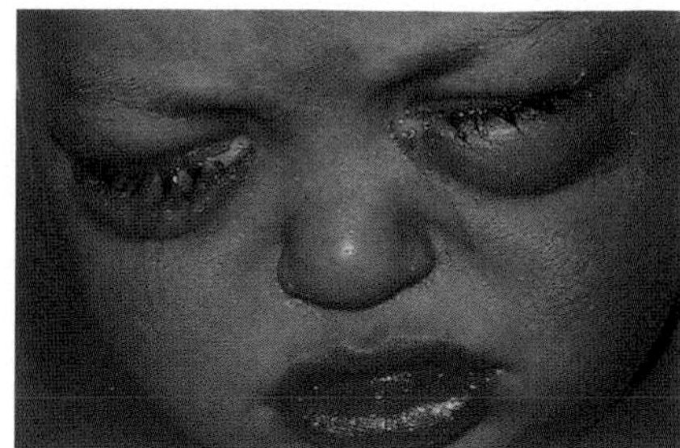

B

Figure 15.15.

Red eye. **A.** Serous conjunctivitis; here, a viral cause. **B.** Purulent conjunctivitis; here, a bacterial cause. (From Zitelli, B, Davis, H. *Atlas of Pediatric Physical Diagnosis*, 2nd. ed.

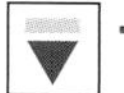 TIPS

- Serous conjunctivitis **(A):** watery discharge, diffuse conjunctival injection, often unilateral; may spread to other side
- Atopic conjunctivitis: mucous-type tearing with diffuse conjunctival injection
- Acute purulent conjunctivitis **(B):** yellow-green discharge, diffuse conjunctival injection, often unilateral

internal surface of the lid, usually in the upper lid, which is caused by an acute inflammation of a meibomian gland. A **chalazion** manifests with a nontender papule or even nodule in the upper eyelid, which is caused by chronic inflammation of a meibomian gland. (Fig 15.14B).

Serous conjunctivitis (Fig. 15.15) manifests with clear watery discharge, no decrease in visual acuity; and a diffuse conjunctival injection, often unilateral, but can spread to the contralateral side. There is associated crusting, rhinorrhea, scratchy sore throat, cough, and palpable preauricular nodes. The company it keeps is specific to the underlying etiology. If caused by **adenovirus**, there is a punctate fluorescein uptake; if caused by **herpes simplex virus**, may have a dendritic pattern of corneal uptake; if a rhinovirus, i.e., common cold, there is little if any corneal uptake. **Atopic conjunctivitis** manifests no decrease in visual acuity but a thick, mucouslike discharge, diffuse conjunctival injection, often bilateral. The company it keeps includes significant crusting of the eyelids, serous rhinorrhea, scratchy sore throat, and sneezing, but no palpable preauricular nodes. **Acute purulent conjunctivitis** manifests with a mild decrease in visual acuity, a yellow-green discharge, and diffuse conjunctival injection; often unilateral, but can spread to the contralateral side. No palpable preauricular nodes unless the cause is gonococcal. A variant of acute purulent conjunctivitis is a hyperacute form, in which there is chemosis, swelling, and rapid spread to involve the cornea. Acute purulent conjunctivitis must be evaluated with Gram's stain and culture.

Trachoma manifests with early on, no decrease in visual acuity, a minimally purulent discharge and a thickened, papular and follicular conjunctiva, especially involving the superior conjunctival fold **(Fig. 15.16)**. Conjunctival and corneal scarring are noted and, in severe cases, depressed areas on the peripheral cornea at the limbus (Herbert's pits). A sequela of this is eversion or inversion of the eyelids with the eyelids rubbing the surface of the cornea, i.e., trichiasis. Ultimately, the cornea is effectively destroyed and replaced with white, opaque connective tissue with marked impact on vision. Trachoma is caused by a chlamydial infection of the conjunctiva.

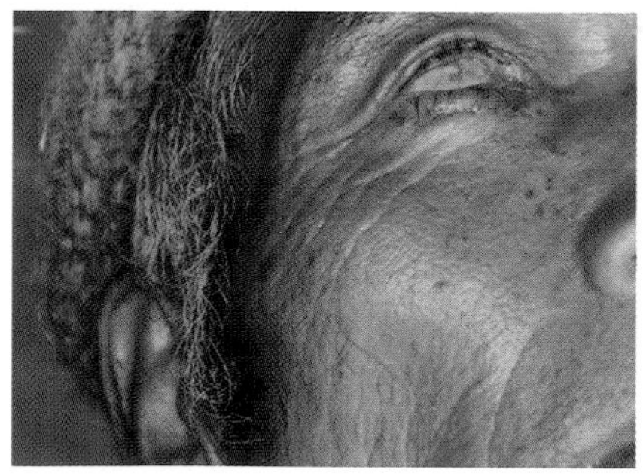

Figure 15.16.

Trachoma, end-stage with keratopathy.

 TIPS

- Trachoma: minimally purulent discharge with a thickened, papular and follicular conjunctiva, especially involving the superior conjunctival fold with scarring
- Sequelae include limbic depressions (Herbert's pits), and eversion and inversion of the eyelids with secondary corneal damage

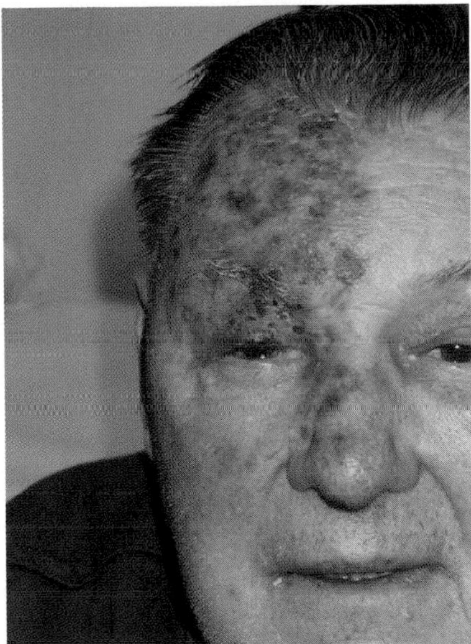

A

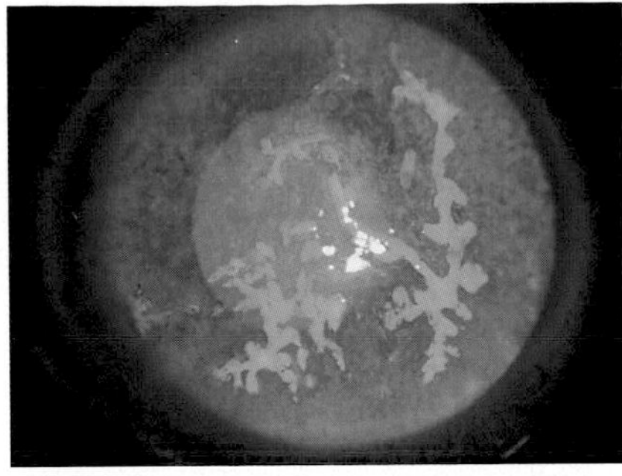

B

Figure 15.17.

Red eye: V1 herpes zoster. **A.** Vesicles in the V1 distribution. **B.** Keratitis. Note psuedodendritic uptake of fluorescein. (From Cohen EJ, Rapuano CJ, Laibson PR. External diseases. In: Tasman W, Jaeger EA, eds. *The Wills Eye Hospital Atlas of Clinical Ophthalmology*, 2nd ed. Philadelphia: Lippincott Williams & Wilkins, 2001:8, with permission.)

TIPS

- Inspect the skin of the head and face
- Herpes zoster, V1: painful clusters of vesicles on the frontal and temporal area superior to the zygomatic arch and the inferior orbital rim; does not cross the midline
- Herpes zoster keratitis: vesicles on the tip of the nose, with involvement of the nasociliary branch of V1 (Hutchinson's sign); sensitivity: 75%
- Concurrent serous conjunctivitis and the branching papular defect, i.e., a pseudodendritic pattern on the cornea

V1 herpes zoster (Fig. 15.17) manifests with painful clusters of vesicles in the V1 distribution that can involve any or all of its branches—supraorbital, lacrimal, or nasociliary—and a red eye. Often noted is a loss of transparency in the cornea and, if keratitis is present, a **pseudodendritic** pattern to the corneal defects. Pseudodendritic is defined as branching papular structures that take up fluorescein. Of great interest is that the presence of vesicles on the tip of the nose (Hutchinson's sign) indicates a 75% probability that keratitis will develop. **Herpes simplex keratitis** manifests with a red eye, a loss of transparency in the cornea caused by edema in the cornea, ulcers on the cornea that have a **dendritic** pattern, and the branching ulcers take up the fluorescein. A concurrent or antecedent cold sore, i.e., a cluster of vesicles in the lip may be seen or reported by the patient in the history.

Corneal abrasion (Fig. 15.18) manifests with acute onset of severe eye pain, tearing, and decrease in visual acuity, often with a discernable event of trauma. There is diffuse conjunctival injection, fluorescein uptake in a discrete area, either with a linear or patch pattern. **Corneal ulcer** manifests with decreased visual acuity, severe eye pain, a ring-shaped corneal opacity, fluorescein uptake in the area, and often anterior uveitis and hypopyon.

Anterior uveitis manifests with a painful red eye, photophobia, decreased visual acuity and cloudy infiltrate and even a pus level in the anterior chamber (hypopyon) **(Fig. 15.19)**. This is caused by infection with *Pseudomonas, Staphylococcus,* or *Streptococcus* organisms or by autoimmune disorders, sarcoid or inflammatory bowel disease.

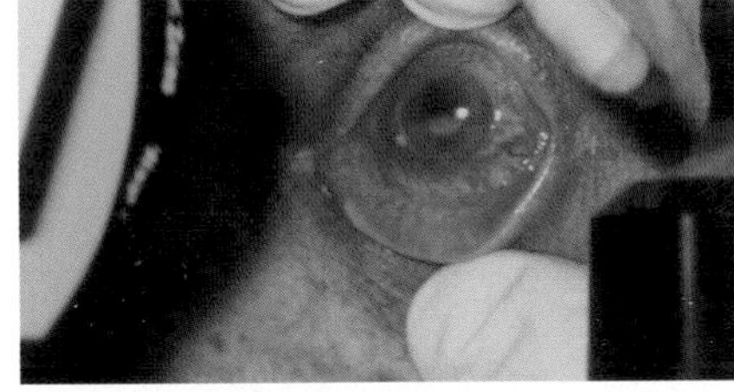

Figure 15.18.

Red eye: Corneal abrasion. Note patch of fluorescein uptake.

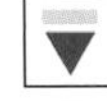

TIPS

- Corneal abrasion: a patch or linear area; has fluorescein uptake in the area

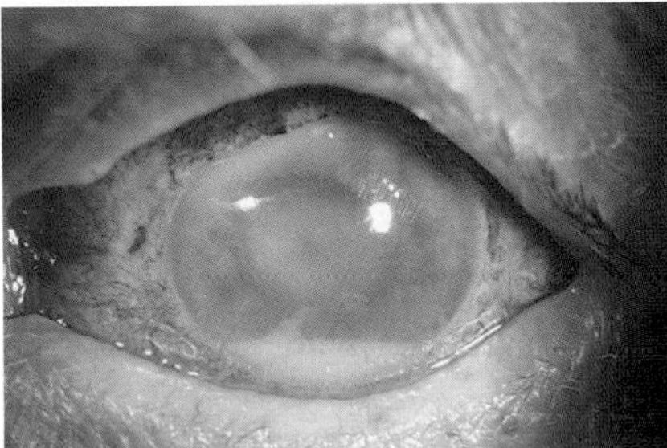

Figure 15.19.

Red eye: Anterior uveitis with secondary hypopyon. (From Eagle RC, Jaeger EA, Tasman W. Lens. In: Tasman W, Jaeger EA, eds. *The Wills Eye Hospital Atlas of Clinical Ophthalmology*, 2nd ed. Philadelphia: Lippincott Williams & Wilkins, 2001:90, with permission.)

TIPS

- Anterior uveitis: note the cloudy infiltrate in anterior chamber
- Hypopyon: pus level present in the anterior chamber

TEACHING POINTS

RED EYE

1. Acute purulent conjunctivitis must be evaluated with Gram's stain and a culture.
2. Preauricular lymph node enlargement indicates a viral conjunctivitis.
3. Dry eyes, dry mouth, and enlargement of parotid and lacrimal glands, consistent with Sjögren's syndrome.
4. In any case of red eye with photophobia, strongly consider performing a slit lamp examination and applying fluorescein dye to look for corneal abrasions or for keratitis.
5. V1 zoster with involvement of the tip of the nose: high likelihood of herpes zoster keratitis.
6. Dendritic pattern of erosion or ulceration: herpes simplex.
7. Subconjunctival hemorrhage is benign.
8. Evert the upper lid to fully assess the conjunctiva.
9. Blepharitis is a common cause of mild red eye.
10. Atopic-related conjunctivitis has the company of serous rhinorrhea, scratchy throat, and sneezing.
11. Chemosis is a thickening of the conjunctiva due to severe atopic conjunctivitis.

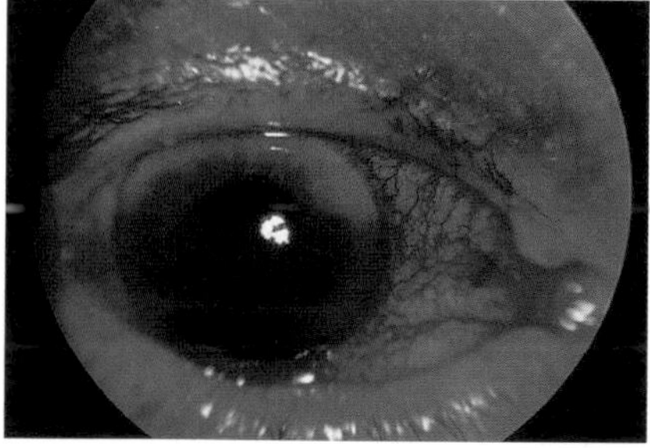

Figure 15.20.

Trauma-related hyphema. (From Azuara-Blanco A, Henderer JD, Katz LJ, et al. Glaucoma. In: Tasman W, Jaeger EA, eds. *The Wills Eye Hospital Atlas of Clinical Ophthalmology*, 2nd ed. Philadelphia: Lippincott Williams & Wilkins, 2001:134, with permission.)

 **TIPS**

- Hyphema: blood level in anterior chamber; most often trauma-related,e.g., a firecracker to the eye
- Recurrence occurs 3–5 days after initial trauma

Hyphema manifests with an acute decrease in vision, marked discomfort, and a collection of blood in the anterior chamber. There is antecedent trauma and, if tense, an "eight-ball" appearance of the cornea. Most hyphemas are trauma-related, e.g., a firecracker to the face **(Fig. 15.20)**; however, spontaneous hyphema can be caused by malignant melanoma of the iris.

Chemosis manifests with a thickened, itchy red conjunctiva **(Fig. 15.21)**. Often there is a history of atopic disease with resultant significant rubbing of the eyes.

Subconjunctival hemorrhage manifests with a painless, asymptomatic bright red macule or patch beneath the conjunctiva, which can be large without any decrease in visual acuity **(Fig. 15.22)**. Most are benign; if recurrent and large or if hemorrhage is found at multiple sites, evaluate for coagulopathy. It may be useful as a clue to diagnose a basilar skull fracture in a patient with a history of head trauma.

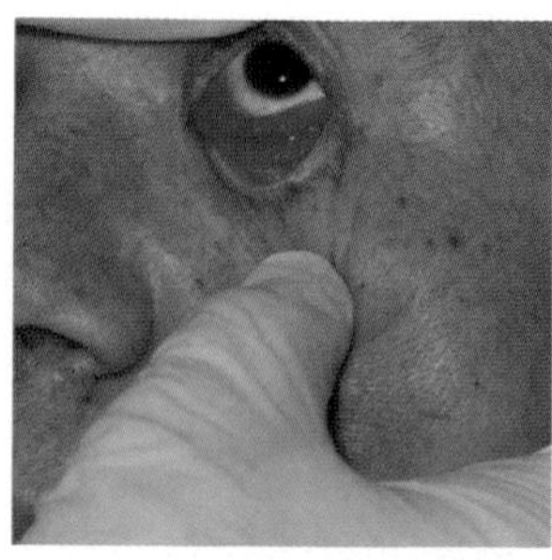

Figure 15.21.

Red eye: Chemosis or marked thickening of the conjunctiva; usually due to severe atopic disease.

 **TIPS**

- Chemosis: thickened itchy red conjunctiva, often bilateral; almost meaty in appearance
- Concurrent findings of hayfever common

Sjögren's disease manifests with bilateral conjunctival injection. Early in course on fluorescein assessment, no uptake is noted but, in severe cases, there is a superficial punctate uptake. *Schirmer's maneuver* reveals <5 mm of wetness on a piece of sterile filter paper placed into the lower eyelid sulcus for 30 seconds, which effectively confirms the diagnosis. In advanced disease the company it keeps includes bilateral lacrimal and parotid gland enlargement, dry mouth, and a marked increase in number of dental caries. Due to lymphoproliferative infiltration of glands; related to long-standing rheumatoid arthritis.

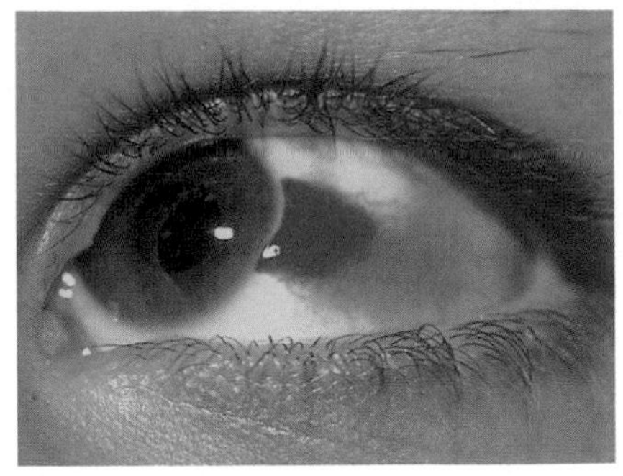

Figure 15.22.

Red eye: Subconjunctival hemorrhage; red macule on visceral conjunctiva. (From Zitelli, B. *Atlas of Pediatric Physical Diagnosis*, 2nd. ed.)

 **TIPS**

- Subconjunctival hemorrhage: red stain as a macule or patch on the conjunctiva
- Most are benign; if recurrent and large, multiple other sites of hemorrhage are seen
- Evaluate for coagulopathy if indicated

SCLERAL AND CONJUNCTIVAL ENTITIES

Pterygium manifests with asymptomatic, thickened, yellow fibrous tissue in the conjunctiva, bilaterally; invariably on the nasal side **(Fig. 15.23)**. It causes mischief only if it grows over the cornea. Because of chronic exposure to UV light, pterygium is prevalent in the people of the Himalayas and Andes and older farmers of the Midwest. **Pinguecula** manifests with an asymptomatic, yellow papule in the conjunctiva on the nasal or temporal side of the cornea. Benign process; common in elderly.

Icterus manifests with yellow discoloration of the conjunctiva; it is caused by elevated bilirubin, usually a total bilirubin that exceeds 4 mg%. Other reasons for yellow-orange color to the conjunctiva include the recent administration of fluorescein dye to the external eye structures or the use of the antibiotic rifampin, which stains all body secretions orange-yellow. **Arcus senilis** manifests with a pale to creamy white rim around the circumference of the cornea; it is caused by the deposition of amyloid protein or lipid adjacent to the limbus that is present in individuals of increasing age **(Fig. 15.24)**. If present in a young individual, it is called "arcus juvenilis" and may be associated with hyperlipidemia.

Blue sclera of osteogenesis imperfecta and connective tissue disorders manifests with diffuse blue color of the sclera as the result of diffuse scleral

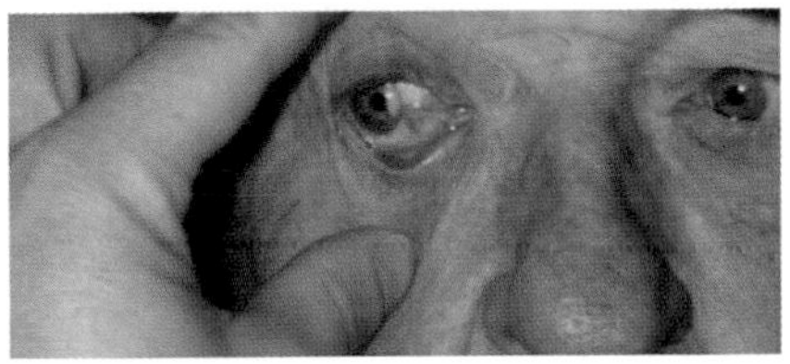

Figure 15.23.

Pterygium; usually bilateral. This is a dairy farmer from Wisconsin.

 **TIPS**

- Pterygium: asymptomatic, thickened yellow fibrous tissue in the nasal conjunctiva bilaterally

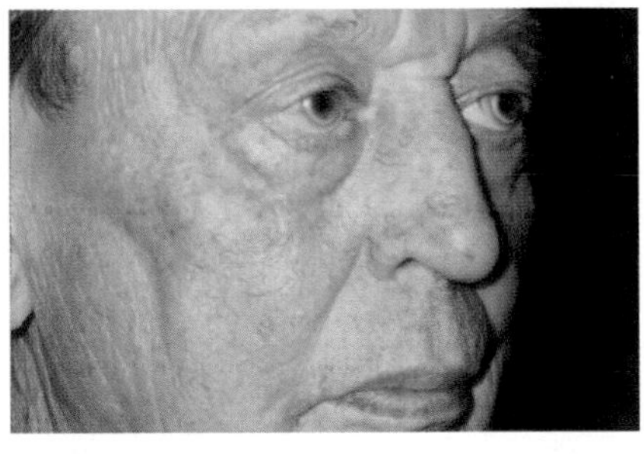

Figure 15.24.

Arcus senilis.

 **TIPS**

- Arcus senilis: a pale colored rim of material around the limbus
- Normal variant in geriatric population

TEACHING POINTS

SCLERAL AND CONJUNCTIVAL EXAMINATION

1. Blue sclera indicates diffuse thinning of the scleral connective tissue.
2. Episcleritis: associated with active rheumatologic disease.
3. Icterus is bilirubin in the conjunctiva, not the sclera.
4. Arcus senilis is a rim of material around the limbus.
5. The conjunctiva ends at the limbus; it does not cover the cornea.
6. Pterygium: bilateral, nasal conjunctiva usually caused by exposure to wind or ultraviolet (UV) light. Commonly found in individuals who live at high altitudes.

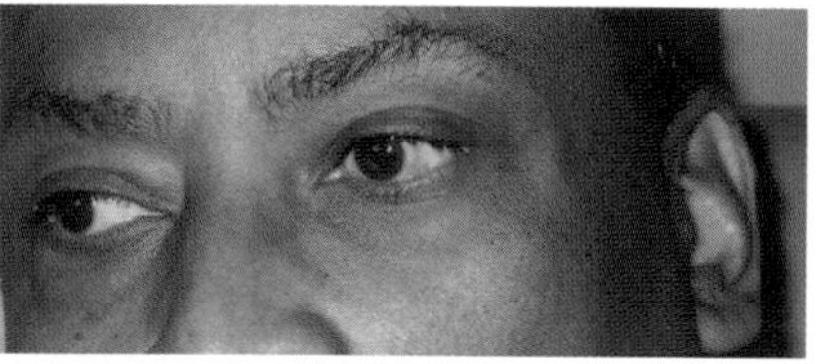

Figure 15.25.

Blue sclera.

 **TIPS**

- Osteogenesis imperfecta: diffusely blue sclera, caused by thinning of the sclera connective tissue
- Any diffuse thinning of sclera causes a bluish-hue to be present

thinning **(Fig. 15.25)**. Other reasons for blue sclerae are profound malnutrition and any collagen-type disorder.

Episcleritis manifests with a mildly tender red macule or papule on the sclera, usually self-limited and not associated with rheumatologic disease. **Scleritis** manifests with a diffuse or papular tender red lesion on the sclera and conjunctiva with one or more areas of bluish hue, i.e., thinned sclera. Scleritis is associated with active Wegener's or rheumatoid arthritis. **Wilson's disease** manifests with a 1- to 2-mm brown-green band of copper in the peripheral cornea immediately internal to the limbus (Kayser-Fleischer ring). The copper is abnormally deposited in Descemet's membrane of the cornea. The company it keeps includes liver damage and choreiform movements (Table 7.15) caused by basal ganglia damage, as the result of the excess copper.

IRIS

Neurofibromatosis (NF-1) manifests with clumps of pigment in the iris called "Lisch nodules" **(Fig. 15.26)**. Other manifestations include café au lait spots, cutaneous neurofibromata, increased pigment in the axilla (Crowe's sign), and the potential to develop pheochromocytoma or neurofibromata of the nerve roots or peripheral nerves.

Iridectomy manifests with a dark column through the iris extending from the pupil to the limbus, usually after and due to cataract surgery. **Iridotomy** manifests with a dark, diamond-shaped area in the iris, usually after

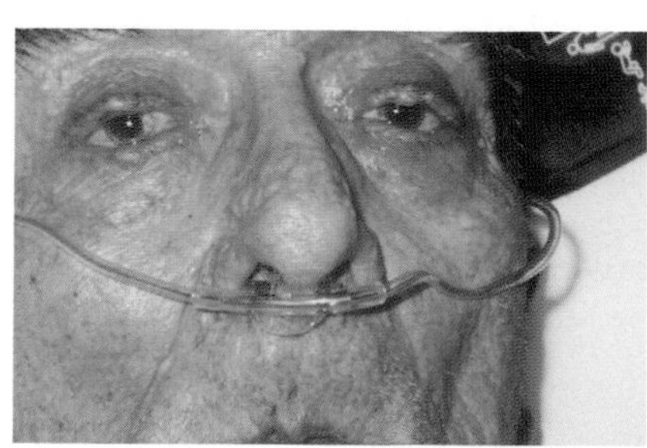

Figure 15.26.

Lisch nodules in iris of neurofibromatosis.

 **TIPS**

- Visually inspect iris; may use a slit lamp
- Neurofibromatosis: clumps of pigment in the iris (Lisch nodules); no concurrent poikiloscoria or anisocoria

TEACHING POINTS

IRIS ENTITIES

1. Clumps of material in the iris: Brushfield spots of Down Syndrome, Lisch nodules of neurofibromatosis, iris adenoma, or iris melanoma.
2. A clump of pigment with deformity of pupil or associated neovascularization; think of the rare diagnosis, iris melanoma.
3. Diabetes mellitus can manifest with neovascularization of the iris (i.e., rubeosis iridis).
4. Iridotomy and iridectomy, which are related to a surgical procedure, are common.

laser therapy performed for glaucoma. Both are common postintervention findings that are important to know. **Malignant melanoma** manifests with a solitary, pigmented entity in the iris that causes poikiloscoria, neovascularization, and even a hyphema. **Rubcosis iridis** manifests with neovascularization in the iris but with no associated pigmented nevi; it is often caused by uncontrolled diabetes mellitus.

Brushfield spots manifest with hypopigmented fine structures in the iris itself; distribution is akin to that of the spokes on a wheel **(Fig. 15.27)**. Concurrent features of Down syndrome are present, including epicanthal fold increase, low set auricles, and cognitive delay.

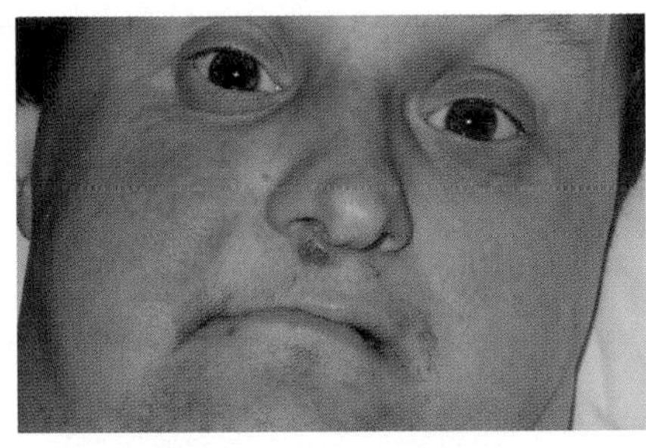

Figure 15.27.

Brushfield spots in iris of Down syndrome. Patient presented with erysipelas on right.

TIPS

- Visually inspect iris; may use a slit lamp
- Brushfield spots: hypopigmented fine structures in the iris itself, distribution akin to spokes on a wheel
- Note the widened epicanthal folds of this patient with Down syndrome

RETINAL EXAMINATION FINDINGS

Drusen manifests with small, pale yellow points that can be at any location in the fundus, including over the macule or fovea. The quantity of drusen increases with age. Drusen is caused by material in the retinal layer about Bruch's membrane. If due to macular degeneration, the company it keeps includes a decreased central vision and wavy lines on the Amsler grid assessment.

Hard exudates manifest with collections of discrete, small yellow, quite bright structures about the retinal vessels **(Fig. 15.28)**. They result from abnormal loss of protein into the retina from abnormally permeable retinal vessels. This is an early manifestation of diabetic nonproliferative retinopathy or of hypertensive retinopathy.

Cotton-wool spots (soft exudates) manifest with large (0.25 to 1 disc diameter) white-yellow areas adjacent to arteries **(Fig. 15.29)**. They have soft edges and can be single or multiple. This is a late manifestation of preproliferative diabetic retinopathy or of ischemic or embolic problems. If caused by endocarditis, these are specifically called Roth or Litten's spots. The company they keep include fevers, Osler's nodes, Janeway lesions, and new heart murmur. If caused by vasculitis, e.g., lupus erythematous these are specifically

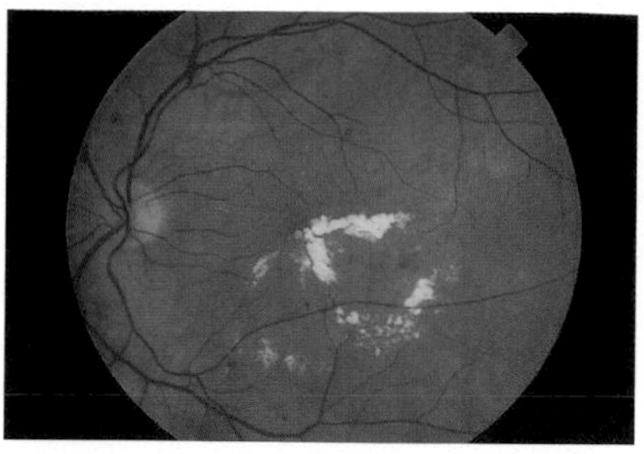

Figure 15.28.

Funduscopic examination. Hard exudates. Note size, each less than caliber of adjacent retinal vessels. (From Tasman W. Retinal vascular disease. In: Tasman W, Jaeger EA, eds. *The Wills Eye Hospital Atlas of Clinical Ophthalmology*, 2nd ed. Philadelphia: Lippincott Williams & Wilkins, 2001:221, with permission.)

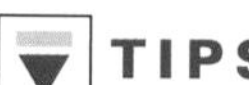

TIPS

- Clusters of discrete, small, yellow, bright structures near the vessels
- Diabetic nonproliferative retinopathy: hard exudates
- Hypertensive retinopathy: hard exudates
- Leakage of protein into the retina

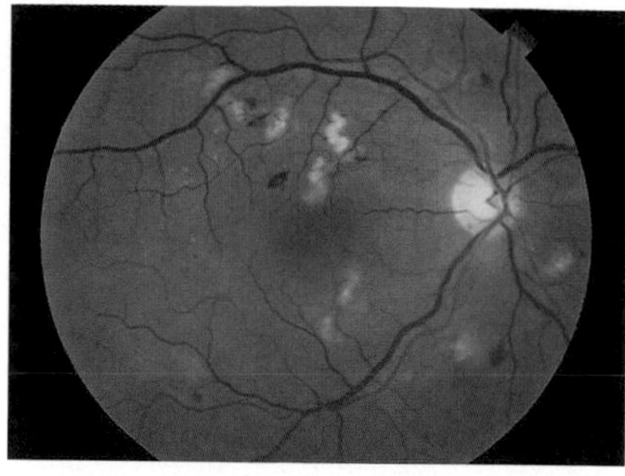

Figure 15.29.

Funduscopic examination. Soft exudates. Note size, each up to 1 optic disc diameter. (From Tasman W. Retinal vascular disease. In: Tasman W, Jaeger EA, eds. *The Wills Eye Hospital Atlas of Clinical Ophthalmology*, 2nd ed. Philadelphia: Lippincott Williams & Wilkins, 2001:222, with permission.)

TIPS

- Soft exudates: large (0.25 to 1 disc diameter) areas adjacent to arteries are pale, have soft edges, and can be single or multiple
- Preproliferative diabetic retinopathy, endocarditis (Roth or Litten spot), vasculitis, or lupus erythematous (cytoid body)
- Soft exudate = cotton-wool spots
- In vasculitis, occurs adjacent to vessels

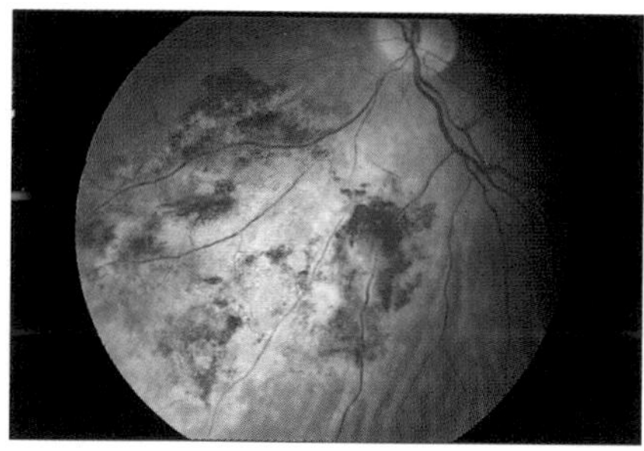

Figure 15.30.

Funduscopic examination. Chorioretinitis.

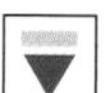

TIPS

- Chorioretinitis: hard exudates at the periphery of one or more vessels and one or more soft exudates
- Toxoplasmosis: multiple yellow and pigmented soft exudates
- Cytomegalovirus (CMV): multiple clusters of yellow and pigmented soft exudates

called cytoid bodies. The company they keep include arthritis, stomatitis, and a malar facial rash.*

Chorioretinitis manifests with both hard and soft exudates. The hard exudates are at the periphery of one or more vessels; there are often multiple soft exudates **(Fig. 15.30)**. The company they keep is specific to the underlying cause. **Toxoplasmosis** manifests with multiple, yellow and pigmented soft exudates, and the patient may have significant visual field deficits. **Cytomegalovirus** (**CMV**) manifests with multiple clusters of yellow and pigmented soft exudates, and the patient may have significant visual field deficits. CMV is most common in severe immunocompromised, e.g., advanced AIDS, patients.

Choroidal melanoma manifests with a pigmented area in the retina, often with concurrent local bleeding and deformity of the retina. **Bull's-eye maculopathy** manifests with a target-shaped area of pigment changes in the area of the macule and fovea centralis, a decreased central vision, and decreased color vision as measured using the Ishihara charts. Concurrent is wavy perception of the lines on the Amsler grid. This is a potential drug side effect (e.g., of the agent hydroxychloroquine or chlorpromazine).

Microaneurysms manifest with outpouchings from the retinal arteries, particularly evident at branch points in the arterioles **(Fig. 15.31)**. The company they keep includes hypertension and diabetes mellitus. **Blot and flame hemorrhages** manifest with small dot or flame-shaped hemorrhages in the

*Recall renal failure and serositis are also common in lupus.

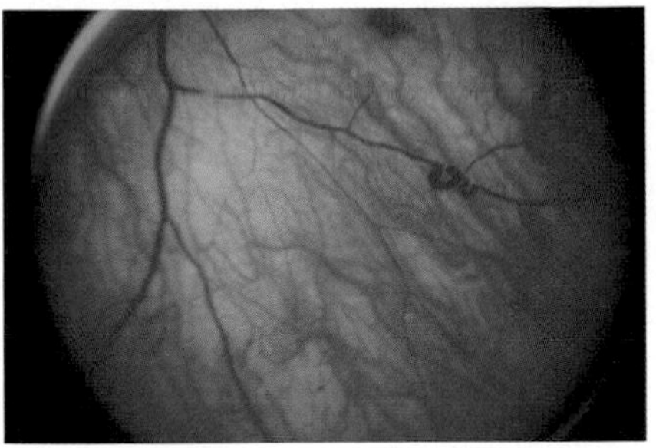

Figure 15.31.

Funduscopic examination: microaneurysms and blot and dot hemorrhages. (From Tasman W. Retinal vascular disease. In: Tasman W, Jaeger EA, eds. *The Wills Eye Hospital Atlas of Clinical Ophthalmology*, 2nd ed. Philadelphia: Lippincott Williams & Wilkins, 2001:223, with permission.)

 **TIPS**

- Microaneurysms: outpouchings from the retinal arterioles, particularly evident at branch points in the arterioles
- Hypertensive or diabetic retinopathy, early: small dot or flame-shaped hemorrhages in the retina, adjacent to the vessels, usually multiple

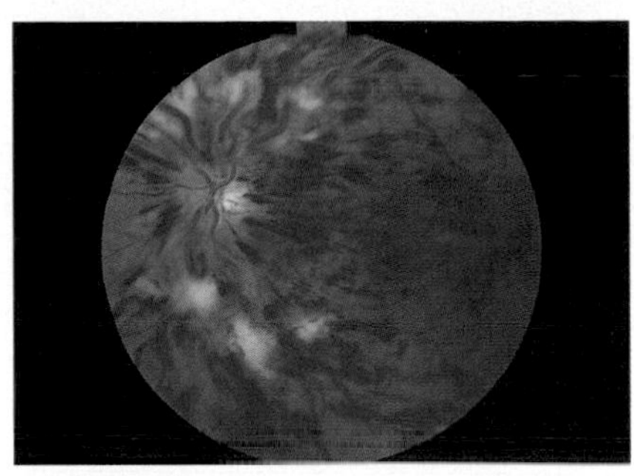

Figure 15.32.

Funduscopic examination: central retinal vein thrombosis. Note the dialated veins, suffused background, and "blood and thunder" appearance. (From Tasman W. Retinal vascular disease. In: Tasman W, Jaeger EA, eds. *The Wills Eye Hospital Atlas of Clinical Ophthalmology*, 2nd ed. Philadelphia: Lippincott Williams & Wilkins, 2001:211, with permission.)

 **TIPS**

- Central retinal vein thrombosis: dilated and tortuous retinal veins, a swollen optic disc, and multiple flame hemorrhages
- Associated with severe uncontrolled hypertension
- Cause of mono-ocular blindness

retina, adjacent to the vessels; these are usually multiple. The company they keep includes uncontrolled hypertension and/or diabetes mellitus.

Central retinal vein occlusion (Fig. 15.32) manifests with a marked decrease in vision in one eye; the patient is often more than 60 years of age and has long-standing, uncontrolled hypertension. Funduscopic examination reveals dilated and tortuous retinal veins, a swollen optic disc, hemorrhages, and neovascularization of the iris in 20% of cases. This was first described by Michel in 1878 as a cause of monocular blindness.

Cherry red macule of *central retinal artery occlusion* manifests with a sudden loss of vision in one eye. The fundus is diffusely pale; the arteries are small and often have intraarterial yellow dots (Hollenhorst plaques), which are emboli of cholesterol. Noted are a deep cherry-colored macule (**Fig 15.33**), a marked decrease in vision except for the central vision, and normal color vision. The fovea and macule are spared because of a different blood supply to the macule. There is an 18% concurrence of iris neovascularization.

Hypertensive changes manifest with arteriovenous (AV) nicking, retinal arterial changes, blot and flame hemorrhages, and, in severe forms, papilledema and edema of the macule—macular star **(Fig. 15.34)**. One of the

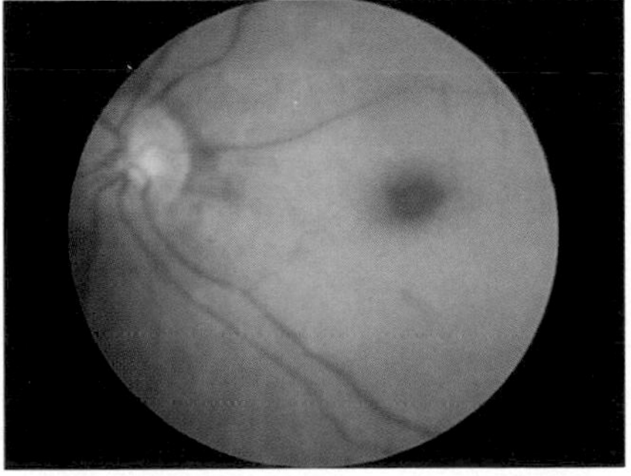

Figure 15.33.

Funduscopic examination. Cherry red macule. Due to central retinal artery occlusion. (From Tasman W. Retinal vascular disease. In: Tasman W, Jaeger EA, eds. *The Wills Eye Hospital Atlas of Clinical Ophthalmology*, 2nd ed. Philadelphia: Lippincott Williams & Wilkins, 2001:216, with permission.)

 **TIPS**

- Central retinal artery occlusion: diffusely pale retina, small retinal arteries, and a deep cherry-colored macule; Hollenhorst plaques are often present
- Associated with emboli: endocarditis, atrial fibrillation, or cholesterol

TEACHING POINTS

RETINAL EXAMINATION

1. Always perform the retinal examination in a darkened room, preferably with a dilating agent instilled in the patent's eye.
2. Describe retinal findings: for size, disc diameter, or for location, by disc diameter from the disc.
3. Concurrent neovascularization of the iris: can be seen the central retinal vein thrombosis, severe proliferative diabetes mellitus, or sickle cell disease.
4. Blot and dot hemorrhages are associated with hypertension and diabetes mellitus, thus are specific for pathology but not to diagnosis.
5. Microaneurysms are associated with diabetes mellitus.
6. The Keith-Wagner-Barker system of classifying hypertensive retinopathy is excellent for target organ damage and may well assist in hypertension prognosis: untreated stage 3 survival rate at 3 years is 22%, stage 4 is 6%.
7. Hard exudates are lipid and plasma protein; soft exudates (cotton-wool spots) are larger areas of retinal ischemia.
8. Damage to the macula and fovea centralis results in decreased central vision, decreased color vision, and a wavy contour of lines when assessing using the Amsler grid.
9. Drugs, including hydroxychloroquine and chlorpromazine (Thorazine), can lead to macular damage, including the classic bull's-eye maculopathy.
10. The Roth spots of endocarditis and the cytoid bodies of lupus are examples of soft exudates.
11. Papillederma indicates increased intracranial pressure.

best categorizations of these findings is from the paper by Keith, Wagner, and Barker in 1939 in which **group I** had diffuse arteriolar narrowing; **group II** had AV nicking; **group III** had retinal hemorrhages, hard and soft exudates, including the hard exudates related to macular star that is a stellate appearing collection of exudates at macule; and **group IV** had swelling of the optic head and cup. Of significant interest is that they studied the prognosis of such pa-

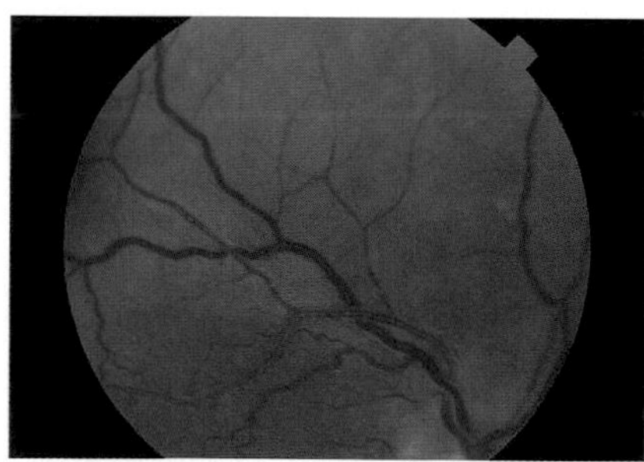

A

B

Figure 15.34.

Retinal changes in uncontrolled hypertension. **A.** Early changes-diffuse narrowing (stage I), arteriovenous (AV) nicking (stage II). **B.** Advanced changes: hard exudates with a macular star (stage III), and edema of the optic nerve "papilledema" (stage IV). (From Tasman W. Retinal vascular disease. In: Tasman W, Jaeger EA, eds. *The Wills Eye Hospital Atlas of Clinical Ophthalmology,* 2nd ed . Philadelphia: Lippincott Williams & Wilkins, 2001:227, with permission.)

TIPS

- Hypertensive retinopathy: Keith-Wagner-Barker stages: I. Diffusely narrowed arteries; II. arteriovenous (AV) nicking; III. hard exudates, including a macular star and dot and blot hemorrhages; a macular star indicates macular edema; and IV. edema of optic nerve
- Useful to diagnosis and in prognosis of hypertension

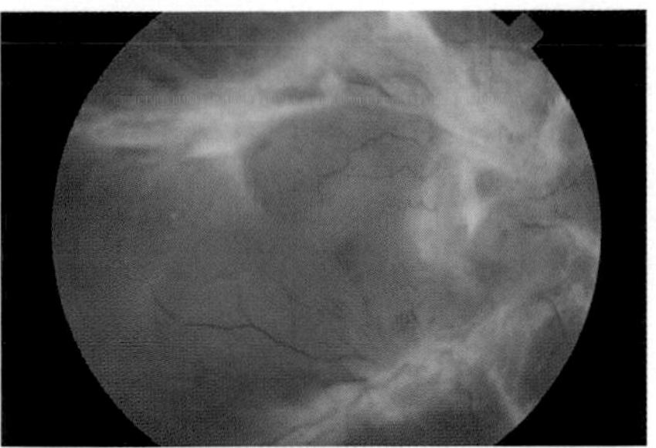

Figure 15.35.

Funduscopic examination: retinal detachment. Note the free floating flap of retina; there was a decrease in visual acuity and a shower of floaters reported by patient. (From Tasman W. Retinal vascular disease. In: Tasman W, Jaeger EA, eds. *The Wills Eye Hospital Atlas of Clinical Ophthalmology*, 2nd ed. Philadelphia: Lippincott Williams & Wilkins, 2001:226, with permission.)

 **TIPS**

- Retinal detachment: free-floating edge or a wrinkle in the retina

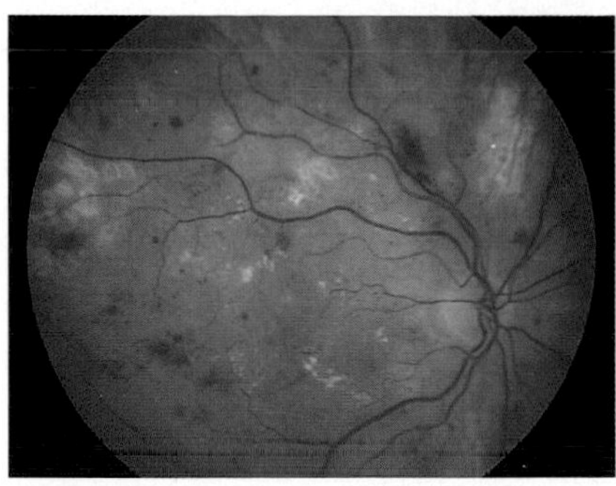

Figure 15.36.

Funduscopic examination: early diabetic retinopathy. Note microaneurysms, blot and dot hemorrhages, hard exudates, and then soft exudates. (From Tasman W. Retinal vascular disease. In: Tasman W, Jaeger EA, eds. *The Wills Eye Hospital Atlas of Clinical Ophthalmology*, 2nd ed. Philadelphia: Lippincott Williams & Wilkins, 2001:221, with permission.)

 **TIPS**

- Nonproliferative changes, diabetes mellitus: microaneurysms in the retinal arterioles, dot and blot hemorrhages
- First hard, then soft exudates develop in this phase

tients and survival rates at 3 years for each group were as follows: group I: 70%; group II: 62%; group III: 22%; and group IV: 6%. The optic disc swelling is called papilledema and is indicative of marked increase in intracranial pressure (Fig. 15.34B).

Hollenhorst plaques manifest with multiple, small, glistening yellow-colored structures in the retinal arteries themselves, which are caused by cholesterol emboli from the carotids or the aortic arch. The company they keep includes carotid bruits, strokes, and acute monocular blindness caused by acute arterial occlusion.

Retinal detachment manifests with a rapid decrease in visual acuity, new defects in the visual field, and the patient complaining of seeing flashes of light and a shower of floaters **(Fig. 15.35)**. Funduscopic examination reveals a free-floating edge of, or a wrinkle in, the retina.

Diabetic retinopathy manifests with a progressive, significant decrease in visual acuity and visual field size. On funduscopic examination are seen the **nonproliferative** changes (**Fig. 15.36**) of microaneurysms in the retinal arterioles, dot and blot hemorrhages in the outer plexiform layer of the retina, splinter hemorrhages in the nerve fiber layer of the retina, soft exudates, and even macular edema. **Proliferative** changes (**Fig. 15.37**) develop and manifest with neovascularization of the vessels about the optic disc (NVD) or

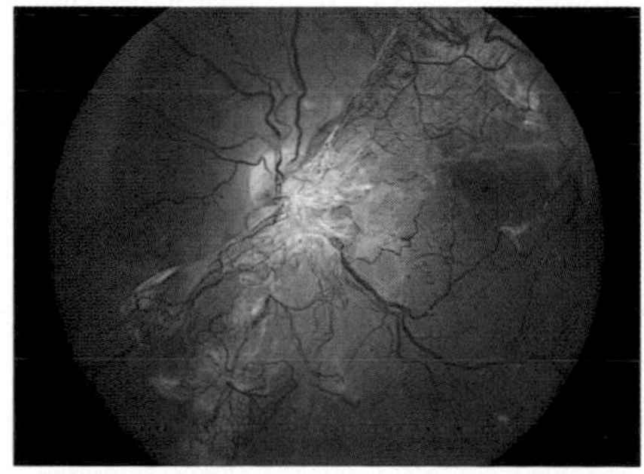

Figure 15.37.

Funduscopic examination: late diabetic retinopathy. Note all of the findings of early retinopathy and new vessels and bleeds. (From Tasman W. Retinal vascular disease. In: Tasman W, Jaeger EA, eds. *The Wills Eye Hospital Atlas of Clinical Ophthalmology*, 2nd ed. Philadelphia: Lippincott Williams & Wilkins, 2001:223, with permission.)

 **TIPS**

- Proliferative changes, diabetes mellitus: neovascularization of the vessels about the optic disc (NVD) or in vessels elsewhere (NVE)
- May have vitreous bleeding because these vessels are fragile

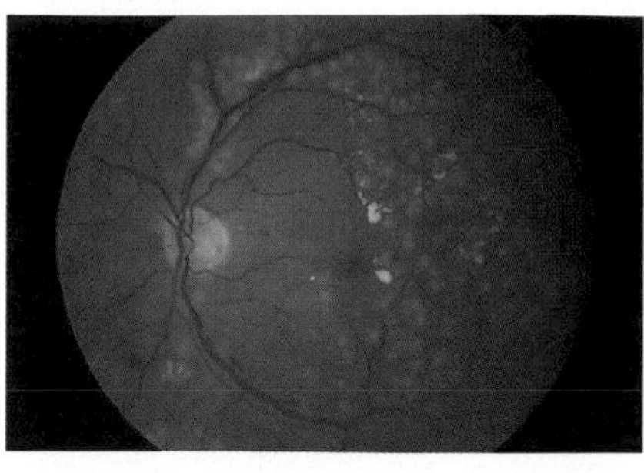

Figure 15.38.

Photocoagulation for diabetic retinopathy. Note multiple dots; these are due to laser treatment for proliferative retinopathy changes. (From Tasman W. Retinal vascular disease. In: Tasman W, Jaeger EA, eds. *The Wills Eye Hospital Atlas of Clinical Ophthalmology*, 2nd ed. Philadelphia: Lippincott Williams & Wilkins, 2001:226, with permission.)

TIPS

- Laser photocoagulation: proliferative diabetic retinopathy and multiple, large, round yellow areas of laser photocoagulation

in vessels elsewhere (NVE). Always recall, visual loss from diabetes is caused by multiple factors, including vitreous bleeds, retinal detachment, soft exudates, hard exudates, and edema in the retina. **Vitreous hemorrhage** manifests with a marked decrease in visual field in one eye; on funduscopic exam there is a collection of nebulous appearing blood in the area anterior to the retina, which prevents effective visualization of the retina. This is caused by diabetic retinopathy or a retinal detachment.

Photocoagulation for diabetic retinopathy **(Fig. 15.38)** manifests with a background of proliferative diabetic retinopathy and one or more, usually multiple, large (about one optic disc diameter size) round yellow areas. These are sites of laser photocoagulation, usually on the periphery of the fundus, used to treat NVE. These are actually, by definition, soft exudates.

NVD=neovascularization disc; NVE=neovascularization elsewhere.

PERIORBITAL ENTITIES

Xanthelasma manifests with one or more yellow plaques or patches on the eyelids and periorbital skin (Fig. 14.73). The company it keeps includes recurrent abdominal pain caused by pancreatitis and eruptive xanthomas on the skin. Underlying etiology includes familial hyperlipidemia (type 1, 4, or 5) or is secondary to diabetes mellitus or hypothyroidism.

Ptosis manifests with the eyelid drooped over the upper cornea so that it covers >10% of the cornea. If congenital, the ptosis may lessen on performing the Marcus-Gunn jaw-wink reflex (Fig. 15.6). **Horner's syndrome** manifests with a miotic pupil, ipsilateral ptosis, upward migration of the lower lid, and an absent Marcus-Gunn jaw-wink reflex (Fig. 15.6). Horner's syndrome is caused by a loss of function of the superior cervical sympathetic chain, due to tumor or trauma. **Stye** manifests with a papule or pustule at the eyelid mar-

TEACHING POINTS

PERIORBITAL STRUCTURES

1. A swollen red eye with decreased range of motion (ROM) and/or proptosis, consider orbital cellulitis.
2. Medial canthus swelling suggests dacrocystitis.
3. Assessment of the ROM of the eyes is extremely important in the setting of proptosis, potential orbital cellulitis, and any facial trauma.
4. External hordeolum = stye = pustule in an eyelash gland (Moll or Zeis).
5. Internal hordeolum = acute infection of a meibomian gland deep to the eyelid surface.
6. Chalazion = chronic enlargement of a meibomian gland.
7. Xanthelasma is a peripheral marker for markedly elevated lipids.

gin, and may be multiple (Fig. 15.14). Often with concurrent blepharitis. This is caused by inflammation of the eyelash gland of Moll or Zeis. An **internal hordeolum** manifests with a tender papule on the internal surface of the lid, usually in the upper lid, is caused by acute inflammation of a meibomian gland. A **chalazion** manifests with a nontender papule or even nodule in the upper eyelid, and is caused by chronic inflammation of a meibomian gland. **Lid lag** manifests with a rim of the sclera present between the cornea and the upper eyelid (Fig. 1.67); caused by either increased sympathetic discharge or hyperthyroidism. **Profound anemia** (Hb <8 g) manifests with pale conjunctiva; pale palmar creases; and often the company of tachycardia, hypotension, and orthostasis. **Vogt-Harada-Koyanagi** syndrome manifests with recurrent uveitis; **poliosis**, i.e., progressive whitening of the eyelashes; and **madarosis**, i.e., loss of the eyelashes. Due to an autoimmune process.

Orbital cellulitis manifests with a diffuse erythematous swelling of the periorbital structures **(Fig. 15.39)**. Proptosis, a marked decrease in ROM to extraocular movements and fever are present. The infection, usually bacterial has spread to the deep orbital structures; urgent if not emergent problem. **Preseptal cellulitis** manifests with diffuse swelling and erythema specific to the eyelid(s) without any decrease in ROM of the eye or proptosis and with minimal fever. **Acute dacrocystitis** manifests with marked swelling in the medial canthus area, especially the inferior punctum area, with increased tearing. There may even be a fluctuant nodule at the medial canthus; it can develop into a draining sinus tract at the site. This is due to inflammation and obstruction of the nasolacrimal duct.

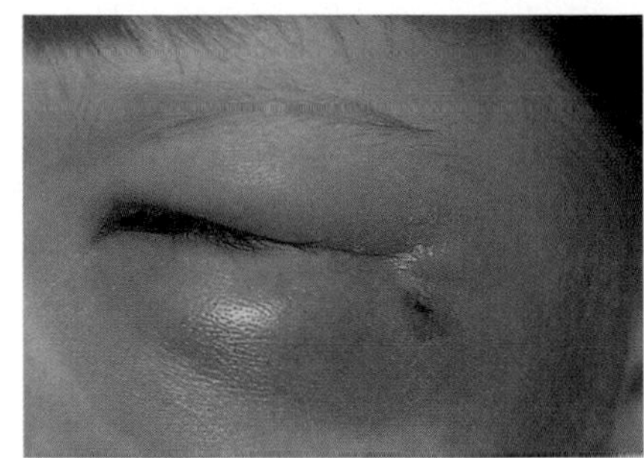

Figure 15.39.

Orbital cellulitis. Note here the proptosis of the affected eye; the patient also had significant strabismus.

TIPS

- Orbital cellulitis: diffuse warm erythematous swelling around the eye
- Patient unable to open the lids
- Proptosis and decreased range of movement of the eye
- Fever is common and expected
- Preseptal cellulitis: swelling and erythema located in the eyelid(s); may have decreased ability to open eye, minimal fever

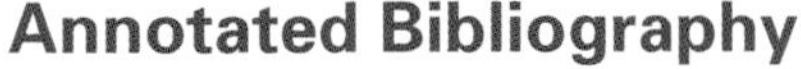

Annotated Bibliography

Overall

Garcia GE. Management of ocular emergencies and urgent eye problems. *Am Fam Phys* 1996;53(2):565–574.

Discusses the evaluation, manifestations, and early treatment of several entities that a primary care physician will likely see. These include subconjunctival hemorrhage, most of which resolve in 5 to 10 days; herpes keratitis, usually simplex, with unilateral limbic injection, photophobia, pain; usually limited to the epithelium, but if stroma is involved, more complex. Zoster is associated with V1 and is more benign. The sequelae of corneal scratches and dry eyes in Bell's palsy are discussed; management includes wearing protective eyewear and patching at light. The importance of using fluorescein strips is discussed because the solution is susceptible to contamination with Proteus and Pseudomonas organisms. Procedure for upper lid eversion is also discussed. Treatment of the abrasion should include a mydriatic or cycloplegic, tropicamide, and tobramycin. Discusses trauma-related and splash-related injuries and complications of lid trauma and orbital bone trauma, including tears of the canaliculus of the lower medial lid and trichiasis. The complications of an orbital blow-out fracture, inferior and medial, with entrapment of muscles, and even lid emphysema if a medial fracture. In cases of hyphema, a high risk exists of rebleeding in the first 5 days; management includes bedrest, no aspirin. Excellent review, good images.

Small RG. Ophthalmology in primary care. *Consultant* 1995;(March):321–327.

Brief review of common entities that cause red eye. Excellent images and then a good overview of the technique to perform Shiotz tonometry.

Michaelson SB. *Color Atlas of Uveitis Diagnosis*, 2nd ed. St Louis: Mosby; 1992.

Excellent reference for this topic, with great color images of specific manifestations and syndromes.

Shields JA, Shields CL. *Atlas of Intraocular Tumors.* Philadelphia: Lippincott Williams & Wilkins; 1999.

Excellent reference for this topic, with great images of specific manifestations and syndromes.

Red Eye

Hara JH. The red eye: diagnosis and treatment. *Am Fam Phys* 1996;54(8):2423–2430.

Excellent practical review of the approach to a patient with a red eye. Mucoid discharge that indicates allergic conjunctivitis; photophobia indicates iritis, keratopathy, acute glaucoma, and corneal abrasions; watery discharge indicates viral conjunctivitis or chemical irritation; purulent discharge indicates a bacterial source. Discusses the pathogenesis and manifestations of stye, chalazion, conjunctivitis (viral, atopic, and bacterial), and chemosis. Also discusses various underlying causes such as dry eye; subconjunctival hemorrhages; corneal abrasions; and keratitis. Describes uveitis with a miotic pupil and ciliary flush and no defect on fluorescein. With episcleritis and scleritis, chronic destruction of collagen is caused by vasculitic changes in the sclera. Acute-angle glaucoma risks include far-sightedness (hypermetropia) and red eye with a dilated pupil. Excellent illustrations and images.

Morrow GL, Abbot RL. Conjunctivitis. ***Am Fam Phys*** **1998;57(4):735–746.**

A primary care review of this common problem. Anatomy and historical clues are reviewed; highly satisfactory, albeit at times wordy, discussion of the various types of conjunctivitis.

Torok PG, Mader TH. Corneal abrasions: diagnosis and management. ***Am Fam Phys*** **1996;53(8):2521–2529.**

Nice overview of this common entity. Reviews the symptoms: sensation of foreign body, lacrimation, photophobia, blepharospasm, and blurred vision. Defects through Bowman's membrane can result in corneal scarring; erosion is in the epithelium. Reviews the underlying causes of the injury: if a fingernail, can become infected; if wood or tree branch, fungal infection; if metal shavings, a deeper wound. Examination features discussed include a ciliary flush (dilation of capillaries in a 1-mm ring about the cornea), and lacrimation. Emphasizes manifestations of direct ophthalmoscopy—translucent: erosion, opaque ulcer or scar; and tangential light—tangential for illuminating foreign bodies and for opacifications. Also need for cobalt blue direct or slit lamp with cobalt blue filter for fluorescein examination which stains the erosion. Differential diagnosis of an erosion includes herpes simplex and UV keratitis, which has a punctate superficial uptake; and chemical burns (alkaline is worse than acid). A tear-drop pupil is ominous for perforation as is the dilution of the fluorescein staining on application of the fluorescein over a suspected perforation (Seidel' test). Reviews the management of cycloplegia: topical antibiotics and patching; and when to refer to an ophthalmologist. Good images.

Retina and Funduscopic Examination

Brown GC, Magargal LE. Central retinal artery obstruction and visual acuity. ***Ophthalmology*** **1982;89:14.**

Demonstrates the severe disability that this entity can and does cause.

Diabetes Control and Complications Trial Research Group. The effect of intensive treatment of diabetes on the development and progression of long-term complications in insulin-dependent diabetes mellitus. ***N Eng J Med*** **1993;329:977.**

Seminal paper that demonstrates a positive impact of glycemic control on primary and secondary prevention of diabetic retinopathy in type 1 diabetics. Tremendous paper.

D'Amico DJ. Diseases of the retina. ***New Engl J Med*** **1994;331(2):95–107.**

Excellent review of the anatomy, histology, and basic physiology of the retina; reviews the pathogenesis and manifestations of several common retinal diseases: diabetic retinopathy, retinal detachment, acquired immunodeficiency syndrome (AIDS)-related retinal disease, and age-related macular degeneration,. Excellent color images. A great paper for this set of retinal disorders. Macular degeneration discussed, including prevalence of MD in the Beaver Dam study: 36.8% in patients >75 years of age had manifestations, including drusen (pale yellow dots single or in clusters). Overall excellent, especially for the AIDS-related disorders. A robust bibliography.

Hollenhorst RW. Significance of bright plaques in the retinal arterioles. ***JAMA*** **1961; 178:23–29.**

Original paper describing the finding of cholesterol emboli in branches of the retinal artery, which can cause complications and are the result of a systemic disorder, including blue toe syndrome.

Keith NM, Wagener HP, Barker NW. Some different types of essential hypertension: their cause and prognosis. ***Am J Med Sci*** **1939;197:332.**

A tremendous paper that contains a classification of hypertensive-related retinopathy: (I) arterial narrowing; (II) AV nicking; (III) hemorrhages and hard exudates (with a macular star); and (IV) disc and retinal edema. Also studied natural history and prognosis: 3-year survival: (I) 70%; (II) 66%; (III) 22%; and (IV) 6%. A study that must be included in any paper on hypertension.

Kohner EM, Dollery CT, Bulpitt CJ. Cotton-wool spots in diabetic retinopathy. ***Diabetes*** **1969;18:691.**

An important paper describing this phenomenon in patients with diabetes mellitus. Established scientific underpinnings for future interventional studies.

Michel J. Die spontane thrombose der vena centralis des opticus. ***Graefs Arch Ophthalmol*** **1878;24:37.**

The original description of central retinal vein thrombosis.

Reichel E. Vitreoretinal emergencies. ***Am Fam Phys*** **1995;52(5):1415–1419.**

Practical discussion of the manifestations and first-line treatment of central retinal arterial occlusion, retinal tears, and posterior vitreous gel detachment. Discussion and excellent images of cherry red macula of central retinal artery occlusion; and features of tears, detachments, and penetrating trauma syndromes are included.

Sapira JD, Olofinboba KA, Schnidemann H. The funduscopic examination. *Consultant* 1995;(Oct):1443–1453.

A good overview of findings on funduscopic examination, with image of a shadow ("nipple sign") of a narrow angle in the anterior chamber; retinal images of diabetic retinopathy, including microaneurysms, hard exudates, cotton-wool spots or soft exudates, Roth (Litten spots). The findings of hypertensive retinopathy include AV nicking or crossing abnormalities (venule under the arteriole). One image of human immunodeficiency virus (HIV)-related retinal disease presented. A nice first level paper.

Sarks SH. Drusen and the relationship to senile macular degeneration. *Australian Journal of Ophthalmology* 1980;8:117.

Shows the relationship between druse and macular degeneration.

Uwaifo GI, Schniederman H. Angioid streaks. *Consultant* 1999;39:179–180.

Case-based discussion of this rare entity. Bilateral, does not branch; yellow, reddish-brown, wider than vessels, and problems with Bruch's membrane. Discusses the causes, including those mentioned but virtually never seen (except when taking Board Exams) pseudoxanthoma elasticum. Also seen in sickle cell and Paget's disease. Discusses sequelae, including macular degeneration.

Periorbital

Char DH. Thyroid eye disease, 2nd ed. New York: Churchill-Livingstone, 1990.

Excellent resource on the manifestations and pathophysiology behind these common and often clinically significant findings.

Jones DB, Steinkuller PG. Microbial preseptal and orbital cellulites. In: Duane TD (ed.). *Clinical Ophthalmology*, Vol. 4: Philadelphia: JB Lippincott, 1989.

Great resource on the manifestations and pathophysiology behind these common and often clinically significant findings.

Olofinboba KA, Ramakrishnan N, Schneiderman H. Ectropion (everted eyelid). *Consultant* 1995;35:839–840.

Case-based discussion of this common problem, usually of the lower eyelid. The sequelae, including dry eye, superficial punctate keratitis, and even paradoxic epiphora, i.e., excessive lacrimation caused by the medial punctum being blocked, is discussed.

Smith B, Regan WF Jr. Blowout fractures of the orbit: mechanism and correction of internal orbit fracture. *Am J Ophthalmol* 1957;44:733.

Seminal paper in which the term blowout fracture was coined.

Anterior Chamber and Lens

Kobryn JL, Blodi FC, Weingeist TA. Ocular and orbital manifestations of neurofibromatosis. *Surv Ophthlamol* 1979;24:45.

Excellent resource on this topic.

Lam BL, Thompson HS, Corbett JJ. The prevalence of simple anisocoria. *Am J Ophthalmol* 1987;104:69.

Wonderful paper with the observation that 20% of normal individuals have anisocoria as a physiologic finding.

Olofinboba KA. Lens subluxation and the bedside recognition of Marfan's syndrome. *Consultant* 1995;35:513–518.

Case-based discussion of this rare finding that demonstrates the importance of examining the anterior chamber structures. The lens upward dislocated in Marfan syndrome (the zonular fibers that suspend the lens are fractures, thus the lens migrates upward). Other manifestations include a large cornea (corneomegaly), pupil tremor, and the systemic disorders of arachnodactyly: the arm span exceeds the person's height and the lower extremity height (pubis to sole) exceeds the upper (pubis to vertex), pes planus, genus recurvatum, and aortic regurgitation.

Appendix

Tools for Teaching Students, and Items for the Teacher's Library and Classroom

Bailey Hamilton: Demonstrations of Physical Signs in Clinical Surgery, 13th edition, Bristol (UK): John Wright, 1960.

Perhaps the best textbook written on physical examination. The text is excellent, the images are of adequate (for the time superb) detail, the descriptions of the examination and use are splendid. The disease processes described are mildly dated: for example there is emphasis on syphilis and tuberculosis, with less emphasis on disease processes more prevalent in US and Western Europe today. The text is particularly singular in the demonstration of the more "nontraditional" medical physical examination. The topics of ENT, abdomen, musculoskeletal examination are extremely well written and useful to clinicians and teachers today. Subsequent and antecedent editions, while very good, do not approach the quality of this edition.

Berg D: Advanced Clinical Skills, 2nd edition, Malden: Blackwell-Science, 2003.

A pocket handbook designed a a companion to our Advanced Physical Diagnosis Course for junior and senior medical students. Nice illustrations complement the text. Excellent resource for students on clinical rotations.

Bickley LS and Szilagyi PG: Bates' Guide to Physical Examination and History Taking, 8th edition, Philadelphia: Lippincott, Williams and Wilkins, 2003.

A well written edition of a solid fundamentally sound and useful textbook. Quite useful as a text for teaching medical students, nurses and health care providers the fundamental aspects of physical examination and history taking. Highly satisfactory images are in the text. A useful and recommended text.

Birrer RB and O'Connor FG: Sports Medicine for the Primary Care Physician, Boca Raton: CRC Press, 2004.

Highly satisfactory overview of sports medicine injuries and their treatment. Physical examination is integral to the effective and efficient diagnosis of many of these problems.

Cabot RC: Physical Diagnosis, 6th edition, New York: William Wood, 1915.

One of the best textbooks on the more traditional aspects of physical examination and diagnosis. He has extremely well written sections on cardiovascular, pulmonary and to a lesser extent, abdominal examination. He set in print some of the basic tenents used in teaching these skills. One particularly useful metaphor that I believe he coined was, "a thrill is akin to the purring of a cat." He also used the state of the art physiology to translate to the bedside-used the work of Thomas Lewis and McKenzie in his discussion of cardiac exam. He described tools and procedures that were of use to him as a practicing physician thus making it practical. Finally, he attempted to use gold standards (in his time autopsy) and evidence to support his text. Any edition of this work by this esteemed teacher from Harvard is of great interest and benefit to student and teacher alike.

Moore KL and Dalley AF. Clinically Oriented Anatomy, 5th edition, Philadelphia: Lippincott Williams and Wilkins, 2005.

An excellent resource for physical examination. It provides the anatomic foundation for physical examination, especially the musculoskeletal, ENT and neurologic examinations. Useful for both first year students in gross anatomy to see potential clinical correlations and useful for those who learn and teach physical examination and diagnosis. Clearly every physician needs an anatomy text for reference in her/his office; this would be an excellent choice.

Sapira JD: The Art and Science of Bedside Diagnosis, 1st edition, Baltimore: Williams and Wilkins, 1990.

An encyclopedic textbook of physical examination. In many areas of the rational physical examination, i.e. cardiac, pulmonary, abdomen, it is exhaustive in detail. Written by an individual who is a professor in all areas, it is in some places authorities whereas in some others modestly authoritative and anecdotal. He brought a force of intellect and enthusiasm to the teaching of physical examination and this work, like the author himself, is a pioneer in the current renaissance of clinical skills. The text although at times irregular in editing and modestly dense/difficult to read, is an important work for all students and teachers to have. Although there is a paucity of useful images in it, the out of print first edition is in my view the best.

Schneiderman Henry: Bedside Diagnosis: An Annotated Bibliography of Literature on Physical Examination and Interviewing, 2nd edition, Philadelphia: Amer Coll of Phys, 1992.

A pocket sized handbook in which a splendid effort is made to review the literature extant regarding history taking and physical examination. This pioneer work by an accomplished scholar and distinguished teacher is a delight to read. Dr Schneiderman in essence lead the way for this generation of teachers. The second edition is the best edition for clinical use.

Seidel HM, Ball JW, Dains JE and Benedict GW: Mosby's Guide to Physical Examination, 5th edition, St. Louis: Mosby, 2003.

An excellent textbook for learning history and physical diagnosis as a student. Richly illustrated; contains a wealth of diverse information from examaintion of a child to the assessment of pain.

Swartz MH: Textbook of Physical Diagnosis, 2nd edition, Philadelphia: WB Saunders, 1994.

Well written and quite complete textbook predominately written for medical students. Has a highly satisfactory set of images. The prose is deftly written and is strong in primary care. Nice integration of history taking into the physical examination. We enjoy reading and using this work.

Zetelli BJ and Davis HW: Atlas of Pediatric Physical Diagnosis, 2nd edition, Philadelphia: JB Lippincott, 1992.

Perhaps the best pediatric physical examination textbook yet written. A tremendous number of excellent images put into clinical context for a primary care pediatrician or emergency room physician, yet written with such depth and with emphasis on pathophysiology, that it is excellent for faculty. Minimal discussion on evidence basis of the physical examination, but overall an amazing work.

Tools for Teaching:

Simulated Male Pelvis; Gaunard.

Simulated anus, rectum and prostate for teaching the rectal and prostate examination. This life sized model predominately of plastic material comes with various sized prostates and prostates with various forms of pathology. It affords the junior level student a chance to learn the techniques of rectal exam and prostate exam the classroom. This in conjunction with standardized trained patients, allows the student to learn the fundamentals of this invasive and potentially challenging examination. The model is adequate but is really useful only for the beginning examiner.

Heartman Infrared Stethoscope, Cardionics Houston Texas.

Portable receivers for an infrared transmitter. The transmitter may be attached to a mannequin with sounds or to a stethoscope that transmits the ausculatory sounds from a real patient. These are of some use on bedside teaching rounds, especially when the group is larger than 5 students. The sound reception is very good. Highly satisfactory method to increase the efficiency of bedside teaching rounds for heart and lung sounds.

Sim-Man: Laerdal: Simulated patient:

Excellent tool for teaching clinical skills. This life sized and full body model and its accompanying equipment provides an excellent format for teaching clinical skills like NG tube insertion, Intubations, pericardiocentesis, Foley catheter placement, sterile technique, peripheral line placement, pulmonary and cardiac physical examination. It affords the user to teach scenarios in the emergency room, the trauma room, the recovery room and the surgical suite. Computer software allows the user to develop a clinical scenario in which the patient presents with a specific complaint (the manikin states the complaint), has a rhythm present on the monitor, breathes at a specific rate, has specific types of breath sounds. Furthermore, there is anesthesia equipment for teaching of ventilator and intraoperative anesthesia care. This is a useful piece of equipment for teaching scenarios and the use of physical examination in acute medical problems. It is not used primarily to teach physical examination skills.

Pugh, CM and others: E-pelvis:

Simulated pelvis for teaching pelvic examinations. This life sized model predominately of plastic material has built in sensors and a lap top computer used for teaching a practice of the pelvic examination in a woman. It comes with various sized cervices and uteruses. It affords the junior level student a chance to learn the techniques of speculum insertion and bimanual palpation of structures in the classroom. This in conjunction with standardized trained patients, allows the student to learn the fundamentals of this invasive and potentially challenging examination. The model is adequate in texture and is really useful only for the beginning examiner.

Gordon, M: The Harvey Cardiac Finding Simulator: University of Miami

A useful tool in the teaching of cardiovascular examination. The manikin is life-sized, has a plastic type coating that is not unrealistic. The manikin has the ability to produce blood pressure readings, jugular venous pulse waves, carotid and femoral pulse waves, respiratory movements, precordial impulses including PMI, heaves, gallops and of course classic heart sounds. The equipment can easily be attached to an infrared transmitter so that small or large groups may use for teaching and learning. The teacher/operator calls up specific diagnoses, like mitral regurgitation or aortic insufficiency and all manifestations of the process are demonstrable. We use this for basic teaching of skills to M1 and M2 students, and also as an adjunct to bedside (never a replacement for bedside) teaching of cardiac sounds. One novel method we use is to start with patients with a real murmur, discuss it over the Harvey findings, then send students back to the bedside on their own to listen again. The advantages of Harvey, reproducible, allows practice, good for basic teaching and includes the company, not just the murmur. Overall quite durable (beware no ink allowed-stains the skin), but modestly expensive. Deficits include, no right sided findings (e.g., tricuspid regurgitation) and Harvey is always supine, thus orthopnea is not possible.

Index

Note: Page numbers followed by f indicate figures; those followed by t indicate tables; and those followed by b indicate boxed material.